CHILD AND ADOLESCENT THERAPY

CHILD and ADOLESCENT Therapy

Cognitive-Behavioral Procedures

THIRD EDITION

Edited by **PHILIP C. KENDALL**

THE GUILFORD PRESS
New York   London

© 2006 Philip C. Kendall and The Guilford Press
Published by The Guilford Press
A Division of Guilford Publications, Inc.
72 Spring Street, New York, NY 10012
www.guilford.com

Printed in the United States of America

This book is printed on acid-free paper.

Last digit is print number: 9   8   7   6   5   4   3   2   1

Library of Congress Cataloging-in-Publication Data

Child and adolescent therapy : cognitive-behavioral procedures / edited by Philip C.
Kendall.—3rd ed.
    p. cm.
   Includes bibliographical references and index.
   ISBN 1-59385-113-8 (hardcover)
     1. Cognitive therapy for children.   2. Cognitive therapy for teenagers.   3. Child
psychotherapy.   4. Adolescent psychotherapy.   5. Clinical child psychology.
I. Kendall, Philip C.
   RJ505.C63C45 2006
   618.92'89142—dc22

                                                                    2005012858

To all the mental health professionals who not only have displayed the intellectual curiosity to read about empirically supported approaches to treatment, but also take the initiative to give them a try.

About the Editor

Philip C. Kendall, PhD, ABPP, is the Laura H. Carnell Professor of Psychology and Director of the Child and Adolescent Anxiety Disorders Clinic at Temple University. An internationally recognized expert on clinical child and adolescent psychology and clinical psychological research, Dr. Kendall has published widely on many topics but is perhaps best known for his development and evaluation of cognitive-behavioral treatments for anxiety in youth. Author or coauthor of over 350 research publications and books, he has twice been a Fellow at the Center for Advanced Study in the Behavioral Sciences, Stanford, California, and is a Fellow of the American Association for the Advancement of Science, the American Psychological Association, and the American Psychological Society. Dr. Kendall has served on the Child and Adolescent Mental Disorders Task Force for the National Academy of Sciences, Institute of Medicine; the William T. Grant Foundation Consortium for "School-Based Promotion of Social Competence"; and the Examination Committee of the American Association of State and Provincial Psychology Boards (overseeing the national licensure examination). He has also been a consultant to the World Health Organization and a Distinguished Visiting Professor to the United States Air Force.

Dr. Kendall has served several professional organizations and publications, including, as Editor, the *Journal of Consulting and Clinical Psychology* (1997–2002), *Cognitive Therapy and Research* (1986–1996), and *Clinical Psychology: Science and Practice* (2004–present). He currently serves on Pennsylvania Governor Edward G. Rendell's Commission on Children and Families and on the Board of Trustees of the American Board of Professional Psychology. He is a past president of Division 53 (Clinical Child and Adolescent Psychology) of the American Psychological Association and of the Association for Advancement of Behavior Therapy. He has served as a member of the Board of Directors of the Council of University Directors of Clinical Training Programs, as a Diplomate Examiner for the American Board of Professional Psychology, and as a member of the Scientific Program Committee for the World

Congress on Cognitive and Behavioral Therapy. Dr. Kendall has been the recipient of several research grants from the National Institute of Mental Health for the study of the nature and treatment of youth. Among his other awards are the Outstanding Alumnus Award from the Phi Kappa Phi Honor Society of Old Dominion University, the Psychology Department's Outstanding Alumnus Award from Virginia Commonwealth University, the State of Pennsylvania Distinguished Contribution to the Science and Profession of Psychology Award, the "Great Teacher Award" from Temple University, and the inaugural Research Recognition Award for anxiety research on children and adolescents from the Anxiety Disorders Association of America.

Contributors

Mona Abad, MA, Department of Psychology, Loyola University, Chicago, Illinois

Leah E. Behl, PhD, New Jersey CARES Institute, University of Medicine and Dentistry of New Jersey, Stratford, New Jersey

Bruce F. Chorpita, PhD, Department of Psychology, University of Hawaii, Honolulu, Hawaii

Craig Colder, PhD, Department of Psychology, State University of New York at Buffalo, Buffalo, New York

Jordana Cooperberg, BA, Departments of Psychology and Psychiatry, Washington University, St. Louis, Missouri

Gilbert Custer, MD, private practice, Austin, Texas

Esther Deblinger, PhD, New Jersey Child Abuse, Research, and Education Services Institute, School of Osteopathic Medicine, University of Medicine and Dentistry of New Jersey, Stratford, New Jersey

Christianne Esposito-Smythers, PhD, Department of Psychiatry and Human Behavior and Center for Alcohol and Addiction Studies, Brown University, Providence, Rhode Island

A. J. Finch, Jr., PhD, ABPP, School of Human and Social Sciences, The Citadel, Charleston, South Carolina

David P. FitzGerald, PhD, Department of Medical Psychiatry, Duke University Medical Center, Durham, North Carolina

Martin E. Franklin, PhD, Department of Psychiatry, University of Pennsylvania School of Medicine, Philadelphia, Pennsylvania

A. Cash Ghee, PhD, Department of Psychology, Xavier University, Cincinnati, Ohio

Alissa R. Glickman, PhD, Center for Children's Support, University of Medicine and Dentistry of New Jersey, Stratford, New Jersey

Jennifer Hargrave, PhD, Department of Educational Psychology, University of Texas, Austin, Texas

Stephen P. Hinshaw, PhD, ABPP, Department of Psychology, University of California, Berkeley, California

Grayson N. Holmbeck, PhD, Department of Psychology, Loyola University, Chicago, Illinois

Marc Karver, PhD, Department of Psychology, University of South Florida, Tampa, Florida

Philip C. Kendall, PhD, ABPP, Department of Psychology and Child and Adolescent Anxiety Disorders Clinic, Temple University, Philadelphia, Pennsylvania

Neville J. King, PhD, Faculty of Education, Monash University, Clayton, Victoria, Australia

Annette M. La Greca, PhD, Department of Psychology, University of Miami, Coral Gables, Florida

John E. Lochman, PhD, ABPP, Department of Psychology, University of Alabama, Tuscaloosa, Alabama

John S. March, MD, Department of Child and Adolescent Psychiatry, Duke University, Durham, North Carolina

Johanna Molnar, MA, Department of Educational Psychology, University of Texas, Austin, Texas

W. Michael Nelson III, PhD, ABPP, Department of Psychology, Xavier University, Cincinnati, Ohio

Thomas H. Ollendick, PhD, ABPP, Department of Psychology and Child Study Center, Virginia Polytechnic Institute and University, Blacksburg, Virginia

Kerry O'Mahar, MA, Department of Psychology, Loyola University, Chicago, Illinois

Vandana A. Passi, BA, Departments of Psychology and Psychiatry, Washington University, St. Louis, Missouri

John C. Piacentini, PhD, ABPP, Department of Psychiatry and Biobehavioral Sciences, University of California, Los Angeles, California

Nicole R. Powell, PhD, Department of Psychology, University of Alabama, Tuscaloosa, Alabama

Janay Sander, PhD, Department of Educational Psychology, University of Texas, Austin, Texas

Sarah Schnoebelen, MA, Department of Educational Psychology, University of Texas, Austin, Texas

Stephen Shirk, PhD, ABPP, Department of Psychology and Child Study Center, University of Denver, Denver, Colorado

Wendy K. Silverman, PhD, ABPP, Department of Psychology and Child Phobia Center, Florida International University, Miami, Florida

Jane Simpson, MA, Department of Educational Psychology, University of Texas, Austin, Texas

Anthony Spirito, PhD, ABPP, Department of Psychiatry and Human Behavior and Center for Alcohol and Addiction Studies, Brown University, Providence, Rhode Island

Kevin D. Stark, PhD, Department of Educational Psychology, University of Texas, Austin, Texas

Richard I. Stein, PhD, Department of Internal Medicine, Washington University School of Medicine, St. Louis, Missouri

Cynthia Suveg, PhD, Child and Adolescent Anxiety Disorders Clinic, Temple University, Philadelphia, Pennsylvania

Anne Updegrove, PhD, private practice, Chicago, Illinois

Janet M. Whidby, PhD, Department of Medical Psychiatry, Duke University Medical Center, Durham, North Carolina

Denise E. Wilfley, PhD, Department of Psychiatry, Washington University School of Medicine, St. Louis, Missouri

Preface

The science and practice of mental health services for children and adolescents have experienced noteworthy developments and forward advances. If you are involved with the mental health of children and adolescents, then you are probably already aware of at least some of these changes and examples of progress. It is my hope that after reading about a selected topic in this book, you will be current on the nature and treatment of a specified condition and that, after completing this volume, you will be on top of the field.

"Youth," used here to refer to children and adolescents, is a topic that has emerged as a fundamental focus for mental health. For example, the Annenberg Foundation invested heavily in gathering scholars for discussion and coordinating their work to produce a state-of-the-art document about the mental health needs of youth. Similarly, the renewed interest in investigations involving youth is evident at the National Institute of Mental Health, where programs of research are evaluated for potential funding—so much so that there is the new requirement that investigators/applicants include or justify why they are not including children and adolescents in their proposed research. This laudable initiative is not well served by rash efforts by a few to try to apply adult treatments to children without proper attention to developmental factors. Nevertheless, the emphasis placed on children and adolescents by such a prestigious institution as the National Institute of Mental Health will favorably affect the research and the clinical services available in the coming decades.

Psychologists have increased their focus on contexts, and "families" are a key context for youth. Families have long been seen as important in the psychological treatment of youth, but early applications of family therapy were not empirically based; some researchers have suggested that the development of family therapy may have been delayed for this reason. In contrast, many of the contemporary family and parent training therapies that are receiving applied attention are emerging from an empirical background, being subjected to empirical evaluations, and receiving empirical support. Several versions of "family" treatment have moved into the family of empirically evaluated interventions for children and adolescents.

In a trend that has continued over the years, the field has placed increased attention on those psychological treatments that have experienced empirical examination. The curious reader will want to know, "What treatments have been tested and which have been found to produce beneficial gains?" Several therapies have emerged as having received empirical support, and it is these treatments that are not only the nucleus of this book but also the themes for the next decade of evaluation. Doctoral, intern, and residency training programs are making decisions with regard to the types of therapy they wish to teach to their trainees, funding and health management agencies are considering which treatments to fund and/or reimburse, and the educated consumer is increasingly seeking out those services that have been supported by science. This book includes detailed descriptions of some of the very programs, often manual-based, that have been identified as empirically supported.

Manual-based treatments are not cookie-cutter operations. Indeed, I have elsewhere argued for "flexibility within fidelity" (Kendall, 2001), where manual-based interventions are not conducted exactly the same way for everyone. The designation "manual-based" indicates that the goals and strategies for the treatment sessions are prepared in advance and can be monitored along with progress. But the written word can be lifeless, and one needs to breathe life and energy into the manuals (Kendall, Chu, Gifford, Hayes, & Nauta, 1998).

The opening chapter provides a description and discussion of the guiding theory for work with children and adolescents. Consideration is given to the need to consider problem solving, cognitive information processing, emotions, and interpersonal relations while at the same time staying performance-based. The chapter also addresses a conceptualization of the therapist as a coach, a temporal model for the development of coping, the role of normal development in youth, and the nature of rational therapist expectations for change. The chapters that follow represent major contributions by leading clinicians/researchers. Each chapter summarizes the background research, the assessment procedures, and the treatment process. Along with the description of the in-session treatment procedures is a review of the empirical evaluations of the intervention. My intent from the outset has been to direct the work toward the practitioner and the researcher. Not surprisingly, therefore, whereas most chapters provide hands-on descriptions for the practitioner, the closing chapter considers the current status of numerous treatments in terms of their empirical support.

I wish to thank each of the contributors for his or her participation in the present volume. Without them, the book would lack the diversity of applications and the needed breadth of perspective; with them, the book is an impressive representation of the field. I also wish to thank my graduate students and colleagues. To the many children who have been part of the research and clinical programs described in this book and to the universities, medical schools, school systems, and other settings that have cooperated over the years, I offer a collective thank-you. I also acknowledge and thank the National Institute of Mental Health for its support of research, some of which is the basis for the work in the book. Preparation of this edition was facilitated by such support (Grant Nos. MH63747, MH59087, and MH64484). Last, for her encouragement and understanding, I thank my spouse, Sue, and for their opening my eyes to new ways to see things, I thank my children, now young men, Reed and Mark.

PHILIP C. KENDALL, PhD, ABPP

REFERENCES

Kendall, P. C. (2001). Flexibility within fidelity. *Clinical Child and Adolescent Psychology Newsletter, 16*(2), 1–5.

Kendall, P. C., Chu, B., Gifford, A., Hayes, C., & Nauta, M. (1998). Breathing life into a manual. *Cognitive and Behavioral Practice, 5*, 177–198.

Contents

PART I

GUIDING THEORY

CHAPTER 1

Guiding Theory for Therapy with Children and Adolescents

PHILIP C. KENDALL

The days when a single megatheory was proposed and expected to explain all of psychopathology or psychotherapy are gone. Rather, it is accepted that no one theory accounts for or explains all human emotion, thought, and action. There are, however, specifiable and useful theories to guide the design, implementation, and evaluation of treatments, and specifically treatment programs for children and adolescents. Theory provides proper initial guidance for clinical endeavors.

Even basic descriptions of any one of the various psychological therapies are related, in large measure, to some form of a guiding theory. For some therapies, the theory is an extrapolation from clinical experiences; for others, the applied theory is an adaptation of a complementary theory from a more basic area of psychology, and in still others, the theory is built upon and extended from empirical research. Theory guides empirical evaluation, and the resulting data guide further applications.

Theories of stable traits are interesting and important, but for clinical work the most direct and useful theories are those that propose to explain the processes of change. Given our special attention to children and adolescents (i.e., youth), we can benefit greatly from consideration of theories that deal with psychological change in youth and that address aspects of human development. What may be alarming, especially to those well versed in either theories of behavior change or those of development, is that until recently there has been precious little connection in applied work between these two arenas. As will be evident in the chapters in this volume, cognitive–behavioral approaches to treating behavioral and emotional problems in youth are both guided by theory and evaluated using rigorous methodologies.

In this chapter, along with consideration of other related themes, I outline a cognitive–behavioral theory in which behavioral events, associated anticipatory expectations and postevent attributions, and ongoing cognitive information processing and emotional states combine to influence behavior and behavior change. Relatedly, the theory adapts to the different challenges facing different levels of development. The theory is problem solving in its orientation, deals directly with the cognitive forces that impact social information processing, incorporates emotional and social domains, addresses matters associated with parenting and families, and emphasizes performance-based interventions. The applications of the guiding theory employ structured and manual-based procedures. A closer look at each of these features is informative.

Why adopt a problem-solving orientation? Without exception, humans routinely experience problems that require solutions. Quite simply, problems occur! The ability to recognize a problem and address it (problem solving) is an essential ingredient to adequate adjustment in childhood, adolescence, and across one's life span. Different developmental challenges face youth as they move through childhood and adolescence, and these youth differ in their ability to recognize a problem and to generate and consider possible solutions. Importantly, their ability to generate alternative solutions and competently evaluate each option will form an important basis for the quality of their psychological health. A problem-solving orientation is seen in many of the empirically supported psychological treatments (see Lonigan, Elbert, & Johnson, 1998) for disorders of youth (Hibbs & Jensen, 2005; Kazdin & Weisz, 2003; Ollendick, King, & Chorpita, Chapter 14, this volume).

Why emphasize cognitive information processing? As we all know from our own lives as well as from the research literature, problems of all sorts can occur, without provocation or effort. Optimal solutions to problems, in contrast, do not materialize from thin air, nor are they handed to someone carte blanche. And, in instances when solutions appear to jump out or be provided by someone else, they are not always the optimal solutions. A child who has someone else solve his or her problems is not him- or herself benefiting. Rather, successful solutions often require some time and effort and then emerge from an individual's active use of thinking—or, as we call it, involvement with cognitive strategies.

Cognitive problem-solving strategies are not transmitted magically from parents to children, but they are acquired through experience, observation, and interaction with others. For our purposes, the use of cognitive strategies can be maximized through intentional and planned intervention. Varying styles of information processing have profound effects on how one makes sense of the world and one's experiences in it, and dysfunctional information processing requires attention and modification (e.g., Ingram, Miranda, & Segal, 1998). Correcting faulty information processing (i.e., changing distorted thinking) and/or teaching strategies to overcome a deficiency in information processing (i.e., overcoming deficiencies in thinking) (Kendall, 1985, 1993) are both valuable steps in the treatment of psychological disorders of youth.

Why be concerned with emotions? Our emotional states, both positive (Diener & Lucas, 1999) and negative, influence our cognitive and behavioral abilities. The absence of positive emotions can have unwanted effects, and a sensitivity to dwelling on negative emotions can be distressing as well. What is especially interesting is that positive and negative emotions are not opposite ends of a single continuum, but rather each is a continuum of its own. Learning about the nature and regulation of our emotions (e.g., emotion management skills) can provide a solid building block for advancing one's well-being. It simply is not enough to know how to think through problems; conditions of persistent emotional arousal, as well as transient but impactful emotions, can interfere with efforts to think reasonably! Effective cognitive problem solving requires an understanding of the experience and modification of emotions (Southam–Gerow & Kendall, 2000), and effective interventions require a recognition and consideration of, and therapeutic attention to, emotional states.

Why focus on social and interpersonal domains? The important psychological problems in need of solutions are not *imp*ersonal problems (e.g., how to distribute weight when loading a trailer) but are *inter*personal (social) ones (e.g., how to adjust to changing physiology and family roles). Mental health professionals are interested in effective adaptation and adjustment (coping) in social situations. Note that developmental theory has uniformly underscored the importance of social relationships (peers [see Hartup, 1984] and family) to psychologically healthy adjustment. Therapy is an interpersonal process, and the child's involvement in therapeutic interactions is associated with favorable outcomes (Chu & Kendall, 2004). Social/interpersonal domains take on special importance in clinical interventions.

Not surprisingly, theory must address matters associated with parenting and families. Indeed, it is common lore, and partially supported empirical practice, that the inclusion of parents in the treatment of youth with behavioral and emotional problems adds to the benefits gained by treatment. What may be surprising, however, is that the nature of this involvement varies across child problems and varies with development. Parents of conduct-disordered youth will likely be shaped to increase their monitoring of their children's activities, whereas parents of anxious youth would likely be shaped to be less vigilant and overseeing of their children. Improvements in children's adjustment may be better when parents are included in sessions—or better when parents are intentionally separated from their children (e.g., Barmish & Kendall, 2005). Younger children, such as a separation-anxious child, may benefit more when parents are included from the start, whereas an adolescent with depression may want to be separate from a parent and benefit more when the parent is not included in treatment sessions.

Why follow a manual-based or structured approach to treatment? This matter has generated lively discussion (see *Clinical Psychology: Science and Practice*, Vol. 5, 1998) and promoted efforts to "breathe life into a manual" (e.g., Kendall, Chu, Gifford, Hayes, & Nauta, 1998). Like theory, structure provides an organization and guides the treatment: an understanding of the target problem and the nature of its experience for the youth, as well as an arranged set of progressive experiences that build on what we know about the disorder—its cognitive, emotional, behavioral, social, and familial features. Having these empirical bases folded into the content of the treatment manuals optimizes the beneficial gains attained by the youth. In addition, a manual-based approach helps focus on explicit goals, offers a suggested pace, and provides sequenced steps for movement toward the goals. Manual-based treatments are *not* inflexible or rigid blueprints—they are intended to be applied with "flexibility within fidelity" (Kendall, 2001). Likewise, workbooks for the child-client to use in treatment provide opportunities to learn new skills and allow for structured practice. For example, the *Taking ACTION Workbook* (see Stark et al., Chapter 5, this volume) provides training materials for use of cognitive-behavioral strategies to overcome depressed mood, whereas the *Coping Cat Workbook* and the *C.A.T. Project* workbook (see Kendall & Suveg, Chapter 7, this volume) provide sequenced tasks for the management of unwanted and disturbing anxious arousal. Manuals and workbooks provide organization and structure to guide treatment; they are not inflexible boundaries.

Why should a guiding theory place an emphasis on performance-based interventions? Some interventions, often targeting adults and of historical interest, may be geared toward helping the client gain insight or understanding. In contrast, interventions focused on youth typically intend to remediate skills deficits or correct distortions in thinking, emotions, or action. It is through performance-based procedures that such goals are best accomplished. Practice, with encouragement and feedback, leads to further use and refinement of social and cognitive skills. Involvement in these performance-based activities is encouraged and shaped, to firm up intrinsic interest or to promote motivation in otherwise disinterested participants. For youth, it simply is not enough to try to talk about what changes may be needed; their level of cognitive development may not be sufficient, and without opportunities to practice their skills will not be honed. Not unlike schoolwork, sports, or musical expression, practice is a crucial part of the optimal intervention.

This third edition of *Child and Adolescent Therapy* is a collection of the refined and advanced treatments for specific youth problems that have been designed and developed by leading therapists. Interestingly, the approaches hold together very well in terms of the dimensions discussed thus far. That is, as will become even more evident throughout the book, the guiding cognitive-behavioral theory has more than one facet and is appropriate in multiple applications. The theory places greatest emphasis on helping youth to advance their cognitive information processing in current (and past) social contexts by using structured, behaviorally oriented practice while concurrently paying attention to the participant youth's emotional state and involvement in the tasks of the treatment. As needed, members of social groups (e.g., parents) can be included. As central as a guiding theory is to the provision of interventions, it is nevertheless crucial that the intervention be examined and evaluated for efficacy and effectiveness (see Chambless & Hollon, 1998; Ollendick et al., Chapter 14, this volume). A guiding theory is necessary but not sufficient. Empirical support for an intervention is a priceless key to the choice of one intervention over another and to the assignment of the label "best practice" or "empirically supported" (see Kendall, 1998). Also included throughout this book are mentions of the empirical evaluations that guided the content of the treatments as well as those that examined the outcomes associated with treatment implementation.

TOWARD A WORKING DEFINITION

The child and adolescent therapies described in this volume are labeled cognitive-behavioral. How is cognitive-behavioral therapy (CBT) defined? There are numerous forms of psychosocial intervention designed to facilitate child and adolescent adjustment and remediate their psychological distress, but they overlap to various degrees and they are not independent of one another. It is easy to speculate about the similarities and differences that actually exist among the different treatment philosophies (for an interesting and informed look inside four different child therapies, see Fishman, 1995), but until a series of empirical studies of the specific therapies is undertaken we can only speculate about the distinct and overlapping features. In an effort to provide a working definition of CBT for youth, consider the following: CBT is a rational amalgam, a purposeful attempt to preserve the demonstrated positive effects of behavioral procedures within a less doctrinaire context and to incorporate the cognitive activities and emotional experiences of the client into the process of therapeutic change (Kendall & Hollon, 1979). Accordingly, CBT uses enactive performance-based procedures and structured sessions (e.g., it is manual-based and uses workbooks) as well as strategies designed to produce changes in thinking, feeling, and behavior.

The cognitive-behavioral perspective on child and adolescent disorders, and related treatment-produced gains, includes consideration of the youth's internal and external environment. A CBT model places greatest emphasis on the learning process and the influence of the models in the social environment while underscoring the centrality of the individual's mediating/information-processing style and emotional experiencing. The hyphenated term "cognitive-behavioral" is not intended as a direct insult to the role of emotions or the impact of the social context. Rather, it is a hybrid representing an integration of cognitive, behavioral, emotion-focused, and social strategies for change. Abandoning an adherence to any singular model, the cognitive–behavioral model recognizes and embraces the relationships of cognition and behavior to the emotional state and the overall functioning of the organism in a larger social context.

"Emotions" have been assigned to both primary and ancillary roles in childhood psychopathology and therapy. Emotions were given a primary role by Bernard and Joyce (1984); child psychopathology was said to be caused by emotional problems. In other writings (e.g., Santostefano & Reider, 1984), cognition and emotion were considered "one and the same" (p. 56) and thereby given comparable status. I argue that although cognition and emotion are interrelated, the variance in the etiology and treatment of some disorders may be best accounted for by a cognitive analysis, whereas some other disorders may be best understood in terms of a more direct focus of emotions. Still other disorders may be best viewed as largely behavioral. Anxious children, for example, behave in frightened ways (they avoid distressing situations), and they not only misperceive threat and danger in an otherwise routine environment but also fail to recognize and understand the modifiability of their own emotions (Southam-Gerow & Kendall, 2000); often they have parents who may facilitate their avoidance. It is not that any one domain is always primary or uniformly accounts for the most variance. Rather, cognition, emotion, action, and social environment are all involved but may vary in their potency across the different types of psychological difficulties and disorders.

Because behavioral patterns in the external world and cognitive interpretations in the internal world pertain to social/interpersonal contexts (peers and family), CBT addresses the social context. For instance, social/interpersonal factors play a crucial role in the design of strategies for treatment. For children and adolescents, the centrality of the social context must be underscored. Indeed, a satisfactory relationship with peers is a crucial component of a child's successful adjustment, and an understanding of peer and social relationships (even if appearing evanescent to the therapist) is required for a meaningful assessment of a child's needs and for accomplishing an effective intervention. Similarly, the role of the family cannot be neglected, for this social microcosm sets many of the rules and roles for later social interaction.

PARENTS: CONSULTANTS, COLLABORATORS, OR CO-CLIENTS?

Acknowledgments of peer and family contributions to child and adolescent psychopathology, however, far outweigh the research database that is currently available, and the need for further inquiry in these areas cannot be overemphasized. This statement is especially true with regard to treatment (e.g., Barmish & Kendall, 2005): Parents are regularly involved in many of the programs designed for their children in spite of the fact that there is a tremendous need for a larger empirical database on the optimal nature of their involvement. Yes, CBT does recommend that treatment involve parents, but how best to do so? For example, parents can serve as *consultants* when they provide input into the determination of the nature of the problem. When parents are seen as contributing to or maintaining some aspect of the child's problem, the parents may become *co-clients* in the treatment itself. Parents may also be involved as *collaborators* in their child's treatment when they assist in the implementation of program requirements. Cognitive-behavioral interventions assess, consider, and incorporate social/interpersonal matters into their programs. Involvement of parents and changing the family system should be used in conjunction with the nature of the treatment and the needs of the child. Research is needed (e.g., studying parents as consultants, co-clients, or collaborators) to further inform the ideal involvement of parents and to examine the different parent roles relative to such factors as the child's age and the principal disorder.

THERAPIST AS COACH: THE POSTURE OF THE THERAPIST

"Basketball as life" is the hypothetical title of an unwritten book. If written, it would highlight how aspects of what children learn through rule-governed activities (e.g., sport, social services, acting, computers) provide valuable life lessons that have broader application. For the past 25 years, I have struggled when searching for the words to try to describe the mental attitude that is recommended for therapeutic work with youth. Using the term "posture" to refer to one's mental attitude, although not exact or ideal, can help to describe a therapist working with youth. The word "coach," too, carries useful connotations. A coach is there because of prior experience, to enhance the participant's abilities, to guide development, to further a common goal, and to have fun in the process. By the way, I recognize that not all coaches conform to this ideal.

I choose to describe three characteristics of the posture of the "therapist as coach," using the terms "consultant/collaborator," "diagnostician," and "educator," all within the umbrella of a supportive yet exacting coach who can bring the best out of someone with opportunities and feedback. After years of using the terms in a certain way, I am now very comfortable with the therapist as "coach."

By referring to the therapist as a consultant/collaborator, I am referring to the therapist as a person who does not have all the answers, but one who has some ideas worthy of trying out and some ways to examine whether the ideas have value for the individual. Telling a child and/or adolescent exactly what to do is *not* the idea; giving the client an opportunity to try something and helping him or her to make sense of the experience is the idea. The therapist as consultant collaborates with the client. The therapist as consultant strives to develop skills in the client that include thinking on his or her own and moving toward independent, mature problem solving. The consultant (therapist) is a problem-solving model working with the client. When the client asks, "Well, what am I supposed to do?," the therapist might reply, "Let's see, what do you want to accomplish here?," and then, "What are your options?" or "What's another way we could look at this problem?" The exchange is geared toward facilitating the process of problem solving, but without forcing a specific solution. The youngster and therapist interact in a collaborative problem-solving manner. In-session activities are practice; life outside a session is the game, and coaches provide practice opportunities for the very skills needed in the real arena.

"Diagnostician" is a term that might suggest the process of labeling within a diagnostic system (e.g., DSM-IV, ICD-10), but although this process is not here criticized, it is not the thrust of the meaning of the term when used here to describe the therapist's mental posture. The mental attitude associated with "diagnostician" is one of being confident to go beyond the verbal report of the client and his/her significant others. A diagnostician is one who integrates data and, judging against a background of knowledge of psychopathology, normal development, and psychologically healthy environments, makes meaningful decisions. This aspect of the term "diagnostician" is that which I underscore. Consider the following example. Suppose that you win a brand-new Jaguar automobile. You are driving it around for 2 days, and you notice a "clug-clug" sound in the front end when you make a right-hand turn. There is no noise when you go straight or when you turn left. The noise has you perplexed, so you contact a mechanic and tell him that the front tie-rod ends need repair. You leave the car for repair and pick it up at the end of the day. Your tie-rod ends have been replaced. Would you be satisfied? My answer is a definite "no." Why should I be satisfied when the mechanic relied on me as the diagnostician? What do I know about tie-rod ends? I just won the car—I am not a mechanic, and I should not be diagnosing the problem. The auto mechanic is the expert who should be making the determination. He should ask for a description of the problem and look under the hood! The mechanic should not fix what I say is wrong, because I am not the Jaguar expert. He can use my descriptions of the problem and consider my ideas as helpful information, but he should nevertheless make his own determination.

Similarly, we (mental health professionals/educators) cannot let others tell us what is wrong and what needs to be fixed when we are working with children and adolescents with psychological problems. That a parent says an adolescent has an anxiety disorder is not, alone, sufficient reason to undertake an anxiety treatment program. That a parent or teacher says that a child is hyperactive is not sufficient reason to initiate a medication regimen and/or cognitive-behavioral therapy. The fact that a parent or teacher suspects or suggests hyperactivity in a child is a valuable piece of information, but there are several rival hypotheses that must be considered. For example, the child's behavior may be within normal limits but appear as troubled when judged against inappropriate parental (teacher) expectations about child behavior. When the parent expects too much "adult-like behavior" from a child, the essential problem does not lie within the child. There is also the possibility of alternative disorders: "Hyperactivity" may be the term used by the referring parent, but aggressive noncompliance may be a better description in terms of mental health professionals' communications and target-ing the treatment. Also, the child's identified problem may be a reflection of a dysfunctional family interaction pattern, with the parenting styles needing the greatest attention, not the child per se. In a nutshell, the cognitive-behavioral therapist serves as a diagnostician by taking into account the various sources of information and, judging against a background of knowledge, determines the nature of the problem and the optimal strategy for its treatment.

The therapeutic posture of a cognitive-behavioral therapist entails being an educator. The use of "educator" here is intended to communicate that I am talk-ing about interventions for learning behavior control, cognitive skills, and emo-tional development, and about optimal ways to communicate to help someone to learn. A good educator stimulates the students to think for themselves. An active and involved coach is a good educator. Let us consider the following sports story. You are off to a week-long golf camp for adults. You arrive and learn that for your $2,600 fee you will lie on the couch and tell your instructor how you feel about golf, about the clubs, hitting the ball, and your early experi-ences with golf. How would you respond? Your answer might be, "Excuse me, but I'd like to improve my golf game. My short irons are weak, and my driving is terrible." The instructor might then reply, "What is it about driving that you don't like? Does it make you feel uneasy to be the driving force?" "No—no," you reply. "My drive is weak—I think my backswing is too quick." "Aha," he mumbles, "backswing. Is there any meaning to that? Are you nervous about your back, or backside perhaps?" An interpretive approach is not seen as optimally instructive toward an improved game of golf. Some observation and comment about what needs to be changed (the role of a diagnostician) is needed, but the week will prove more successful following opportunities for practice with feed-back.

In contrast to the scenario just described, what would a good educator (coach) do? He or she would first get you out on the links and watch you play, not taking your self-report as perfect truth but instead observing how you hit the ball and determining for him- or herself (diagnostician) whether your backswing is or is not too quick. The observations would take place on different occasions, using different clubs, and approaching long and short holes. Then, there would be some feedback about strengths and weaknesses, and some discussion of alter-natives and options (acting as a consultant). For example, the educator might inform you that your drives are inconsistent because your waist is shifting when it should not—and it may be that you need to practice with a pole in the ground at your side to get feedback about when your waist is moving. Videotaping might be used, along with modeling by the expert, and group lessons could be integrated as well—before you play the course and keep score. Importantly, a good educator/coach does not make all players play the game the same way! A good coach observes how each student is playing and helps to maximize strengths while reducing hindrances. If a player uses a cross-finger grip for driving but a noncrossed grip for putting, there is no reason to force the player always to cross fingers—if the putting is effective, there is no need to force conformity. Individualized educational attention means that individuals can and should do things a bit differently.

A good educator/coach also pays attention to what the learner is saying to him- or herself, as this internal dialogue can be interfering with performance. Walking up to address the ball and thinking "I can't hit this low iron—the ball's going to go into the rough" is not a preferred internal dialogue. An effective therapist, just like an effective teacher/coach, is involved in the cognitive and behavioral process. More on this later in this chapter.

The posture, or mental attitude, of the cognitive-behavioral therapist working with children and adolescents is one that has a collaborative quality (therapist as consultant), integrates and decodes social information (therapist as diagnostician), and teaches through experiences with involvement (therapist as educator). A quality coach has many of these characteristics, and it is not difficult to suggest that the child therapist view him- or herself somewhat as a mental health coach. A high-quality intervention, be it provided by a psychologist, psychiatrist, school counselor, special educator, classroom teacher, or parent, is one that alters how the client makes sense of experiences and the way the client will behave, think, and feel in the future. Such coaching and correction in thought and action places the client on track toward improved adjustment.

COGNITIVE FUNCTIONING AND ADJUSTMENT IN YOUTH

Although it is not uncommon for some to infer that cognitive functioning has to do with intellectual skills and related assessments, such is not the theme of our discussion. Rather, cognitive functioning within psychopathology and psychotherapy has more to do with complex information processing than with intelligence. As the term is used here, "cognition" refers to a highly complex system, but one that can nevertheless be subdivided for added access and increased understanding. For instance, it has been suggested (Ingram & Kendall, 1986; Kendall & Ingram, 1989) that cognitive content (events), cognitive processes, cognitive products, and cognitive structures can be meaningfully distinguished. Considering these various facets of cognitive functioning permits a more detailed examination of the nature of change sought through treatment.

Cognitive structures can be viewed as memory, and the manner in which information is internally represented in memory. Cognitive content refers to the information that is actually represented or stored: the contents of the cognitive structures. Cognitive processes are the procedures by which the cognitive system operates: how we go about perceiving and interpreting experiences. Cognitive products (e.g., attributions) are the resulting cognition that emerges from the interaction of information, cognitive structures, content, and processes. Psychopathology may be related to problems in any or all of these areas, and effective therapy includes consideration of each of these factors as relevant for and related to each individual client. Although these concepts are complex, a simple, though not everyday, example can help to illustrate their meaningful interrelationships.

Consider the experience of stepping in something a dog left on the lawn. Have you ever had such an experience? If this were to happen to you now, what would you say to yourself? The typical first reaction ("Oh, sh____!") is a self-statement that reflects dismay. This self-statement may be made by most of the people having just made such a misstep, and reflects an initial cognitive content. But these same people then proceed to *process* the experience quite differently, and it is important to understand how these individuals process the same experience differently. For example, some people might process the event by beginning to think about the potential for social embarrassment ("Did anyone see me?"), some might become self-denigrating ("I can't even walk"), while others might be inattentive to the processing of environmental cues and might simply keep walking! The manner of processing the event contributes meaningfully to the behavioral and emotional consequences for the individual.

After the unwanted experience (i.e., stepping in it) and a processing of the event, conclusions are reached regarding the causes of the misstep—cognitive products, such as causal attributions, which also vary across individuals. Some

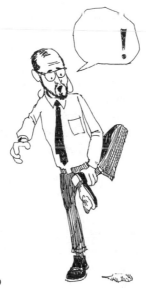

Artist: Peter J. Mikulka, PhD

may attribute the misstep to their inability to do anything right: Such a global internal and stable attribution often characterizes depression (Abramson, Seligman, & Teasdale, 1978; Stark et al., Chapter 5, this volume), and there are related implications for suicidality (see Spirito & Esposito-Smythers, Chapter 6, this volume). An angry individual, in contrast, might see the experience as the result of someone else's provocation ("Whose dog left this here?—I bet the guy knew someone would step in it!"); attributing the mess to someone else's intentional provocation is linked to aggressive retaliatory behavior (see Lochman, Powell, Whidby, & FitzGerald, Chapter 2, and Nelson, Finch, & Ghee, Chapter 4, this volume). Cognitive content, processes, and products are involved in each individual's making sense of environmental events.

Cognitive structures, or templates, are an accumulation of experiences in memory and serve to filter or screen new experiences. The anxious child, for instance, brings a history to upcoming events: the memory of the past. Also referred to as a cognitive schema, a theme of this structure for anxious children/adolescents is threat—threat of loss, threat of anticipated criticism, or threat of physical harm (see Kendall & Suveg, Chapter 7, and Piacentini, March, & Franklin, Chapter 8, this volume). An individual who brings an anxiety-prone structure to the misstep experience noted earlier would see the threat of embarrassment and the risk of germs, and process the experience accordingly. Anxious cognitive processing of the misstep experience might include self-talk such as "What if somebody notices the bad smell; they'll think I'm dirty" or "What if germs get into my shoes and then to my socks, and my feet? Should I throw these shoes away?" Anxiety, as seen in this example of cognitive processing of an event, is laced with perceptions of threat and social evaluation.

Cognitive structures can serve to trigger automatic cognitive content and information processing about behavioral events. That is, after several real or imagined experiences, the person can come to have a characteristic way of making sense of events. Attributions (cognitive products) about the event and its outcomes reflect the influence of the preexisting structure. Therapeutically, cognitive-behavioral interventions seek to provide meaningful and real experiences while intentionally attending to the youth's cognitive content, process, and product (paying attention to the child's self-talk, processing style, and attributional preferences), so that the child/adolescent can be helped to build a cognitive structure that will have a beneficial influence on future experiences.

Does this theoretical approach make too much of too little? After all, stepping in a dog mess is not psychopathology. True, but the example illustrates cognitive processing variations that are linked to maladaptive emotional adjustment. Indeed, the same experience may be linked to reasonable adjustment. What is a healthy way to think about and deal with having just made such a misstep? It would certainly be detrimental if one were to think "It's good luck to step in sh____!," because that might lead one to seek out and intentionally step in it more frequently. Good luck is not likely to accrue, and this would not be healthy thinking. To think (say to oneself) "Good thing I had my shoes on" might be reasonable, as it reflects the absence of self-punitiveness and has an accepting quality. Likewise, "Good thing it was a small dog" reflects self-talk that is not overly harsh. The person might then process the experience by thinking/accepting that cleaning is necessary, that some time will be needed to do an adequate job, and that, next time, one might be more careful and look where one is walking. With regard to an attribution, a person might conclude: "I made a mistake— maybe rushing too much" or "I haven't stepped in it for over a year. Maybe I can go for over 2 years before the next misstep." Such an attribution reflects acceptance of a minor error and hints that increasing the time between mistakes (not never doing it again) is a reasonable goal.

Cognitive-behavioral interventions provide an organized set of treatment activities that challenge the youth's existing structures. Knowing that we all, figuratively, step in it at times, what is needed is a structure for coping with these unwanted events when they occur. In-session role-playing experiences are ideal opportunities for learning, as are out-of-session activities, and with the focus on cognition and emotion during the experience, the experiences make an impression on the client's current and future information processing.

Recall that a goal of treatment is to alter the cognitive structure of the child/adolescent such that he or she will think, feel, and behave differently in the future. Might I be so bold as to now suggest that I have already altered your cognitive structure for the rest of your life! Indeed, I am confident that I have done so. When you next step in a dog mess, you will think of me (this chapter). You will step in it and have a self-statement that reminds you of this passage. Even if I would like for you not to think of me, I probably cannot stop it. I cannot chemically or surgically remove the memory, and I cannot, effectively, ask you not to think of me. I am, as a result of your reading this passage, inextricably linked to dog mess. Paul Salkovskis, himself a cognitive therapist in London, England, has himself been impacted by my earlier telling of this example—so much so that he has adopted it in his own lectures. The story of your misstep has altered your cognitive structure in such a way that you will think differently the next time you step in it. So, too, the therapeutic activities in the CBT interventions described in this book, when accompanied by careful attention to the child's thinking, result in a major alteration in the child's view of future events and experiences.

DISTORTIONS AND DEFICIENCIES

Dysfunctional cognition is maladaptive, but not all dysfunctional cognition is the same. Understanding the nature of the cognitive dysfunction has very important implications for the optimal design of treatment. One central issue for children and adolescents concerns cognitive processing and the differentiation between *cognitive deficiency* in processing and *cognitive distortion* in processing. Processing deficiencies refer to an absence of thinking (lacking careful information processing where it would be beneficial), whereas distortions refer to dysfunctional thinking processes. I have elsewhere (Kendall, 1981) made this distinction to highlight the differences between the forerunners of cognitive-behavioral therapy with adults who focused on modifying distorted thinking (e.g., Beck, 1976; Ellis, 1971) and early cognitive-behavioral training with children that dealt mostly with teaching to remediate deficiencies in thinking (e.g., self-instructions; Kendall, 1977; Meichenbaum & Goodman, 1971). This processing distinction can be furthered when other childhood and adolescent disorders are considered. Anxiety and depression, for example, are typically linked to misconstruals or misperceptions of the social/interpersonal environment. There is active information processing, but it is distorted (e.g., illogical, irrational, crooked). In a series of studies of depressed children, for example, depressed youngsters reported viewing themselves as less capable than did nondepressed children when, in fact, teachers (an objective outsider's judgment) saw the depressed and nondepressed groups of children as nondistinct on the very dimensions that the depressed youth saw themselves as lacking (Kendall, Stark, & Adam, 1990). In the teachers' eyes, the depressed children were not less competent across social, academic, and athletic dimensions. It was the depressed children who evidenced distortion through their misperception (underestimation) of their competencies.

Impulsive children, in contrast to anxious and/or depressed youngsters, are often found to act without thinking (Kendall & Braswell, 1993) and perform poorly due to the lack of forethought and an absence of planning (see also Hinshaw, Chapter 3, this volume). The same can be said for children with attention-deficit/hyperactivity disorder (ADHD). Here, cognitive deficiencies are implicated. These children are not engaging in careful information processing, and their performance suffers as a result. Consider an example where a small group of youngsters is playing soccer. Twelve players are on the soccer field; some are kicking at the ball, others are looking around and talking, while others are standing still. A nonparticipating child sits on the sidelines and, when asked why he is not playing, replies, "I can't play. I'm not good at soccer." In reality, the child can stand, talk, kick at a ball, and so on, and could easily participate in this game being played at a modest skills level. The child's comment reflects mistaken perceptions of the demands in the situation and suggest that he thinks he could not play as well as the others—that they are good players, but he is not. This perception is distorted, and such thinking is tied to feelings of inadequacy, isolation, and withdrawal. Contrast this overly self-critical and isolating style of the withdrawn and depressive child to the impulsive child who, when seeing the soccer game, runs directly onto the soccer field and starts chasing after the ball. He is kicking and running but does not yet know what team he is on, who is on his team with him, or which goal he is going to use. His difficulties emerge more from failing to stop and think (cognitive deficiency) than from active but distorted processing of information.

The terms "deficiency" and "distortion" have been used in the extant literature to describe features of cognitive dysfunction (Kendall, 1993, 2000). In the many instances where the terms have been employed, their use has been, even if unwittingly, consistent with my distinction. For instance, Prior (1984; often citing Hermalin & O'Connor, 1970) described the considerable evidence concerning "the nature of the cognitive deficits in autism" (p. 8) (e.g., suggested inability to use meaning to aid recall). The dominant role assigned to distortions (errors) by rational–emotive theory is evident in DiGiuseppe and Bernard's (1983) comment that "emotional disturbance develops because of one of two types of cognitive errors: empirical distortions of reality that occur . . . (inferences) and exaggerated and distorted appraisals of inferences" (p. 48). In contrast, Spivack and Shure (1982) contend that deficits in interpersonal cognitive problem-solving skills carry etiological clout, and Barkley (1997) has described impulsivity as a disorder resulting from mediational deficits.

To further illustrate the differences between distortions and deficiencies, consider the role of cognition in overcontrolled and undercontrolled (Achenbach, 1966) childhood disorders. Anorexia, most often observed in adolescent females, is related to setting perfectionist goals and demands, carrying an inaccurate view of the self (e.g., self-perception of body), and being "too good" behaviorally. These features of an *overcontrolled* problem reflect cognitive distortions. Anxiety and depression are also considered internalizing problems, and they, too, evidence cognitive distortions that are dysfunctional—misperceptions of demands in the environment, misperceptions of threat and danger, attributional errors (e.g., depression: Hammen & Zupan, 1984; Prieto, Cole, & Tageson, 1992; anxiety: Daleiden, Vasey, & Williams, 1996; Kaslow, Stark, Printz, Livingston, & Tsai, 1992; see also chapters in this volume). In contrast, impulsive acting-out and aggressive behavior, often more characteristic of young boys, is in part related to a lack of self-control, a failure to employ verbal mediational skills, and a lack of social perspective taking. The *undercontrolled* problem child seems to evidence a deficiency in activating and following careful and planful cognitive processing. In aggression, there is evidence of both cognitive deficiency and cognitive distortion (Kendall, Ronan, & Epps, 1990). There are data to suggest that aggressive youth have deficiencies in interpersonal problem solving and data to document that they also show distortions in their processing of information (e.g., Edens, Cavell, & Hughes, 1999; Lochman & Dodge, 1998; see also Lochman et al., Chapter 2, and Nelson et al., Chapter 4, this volume). Limited ability to generate alternative, nonaggressive solutions to interpersonal problems is an example of their deficiencies, while misattribution of the intentionality of others' behavior (Dodge, 1985) demonstrates a tendency toward distorted processing.

My position, emerging from and consistent with the empirical literature, is that (1) undercontrol versus overcontrol is an important behavioral differentiation; (2) distortions versus deficiencies is an important cognitive differentiation; and (3) there are meaningful relationships between the two (Kendall & MacDonald, 1993). Internalized problems are linked more to maladaptive, distorted processing, whereas externalizing problems reflect, in part, deficiencies in processing. Moreover, recognition of this distinction and use of interventions that direct themselves appropriately to the needed arena have benefits for participating youth.

DEVELOPING COPING OVER TIME: A TEMPORAL MODEL

Both empirical research and clinical theory continue to document and emphasize the role of cognitive concepts such as expectations, attributions, self-statements, beliefs, distortions and deficiencies, and schemata in the development of both adaptive and maladaptive behavioral and emotional patterns. Interestingly, these same concepts play important roles in the process of behavioral change. However, the interrelationships of these and other cognitive factors themselves have yet to be fully clarified. How are the functional effects of self-statements similar to or different from those of attributions? How does an individual's maladaptive cognitive structure relate to his or her level of irrational beliefs? Do inconsistent or anxious self-statements reduce interpersonal cognitive processing and problem solving? Quite simply, we know only a modest amount about the organization and interrelations of the cognitive concepts receiving theoretical, research, and clinical attention.

A model with some potential utility is one built on development and organized along a temporal dimension. The developmental model must take into account and be able to reflect the role of cognition associated with behavior across time (e.g., the cognition that occurs before, during, and after events). Because events do not occur in a vacuum (they are typically social and have associated emotional components), and because behavior is determined by multiple causes, the model must allow for the feedback that results from multiple sequential behavioral events and the associated emotional reactions. Again, this involves development over time; that is, a person's cognitive processing before an event varies, depending on the outcomes (behavioral and emotional) of previous events. Thus, the model must allow for fluctuations in preevent cognition associated with the different outcomes (e.g., successful, unsuccessful) of prior events. Moreover, because repetitions of cognitive-event sequences will eventually result in some consistency in cognitive processing, the model highlights the eventual development of more regularized cognitive processing (e.g., cognitive structures, cognitive styles).

Figure 1.1 offers an illustration of the proposed model. The figure depicts the flow of cognition across multiple behavioral events that vary in their emotional intensity. The starting point is a hypothetical initial behavioral event (BE), and the model moves from the initial BE point at the left in Figure 1.1 to the cognitive consistency that results (at the right of the figure).

How do children disambiguate the causes of their behavior once it has already taken place? Stated differently, of all the possible explanations for behavior that can be proposed, how do youth explain their own and others' behavior to themselves? Attributions are temporally short-lived in that their occurrence is at the termination of an event. Nevertheless, their effects can be long-lasting. One could assess an attribution long after an event, although numerous factors (e.g., recall from memory) may interfere with accurate recall. Typically, attributions are preferably assessed immediately after the behavioral event has taken place.

Repetition of behavioral events (multiple BEs in Figure 1.1), especially those with heightened emotional impact, and repetition of the related cognitive processing will result in some degree of consistency. The figure illustrates that cognitive consistency (i.e., a cognitive structure, beliefs, an attributional style) results after multiple events. These cognitive variables (consistencies over time) are more stable than a single attribution. More stable cognitive style variables may be more predictive in a general sense but are less predictive in specific situations than the actual cognition at the time of the specific behavioral event. Upon the accumulation of a history of behavioral events and event outcomes, the child or adolescent entertains more precise anticipatory cognition (i.e., expectancies).

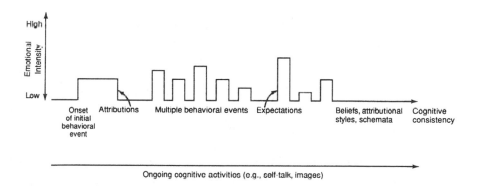

FIGURE 1.1. A temporal model of the flow of cognition across behavioral events of different emotional intensity. Self-statements and images occur at any point and can be studied at various points in the temporal flow. Problem-solving processes also occur at various points, especially where conflicts arise.

Expectancies have been described, for example, as outcome expectancies and self-efficacy expectancies (Bandura, 1977). Other anticipatory cognition includes intentions, plans, and commitments. These latter variables may be more stable and consistent over time than situationally specific expectancies. A generalized expectancy (e.g., locus of control), by its very general transsituational nature, can also be seen as an attributional style. For instance, the generalized expectancy of an external locus of control could be present both before (expectancy) and after (attribution) an event. Before the event, the person's externality leads to an anticipation of having a minimal effect: "Why bother to speak up? No one listens to me." After the event, when a decision has been reached without the individual's input, the event is attributed to powerful others: "See, the big mouths always get their way."

In addition to the cognitive factors mentioned thus far, other cognitive variables have been demonstrated to be important in a cognitive-behavioral analysis—variables such as imagery, self-statements, and cognitive problem-solving skills. These factors occur at all points along the temporal flow depicted in Figure 1.1, and assessments of these factors (e.g., self-talk) can prove valuable in understanding and treating children and adolescents.

Emotional forces are crucial in the design and conduct of interventions, and in the eventual permanence of effective intervention outcomes. The intensity of emotion is represented vertically in Figure 1.1. The higher the bar, the higher the emotionality: A high bar indicates a behavioral event that is more emotionally intense. Emotional intensity contributes because the more intense the experience, the greater the impact on the development of a cognitive structure (schema). Accordingly, minor events, in terms of emotional involvement, may have a limited influence of attributions, future expectations, and behavior, whereas an emotionally significant event has greater impact on the development of a cognitive structure and on future thinking and action. One strives to design and implement therapy as an emotionally positive and involving experience, leading to coping and adaptive cognitive processing. As will be discussed in more detail later in this chapter and in other chapters throughout this book, therapy can help to reduce the client's support for dysfunctional thinking/schemata, and it can help to construct a new schema through which the client can identify and solve problems—movement toward coping.

With specific reference to therapy for children and adolescents, an effective program is one that intentionally plans and capitalizes on creating behavioral experiences with intense positive emotional involvement while paying attention to the anticipatory and after-the-fact cognitive activities of the participants. The therapist guides both the youngster's attributions about prior behavior and emotions and his or her expectations for future behavior and emotions. Thus, the youngster can acquire a cognitive structure for future events (a coping template) that includes the adaptive skills and accurate cognition associated with adaptive functioning.

REASONABLE ASPIRATIONS

To what end does the cognitive-behavioral therapist aspire? What goals are set before us as worthy of conscientious effort? To answer these questions, we will consider (1) the trajectory of normal development, (2) rational therapist expectations about change, and (3) theoretical models that detail the nature of our goals.

Normal Developmental Trajectory

The human organism is on a course of development that, in general, moves toward the acquisition of skills, self-direction, autonomy, and happiness in life; that is, when developmental trajectories are not deflected, an organism moves toward a satisfying self-determined role. Assuming such a trajectory, what place do cognitive-behavioral interventions serve?

Interventions for children and adolescents can be therapeutic, preventive, or enhancement-focused. Ameliorative interventions (therapy) are designed to help youth overcome problems that already exist, whereas prevention attempts to forestall problems before they emerge. Enhancements are aimed at the improvement of the quality of life for individuals not currently in distress (not meeting diagnostic criteria). The clear majority of cognitive-behavioral interventions are therapeutic, with a substantial number being currently or potentially preventive and fewer still serving to enhance an adequate adjustment. Some, such as those intended for victims of disaster (see La Greca and Silverman, Chapter 10, this volume), are designed for otherwise adapting individuals who are victims of natural and other crises. It is considered advantageous to work to both serve currently suffering individuals as well as to prevent future suffering by intervening to help build self-determined persons.

Children and adolescents, as clients, require that the therapist give special consideration to treatment goals. To what extent does the therapist want to help the client make a better adjustment to the present life situation? To what extent does the therapist want to help the client to alter his or her life situation? When family members, school personnel, and other adult authorities are involved, the matter becomes even more complicated. Adjusting to a life situation that is psychologically unhealthy may not be advised (see Deblinger, Behl, & Glickman, Chapter 11, this volume); yet, one cannot always alter a life situation as dramatically as might be construed when thinking of optimal adjustment for the client. The resolution offered by the cognitive-behavioral approach is one that focuses on individual problem solving. The client is given skills that can be used to make self-determinations—skills that are in natural agreement with the developmental move toward autonomy.

Problem-solving skills allow for individual choices, unique to the client, that are optimal for the individual at the time. A child or adolescent client is supported through the thinking processes, encouraged to consider alternative solutions, rewarded and encouraged for effort, and helped to practice the skills needed for future challenges to adjustment. In this manner, the child or adolescent is guided through the process of becoming an active participant in a problem-solving process that, while it does not dictate which answers to choose, does allow for some choice and self-determination. Adolescence may be an especially opportune time for applications of problem-solving (see Holmbeck, O'Mahar, Abad, Colder, & Updegrove, Chapter 12, this volume). Helping to identify options, think through options in a careful manner, and guide the testing and evaluation of options is a goal of cognitive-behavioral therapy.

To return to the notion of a natural developmental trajectory, psychologically healthy adjustment, as it unfolds in nature, builds on resolutions to prior challenges. No one passes directly through. Managing frustration contributes to competence. When one is on a fault-free course of adjustment, interventions may appear to be unnecessary. However, when challenges do not present themselves, or when prior challenges have not been met successfully, new skills are needed and, to the extent possible, the acquisition of those general skills that can be applied to a multitude of new challenges is most promising. By demonstrating, teaching, and honing problem-solving skills, the cognitive-behavioral therapist's efforts coincide with changes to adjustment. The goal is a better-prepared individual—prepared for the inevitable difficulties of life with a set of skills that can facilitate problem resolution.

Rational Therapist Expectations

The best hitter in major league baseball hits approximately .340, professional bowlers do not bowl 300 routinely, and not every play in football leads to a touchdown or even a first down. Perhaps even more striking, Michael Jordan—consensually the best basketball player ever—has a lifetime shooting percentage of approximately 49%. Yet we, as mental health professionals, often carry expectations that we (and our therapies by implication) are expected to help all or almost all of our clients. To expect such a success rate is irrational, maladaptive, and likely to be associated with other distressing problems.

Rational therapist expectations include the belief that interventions will be helpful in the movement toward successful adjustment and that individuals who acquire the skills communicated in therapy will at some time experience the benefit of those skills. What is irrational is to expect that any child, with any problem, can be "fixed" using psychotherapy—cognitive-behavioral or otherwise. The notion that therapy provides a "cure" is a troublesome and misleading belief (see Kendall, 1989).

Children and adolescents do not, automatically, evidence benefit from psychological forms of therapy or health-enhancing programs. And, even in cases where some success is obvious, the chance of relapse remains ever present. If relapse does occur, was the therapy ineffective? Should therapy be expected to prevent all relapses as a part of the "cure" of psychopathology? A reasonable and rational expectation for therapists to hold is that therapy does not cure maladaptation. Therapy does provide help, but the help is more in the form of a strategy for the *management* of psychopathology. The anxiety-disordered adolescent, for example, will not receive a treatment that will totally remove all perceptions of situations as anxiety-provoking or totally eliminate self-evaluative concerns, but the treated youth will be able to employ newly acquired strategies in the management of anxious arousal when it does occur. The angry–aggressive child may not erase all impulses for immediate retaliatory action, but he or she will have available skills that can be implemented when more cautious, thoughtful action and emotion management are needed. To expect cures is irrational; to expect to impart the wisdom that, through experience, will facilitate adjustment is sage.

Dealing with relapse, or relapse temptations, is part of life, as evident in efforts to maintain healthy eating habits (see Wilfley, Passi, Cooperberg, & Stein, Chapter 9, this volume). Even our most successful clients will be challenged by the many opportunities for decisions that are less than optimal. Our goal is not to "have all go well forever," but to improve upon the trajectory that was evident before treatment began. To alter a nonadaptive trajectory is to produce therapeutic gains, and such an expectation is rational.

Social anxiety and depressive symptomatology are common emotional difficulties. Many therapists working with children and adolescents deal with problems of detrimental anxiety and unwanted depression. Youth with these emotional problems have, as part of their distress, a maladaptive way of processing their world that requires intervention. As is true with adult clients suffering from these same disorders, cognitive–behavioral interventions strive to rectify the distorted information processing that is linked to the emotional distress. Unfortunately, the popular press has overpromoted an idea that has been labeled the "power of positive thinking." Do we want our clients to become big-time positive thinkers? Is such a goal a rational and desired outcome of treatment? As it turns out, theory suggests, and research evidence supports, the notion that it is *not* so much the power of positive thinking that is related to emotional adjustment or improvement in treatment as it is the reduction in negative thinking. I have elsewhere referred to this as "the power of nonnegative thinking" (Kendall, 1984). As we achieve reductions in overly negative and harsh cognitive processing, we reduce negative thinking and we reduce associated psychological distress (Kendall & Treadwell, 2005; Treadwell & Kendall, 1996).

Would you want to be someone who always thinks positively? Individuals who think or talk to themselves in only positive terms are not psychologically healthy. Rather, we all experience life events that have negative features, and a rational individual accepts these inevitabilities. One would not want to be thinking only positive thoughts when in a difficult situation. For example, imagine that you are on an intercontinental airplane trip. During excessive air turbulence, you find yourself sitting next to someone who sees everything positively. The turbulence causes the plane's door to open, and the person next to you says, "Ah, fresh air!" Not exactly a rational response! There are times when a negative thought or two is quite reasonable. Purely positive information processing is, when judged against reality, somewhat distorted. If purely positive thinking is not the goal, and adjustment is related to a reduction in negative thinking, what then should therapists hold as a rational expectation for the outcome of interventions?

Should treatments be designed to reduce the negative, self-critical styles of thinking of the anxious and depressed youth? An answer lies in the ratio of positive to negative thinking. The ratio of positive to negative thinking that has been found to be associated with adjustment is 0.62:0.38 (see Kendall, Howard, & Hays, 1989; Schwartz & Garamoni, 1989). These findings are reported for older adolescents, but the concept holds true for younger persons as well. Generally speaking, this 2:1 ratio suggests that positive thinking occupies two-thirds of the thinking, whereas negative thinking occupies one-third of the thinking in individuals who are not maladjusted (see also Treadwell & Kendall, 1996). Depressed cases, identified psychometrically and clinically, show a 1:1 ratio: the 50–50 split reflecting an equal frequency of positive and negative thinking—an internal dialogue that evidences conflict between the positive and the negative.

Let me suggest that knowing an optimal ratio of positive to negative thinking is 2:1 serves as a guide for the therapist. Overly optimistic thinking is not necessarily healthy, and shifting too much toward a 1:1 ratio is unhealthy as well. It is healthy to acknowledge certain unwanted situations, accept a negative thought or two, and then proceed to counter the negative aspects with some positive thinking. Positive thinking helps overrule negative thinking, but negative thinking should not be totally eliminated.

Although we all have our share of successful child clients, is it the case that children and adolescents typically strive to (1) display their newly acquired skills and (2) thank the therapist for the help? Sometimes, as the many fortunate therapists can attest, children and/or their parents do offer a warm and genuine "thanks." However, it is also quite possible (even likely) that children and adolescents learn from their therapeutic interactions but, for a variety of reasons, do not want to let us know. They sometimes act as if they were right all along and did not need nor benefit from therapy. It is irrational for therapists to expect that all clients will, at posttreatment, demonstrate that they have benefited from our interventions.

It is possible that there will be beneficial effects, but that these effects will not be readily evident immediately at the end of treatment. I refer to this, admittedly optimistically, as "sleeper effects." Beneficial learning took place, but the evidence of the learning does not appear until a later point in development, or until a different situation emerges. For example, completion of a therapy that provides an opportunity for learning social problem-solving skills might not produce immediate use of these skills. It may be that after the passage of time, the percolation of the ideas at various times, and the successful use of parts of the problem-solving process, the child/adolescent client comes to employ and recognize the benefits of a problem-solving approach. It has been my experience, for instance, that interpersonal skills learned by a child during early childhood take a temporary backseat to the social pressure of peers. After further developmental changes, the skills acquired earlier can emerge without conflict and better serve the individual's current adjustment.

Continuing an optimistic line of thought, it is also possible for "spillover" effects to occur. Spillover effects refer to the beneficial gains associated with a child's treatment that may be evident in the parents, siblings, or other nontarget participants in the treatment. For example, a child participates in and successfully completes a cognitive-behavioral treatment for an anxiety disorder (see Kendall & Suveg, Chapter 7, this volume). At the end of treatment he or she is less avoidant and more participatory in the activities of his or her peers. As a result, the child is spending less emotionally draining time with the parents and is less demanding and troublesome to them. The tension between the parents, which had been in part linked to the child's anxious distress, diminishes in conjunction with the child's overcoming the unwanted anxiety. The effects of the treatment spill over onto other nontarget arenas. In this example, although such effects may occur, it is likely that they will be more likely and more pronounced with increased involvement of the child's parents. Some optimism is justified, given the frequency with which CBT appears among the list of empirically supported treatments. However, there are challenges remaining (Kendall & Choudhury, 2003; Kendall & Ollendick, 2004), and the authors contributing to this volume add to our knowledge of not only what to do and how to do it but also what remains to be done.

Conceptualization of Change

Children and adolescents with behavioral and emotional difficulties have associated maladaptive qualities in their social information processing. For the depressed adolescent who is misattributing negative outcomes to internal–global–stable features, as well as for the impulsive/hyperactive child who is active in behavior but deficient in planful forethought, modifications of the cognitive processing are in order. Theoretically speaking, how might we conceptualize the needed changes? How best to describe the nature of the cognitive changes that are a part of the goals of treatment?

Some cognitive distortions, as noted in earlier discussion, require modification. New experiences, with guided processing both before and after the experiences, will help to straighten out crooked thinking. What is being suggested is that the existing cognitive structure is not erased but that new skills and means of construing the world are built, and these new constructions come to serve as new templates for making sense of future experiences. Therapy does not provide a surgical removal of unwanted cognitive structures or emotional histories, but it helps to build new schemata with new strategies that can be employed in place of the earlier dysfunctional ones.

Therapy offers exposure to multiple behavioral events with concurrent cognitive and emotional processing, such that new cognitive structures can be built over time (recall the discussion tied to Figure 1.1). Positive emotional tones can increase the potency of the experience and add to its impact on the youth's developing new views. As these new perceptions are incorporated into the child's more overarching view of the world and his or her place in it, future experiences are construed differently (less maladaptively). Using these "revised views" (newly acquired skills and constructed schemata), the individual moves forward to face and confront new challenges in ways that manage former maladaptive tendencies.

CLOSING

Children and adolescents typically do not call or refer themselves for services from a mental health professional. Quite the contrary, individuals other than the child or adolescent, such as parents, teachers, or guardians, are often the initiators of psychological services. The receipt of mental health services as youth is special: Seeking help for oneself is very different than being sent for services by someone else! Adults, who themselves are in personal suffering, seek their own mental health services.

The fact that children are sent for treatment, whereas adults often seek it, is an important distinction that has clinical implications. Children and adolescents must, on their own, enjoy the experience, want to be there, and even come to see the potential benefits of therapy. Accordingly, efforts to create a pleasant affective environment and a motivation for further participation are essential.

One of the main challenges facing the developing organism is the movement toward autonomy and independence. Central to this movement is the family, specifically, the parents, and their supportive or constraining styles. Child and adolescent clients are not fully capable, as yet, of being entirely independent, and family, school, and other contextual influences must be considered. Indeed, although the thrust of the present theory is on individual change, multiple influences have been considered and incorporated.

In the analysis thus far, little discussion has been devoted to factors such as trust, respect, and the child–therapist relationship as part of the therapeutic process. It is not because these matters are unimportant, but rather because they are *essential* to all forms of therapeutic interventions. The relationship, for example, is a common factor across treatment approaches that can contribute to favorable outcomes (see Shirk & Karver, Chapter 13, this volume). Factors that contribute to a strong relationship, such as "flexibility" (Chu & Kendall, 2004), are to be encouraged, as are behavioral and emotional patterns that clearly communicate mutual respect and trust. As an illustration, independent raters' judgments about the therapists' degree of "collaboration" has been found to be predictive of the child's assigning a favorable rating to the therapeutic relationship (Creed & Kendall, 2005). It is my position that optimal treatment outcomes are linked to the implementation of empirically supported procedures in a manner that evidences "flexibility within fidelity" and in a context that is based on a supportive environment.

ACKNOWLEDGMENTS

I express gratitude to the many graduate students and faculty of the clinical psychology doctoral training program at Temple University for their thoughtful discussions and meaningful collaborations. Portions of this chapter were prepared with the help of research grant support from the National Institute of Mental Health (Grant Nos. MH59087, MH64484, and MH63747).

REFERENCES

Abramson, L. Y., Seligman, M. E. P., & Teasdale, J. D. (1978). Learned helplessness in humans: Critique and reformulation. *Journal of Abnormal Psychology, 87,* 49–74.
Achenbach, T. M. (1966). The classification of children's psychiatric symptoms: A factor analytic study. *Psychological Monographs, 80*(Whole No. 615)
Bandura, A. (1977). Self-efficacy: Toward a unifying theory of behavior change. *Psychological Review, 84,* 191–215.
Barkley, R. A. (1997). Behavioral inhibition, sustained attention, and executive functions: Constructing a unifying theory of ADHD. *Psychological Bulletin, 121,* 65–94.
Barmish, A., & Kendall, P. C. (2005). Should parents be co-clients in cognitive-behavioral therapy with anxious youth? *Journal of Clinical Child and Adolescent Psychology, 34,* 569–581.
Beck, A. T. (1976). *Cognitive therapy and the emotional disorders.* New York: International Universities Press.
Bernard, M. E., & Joyce, M. R. (1984). *Rational emotive therapy with children and adolescents: Theory, treatment strategies, preventive motives.* New York: Wiley
Chambless, D., & Hollon, S. (1998). Defining empirically supported treatments. *Journal of Consulting and Clinical Psychology, 66,* 5–17.
Chu, B. C., & Kendall, P. C. (2004). Positive association of child involvement and treatment outcome within a manual-based cognitive-behavioral treatment for children with anxiety. *Journal of Consulting and Clinical Psychology, 72,* 1–11.
Creed, T., & Kendall, P. C. (2005). Therapist alliance-building behavior within a cognitive-behavioral treatment of anxiety in youth. *Journal of Consulting and Clinical Psychology, 73,* 498–505.
Dalciden, E. L., Vasey, M. W., & Williams, L. L. (1996). Assessing children's state of mind: A multitrait, multimethod study. *Psychological Assessment, 8,* 125–134.

Diener, E., & Lucas, R. (1999). Personality and subjective well-being. In D. Kahneman, E. Diener, & N. Schwarz (Eds.), *Well-being: The foundations of hedonic psychology* (pp. 213–239). New York: Russell Sage Foundation.

DiGiuseppe, R., & Bernard, M. E. (1983). Principles of assessment and methods of treatment with children: Special consideration. In A. Ellis & M. E. Bernard (Eds.), *Rational–emotive approaches to the problems of childhood* (pp. 45–88). New York: Plenum Press.

Dodge, K. (1985). Attributional bias in aggressive children. In P. C. Kendall (Ed.), *Advances in cognitive-behavioral research and therapy* (Vol. 4, pp. 75–111). New York: Academic Press.

Edens, J., Cavell, T., & Hughes, J. (1999). The self-systems of aggressive children: A cluster-analytic investigation. *Journal of Child Psychology and Psychiatry, 40*, 441–453.

Ellis, A. (1971). *Growth through reason*. Hollywood, CA: Wilshire Books.

Fishman, K. D. (1995). *Behind the one-way mirror: Psychotherapy with children*. New York: Bantam Books.

Hammen, C., & Zupan, B. (1984). Self-schemas, depression, and the processing of personal information in children. *Journal of Experimental Child Psychology, 37*, 598–608.

Hartup, W. W. (1984). Peer relations. In P. Mussen (Ed.), *Handbook of child psychology*. New York: Wiley.

Hermalin, B., & O'Connor, W. (1970). *Psychological experiments with autistic children*. Oxford, UK: Pergamon Press.

Hibbs, E. D., & Jensen, P. S. (Eds.). (2005). *Psychosocial treatments for child and adolescent disorders: Empirically based strategies for clinical practice* (2nd ed). Washington, DC: American Psychological Association.

Ingram, R. E., & Kendall, P. C. (1986). Cognitive clinical psychology: Implications of an information processing perspective. In R. E. Ingram (Ed.), *Information processing approaches to clinical psychology* (pp. 3–21). New York: Academic Press.

Ingram, R. E., Miranda, J., & Segal, Z. V. (1998). *Cognitive vulnerability to depression*. New York: Guilford Press.

Kaslow, N., Stark, K., Printz, B., Livingston, R., & Tsai, S. (1992). Cognitive Triad Inventory for Children: Development and relation to depression and anxiety. *Journal of Clinical Child Psychology, 21*, 339–347.

Kazdin, A. E., & Weisz, J. R. (Eds.). (2003). *Evidence-based psychotherapies for children and adolescents*. New York: Guilford Press.

Kendall, P. C. (1977). On the efficacious use of verbal self-instructional procedures with children. *Cognitive Therapy and Research, 1*, 331–341.

Kendall, P. C. (1981). Assessment and cognitive-behavioral interventions: Purposes, proposals and problems. In P. C. Kendall & S. D. Hollon (Eds.), *Assessment strategies for cognitive-behavioral interventions* (pp. 1–12). New York: Academic Press.

Kendall, P. C. (1984). Behavioral assessment and methodology. In G. T. Wilson, C. M. Franks, K. D. Brownell, & P. C. Kendall, *Annual review of behavior therapy: Theory and practice* (Vol. 9, pp. 39–94). New York: Brunner/Mazel.

Kendall, P. C. (1985). Toward a cognitive-behavioral model of child psychopathology and a critique of related interventions. *Journal of Abnormal Child Psychology, 13*, 357–372.

Kendall, P. C. (1989). The generalization and maintenance of behavior change: Comments, considerations, and the "no-cure" criticism. *Behavior Therapy, 20*, 357–364.

Kendall, P. C. (1993). Cognitive-behavioral therapies with youth: Guiding theory, current status, and emerging developments. *Journal of Consulting and Clinical Psychology, 61*, 235–247.

Kendall, P. C. (1998). Empirically supported psychological therapies. *Journal of Consulting and Clinical Psychology, 66*, 3–7.

Kendall, P. C. (2000). *Childhood disorders*. London: Psychology Press.

Kendall, P. C. (2001). Flexibility within fidelity. *Clinical Child and Adolescent Psychology Newsletter, 16*(2), 1–5.

Kendall, P. C., & Braswell, L. (1993). *Cognitive-behavioral therapy for impulsive children* (2nd ed.). New York: Guilford Press.

Kendall, P. C., & Choudhury, M. (2003). Children and adolescents in cognitive-behavioral therapy: Some past efforts and current advances, and the challenges in our future. *Cognitive Therapy and Research, 27,* 89–104.

Kendall, P. C., Chu, B., Gifford, A., Hayes, C., & Nauta, M. (1998). Breathing life into a manual. *Cognitive and Behavioral Practice, 5,* 177–198.

Kendall, P. C., & Hollon, S. D. (1979). Cognitive-behavioral interventions: Overview and current status. In P. C. Kendall & S. D. Hollon (Eds.), *Cognitive behavioral interventions: Theory, research and procedures* (pp. 1–13). New York: Academic Press.

Kendall, P. C., Howard, B. L., & Hays, R. C. (1989). Self-referent speech and psychopathology: The balance of positive and negative thinking. *Cognitive Therapy and Research, 13,* 583–598.

Kendall, P. C., & Ingram, R. E. (1987). The future for cognitive assessment of anxiety: Let's get specific. In L. Michelson & L. M. Ascher (Eds.), *Anxiety and stress disorders: Cognitive-behavioral assessment and treatment* (pp. 89–104). New York: Guilford Press.

Kendall, P. C., & Ingram, R. E. (1989). Cognitive-behavioral perspectives: Theory and research on depression and anxiety. In P. C. Kendall & D. Watson (Eds.), *Anxiety and depression: Distinctive and overlapping features* (pp. 27–54). New York: Academic Press.

Kendall, P. C., & MacDonald, J. P. (1993). Cognition in the psychopathology of youth, and implications for treatment. In K. S. Dobson & P. C. Kendall (Eds.), *Psychopathology and cognition* (pp. 387–430). San Diego, CA: Academic Press.

Kendall, P. C. & Ollendick, T. (2004). Setting the research and practice agenda for anxiety in children and adolescents: A topic comes of age. *Cognitive and Behavioral Practice, 11,* 65–74.

Kendall, P. C., Ronan, K., & Epps, J. (1990). Aggression in children/adolescents: Cognitive-behavioral treatment perspectives. In D. Pepler & K. Rubin (Eds.), *Development and treatment of childhood aggression* (pp. 341–360). Hillsdale, NJ: Erlbaum.

Kendall, P. C., Stark, K., & Adam, T. (1990). Cognitive deficit or cognitive distortion in childhood depression. *Journal of Abnormal Child Psychology, 18,* 267–283.

Kendall, P. C., & Treadwell, K. R. H. (2005). The mediational role of negative self-talk in treatment outcome for anxiety-disordered youth. *Journal of Consulting and Clinical Psychology.* Manuscript submitted for publication.

Lochman, J., & Dodge, K. (1998). Distorted perceptions in dyadic interactions of aggressive and nonaggressive boys: Effects of prior expectations, context, and boy's age. *Development and Psychopathology, 10,* 495–512.

Lonigan, C., Elbert, J., & Johnson, S. B. (1998). Empirically supported psychosocial interventions for children: An overview. *Journal of Clinical Child Psychology, 27,* 138–145.

Meichenbaum, D., & Goodman, J. (1971). Training impulsive children to talk to themselves: A means of developing self-control. *Journal of Abnormal Psychology, 77,* 115–126.

Prieto, S., Cole, D., & Tageson, C. (1992). Depressive self-schemas in clinic and nonclinic children. *Cognitive Therapy and Research, 16,* 521–534.

Prior, M. (1984). Developing concepts of childhood autism: The influence of experimental cognitive research. *Journal of Consulting and Clinical Psychology, 52,* 4–16.

Santostefano, S., & Reider, C. (1984). Cognitive controls and aggression in children: The concept of cognitive-affective balance. *Journal of Consulting and Clinical Psychology, 52,* 46–56.

Southam-Gerow, M., & Kendall, P. C. (2000). A preliminary study of the emotional understanding of youths referred for treatment of anxiety disorders. *Journal of Clinical Child Psychology, 29*, 319–327.

Spivack, G., & Shure, M. B. (1982). The cognition of social adjustments: Interpersonal cognitive problem-solving thinking. In B. B. Lahey & A. E. Kazdin (Eds.), *Advances in clinical child psychology* (Vol. 5, pp. 323–372). New York: Plenum Press.

Treadwell, K. R. H., & Kendall, P. C. (1996). Self-talk in anxiety-disordered youth: States-of-mind, content specificity, and treatment outcome. *Journal of Consulting and Clinical Psychology, 64*, 941–950.

PART II
EXTERNALIZING DISORDERS

CHAPTER 2

Aggressive Children
Cognitive-Behavioral Assessment and Treatment

JOHN E. LOCHMAN, NICOLE R. POWELL,
JANET M. WHIDBY, and DAVID P. FITZGERALD

Aggression is a set of primarily interpersonal actions that consist of verbal or physical behaviors that are destructive or injurious to others or to objects (Bandura, 1973). Although almost all children display some of this type of aggressive behavior, it is only when aggression is exceptionally severe, frequent, and/or chronic that it becomes indicative of psychopathology.

Children with high levels of aggressive behavior are most often diagnosed as having conduct disorder or oppositional defiant disorder, but aggressive behavior can be comorbid with other diagnostic categories as well. Children with subclinical conditions or a variety of other primary diagnoses (e.g., attention-deficit/hyperactivity disorder [ADHD]; dysthymia; posttraumatic stress disorder) may have periodic or chronic bursts of aggressive behavior. A common characteristic of all seriously aggressive children is that they have intense negative effects on the people who interact with them. Peers are victimized, teachers are disrupted from their teaching activities, and parents are frustrated with being unable to control these children's coercive and provocative behaviors. Because of these intense, flagrant effects on others, aggressive children are referred for mental health services at higher rates than are children with most other forms of psychopathology.

Longitudinal research has indicated that aggressive behavior is quite stable during childhood and adolescence, and that aggression is more consistent over time than most other behavioral patterns (Hill, Coie, Lochman, Greenberg, & the Conduct Problems Prevention Research Group, 2004). Children who display a wide range of different kinds of aggressive, antisocial behavior and who are highly antisocial in multiple settings (e.g., home, school, community) are at greatest risk for continued disorder (Loeber & Dishion, 1983). These children display a progressive accumulation, or "stacking," of a variety of problem behaviors as they develop further along the trajectory to conduct disorder (Loeber, 1990), and they are at risk for a wide range of negative outcomes, including adolescent drug and alcohol use, cigarette smoking, school truancy and dropout, early teenage parenthood, delinquency, and violence (e.g., Lochman & Wayland, 1994; Miller-Johnson et al., 1999; Windle, 1990).

Problem youth typically do not differ from their peers on just one dimension, such as aggressiveness, but instead vary on multiple behavioral dimensions related to poor self-control, leading to the high correlation among delinquency, substance use, and depression (Wills & Filer, 1996). These self-control difficulties may be the result of deficits in children's executive cognitive functioning, which controls children's self-regulation of goal-directed behavior (Giancola, Martin, Tarter, Pelham, & Moss, 1996; Seguin, Pihl, Harden, Tremblay, & Boulerice, 1995). As individuals accumulate an increasing number of risky problem behaviors, their odds for violent behavior increase (Lochman, 2003). By age 14, risk taking, drug selling, gang membership, early initiation of violence, and peer delinquency all combine to become the strongest predictors of later violence (Herrenkohl et al., 1998). Thus, it is important to anticipate co-occurring negative outcomes and comorbidity of risk factors. For example, aggressive children who are also socially rejected by their peers have twice the risk rate for middle school adjustment problems than do aggressive-only children (Coie, Lochman, Terry, & Hyman, 1992); conduct-disordered adolescents who are also depressed have an earlier onset of alcohol use than do conduct-disordered-only adolescents (Miller-Johnson, Lochman, Coie, Terry, & Hyman, 1998); and aggressive children who also have ADHD have more violent offending and greater substance use than do aggressive-only children (Thompson, Riggs, Mikulich, & Crowley, 1996). Because aggression is a broad risk factor, it has become an important focus for intervention.

In this chapter, we present a cognitive-behavioral (social-cognitive) model for aggression, and discuss the cognitive-behavioral assessment techniques and intervention strategies associated with this model. The Coping Power Program, a multifaceted intervention program for aggressive children, will be described. We will review only cognitive-behavioral therapy (CBT) results and procedures with aggressive children and will not cover adolescence or impulsive, hyperactive behavior. Another chapter in this volume addresses related topics.

CONCEPTUAL FRAMEWORK FOR COGNITIVE-BEHAVIORAL THERAPY: IDENTIFYING MEDIATIONAL PROCESSES

CBT focuses upon the perceptions and thoughts of aggressive children as they encounter perceived threats and frustrations. The techniques and goals of CBT are directed at children's deficiencies and distortions in their cognitive processing of events, and at their regulation of emotions, especially anger. Anger is the mood that people have most difficulty controlling (Goleman, 1995), and intense uncontrolled anger arousal can be a central component of aggression and externalizing behavior problems (Lochman, Dunn, & Wagner, 1997). Anger corresponds to the "fight" response in the fight–flight arousal mechanism; this innate action tendency involves an attack on the agent perceived to be blameworthy (Lazarus, 1993). Refinements in CBT techniques have arisen largely because of new research and models of these deficiencies in children's self-regulation and processing of social conflicts, and of the parent and community contextual factors that influence these dysfunctional cognitive-affective processes. Before examining CBT with aggressive children, we will first review the social-cognitive model used as a foundation for our Coping Power program. As described elsewhere (e.g., Lochman, Whidby, & FitzGerald, 2000), this social-cognitive model is rooted historically in earlier research on social learning theories (Bandura, 1977; Rotter, Chance, & Phares, 1972) and on the development of children's self-regulation abilities (Meichenbaum & Goodman, 1971). These self-regulation abilities are affected by children's executive cognitive functioning abilities (Giancola, Zeichner, Yarnell, & Dickson, 1996) and are shaped by children's relationships with their caregivers into "working models" of their interpersonal environment (Lochman & Dodge, 1998; Shaw & Bell, 1993).

Contextual Social-Cognitive Model of Anger and Aggression

The Coping Power Program we use with aggressive children is based on an evolving, empirically based social-cognitive model (Lochman & Wells, 2002b) of how anger develops in children and results in aggressive responses. In these types of information processing models, Kendall and MacDonald (1993) differentiated cognitive deficiencies, which involve an insufficient amount of cognitive activity, from cognitive distortions, which involve misperceptions. Both types of cognitive dysfunctions can be seen in aggressive children's social-cognitive dysfunctions.

The model presented here originally derived in large part from Novaco's (1978) conceptualization of anger arousal in adults, and has been substantially affected by Dodge's (Crick & Dodge, 1994) social information-processing model. In the social-cognitive model the child encounters a potentially anger-arousing stimulus event, but the emotional and physiological reaction is due to the child's perception and appraisal of the event rather than due to the event itself. These perceptions and appraisals can be accurate or inaccurate, and are derived from prior expectations that filter the event and from the child's selective attention to specific aspects, or cues, in the stimulus event. If the child has interpreted the event to be threatening, provocative, or frustrating, he or she can then experience physiological arousal and also will become engaged in another set of cognitive activities directed at deciding upon an appropriate behavioral response to the event. The internal arousal has a reciprocal interaction with the individual's appraisal processes, because the child has to interpret and label the emotional connotations of the arousal, and the increased arousal narrows the child's attention to certain types of cues associated with possible threat. These three sets of internal activities—(1) perception and appraisal, (2) arousal, and (3) social problem solving—contribute to the child's behavioral response and to the resulting consequences the child receives from peers and adults and experiences internally as self-consequences. These consequent reactions from others can then become stimulus events, which feed back into the model, becoming recurrent, connected behavioral units.

We overview the social-cognitive deficiencies and distortions that have been found in research with aggressive children (e.g., Dodge, Laird, Lochman, Zelli, & the Conduct Problems Prevention Research Group, 2002) and propose how other cognitive, physiological, and familial factors could affect these social-cognitive products. The social-cognitive processes we have described account for sequential activation of situational moment-to-moment processes, but they do not specify the structural relationship of more basic cognitive activities to social cognitions. Social information-processing models have begun to indicate how enduring, cross-situational cognitive schemata affect immediate momentary processing (Lochman & Dodge, 1998). Similarly, the effects of psychophysiological processes and family influences on children's social information-processing have only become an active area of investigation in the past decade.

In this chapter, we use an adaptation of the cognitive taxonomic system (Kendall & Ingram, 1989) to organize the relevant sets of cognitive activities into three clusters, which will then be integrated into our model. Schematic propositions are the stored information in cognitive structures in memory. Cognitive operations are various procedures that process stored and incoming information (e.g., attention, encoding, retrieval), and, in our case, can be separated from the content of social-cognitive products. Social-cognitive products are the results of interaction between stored schematic propositions, cognitive operations, and incoming sensory data about stimulus events. Social-cognitive products include social-cognitive appraisals, social problem solving, and cognitive-emotional linkage (see Table 2.1). Finally, the role of key social influences, especially parents and peers, will be noted.

TABLE 2.1. Cognitive Characteristics of Aggressive Children

Social-cognitive products

Social-cognitive appraisals
  Overly sensitive to hostile cues
  Bias in attributing hostile intentions to others
  Underestimate own aggressiveness
Social problem solving
  Limited repertoire of solutions for the most aggressive youth
  For preadolescent aggressive children: few verbal assertion solutions and excess
    direct-action solutions
  For aggressive adolescents: few cooperative solutions
  Aggressive backup solutions
Appraisal of internal arousal
  Overlabeling of affective arousal as anger
  Associated with increased hostile attributional biases
  Low levels of empathy

Cognitive operations

Difficulty in sustaining attention
Retrieval of salient, less competent solutions when automatically retrieving solutions
  from long-term memory

Schematic propositions

Higher value on social goals of dominance and revenge rather than affiliation
Less value placed on outcomes such as victim suffering, victim retaliation, or peer
  rejection
Expectation that aggressive behavior will produce tangible rewards and reduce aversive
  reactions
Bias in expecting that others will be excessively aggressive in upcoming interactions
Low self-esteem in the preadolescent period

Social-Cognitive Products

Social-Cognitive Appraisals

These social-cognitive products consist of the first two stages in Crick and Dodge's (1994) reformulated social information-processing model: cue utilization and attributions about others' intentions. Aggressive children have been found to perceive and encode cues in the environment around them in a different manner than do nonaggressive children, scanning for hostile cues in a hypervigilant manner. Social cognitive researchers have had children listen to a series of audiotaped and videotaped segments in which child actors describe and portray hostile, benevolent, and neutral situations. After listening to, or viewing, the segments, the children were asked to remember as many cues as they could. In comparison with nonaggressive children, aggressive children and adolescents have been found to recall fewer relevant cues (even after controlling for intelligence levels) (Lochman & Dodge, 1994) and to remember more of the last statements they hear, indicating that they had a developmental lag in their cue utilization (Milich & Dodge, 1984).

Another developmental lag has been evident in aggressive boys' tendencies to decide to attend to few cues while attempting to interpret the meaning of others' behavior (Dodge & Newman, 1981). When given an opportunity to listen to as many taped statements about a child's intentions as they wished, nonaggressive boys listened to 40% more cues before making a decision than did aggressive boys. In addition, aggressive children have been found to encode and retrieve significantly more cues that convey hostile connotations than do nonaggressive children (Dodge, Pettit, McClaskey, & Brown, 1986). McKinnon, Lamb, Belsky, and Baum (1990) have suggested that these cue encoding biases can be the result of aggressive children's earlier social interactions with their parents, because children who experience primarily negative or aggressive interactions with their parents will be more likely to attend to cues of hostility and aggression in others.

In the milliseconds after cues are perceived, aggressive children form inferences about others' intentions, and these efforts to decipher the meaning of others' behavior have been found to be significantly influenced by their higher rate of detection of hostile cues and by their prior expectations that others would be hostile toward them (Dodge & Frame, 1982). As a result, aggressive boys have been found to be 50% more likely than nonaggressive boys to infer that antagonists in hypothetical provocations acted with hostile rather than neutral or benign intent (Dodge, 1980). Furthermore, recent research has demonstrated that highly aggressive boys' tendency to make hostile attributions is exacerbated by the induction of negative feelings (Orobio de Castro, Slot, Bosch, Koops, & Veerman, 2003). A recent meta-analytic review has demonstrated that the relation between hostile attribution of intent and aggressive behavior is robust (Orobio de Castro, Veerman, Koops, Bosch, & Monshouwer, 2002), although the size of the effect was found to be largest when certain assessment methods were used (e.g., orally presented vignettes). This hostile attributional bias has been found to be equally evident in both preadolescent and adolescent severely aggressive boys (Lochman & Dodge, 1994), again suggesting that these appraisal difficulties become well established during early socialization experiences in the home, neighborhood, and peer group.

In actual competitive dyadic discussions with nonaggressive peers, aggressive boys not only tend to overperceive the peer's aggressiveness, but they also substantially underestimate their own aggressiveness (Lochman & Dodge, 1998). These distorted perceptions by aggressive children during live interactions have been found to occur on both competitive and cooperative tasks, and have been found to be due to aggressive boys' prior expectations (Lochman & Dodge, 1998). Due to their distorted perceptions of the peer and of themselves, aggressive boys implicitly attribute responsibility for the conflict to the peer. This pattern of distorted perceptions and interpretation of others in the early stages of a conflict sequence can contribute to the boy's subsequently feeling quite justified in responding in an intensely aggressive manner.

Social Problem-Solving

While cognitive distortions are evident in aggressive children's appraisal processes, cognitive deficiencies are more evident in their social problem-solving difficulties. In this chapter social problem solving refers to the last four of Crick and Dodge's (1994) stages, and includes goal selection, generation of alternative solutions, consideration of the consequences of solutions, and behavioral implementation of solutions. Solution generation and consideration of the consequences are social-cognitive products in our model. Boys with the very highest level of aggressive behavior, in comparison with moderately aggressive boys, generate few solutions to the social problems they face (Lochman & Dodge, 1994). Although moderately aggressive children do not have a clear deficit in the number of solutions they generate, both moderately and severely aggressive children have consistent and characteristic deficiencies in the content or quality of the solutions they generate.

Using measures with hypothetical open-middle and open-ended vignettes, aggressive children have been found to generate fewer verbal assertion and compromise solutions than do nonaggressive children (Joffe, Dobson, Fine, Marriage, & Haley, 1990; Lochman & Dodge, 1994), along with more direct-action solutions (Lochman & Dodge, 1994; Lochman & Lampron, 1986) and more physically aggressive solutions (Waas & French, 1989). Aggressive children have been found to consider more of the aggressive responses in their second or third solution to a problem, indicating they have more aggressive ineffective backup solutions to social problems (Evans & Short, 1991). When subtypes of aggressive children have been examined, boys with more severe conduct disorder diagnoses produce more aggressive/antisocial solutions in vignettes about conflicts with parents and teachers, and fewer verbal/nonaggressive solutions in peer conflicts, in comparison to boys with oppositional defiant disorder (Dunn, Lochman, & Colder, 1997). The findings about verbal assertion are particularly important, since nonaggressive children, by verbally labeling what they want in a simple, direct manner, are better able to indicate their intentions to those around them. Aggressive children's nonverbal direct actions, in contrast, can easily lead their peers to assume that the aggressive children's intentions may have been hostile, and can lead to progressive escalations of aggression.

At the next stage of problem solving, children evaluate the solutions they have generated and decide which solution would produce the best outcome for them. Aggressive children evaluate aggressive behavior as more positive (Crick & Ladd, 1990) than do nonaggressive children. Aggressive children expect that aggressive behavior will lead to tangible rewards and have a positive outcome (Hart, Ladd, & Burleson, 1990; Perry, Perry, & Rasmussen, 1986), will reduce others' aversive behavior (Lochman & Dodge, 1994; Perry et al., 1986), and will result in a positive image and not create suffering in others (Slaby & Guerra, 1988). These beliefs about the acceptability of aggressive behavior lead to deviant processing of social cues, which in turn then mediates or leads to children's aggressive behavior (Zelli, Dodge, Lochman, Laird, & the Conduct Problems Prevention Research Group, 1999), underscoring the importance of recognizing that these information-processing steps have bidirectional and recursive effects, rather than strictly linear effects, on one another.

When children attempt to behaviorally enact the solutions they have selected, aggressive children have been found to be less adept at enacting positive or prosocial behaviors (Dodge et al., 1986). Thus, aggressive children's beliefs that they will be less successful in enacting prosocial behaviors than aggressive behaviors (Erdley & Asher, 1993) may reflect reality, and emphasizes the need for social skills training embedded within the cognitive-behavioral intervention for these children.

Appraisal of Internal Arousal and Emotional Reactions

There appear to be important developmental changes that occur in the affect-labeling patterns of aggressive children. As aggressive boys pass into early adolescence, they become even more likely to minimize their endorsement of negative affective states during stressful situations and social conflicts, especially avoiding affective expression of feelings related to vulnerability (e.g., sadness, fear). Instead, aggressive adolescent boys strive to act unconcerned or even to have positive "happy" emotional reactions to threatening events (Lochman & Dodge, 1994).

The relationship between aggression and affective factors such as empathy has also received attention. In an extensive review of the literature (Miller & Eisenberg, 1988), empathy has been found to be positively correlated with prosocial behaviors and negatively correlated with antisocial behaviors. There is stronger evidence for the relationship between empathy and pro- and antisocial behaviors among school-age children and adolescents than preschool children. Slaby and Guerra (1988) have noted that some of the beliefs of antisocial aggressive youth would interfere with their ability to develop appropriate empathy skills. Empathy has been found to be lower among conduct-disordered than comparison youth and to be related inversely to antisocial and aggressive attitudes (Cohen & Strayer, 1996).

Individual Differences among Aggressive Children's Social-Cognitive Processes

When assessing individual children, as we shall soon discuss, it is important to identify the specific patterns of appraisal and problem-solving difficulties of each aggressive child. As noted above, conduct-disordered children have a wider range of social problem-solving deficits than do children with oppositional defiant disorder (Dunn et al., 1997), and in a similar way more severely aggressive, violent boys have poorer social problem-solving skills than do moderately aggressive boys (Lochman & Dodge, 1994). A similar pattern exists for children who are both aggressive and rejected by their peer group in comparison to aggressive children who are relatively accepted by their peer group (Lochman, Coie, Underwood, & Terry, 1993). A particularly useful distinction has been made between reactive and proactive aggressive children (Dodge, Lochman, Harnish, Bates, & Pettit, 1997), with direct implications for information-processing patterns. Reactive aggressive children, who display intense anger and arousal as they impulsively respond with aggression to perceived provocations, have a broad range of social cognition problems, including encoding and attributional distortions as well as social problem-solving deficits. Reactive aggressive children are also more likely to be victimized by their peers (Schwartz et al., 1998) and to have comorbid affective distress, and to come from families who use harsh discipline (Dodge et al., 1997). Reactive aggressive children have been found to have more deficits in executive cognitive functioning and to be more at risk for substance abuse (Giancola, Moss, Martin, Krisci, & Tarter, 1996). Proactive aggressive children, in contrast, engage in aggressive behavior in a more planful, less emotionally aroused way, and have higher levels of psychopathy (Cornell et al., 1996), and their primary social cognition difficulty is their strong belief that aggressive strategies will work for them (Dodge et al., 1997).

Cognitive Operations

The operations used to manipulate information that individuals encounter externally and internally include attention, retrieval processes from short- and long-term memory, and concept formation and problem-solving processing. External information is evident in cues from the environment around the individual, and internal information is present in physiological cues and in images, thoughts, or beliefs accessed from memory. Attention can be conceived as an operation that assists other cognitive operations such as encoding and retrieval (Cohen & Schleser, 1984); thus, the efficiency and quality of the attentional operations can have major effects on the quality of other cognitive operations and products.

There is suggestive evidence that links deficiencies in sustaining and focusing attention to aggression in children. Mirsky (1989) administered a variety of attentional measures, including the Continuous Performance Task (CPT), to adolescents involved in a 10-year follow-up of a population sample. Aggressive adolescents had difficulty concentrating and sustaining attention on the CPT, in comparison to other adolescents. These attentional deficits produce impairments in encoding of information so that individuals do not perceive relevant bits of information (omission errors), and they perceived information that was not present (commission errors, or intrusions). Similar impairments on attention tasks have been found with aggressive children (Agrawal & Kaushal, 1988) and with ADHD children who are comorbid for conduct disorder or oppositional defiant disorder (Werry, Elkind, & Reeves, 1987). Children with ADHD have a basic problem with self-control (Barkley, 1997), and ADHD is the most common comorbid diagnosis in children with conduct disorder. These children who are comorbid for ADHD and conduct disorder are most likely to display these attentional difficulties and to display behavioral activation rather than behavioral inhibition (Matthys, van Goozen, de Vries, Cohen-Kettenis, & van Engeland, 1998); they also have more wide-ranging and intense problems, including earlier age of onset of severe conduct problems, more violent offending, and earlier and greater substance use (August, Realmuto, MacDonald, Nugent, & Crosby, 1996; Thompson et al., 1996).

These attentional impairments may also be related to a distinct pattern of deficiencies in memory retrieval for aggressive children. In addition to deficient retrieval from short-term memory, which has an impact on distortion in appraisal processes, aggressive children have characteristic styles of retrieving known strategies from long-term memory that contribute to social problem-solving deficiencies. Lochman, Lampron, and Rabiner (1989) found children responding to the Problem-Solving Measure for Conflict (PSM-C) in the usual open-middle format, which simulates automatic retrieval processes, had different patterns of responses than children responding to the PSM-C with a multiple-choice format. The multiple-choice format simulated more deliberate comparative retrieval processes, similar to a process of carefully sifting through stored solutions in "memory bins." In the open-middle condition, aggressive elementary school boys produced significantly more direct-action solutions and tended to produce fewer verbal assertion solutions than nonaggressive children, replicating earlier results. In the multiple-choice condition, both aggressive and nonaggressive boys had higher rates of verbal assertion solutions and lower rates of direct action solutions than occurred in the open-middle condition; however, aggressive boys still had lower rates of verbal assertion and higher rates of help-seeking solutions than did nonaggressive boys. Thus, aggressive boys' solutions to social problems seemed to be affected by salience effects during retrieval from long-term memory, as well as by learned patterns stored in memory. In a subsequent study, Rabiner, Lenhart, and Lochman (1990) replicated these findings while using a more direct paradigm in which automatic retrieval processes were forced by requiring children to provide responses immediately, while deliberate processing was facilitated by having children wait 20 seconds after hearing the problem vignette before responding.

Schematic Propositions

In Ingram and Kendall's (1986) cognitive taxonomic system, cognitive propositions are defined as the content of cognitive structures, and essentially are personal information or general knowledge stored in memory (e.g., belief, expectations). Cognitive structure is the architecture of functional psychological mechanisms such as short-term memory, long-term memory, cognitive networks, and memory nodes. Propositions and structure are classified as categories of schema, but only the schematic propositions are relevant for our discussion here. Schematic propositions are also similar to the "cognitive structures" identified by Meichenbaum (1985) and others. Schematic propositions are ideas and thoughts stored in memory that have a direct influence on how new pieces of information, or cognitive products, are processed moment by moment. Schemas are regarded as conservative because preexisting beliefs are accepted over new ones, and they are self-centered because they draw on personal beliefs over information or experiences from other sources (Fiske & Taylor, 1984). With stronger schemas, children's perceptions become more filtered and potentially more distorted (Lochman & Dodge, 1998), and schemas can operate quickly outside of conscious awareness (Erdley, 1990), in a manner similar to the automatic preemptive information processing evident in aggressive children's social problem solving (Lochman, Lampron, & Rabiner, 1989; Rabiner et al., 1990). Children's schemas, acquired through prior socialization, may have powerful effects on how children appraise the meaning of interpersonal behavior and how they decide to respond to perceived social problems (e.g. Crick & Dodge, 1994; Lochman & Dodge, 1998). Classes of schematic propositions that have been found to be related to children's aggressive behavior, and which, therefore, may influence social-cognitive products, are goal values, generalized outcome expectations, beliefs, and perceived competence and self-worth.

In a study of the direct effect of adolescents' social goals on their solutions to social problems, Lochman, Wayland, and White (1993) used a social learning theory framework (Rotter et al., 1972) to examine boys' ratings of (1) the value of four social goals in a conflict situation (avoidance, dominance, revenge, affiliation), (2) the solution they would use to accomplish each goal, and (3) their level of expectations that they could attain the goals with their selected responses. Aggressive boys had significantly higher value ratings for the dominance and revenge goals and lower ratings for an affiliation goal, in comparison to nonaggressive boys. This dominance-oriented pattern of social goals was found to be associated with adolescents' delinquency and substance use rates. Although aggressive and nonaggressive boys endorsed similar patterns of behavioral solutions to attain each of the goals, aggressive boys had substantial differences from nonaggressive boys in solutions they would use to gain their main goal. This suggests the direct effect of goals (schematic proposition) on problem solutions (cognitive products). Due to their overvaluing of dominance and revenge goals, aggressive boys had more aggressive and fewer bargaining solutions than did nonaggressive boys. In a conceptually related study of goals, Rabiner and Gordon (1992) found that aggressive-rejected children were less able to integrate self-oriented and other-oriented concerns than average and popular boys. In another study documenting aggressive children's self-oriented goals for dominance, Boldizar, Perry, and Perry (1989) used the Rotter and colleagues (1972) social learning framework to examine outcome values. In their goal–oriented outcome values, aggressive children were found to place more value on achieving control of the victim and less value on suffering by the victim, retaliation from the victim, peer rejection, or negative self–evaluation. These sets of findings about goals and outcome values are also consistent with moral reasoning research in which children consider the consequences of their hypothetical actions. Aggressive children and adolescents have lower levels of moral reasoning (Jurkovic & Prentice, 1977), generally at a preconventional level. That is, they primarily attempt to avoid punishment by authority figures and do not act cooperatively to bolster the positive consequences for themselves and others.

In addition to their stored schematic representation of their goal and outcome values, aggressive children have certain patterns of expectations of achieving their outcomes/goals. Aggressive children have been found to be more confident that aggressive behavior would produce tangible rewards and would reduce aversive treatment from others, in comparison with nonaggressive children (Lochman & Dodge, 1994). In Slaby and Guerra's (1988) study of beliefs, antisocial aggressive youth similarly believed that aggressive behavior would increase self–esteem, would avoid a negative image, would not cause victims to suffer, and was a legitimate response. This set of expectations could certainly inhibit the formation of cognitive products involving accurate empathy.

In addition to the goals and expectations identified already, it is likely that other generalized expectations (e.g., locus of control) and other types of schematic propositions, such as self–esteem, would have effects on social–cognitive products. Self–esteem weaknesses appear to be most pronounced in certain types of aggressive children and are most clearly detected at certain developmental periods. Lochman and Lampron (1985) found that highly aggressive preadolescent boys who also had low levels of social status with their peers had the most pronounced impairment in self–esteem. Although aggressive preadolescent boys have expressed lower self–esteem and more dysphoric affect than nonaggressive boys, by early adolescence aggressive boys report very high levels of self–esteem and little dysphoria (Lochman & Dodge, 1994). This developmental shift is likely due to aggressive boys' avoidance of being perceived as vulnerable as they enter adolescence. The complex network of associations between stored cognitive representations, physiological arousal, and affective states is only beginning to be understood.

Noncognitive Influences

Psychophysiology and Arousal

Children's initial appraisals of an event can produce immediate increases in arousal, possibly due to a classically conditioned reaction in which a stimulus has become capable of automatically eliciting an aroused psychophysiological state in an individual. In comparison to nonaggressive peers, boys with oppositional defiant disorder have been found to have a low-level heart rate during baseline nonstress periods, but then to have sharp increases in heart rate during provocation and frustration (van Goozen, Matthys, Cohen-Kettenis, Gispen-de Wied, et al., 1998). In the latter study, boys who had high levels of both externalizing behavior problems and anxiety had the sharpest increases in cortisol following provocation, indicating they experienced much more stress in these situations than did aggressive boys who were without anxiety. Once aroused, preemptive cognitive processing becomes likely, as the individual responds quickly and automatically. In this way, it is anticipated that arousal would produce marked influences on social-cognitive products, as well as being influenced by social-cognitive appraisals.

Aggressive children's cognitive processing has been noticeably affected by arousal. Williams, Lochman, Phillips, and Barry (2003) examined the relationship between attributional processes and physiological arousal. As in the van Goozen, Matthys, Cohen-Kettenis, Gispen-de Wied, and colleagues (1998) study, highly aggressive boys had the lowest resting heart rate but the sharpest increase in heart rate following an experimental threat. In this study, boys were told that an unknown peer was in waiting in another room to work with them on a task, but they were then told that the peer was agitated and threatening to initiate a conflict. As boys' heart rate increased during the study, they began to display more hostile attributional biases on vignette measures, indicating that their increasing cognitive distortions were accompanied by increases in physiological arousal.

Although these studies supported the assumption that aggressive children's preemptive cognitive operations can further impair their social-cognitive product, they have not examined the direct effect of biological arousal on cognition. Arousal has been conceptualized as an end product of the activational properties of the neuroendocrine and sympathetic nervous system (Raine, Venables, & Williams, 1990). In this regard, aggressive adolescents have been found to have higher levels of serum and salivary testosterone than nonaggressive adolescents (Dabbs, Jurkovic, & Frady, 1988), although other studies have not found this effect (van Goozen, Matthys, Cohen-Kettenis, Thijssen, & van Engeland, 1998). Testosterone levels have been found to fluctuate in response to provocations, and the testosterone has effects on brain areas associated with the production of aggressive behavior, such as the hypothalamus. Other research has suggested that androgens, involving high levels of DHEAS (dehydroepiandrosterone sulfate) and androstenedione (van Goozen, Matthys, Cohen-Kettenis, Thijssen, & van Engeland, 1998), and measures of serotonergic function (low levels of 5-HIAA and HVA) (Halperin et al., 1997; van Goozen, Matthys, Cohen-Kettenis, Westenberg, & van Engeland, 1999) may be more substantially related to children's levels of attentional problems, aggression and delinquency, and to the history of aggressive behavior in these children's parents. Comparative research with animals has supported the link between low serotonergic functioning and high levels of hyperactivity and impulsivity (Gainetdinov et al., 1999). Continued research on the integrated assessment of biological, psychophysiological, and social–cognitive processes will be critical in the years ahead.

Parental, Peer, and Teacher Influences

We assume that parents and other adult caregivers, and subsequently children's peers, have a formative influence on children's schematic propositions and social–cognitive products. Research on families of aggressive children indicate that parents and siblings display high levels of aversive behavior as well as other maladaptive parental processes, such as vague "beta" commands, inaccurate monitoring of children's behavior, low cohesion, and rigid or chaotic control efforts (Bry, Catalano, Kumpfer, Lochman, & Szapocznik, 1999). Children who have been exposed to more marital conflict have been found to be hypervigilant to hostile words on a laboratory task, making more false positive and fewer false negative memory errors, indicating that marital conflict leads to schemas about interpersonal conflict which then impact children's information processing (O'Brien & Chin, 1998). These results imply that children's social–cognitive products may be affected through modeling of their parents' ways of perceiving and responding to conflicts with spouses and children, and through parents' socialization of their children's schemas and working models (Lochman & Dodge, 1998; Shaw & Bell, 1993).

A more direct test of the transmission of social–cognitive products from parents to children involves assessing the attributional processes of parents. Following findings of attributional biases in child-abusing parents (e.g., Larrance & Twentyman, 1983), Dix and Lochman (1990) found that, in contrast to a nonaggressive group, mothers of aggressive boys attributed the cause of children's misdeeds more to a negative disposition within the children rather than to the external circumstances. Thus, aggressive children's attributional biases appear to mirror the attributional biases of their parents. Parents' behavior and cognitions are closely linked to their children's social–cognitive processes and behavior, and intervention should be directed at both aggressive children and their parents.

Similar investigations can begin to examine the relationship between the social–cognitive products of additional significant others in children's lives (peers, teachers, other relatives) and the aggressive children's appraisal and problem-solving processes. It is clear that children's peer relationships are linked to their aggressive behavior. Children who are both aggressive and rejected by their peer group are at risk for more negative outcomes in adolescence than are children who are aggressive but accepted by their peer group (Coie et al., 1992). Children who gravitate to deviant peer groups by early adolescence (sometimes because of prior rejection from their peer group at large) receive frequent models, reinforcement, and peer pressure to engage in increasingly antisocial behavior, and they then increase their rates of school truancy, delinquency, and substance use

(Dishion, Patterson, & Griesler, 1994; Wills, McNamara, Vacarro, & Hirkey, 1996).

ASSESSMENT OF AGGRESSION IN CHILDREN

Conducting a thorough assessment of the factors related to a child's aggressive tendencies is an extremely important part of designing a comprehensive treatment plan. In this section, a rationale is provided for evaluating children on a number of behavioral and social-cognitive variables. Implications for assessment from empirical research are noted, followed by a proposed model for an in-depth evaluation procedure.

We have used a battery of all these types of assessment tools in clinical research with our school-based Anger Coping and Coping Power programs. In our clinic-based Conduct Disorders program we have used selected subsets of the measures and have often informally assessed for aspects of the social-cognitive deficiencies and distortions during comprehensive structured and unstructured interviews. It is anticipated that the breadth of the assessment battery will be affected by practical factors.

Behavior Presentation of the Child

It is important to look at aggression within the context of all other observable behavior problems, interaction styles, and environmental factors. Often these patterns of behavior problems will vary with respect to the environmental context (e.g., location, home vs. school; person involved, peer vs. teacher). Therefore it is important to obtain information from as many sources as possible.

Behavioral Rating Scales

Probably the best way to easily obtain a "reading" of the breadth and severity of the problem is through the use of behavioral checklists (McMahon & Forehand, 1988). A checklist allows assessment of a broad range of behaviors, including low-frequency behaviors (e.g., aggression, stealing), requires little time to administer, and incorporates the perceptions of significant others (e.g., parents, teachers) in the child's life. One of the most commonly used behavioral rating scales is the Behavior Assessment System for Children (BASC; Reynolds & Kamphaus, 1992). The BASC is appropriate for use with children and adolescents from the age of 2 years, 6 months, through 18 years, 11 months. Different versions of the BASC are available, including Teacher Rating Scales (TRS), Parent Rating Scales (PRS), and Self-Report of Personality (SRP), allowing information to be gathered from multiple informants. Scoring of the BASC yields both broadband composite scores (e.g., Externalizing Problems, Internalizing Problems), and narrowband scale scores (e.g., Aggression, Anxiety). Another advantage of the BASC is that it offers information on adaptive skills (e.g., Leadership, Social Skills) in addition to problem areas. Other useful rating scales include the Child Behavior Checklist (CBCL; Achenbach, 1991; Achenbach & Edelbrock, 1983), the Revised Behavior Problem Checklist (RBPC; Quay & Peterson, 1983), and the Eyberg Child Behavior Inventory (ECBI; Eyberg, 1980).

Interviews

Interviews with aggressive children, their parents, and teachers can be extremely helpful in identifying situational variables related to the occurrence of aggressive behavior. Interview formats with parallel forms for parent and child can be particularly useful, thereby allowing for comparison of different perceptions and convergence of reported problem areas. For these purposes, interviews such as the Child Assessment Schedule (CAS; Hodges, 1987) and the Diagnostic Interview Schedule for Children (DISC; Costello, Edelbrock, Dulcan, & Kalas, 1984) may be most useful, as they allow for important distinctions regarding the setting and objects of aggression (e.g., toward peers and siblings, cruelty toward animals). The CAS and DISC and other similar diagnostic interviews provide information about both externalizing (e.g., overactivity) and internalizing (e.g., depression, anxiety) symptoms, the presence of which may provide critical information in developing a comprehensive understanding of the context in which the aggressive behavior occurs. The interview of antisocial behavior (Kazdin & Esveldt-Dawson, 1986) may be particularly useful in determining patterns of covert–overt symptomatology. We have found that with children who have fairly serious problems with aggression, the use of a less-structured clinical interview may also be helpful, especially in uncovering a child's attributions and reasoning about a particular incident. For instance, some children and young adolescents attribute their poor reasoning in aggressive interactions to the use of drugs or associating with a particular set of peers. Their descriptions of relatively extreme acts of violence (e.g., muggings) may provide important clinical "hunches" about their capacity for empathy, their assessment of their own self-control, and their sense of remorse.

Behavioral Observations

Behavioral observations may yield some of the most useful information about aggressive children (McMahon & Estes, 1997). The aforementioned measures may be subject to perceptual biases or motivation to deny specific behavior problems. Comparing data obtained from direct observation, checklists, and interviews will most likely reveal treatment targets (e.g., school-based intervention with peers, parent–child interaction).

The assessment procedure should include as many opportunities to observe behavior as possible. Conducting screenings in a group format with potential group members has the advantage of allowing clinicians to observe peer interactions as well as to obtain a preview of important group composition and cohesion issues. Parent–child interactions also should be observed during the assessment period. The seating behavior that occurs prior to conducting a parent–child interview often informs clinicians about family structure, especially if the child verbally or behaviorally dictates where the parent should sit. Other important behaviors to observe during a parent–child interview include interrupting, withdrawal, and the affective valence of the interaction. Hostile interactions devoid of affective warmth or humor will require increased treatment attention to the parent–child relationship. Finally, individual child assessments grant clinicians a sample of the child's social and verbal skills as well as the opportunity to establish a personal rapport that will assist in the success of future therapeutic contacts.

Peer Ratings

Not surprisingly, many aggressive children have problematical peer relations. They are often judged as being less socially competent by parents, teachers, and peers (e.g., Coie, Dodge, & Coppotelli, 1982). Use of peer evaluations may be particularly helpful in identifying a subgroup of aggressive socially rejected children who exhibit a combination of risk factors (e.g., attentional and learning problems, low self-esteem, peer-rejected status) that point to possible situational factors related to their experience of frustration and aggressive outbursts (Dodge, Coie, & Brakke, 1982). However, other highly aggressive children are more socially accepted and report higher general self-esteem, even in comparison to socially accepted boys who are less aggressive (Lochman & Lampron, 1985). Since these children enjoy greater social acceptance and self-esteem, they may be less motivated to cooperate with treatment efforts to reduce their aggressive behavior.

Evaluation of Social-Cognitive/Affective Characteristics

As presented in the social-cognitive model of aggression, the current literature on aggressive children clearly indicates that there are particular characteristics of their social-cognitive style that differ in a meaningful way from nonaggressive children. Based upon empirical findings, measures will be proposed for use in a "battery" of assessment techniques for clinical evaluation. It is important to caution that, while meaningful group differences exist on these measures, the psychometric properties are yet to be determined. Therefore, the following procedures are offered for consideration as a means by which to obtain relevant clinical information to be collected along with other measures (e.g., IQ and achievement tests, behavioral checklist) using well-established psychometric properties.

Most researchers and clinicians with any experience with highly aggressive children readily agree that these children seem to perceive the social world in a very different manner than nonaggressive children (see Table 2.1). The goal of a social-cognitive assessment battery is to refine a clinician's understanding of a particular aggressive child's social information processing using the general framework presented in Table 2.1.

Social-Cognitive Products

To answer the question of what a child attends to and encodes when presented with information in a social situation, Dodge (1980) has developed a number of interesting measures to test a series of related hypotheses about aggressive children's skills for encoding different types of social cues. Dodge and Frame (1982) have presented videotaped "hypothetical situations" to children in which a child experiences hostile, benign, or neutral outcomes in a peer interaction. Children's responses to this measure can be used to evaluate their (1) ability to recall cues freely from the interaction, (2) recognition of events that actually occurred, (3) "mistaken" accounts of the event (commission errors, intrusions), and (4) attributions and expectations about a hypothetical peer's intentions of future behavior. Generally, aggressive children tend to attend to and remember hostile cues selectively in interactions with peers, particularly when they are asked to imagine being a participant in the interaction.

A second general question about aggressive children's way of thinking is: What kinds of ideas do they have about how to interact and "solve" social situations? How does their style of information processing influence their strategies (or lack therefore) in social problem solving? In evaluating the actual content of social problem-solving solutions, a number of factors need to be considered: (1) the type of social task (e.g., peer group entry, initiating friendships, resolving conflict situations); (2) the persons involved in the hypothetical situation (peers, teachers, parents); (3) the apparent intentions (hostile, benevolent, ambiguous).

Lochman and Lampron (1986) evaluated aggressive children's social problem-solving strategies to two types of situational variables while holding constant a third variable—the type of social task. The PSM-C presents hypothetical stories involving only interpersonal conflict and systematically varies the type of antagonist (peer, teacher, parent) and the expressed intent of the antagonist (hostile or ambiguous frustration of the protagonist's wishes). On this measure aggressive boys, as compared to nonaggressive boys, had lower rates of "verbal assertion" solutions for conflicts with peers and those involving a hostile antagonist (of any type: peer, parent, teacher). They had higher rates of direct-action solutions for conflicts with teachers and hostile antagonists, and a higher rate of physically aggressive solutions in peer conflicts.

The following examples illustrate deficits in appraisal and problem-solving strategies exhibited by two aggressive boys. These boys' responses to the same stimuli from the PSM-C (Dunn et al., 1997; Lochman & Lampron, 1986) and Dodge's recall test are provided.

M. is a 15-year-old highly aggressive and sociopathic youth referred for evaluation and treatment following adjudication for property offenses and assault

charges. J. is a 12-year-old male referred for treatment to address chronic oppositional behavior in school. J. is particularly prone to respond passive–aggressively
in response to adult authority, and to have trouble labeling emotions. Both boys
responded to the following story from the PSM C:

> Some of Ed's friends borrowed his soccer ball during lunch period but did not
> return it. When Ed came out of school at the end of the day, the other boys had
> already starting playing with it again. Ed was supposed to go right home after school,
> and he wanted to have his soccer ball back. The story ends with Ed walking home
> with his soccer ball. What happens in between Ed not having his soccer ball, and
> later when he walked home with it?

M.'s immediate response represents an attempt to seek help from an authority:

> "They wouldn't let Ed have the ball, right? So Ed went to the principal and
> told him the situation, he went back to the kids and told them to give Ed
> the soccer ball back and if they messed with Ed they would be expelled
> from school. Because Ed is the kind of person who doesn't like violence or
> to fight—he has values and stuff."

M.'s initial backup solution:

> "He could have gone up there, say for instance if he had a knife or some-
> thing, he could have cut one of them up."

M.'s final solution:

> "He could have come over to the school with his mother. His mother could
> have got the ball back."

Thus, after paying lip service to prosocial thinking, M. generated an extremely
antisocial response and then resorted to immature help seeking.

J.'s initial response represents a direct-action solution:

> "Ed went up and act like he was fixing to play with the soccer ball, but took
> the ball and walked away with it."

J.'s backup solutions:

> "He could have just took the soccer ball without playing with them."

> "He could have went home and next morning seen them playing and gone
> up to them and taken it without asking."

> "Next morning if it's in the locker he could have went in the locker and
> took it out."

J. is clearly fixated on direct-action solutions, which characterize each of the four problem-solving strategies he provided. Together, these boys demonstrate aggressive boys' tendency to rely on physically aggressive or direct-action solutions and to be deficient in their use of verbal assertion.

M.'s and J.'s responses to a series of five hostile, benevolent, and neutral audiotaped statements on one segment of Milich and Dodge's (1984) Recall Test (this segment contains two positive, five hostile, and two neutral statements) were as follows:

> M.:"He stole somebody's money. He hit this boy so hard that his nose started bleeding. He hates this boy named Kenny so much that he wishes his arms would fall off."

> J.:"There was this boy who made him so mad that he punched him in the nose. There was this other boy who was crippled, the boy helped him get his lunch. One day he told this boy to beat up this other boy."

Both boys exhibited a tendency to overrecall hostile cues and to include hostile commission errors or intrusions, as they remembered some items in hostile terms rather than in their original positive or neutral form.

Clearly, aggressive children not only perceive social situations in a different light but also tend to generate solutions to problematic situations that are maladaptive. This pattern leads to the question of "Why?" Are there particular beliefs or expectations or goals that aggressive children hold that are related to, or perhaps lead them to, their unskilled handling of social situations? In addition to assessing for the answers to these questions during the interview, several experimental measures can also be useful. The Outcome-Expectation Questionnaire and Self-Efficacy Questionnaire (Perry et al., 1986), measures of beliefs and expectations (Slaby & Guerra, 1988), and a measure of social goals (Lochman, Wayland, et al., 1993) have all been used to distinguish aggressive children and adolescents from less aggressive peers. Assessments of such schematic propositions permit a more detailed and coherent understanding of aggressive children's maladaptive behavior and approaches for intervention with them.

Schematic Propositions

A measure of a child's relative evaluation of social goals such as dominance, revenge, avoidance, and affiliation assists clinicians in determining how consistent a child's social behavior is with his stated goals. A measure adapted from Lochman, Wayland, and colleagues (1993) allows clinicians to view a child's relative ranking of these social goals. These rankings can then be placed in context with the child's other social-cognitive characteristics. For example, some aggressive children with a poor ability to manage their arousal may endorse prosocial goals and adequate problem-solving strategies, but may be unable to exercise behavior consistent with these goals because of their self-control deficits. The knowledge gained from such an assessment profile has clear treatment indications.

Appraisal of Internal Arousal

Aggressive children often have difficulty differentiating their own negative affect, tending to overlabel negative affective arousal (fear, sadness) as anger. An aggressive child's unstructured self-report of his or her negative affect can provide some insight into the child's feeling identification skills. Of course, these feeling identification skills are a prerequisite for understanding the emotions of others. Social perspective taking and empathy are tapped by Bryant's (1982) Empathy Index for Children and Adolescents. Assessing a child's empathic tendencies can also establish how receptive he or she might be to change in general, and to cognitive-behavioral techniques in particular.

Other Domains of Functioning in the Aggressive Child

Assessing familial/parental functioning is necessary so that a complete picture of the behavioral contingencies and influences can be outlined. Parental and marital adjustment can be measured to determine what types of social problem-solving styles are being modeled and to evaluate the degree to which parents are able to be receptive to intervention efforts. Commonly used instruments for which there are adequate psychometric validation include the following: (1) for parental depression, Beck Depression Inventory (BDI; Beck, Rush, Shaw, & Emery, 1979); (2) for parent stress, the Parenting Stress Index (PSI; Abidin, 1983); (3) for marital adjustment, the Dyadic Adjustment Scale (DAS; Spanier, 1976). Measures that can yield an assessment of the child's exposure to marital hostility and experience of direct or indirect use of force include the O'Leary–Porter Scale (Porter & O'Leary, 1980) and the Conflict Tactics Scales (CTS; Straus, 1979). The Child Perceptions of Marital Discord (CPMD; Emery & O'Leary, 1982) has been found to be a useful index of child distress and a correlate of parental report of aggression (Wayland, Schoenwald, & Lochman, 1989). Parent practices are critical areas of functioning to assess, and measures such as the Alabama Parenting Questionnaire (Wootton, Frick, Shelton, & Silverthorn, 1997) have both parent and child forms.

In addition to assessment of familial and parental functioning, it is well known that children with aggressive behavior disorders often have other cognitive/academic deficits (see McMahon & Forehand, 1988). A thorough evaluation of intellectual and academic strengths and weaknesses should be conducted. An accurate assessment of the type of obstacles and frustrations experienced in the learning environment (e.g., specific learning disabilities, especially reading) may shed some light on the reasons why children may be perceived as defensive, defiant, or argumentative by teachers and peers. Also, to streamline the assessment of verbal and nonverbal cognitive skills, a cognitive screening instrument, such as the Kaufman Brief Intelligence Scale (K–BIT; Kaufman & Kaufman, 1990), provides essential information about basic cognitive strengths and weaknesses and a child's readiness for cognitive-behavioral techniques.

Measures of the aggressive child's subjective experience are also important and have implications for response to treatment (e.g., Lochman, Lampron, Burch, & Curry, 1985). The Self-Perception Profile for Children (Harter, 1985) yields self-ratings of competence in a number of areas (e.g., home vs. school, cognitive vs. social). Given the aggressive child's high likelihood of difficulties in multiple areas (e.g., academic achievement, peer relations), it is important to be aware of areas of functioning about which a child may feel particularly sensitive as well as those for which a sense of pride and accomplishment is present. The Piers–Harris Children's Self-Concept Scale (Piers & Harris, 1964) is useful because it provides a gross measure of several affective factors. These factors usually contribute and/or maintain aggressive behavior, such as a child's evaluation of his or her popularity and competency skills. This scale also seems to provide greater insight into depressive symptoms/tendencies in some populations.

Parent Assessment

As indicated earlier, every attempt should be made to include the parent and/or parent surrogate in the assessment process. Along with the previously discussed formal behavioral rating scales completed by parents, less formal behavioral scales are useful. In our clinical work, we devised a CD/ODD Symptom Severity (Disruptive Behavior) Checklist based on the specific diagnostic criteria for conduct disorder and oppositional defiant disorder in DSM-IV (American Psychiatric Association, 1994).

Another extremely important ingredient is the assessment of parental willingness to be involved in the treatment process. To expedite this process, the parents' screening/assessment group is conducted simultaneously with the child's assessment process. This format allows group leaders to discuss a parent's role in the intervention while at the same time gauging a parent's interest, as well as availability, in participating in a weekly parenting group.

COGNITIVE-BEHAVIORAL THERAPY WITH AGGRESSIVE CHILDREN

CBT addresses the deficient and distorted social-cognitive processes in aggressive children including distortions in their perceptions of others' and their own behavior, biases in their attribution of the hostile intention of others, overreliance on nonverbal direct action solutions, and underreliance on verbal assertion and verbal negotiation solutions. CBT programs can include training in self-instruction, social problem solving, perspective taking, affect labeling, or relaxation, and most programs include a combination of several of these techniques.

All of these programs have a common focus on children's social cognitions during frustrating or provocative situations.

Coping Power Program

To provide a sample of the kinds of cognitive-behavioral techniques that can be used with aggressive children, we will describe our Coping Power program, which targets characteristic social-cognitive difficulties demonstrated by aggressive children (see Lochman, Wells, & Murray, in press, for a session-by-session description). The Coping Power program has evolved from our previously developed Anger Coping program (Larson & Lochman, 2002; Lochman, Fitz-Gerald, & Whidby, 1999). We will also address the major content and process issues that constitute the foci of CBT interventions.

The Coping Power program was designed to be implemented in the school setting with fourth- through sixth-grade students. The program comprises a 34-session child component and a 16-session parent component, delivered simultaneously over a 16- to 18-month period. Child sessions are typically 45–60 minutes, including four to six children in a group. Parent sessions span a 90-minute period and may include up to 12 parents or parent dyads. All sessions are highly structured, with specific goals, objectives, and structured exercises outlined for each session. Although our model has more often been implemented in schools, it can easily be adapted for use in clinical settings with only minor procedural modifications (e.g., goals for children's behavior will be home- or community-based rather than school-based). In addition to group sessions, each child receives 6–8 individual half-hour sessions, approximately once per month, to build rapport and to individualize Coping Power concepts and goals for each student.

We believe there are several advantages to the use of group therapy as the modal form of treatment. Peer and group reinforcement is frequently more effective with children than reinforcement provided in a dyadic context, or by adults (Rose & Edelson, 1987). This may be especially true for children with disruptive behavior disorders, who research suggests are relatively resistant to social reinforcement. Additionally, the group context provides in vivo opportunities for interpersonal learning and development of social skills.

Using a variety of instructional strategies and activities, the Coping Power child component is designed to remediate aggressive children's characteristic social-cognitive difficulties. These include increased attention to hostile cues, a tendency to interpret others' intentions as hostile, an orientation toward dominance in social goals, overreliance on action-oriented problem-solving strategies, a relative deficit in the use of verbal assertion or negotiation, and a belief that aggressive behavior will result in personal gratification. Topics addressed in the Coping Power child component include goal setting, organizational and study skills, awareness of arousal and anger, self-regulation of anger and arousal, social problem solving, and dealing with peer pressure and neighborhood problems.

Parent Component

The Coping Power parent component aims to improve the parent–child relationship and facilitate effective parenting practices. The content, derived from social learning theory-based parent training programs, includes rewarding appropriate child behaviors, using effective instructions and rules, applying effective consequences for inappropriate child behaviors, employing constructive family communication practices, and implementing parental stress management strategies. In addition, parents are introduced to the skills their children are learning so that they can identify, coach, and reinforce their children's use of the skills. The sequence of Coping Power parent and child sessions are structured to coincide so that parents and children are introduced to certain topics at around the same time. For example, while children learn about study skills and organization, their parents are instructed in ways to support children's academic success, such as developing a structure for homework completion, monitoring homework completion, and communicating with teachers. Other topics that are timed to correspond in the parent and child groups include conflict resolution skills and problem-solving strategies. Timing the parent and child sessions in this manner enhances the probability that parents will work with their children on these skills, providing additional practice and reinforcement for the children and promoting generalization to the home setting.

Each session of the Coping Power parent component is structured to include an opening period, a topic-based interactive presentation, and a closing period. During each closing period, homework is assigned to encourage parents to put the skills they have learned into practice and to enhance their ability to retain the information learned from session to session. The opening period of each session also promotes continuity between sessions through review of homework assignments and discussion of parents' reactions to the previous session. Other elements of the Coping Power parent component include group cohesion building and encouragement of families' involvement in the community. In-session practices such as encouraging parents to share personal experiences, problem-solve together, and participate in activities such as group potlucks help to build a sense of cohesion among group members, which serves to enhance members' investment and satisfaction. To encourage positive involvement in the community, several sessions also provide information to parents on specific resources for academic assistance, summertime activities, and family outings.

Pragmatic and Logistical Issues

Although group therapy has the advantages discussed above, individual therapy that addresses the components discussed below may be indicated in several instances. First, individual therapy may be indicated to assist a child in preparing to enter a group. This strategy is likely to be helpful if a child is unable to participate in groups either because of his or her disruptive behavior (e.g., ADHD) or perhaps a comorbid anxiety disorder. Second, a child may benefit from individual therapy as a "step-down" from a successful group experience that requires continued practice and skill acquisition.

The Coping Power program can be modified for use with individual clients. In terms of content, few changes are necessary, though some activities require alterations in the absence of peers. For example, the clinician will need to take a more active role in some activities (e.g., being involved in role plays) and will need to provoke discussion with examples and questions that other group members might have raised. More often than in a group setting, clinicians may also need to incorporate appropriate self-disclosures and hypothetical case examples (e.g., "I once worked with a boy your age who . . .") to bring salience to the program content. Currently, our research group is pilot testing an individual version of the Coping Power program, based on the original group program but modified for one to one use.

School-based delivery of services often depends upon the level of support from school administrators and personnel and usually targets children who have a wider range of aggression relative to clinic-referred children. Clinic-based groups often contain children that are experiencing frequent, intense, and problematic levels of aggression, although some children in school-based groups are just as behaviorally disturbed. As such, the clinic groups are typically smaller (4–5 members) than school-based groups (5–7 members).

A large room with an adequate number of chairs and a place to hang posters is highly recommended, regardless of service site. A chalkboard or "dry-erase" marker board are helpful but not necessary, as writing can be done on posterboard. The comorbidity of disruptive behaviors (e.g., ODD and ADHD) creates the need to plan the physical environment. It is best to have as few visual, tactile, and auditory distractions as possible, within the recognized limitation that group rooms often have multiple users/uses. In the first group session a list of group rules will be generated, which include "coming and going to group" rules to encourage expected and appropriate behavior during these transitions.

Self-Management Skills

First, children are taught to become more competent observers of internal states related to affective arousal. As is true of other skills taught, this process occurs throughout the entire course of treatment. Through modeling, observation, structured exercises and group discussion, children are taught to identify physiological and affective cues of anger arousal. For example, they are asked to define the concept of anger in terms of its affective and behavioral concomitants (e.g., "anger is the feeling you have when you think you cannot get something you want, or do something you want to do, or when you feel provoked") (Lochman, Lampron, Gemmer, & Harris, 1987, p. 347). Children are asked to identify environmental cues and precipitants by generating examples of anger-arousing stimuli (e.g., situations at home and at school that make them angry with peers and authority figures). Next, physiological aspects of anger arousal are addressed. A videotaped instruction is used to introduce the topic, showing a boy displaying several overt symptoms of anger arousal. The signal function of these cues is emphasized, and group brainstorming or discussion is used to identify a variety of physiological cues of anger (blood rushing to one's face, quickening pulse, increased muscle tension, affective flooding). Children are asked to identify the specific ways in which they and others experience anger arousal (facial and gestural expression, tone of voice, body posture, thoughts, statements, action). This implicitly communicates that people differ in their internal experience of, and behavioral response to, anger and is intended to help children become better observers of a wide range of cues regarding their own and others' anger. Children may be encouraged to differentiate their affective experience of anger on the dimension of intensity (e.g., to generate situations that make them angry "on a scale of 1 to 10" to label affective states of different intensity such as "simmering, "steaming," and "boiling"). The phenomenological experience of anger can thus be conceptualized as occurring on a continuum, and children can be taught to identify affective and physiological symptoms at lower and more manageable levels of affective arousal. Children can also be taught to link affective states of different intensity to specific environmental events or cues. One such method of helping children concretize their understanding of these issues is use of role plays. Children can be asked to provide "Academy Award portrayals" of anger arousal and anger coping, including nonverbal and verbal cues.

In addition to self-monitoring strategies designed to increase awareness of environmental triggers, and of affective and physiological states related to anger, cognitive self-control strategies are also taught. Instruction in this area attempts to address deficiencies in verbal mediation strategies that help to regulate behavior. Children are helped to appreciate the impact of cognition on subsequent affective arousal and behavior, and are instructed on the role of internal dialogue in enhancing or decreasing the experience of anger arousal. This concept is taught through the construct of "self-talk." Through repeated instruction, children are helped to identify anger-enhancing and anger-reducing cognitions, and to understand the impact of private speech on emotions and behavior. A series of verbal-taunting games is particularly useful in concretizing this concept. In this application, children receive insults or taunts from other group members and discuss their thoughts and feelings in response to this structured provocation. Stimuli are presented in a hierarchical format, progressing from relatively distanced stimuli (e.g., taunting of puppets) to increasingly more threatening stimuli (direct taunting of group members). Instruction on self-talk is combined with exercises designed to increase awareness of individual perceptual processes. For example, group members may be asked to identify the kinds of assumptions they are most likely to make in situations of social conflict, and the kinds of anger-reducing statements that are most likely to facilitate adaptive coping. In this way, children are encouraged to develop a repertoire of coping statements that will work specifically for them. Other self-control techniques are discussed and rehearsed as well, including visualization, distraction, and relaxation. Through discussion of self-monitoring techniques, children are implicitly taught that the triggers for anger arousal vary from individual to individual and from event to event. The awareness of these triggers is then used to prompt children to employ their self-management skills.

Sitting in on Therapy

The following interactions occurred in the context of a self-control exercise that is part of the Coping Power group treatment model. In this exercise, group members taunt a target child under controlled circumstances to develop the target child's ability to respond adaptively to provocation. The child is physically separated by a "safety circle" outlined on the floor and typically begins this "hot-seat" exercise with "coaching" support from a group co-leader who stands with the child in the circle—in this case, Co-Leader 1. A "safe environment" for the child can also be achieved by having the group members sit around a table.

CO-LEADER 1: OK, B., before we begin this first time, is there anything that is "off-limits"?

B. : No.

CO-LEADER 1: You're sure?

B.: Yeah.

CO-LEADER 2: OK, for this first time each person will spend 1 minute in the "hot seat."

MEMBERS: Yeah.

CO-LEADER 1: Are you ready, B.?

B.: Yeah.

CO-LEADER 1: OK, then, go!

MEMBER 1: Look at that hat on his head—all dirty and stuff!

MEMBER 2: Yeah, look at his hat! (*laughing*)

MEMBER 3: Do you ever wash that thing?

B.: Yeah, I wash it! Look at your hat! You . . .

CO-LEADER 1: (*interrupting*) Remember, B., we're practicing our self-control strategies.

B.: OK. OK.

CO-LEADER 2: OK, guys, keep going.

MEMBER 2: Your mama make that hat for you? (*Other members laugh and point.*)

CO-LEADER 1: B., I can see that you're making a fist and your teeth are clenched.

B.: (*He unclenches his fist as he begins to take several deep breaths.*) OK. That's right (*to himself*), "They don't even know my mama. They're just trying to get me mad. There's nothing wrong with my hat."

MEMBER 4: B.'s mama made that dirty, funky hat! (*Members laugh.*)

CO-LEADER 1: Keep your cool, B.

MEMBER 3: He needs the hat to cover up his ugly face!

B.: (*to himself*) I'm gonna stay calm. They just want me to fight, and I'm not going to.

This activity demonstrates the need for leaders to shape and support children's skills acquisition. Group members are reminded that these are *skills*, that they require practice to become effective, and that there will be times when they do not perform them competently. This type of anticipatory guidance validates the children's frustration with learning a difficult and new skill.

One activity in this section includes verbal taunting during a domino-building task. One group member builds a tower for 30 seconds, using one hand, while the others taunt him. Each member receives a turn building a tower, and the highest tower wins. The discussion after the task centers on how hard it was to concentrate on the domino building, how group members kept their concentration focused, if they started to feel angry, if the anger hurt their concentration, if the players used self-talk to help them do well, and how anger management was critical for winning.

In summary, through hierarchical exposure to stimuli of increasing threat, behavioral rehearsal, and group discussion, children are encouraged to develop and practice using cognitive and affective self-reflection and self-monitoring strategies for situations involving interpersonal conflict. To help consolidate their learning of these strategies, children are also provided opportunities to write "scripts" that include the set of skills and coping strategies they have been developing, and to practice these skills by acting out these scripts on a videotape.

Social Perspective-Taking Skills

Research suggests that children with externalizing disorders exhibit egocentric and distorted perceptions of social situations (Lochman & Dodge, 1998). As noted earlier, these social cognitive deficiencies involve difficulty integrating self- and other-oriented concerns, overattribution of hostile intent on the part of others, and deficient perspective-taking skills. Such maladaptive interpersonal processing places aggressive children at high risk for dysfunctional social relationships (for example, a child who quickly assumes hostile intent on the part of others may respond to social conflict based on inaccurately perceived threats; a child who has difficulty adopting others' perspectives may quickly disregard others' views or needs and respond entirely from his or her own vantage point). A series of perspective-taking exercises is presented to address these issues, employing a variety of techniques (structured exercises, role plays, modeling, and group discussion). Perspective-taking instruction attempts to improve children's ability to infer accurately others' thoughts and intentions (cognitive perspective taking) and to enhance their understanding of others' feelings and internal emotional states (affective perspective taking). Children are asked to differentiate individual cognitive and affective processes by identifying similarities and differences between people, by delineating alternative interpretations of social cues; and by generating inferences of what others may be thinking or feeling. For example, a prototypical exercise presents children with an ambiguous picture, asks them to generate, independently, "stories" about the picture, and engages them in a discussion about differences in their perceptions of the same stimulus. Perspective-taking instruction is routinely provided when children present examples of conflict with peers, teachers, and family members, and is used to address interpersonal conflict as it arises in the group. Thus, this component of the intervention continues throughout the course of the group.

Social Problem-Solving Skills

Aggressive children exhibit deficiencies in their ability to resolve interpersonal problems successfully. The Coping Power program addresses the deficient problem-solving strategies exhibited by aggressive children by helping them to identify conflictual situations as problematical and by encouraging them to increase their repertoire for responding to these situations. A sequential step-wise model of handling social conflict is presented, including the following three components: problem identification; generation of multiresponse alternatives; and evaluation and prediction of consequences for their actions. A variety of techniques are used to help children learn and implement this model, including modeling, instruction in divergent and consequential thinking, practice in generating and elaborating solutions, and behavioral rehearsal. The latter is accomplished through role playing and the use of videotaping, in which children develop scripts for handling conflictual situations and enact them on videotape. Children are encouraged to incorporate into these scripts the personalized menu of anger-coping strategies (self-talk, conflict resolution strategies) they have developed over the course of the group. A critical aspect of this instruction involves helping children to identify a potentially problematic situation early on, before it escalates to a point where they are unable to respond adaptively. Children's use of direct-action solutions is discouraged, and their use of verbal expression, discussion, and negotiation solutions is reinforced. Attention is also placed on identifying how solutions are affected by social goals, how solutions can be competently enacted, and how there is a need to have backup solutions when initial solutions fail or when obstacles arise in the implementation of a solution. In summary, the social problem-solving component provides children with a model for responding to social conflicts and encourages qualitative and quantitative improvements in their range of coping solutions.

In addition to structured exercises, children also use social problem solving with the real-life problems they bring into the group. In a recent group session, Bob began talking about an incident that had led to a 5-day suspension from school the prior week. Rather than continue with the scheduled group activity, the bulk of the session was spent in group problem solving about this situation. Bob described how the incident began when he and another boy disagreed over who could sit on a cushion in the library. After a brief exchange of insults took place, the two boys were quiet for the remainder of the library period. However, as the class left the library, Bob got up in the other boy's face and reinitiated the verbal assaults in a more provocative way. When the boy responded with verbal insults, Bob knocked him down and kept hitting him until he was pulled away by the assistant principal. The group discussion included a focus on perspective taking with regard to the other boy's intentions—which did not initially appear to be as purposefully malevolent as Bob had perceived—and with regard to the assistant principal's intentions. In a spirited discussion, the group noted the assistant principal may have been either mean or trying to protect the combatants when he grabbed Bob and swung him around (most group members eventually decided he was trying to be protective). After several ways of handling the initial "cushion problem" were suggested to Bob, Bob asked each of the group members how they would have handled it. When the group member with the most streetwise demeanor suggested a nonconfrontational solution, Bob tentatively decided to try that strategy in the next conflict. Notable aspects of this discussion included how aggressive incidents often escalate from trivial initial problems, how Bob had great difficulty letting his anger dissipate after the initial provocation, how Bob's anger disrupted his ordinarily adequate social cognitions through preemptive processing, and how the group members were instrumental in providing training in social perspective taking and social problem solving.

Process Variables in the Coping Power Program

Three process variables are considered central in the Coping Power program: a behavior management system, in which the social microcosm of the group is used to encourage prosocial behavior and to facilitate group cohesiveness; goal-setting activities, which provide a structured vehicle to encourage generalization of treatment effects; and use of the interpersonal "here-and-now" of the group to encourage development of the context of the group.

Behavior Management System

The primary mechanism for encouraging a "positive peer culture" is early development of group rules and specification of a behavior management system. Children are involved in the process of instituting rules, which allows them to assume psychological ownership of group norms and sensitizes them to aspects of behavior that would interfere with group process. Their participation in developing this shared social contract facilitates group cohesion and helps to minimize the power struggle that can evolve between adults and conduct-disordered children. Contingency management techniques such as response cost or reward systems (Sulzer & Mayer, 1972) are essential to enable group leaders to shape, maintain, and reinforce desired behavior (participation, prosocial behavior). It is helpful to display group rules at each session and to provide children with frequent feedback about their behavior (e.g., review the number of points earned at the end of each session or periodically during the session). It is useful to provide children with corrective feedback early on and to provide such feedback in a neutral, matter of fact manner. This early "detoxification" of corrective feedback helps to defuse aggressive children's tendencies to overpersonalize adult feedback and respond with oppositional or challenging behavior. As children accumulate points to be exchanged for individual and group rewards, they are provided opportunities to delay immediate gratification, often a problem area for children with disruptive behavior disorders. Group contingencies provide an additional vehicle for further developing group cohesion.

Goal Setting

Each week children target a problem behavior, set a goal regarding behavior change, and monitor their ability to meet their goal. Weekly goal sheets are used to help children concretize this process. Goals are selected with input from group leaders, teachers, and parents, and individualized treatment goals are developed for each child based on the particular social-cognitive deficits or distortions exhibited by that child. Teachers or parents provide external monitoring of children's progress by initialing children's daily goal sheets. Goal setting thus provides a structured vehicle to enhance generalization of treatment effects, encourages children to assume responsibility for changing problematic aspects of their behavior, and facilitates the development of self-monitoring skills. Goal setting and monitoring can be enhanced by parents' participation in the Coping Power parent component, which includes behavioral management skills training. Learning these skills enables parents to increase their ability to effectively set and monitor behavioral limits.

Interpersonal Group Process

The spontaneous interaction that occurs among group members throughout the course of treatment provides an excellent opportunity to assess children's interpersonal styles and deficits and to identify peer relationship difficulties. Through the modeling, coaching, and shaping of their behavior, children can be helped to develop listening skills; interact in a prosocial manner; increase their ability to respond in a verbally assertive manner; and better understand the perspectives of their peers. The inevitable tensions that arise among group members, and children's negative reactions to corrective feedback from leaders, provide *in vivo* opportunities to work with children on issues of anger control. Thus, in addition to the "cold" processing that occurs in structured exercises and role plays, "hot" processing provides an excellent opportunity to guide children in the use of newly acquired skills, that is, to label anger arousal as it occurs and to practice the use of anger management techniques. In summary, through the social microcosm of the "here-and-now" group process, there is much opportunity for interpersonal learning through modeling, processing of interpersonal conflict, *in vivo* social skills instruction, and opportunities to practice more adaptive means of interacting with peers.

OVERVIEW OF COGNITIVE-BEHAVIORAL THERAPY OUTCOMES

In this section we overview the results of outcome research using CBT with aggressive children and of studies examining child and treatment characteristics that are predictive of treatment outcomes. These studies have begun to establish that CBT with aggressive children is an empirically supported therapy (Brestan & Eyberg, 1998; Kazdin & Weisz, 2003; Kendall, 1998). More detailed reviews of CBT outcome research with aggressive children and adolescents are available elsewhere (Kazdin, 1995; Kendall & Choudhury, 2003; Southam-Gerow & Kendall, 1997; Sukhodolsky, Kassinove, & Gorman, 2004).

Outcome Effects

Based on promising findings from pre- and poststudies (e.g., Lochman, Nelson, & Sims, 1981), controlled research on CBT with aggressive children has expanded in the past two decades. These studies can be grouped into those that had negative, mixed, or generally positive treatment effects. Three studies have not found changes in aggressive behavior following CBT, although two of these did produce improvements in the cognitive processes that were hypothesized to mediate the behavior (Camp, Blom, Herbert, & van Doornick, 1988; Coats, 1979; Dubow, Huesmann, & Eron, 1987). Five studies with mixed findings have found improvements on some, but not all, behavioral measures (e.g., Forman, 1980; Garrison & Stolberg, 1983; Kettlewell & Kausch, 1983). In a broad-based intervention for black, lower-class, socially rejected children, Lochman, Coie, and colleagues (1993) used a combination of CBT and social skills training with three annual cohorts. Although the first two cohorts of treated children displayed little improvement in comparison to a control condition, the third cohort evidenced more favorable results. Treated aggressive-rejected children had significantly higher peer ratings for social preference and prosocial behavior by posttreatment, and they tended to have reductions in teachers' ratings of aggression. This year-long school-based intervention was progressively revised over the 3 cohort years, with the last and most successful intervention year emphasizing more contingency contracting and reframing of who wins in interpersonal conflicts.

Of greater concern, the Adolescent Transitions Program (ATP) has found evidence for iatrogenic effects on some outcomes. The ATP program, which was designed as a preventative intervention for high-risk adolescents and their families, utilizes both parent-directed and child directed group interventions to curb maladaptive developmental processes (Dishion & Andrews, 1995). Participants who attended the teen-focused group as part of treatment exhibited higher levels of teacher-rated disruptive behavior and tobacco use at the end of treatment in contrast to controls, while families assigned exclusively to the parent-training condition showed improvements in ratings of disruptive behavior in comparison to controls. This seemingly detrimental effect of the peer group training on participants' drug use and ratings of disruptive behavior remained at 1-year follow-up. It is important to note that this finding seems to indicate that, while some cognitive-behavioral interventions targeted at youth may be beneficial in reducing antisocial behavior, certain risk factors for delinquency, such as affiliation with a deviant peer group, may be artificially facilitated by the intervention itself, thereby escalating the development of problematic behaviors rather than reducing them.

Stronger treatment effects have been documented in several programmatic research efforts (Southam-Gerow & Kendall, 1997). Kendall, Ronan, and Epps (1991) adapted their CBT program for use with impulsive children (Kendall & Braswell, 1993) to treat day-hospitalized children with conduct disorder. Comparing 20 sessions of CBT with a "current conditions treatment" in a cross-over design, CBT-treated children had improvements in teachers' ratings of children's self-control and prosocial behavior and in children's perceived social competence. However, reductions in cognitive impulsivity were not noted, and the treatment gains that were present at posttreatment did not persist to a 6-month follow-up. In the second programmatic research effort (Kazdin, 1995), Kazdin, Esveldt-Dawson, French, and Unis (1987b) used a 20-session problem-solving skills training (PSST) program with psychiatric inpatient children, and did find follow-up effects. Relative to two control conditions, PSST produced significant reductions in parents' and teachers' ratings of aggressive behavior at posttesting and at a 1-year follow-up. These results were replicated in several studies that combined PSST with parent behavioral management training (Kazdin, Esveldt-Dawson, French, & Unis, 1987a; Kazdin, Siegel, & Bass, 1992) and in another study using PSST with antisocial children treated in outpatient and inpatient settings (Kazdin, Bass, Siegel, & Thomas, 1989). Treated children in the latter study were behaviorally improved in both home and school settings, indicating the generalization of intervention effects. In addition, the combined child-and parent intervention program (Kazdin et al., 1992) was found to produce the greatest and most long-lasting improvements in children's behavior, in comparison to either intervention alone. These findings argue for the importance of providing cognitive-behavioral intervention to both aggressive children and their parents (Southam-Gerow & Kendall, 1997).

Several studies from other research groups have documented that these combined effects of child-and-parent cognitive-behavioral interventions can also be apparent with younger children in the 4- to 8-year age range (Webster-Stratton, Reid, & Hammond, 2001), producing reductions in aggressive and other externalizing behaviors and improvements in conflict management strategies, and on longer-term outcomes such as delinquency and school adjustment at age 12, over 4 years after intervention (Tremblay, Pagani-Kurtz, Masse, Vitaro, & Pihl, 1995).

Universal Interventions

Universal preventive interventions, directed at entire child populations in communities rather than high-risk groups, have also been found to produce significant effects on adolescent antisocial behavior and substance use (Hawkins et al., 1992; Kellam & Rebok, 1992). Combining universal interventions, directed at classroom teachers, along with comprehensive, long-lasting interventions targeted at high-risk children and their families, has been shown in initial analyses to produce significant improvements even in the highest-risk first graders, suggesting the potential utility of this type of intensive, multicomponent intervention with the "early starting" (Moffitt, 1993) conduct problem children who have the poorest prognosis and the greatest likelihood of negative adolescent outcomes (Conduct Problems Prevention Research Group, 2004). This program, known as Fast Track, has produced clear improvements in children's social relations, social cognitions, reading achievement, and behavior, and in parents' warmth and discipline at the end of the first-grade year, and it is designed to be delivered to these very high-risk children through their tenth-grade year to prevent serious delinquency, substance use, and conduct disorder. Eddy, Reid, Stoolmiller, and Fetrow (2003) have also documented improved outcomes resulting from a multicomponent program involving a universal preventive intervention, behavioral parent management training, and child social and problem-solving skills training. Late-elementary school-age children who participated in the LIFT (Linking the Interests of Families and Teachers) program had a decreased likelihood of police contact and alcohol use during middle school.

Anger Coping Program

Additional evidence for the clinical utility of CBT programs for aggressive children can be found in a programmatic series of controlled studies examining the Anger Coping program, Coping Power's predecessor. In comparison with a minimal treatment and untreated control condition, Lochman, Burch, Curry, and Lampron (1984) found that treated aggressive elementary school boys had reductions in independently observed disruptive-aggressive off-task classroom behavior, reduction in parents' ratings of aggression, and improvements in self-esteem. Other ratings by teachers and peers did not show improvement. The posttreatment behavioral improvements in this study have been replicated in subsequent studies (e.g., Lochman & Curry, 1986; Lochman, Lampron, Gemmer, Harris, & Wyckoff, 1989), and gains in classroom on-task behavior have been found in a 7-month follow-up (Lochman & Lampron, 1988). While some maintenance of treatment effects was evident in a 3-year follow-up, at age 15, these results were mixed (Lochman, 1992). In comparison to an untreated condition of aggressive boys, Anger Coping boys maintained their gains in self-esteem, displayed better problem-solving skills, and had significantly lower levels of substance use. On these measures, the treated boys were in the same range as nonaggressive boys at follow-up, and the results indicated important prevention effects on adolescent substance use. However, continued reduction in off-task behavior and in parents' ratings of aggression were only evident for Anger Coping boys who had received a six-session booster treatment for themselves and their parents during the next school year. Without the booster treatment, the reductions in aggressive behavior were not maintained.

Coping Power Program

Empirical evidence also supports the effectiveness of the Coping Power program. Outcome analyses in randomized, controlled intervention studies indicate that the Coping Power intervention has had broad effects at postintervention on boys' social information processing and locus of control and on parents' parenting practices (Lochman & Wells, 2002a). In analyses of the 1-year follow-up effects of the program, Coping Power produced significant reductions in risks for self-reported delinquency, parent-reported substance use, and teacher-reported behavioral problems, especially for boys who received both the child and parent components (Lochman & Wells, 2004). A second effectiveness study examined whether the Coping Power program effects could be augmented by delivering the program along with a classroom-based intervention involving teacher training. Outcome analyses with 245 aggressive children indicate that Coping Power produced significant postintervention effects on children's social competence and aggressive behavior (Lochman & Wells, 2002b). This study replicated the 1-year follow-up results from the prior study, as Coping Power children had reduced levels of delinquency, substance use, and aggressive behaviors in the school setting (Lochman & Wells, 2003). The program has also been effectively disseminated with aggressive deaf children (Lochman et al., 2001) and has been found to be cost-effective in a Dutch outpatient setting with children diagnosed with oppositional defiant disorder and conduct disorder (van de Wiel, Matthys, Cohen-Kettenis, & van Engeland, 2003).

Clinical and Treatment Characteristics as Predictors of Outcomes

Although efforts to find which aspects of CBT are most effective with which types of aggressive children are still in rudimentary stages, some initial findings have emerged. Kendall and colleagues (1991) have found that CBT with conduct-disordered children has been most effective in reducing conduct problems with children who had initially lower perceived levels of hostility and a more internalized attributional style. Lochman and colleagues (1985) found that boys in the Anger Coping program who had the greatest reductions in aggressive behavior, relative to the control condition, were boys who initially were the poorest social problem solvers. In addition, better outcomes tended to occur for boys with more initial somatization and anxiety behaviors, and lower social acceptance from peers, suggesting that these boys may have been more motivated for treatment because of a desire to alleviate distress and decrease peer rejection. Interestingly, those boys in the untreated condition who improved the most spontaneously had better problem-solving skills and higher self-esteem. The differential correlates of improvement for the treated and untreated conditions suggest that the Anger Coping program was most successful with those boys who were the poorest problem solvers and most in need of intervention. The Coping Power program has been found to be equally effective at the 1-year follow-up with boys and girls, with African American and Caucasian children, and with children from neighborhoods with different levels of neighborhood violence (Lochman & Wells, 2003). However, the Coping Power program's effects on preventing escalation of substance use were most apparent for older children in the sample.

In studies of treatment characteristics that could augment the effects of the Anger Coping program, Lochman and colleagues (1984) have found that inclusion of a behavioral goal-setting component tended to lead to lower aggression and disruptiveness. In this component, boys set weekly goals for themselves in their group meetings, these goals were monitored daily by teachers, and contingent reinforcement occurred for successful goal attainment. Similar evidence for the effectiveness of homework assignments in CBT has been obtained by Kazdin and colleagues (1989). In addition, more widespread improvements in classroom behavior have been noted when the Anger Coping program was offered in an 18-session format instead of the original 12-session format (Lochman, 1985). We have not found that inclusion of limited forms of structured teacher consultation (Lochman, Lampron, Gemmer, et al., 1989) or additional training in self-instruction training on nonsocial academic tasks (Lochman & Curry, 1986) augments the basic Anger Coping program's effects. However, training teachers to implement a classroom-level intervention has been shown to enhance the preventive effects of the Coping Power program on at-risk children's school behavior (Lochman & Wells, 2003).

Mediation of Intervention Effects

Path analyses indicate that the Coping Power intervention effects were at least partly mediated by changes in boys' social-cognitive processes, schemas, and parenting processes (Lochman & Wells, 2002a). Changes in social-cognitive appraisal processes, involving boys' hostile attributions and resulting anger, and decision making processes, involving reductions in the boys' expectations that aggressive behavior would lead to good outcomes for them, contributed to the boys' reduced risk for antisocial behavior. Similarly, changes in boys' schemas involving their beliefs about their degree of internal control over successful outcomes and the complexity of their internal representations of others, and changes in their perceptions of the consistency of the parents' discipline efforts, led to lower levels of delinquency, substance use, and school behavioral problems. Consistent with the assumptions of the contextual social-cognitive model used here, boys' engagement in serious problem behavior in the year following their involvement in the Coping Power intervention was affected in part by improvements in the ways that they perceived and processed their social world and in their expectations of more consistent and predictable responses from their parents.

Implications for CBT Outcome Research

As Kazdin (1995) has noted, these research results present a generally positive and promising view of the effects of CBT with aggressive children. However, because of the mixed posttreatment and follow-up findings, further program development and outcome research are clearly needed. Future outcome research should address the following issues (see also Lochman, 1990): (1) longer-term follow-up assessments in designs that include control conditions and direct behavioral observation measures; (2) further exploration of child and treatment characteristics that predict the outcome; (3) attention to contextual factors in the development and evaluation of intervention programs in this area (Lochman, 2004); and (4) intensive CBT programs for childhood aggression, since research in treatment of chronic behavioral problems should focus on creating clinically meaningful improvement, although research will need to critically examine whether each additional component is necessary and adds to effectiveness. More intensive CBT programs can include behavior modification components in school settings, longer treatment periods with follow-up boosters, and behavioral parent training. The fifth issue to address involves evaluating the effectiveness of our dissemination efforts, using evidence-based CBT programs. It is not clear whether evidence-based CBT programs can be successfully taken to scale in the real world, whether CBT programs can be implemented with high intervention integrity, and whether certain forms of adaptation of programs by clinicians are not only permissible but may actually increase the utility and effectiveness of the programs.

Issues and Recommendations

Ethnic and Community Context

There are several ethnic and community factors that may delimit the transferability and the consistent use of the Coping Power strategies for aggressive boys and adolescents, especially among African American, low-income individuals. First, parents indirectly and/or directly may promote the use of physically aggressive problem-solving strategies by their greater dependence on corporal punishment as well as actively teaching their children to retaliate when confronted with physically or verbally aggressive situations. These covert and overt messages may cause a child or adolescent to underutilize some of his new problem-solving skills and alternatives to aggression. It is important to keep in mind that many of these messages have developed as the result of many urban parents' ongoing struggle to protect their boys, on the one hand, while trying to inculcate responsibility, on the other. Of course, much of this struggle is primarily a result of living in an impoverished neighborhood, along with the long-term effects of racism and discrimination. Another factor, which may also serve to limit the effectiveness of treatment, is conflicting messages about the use of aggression between parents and other authority figures, such as school personnel. Equally important is the fact that there are survival mechanisms within the low-income community that are antithetical to those espoused by the Coping Power program. That is, peers who are assaultive or physically threatening—which a child or adolescent might encounter in their community—may require the use of physically aggressive strategies. Finally, if the child or adolescent has had a traumatizing event occur in his community involving himself, a peer, or family member—which renders these alternative strategies as counterintuitive—then this will significantly limit the long-term use of these alternative problem-solving skills.

One technique, which might serve to offset some of these limitations, is to further investigate the relationship between the duality of roles and the use of a phenomenon called "code switching" (Johnson & Farrell, 1997). This technique serves as a mechanism specifically to train children or adolescents to have a different code of behavior depending on the immediate environment.

Adaptation of CBT to Early Elementary-School-Age Children

The behavioral and social-cognitive characteristics of younger children require group leaders to modify the structure and content of group sessions. Five- to seven-year-olds are active and less skilled in important group behavior such as turn taking, sitting in one's seat, and making relevant comments. Children in this age group also are egocentric in perspective-taking skills and typically do not demonstrate a sequential problem-solving style. Information on how to alter group sessions to accommodate these behavioral and social-cognitive differences can be found in Lochman and colleagues (1999).

Adaptation of CBT to Middle to Late Adolescents

The emotional/behavioral/cognitive development of middle to late adolescents requires group leaders to modify the structure and content of group sessions. The role of peer pressure is an important factor as well. Based on work with adolescents within several settings, a general outline of the various structural and content changes can be found in Lochman and colleagues (1999).

Future Directions for CBT

When we wrote this chapter (Lochman et al., 2000; Lochman, White, & Wayland, 1991) for prior editions of this book, we identified the three most compelling emerging themes for CBT assessment and intervention to be (1) the inclusion of cognitive-behavioral parent assessment and therapy, (2) the intensification and broadening of CBT programs, and (3) an increasing focus on universal (primary) and indicated and selected (secondary) prevention. Clear signs exist that the evolution of CBT with aggressive children has moved in these directions. However, these themes remain an important focus for continued intervention development.

The most striking deficiency in many earlier CBT programs and research with aggressive children has been the neglect of children's caregivers, especially parents. Intervening with these caregivers can be critical in strengthening treatment effects and in maintaining generalization of treatment effects over time. The best-documented effective treatment for childhood antisocial behavior is behavioral parent therapy (Kazdin, 1995; Lochman & van den Steenhoven, 2002). Behavioral parent training can focus on altering the deficient parenting skills and parental aggressiveness that are so often evident in families of aggressive children, thereby reinforcing the behavioral changes children begin to make in CBT. Behavioral training for teachers could be similarly useful. Perhaps more critically, parent treatment can, over time, promote changes in parents' appraisal distortions and social problem-solving deficiencies. As parents change these pathological patterns in thinking, which are shared by their children, the children can begin responding to the parents' and teachers' modeling of more adaptive and competent cognitive processes.

A CBT program can be broadened by including an emphasis on cognitive schemata and operations, and cognitive appraisal and coping with arousal, as well as social-cognitive products. By focusing on children's social goals, expectations of achieving goals, labeling, and coping with affective states and concomitant arousal, we can impact key processes that are critical in successful use of self-instruction or social problem solving. It is in the context of strong therapeutic alliance in individual or group therapy that children can begin to examine, trust, and try out others' perceptions of interpersonal events. These perceptual changes are slow in coming, since they involve revisions in internalized styles of attending to and interpreting events. In contrast, social problem-solving skills can be altered through role playing and discussion more rapidly.

CBT can be easily and effectively adapted for universal, selected, and indicated prevention programs (Conduct Problems Prevention Research Group, 1992; Lochman & Wells, 1996). To facilitate development of these programs, risk markers (e.g., temperament, parenting skills; Colder, Lochman, & Wells, 1997) for childhood aggression will have to be identified during the preschool and early elementary school period. With a preventive orientation, CBT-based services can be provided in settings providing broad access to children (e.g., schools, pediatric clinics, day care and community athletic facilities), as we have successfully done in the Fast Track, Anger Coping, and Coping Power programs Through early identification, and by not having to rely on caregivers' compliance with referrals to clinics, CBT can be provided to children and their caregivers at a time when children's self-regulation processes are being internalized.

REFERENCES

Abidin, R. R. (1983). *Parenting Stress Index—Manual*. Charlottesville, VA: Pediatric Psychology Press.

Achenbach, T. M. (1991). *Manual for the Child Behavior Checklist/4–18 and 1991 Profile*. Burlington: University of Vermont, Department of Psychiatry.

Achenbach, T. M., & Edelbrock, C. S. (1983). *Manual for the Child Behavior Checklist and Revised Child Behavior Profile*. Burlington: University of Vermont, Department of Psychiatry.

Agrawal, R., & Kaushal, K. (1988). Attention and short-term memory in normal children, aggressive children, and nonaggressive children with attention deficit disorder. *Journal of General Psychology, 114*, 335–343.

American Psychiatric Association. (1994). *Diagnostic and statistical manual of mental disorders* (4th ed.). Washington, DC: Author.

August, G. J., Realmuto, G. M., MacDonald, A. W., III, Nugent, S. M., & Crosby, R. (1996). Prevalence of ADHD and comorbid disorders among elementary school children screened for disruptive behavior. *Journal of Abnormal Child Psychology, 34*, 571–595.

Bandura, A. (1973). *Aggression: A social learning analysis*. Englewood Cliffs, NJ: Prentice-Hall.

Bandura, A. (1977). *Social learning theory*. Englewood Cliffs, NJ: Prentice-Hall.

Barkley, R. A. (1997). *ADHD and the nature of self-control*. New York: Guilford Press.

Beck, A. T., Rush, A. J., Shaw, B. F., & Emery, G. (1979). *Cognitive therapy of depression*. New York: Guilford Press.

Boldizar, J. P., Perry, D. G., & Perry, L. C. (1989). Outcome values and aggression. *Child Development, 60*, 571–579.

Brestan, E. V., & Eyberg, S. M. (1998). Effective psychosocial treatments of conduct-disordered children and adolescents: 29 years, 82 studies, and 5,272 kids. *Journal of Clinical Child Psychology, 27*, 180–189.

Bry, B. H., Catalano, R. F., Kumpfer, K. L., Lochman, J. F., & Szapocznik, J. (1999). Scientific findings from family prevention intervention research. In R. Ashery (Ed.), *Family-based prevention interventions* (pp. 103–129). Rockville, MD: National Institute of Drug Abuse.

Bryant, B. K. (1982). An index of empathy for children and adolescents. *Child Development, 53*, 413–425.

Camp, B. W., Blom, G. F., Herbert., F., & van Doornick, W. J. (1977). "Think Aloud": A program for developing self-control in young aggressive boys. *Journal of Abnormal Child Psychology, 5*, 157–169.

Coats, K. I. (1979). Cognitive self instructional training approach for reducing disruptive behavior of young children. *Psychology Reports, 44*, 127–132.

Cohen, R., & Schleser, R. (1984). Cognitive development and clinical implications. In A. W. Meyers & W. E. Craighead (Eds.), *Cognitive behavior therapy with children* (pp. 45–68). New York: Plenum Press.

Cohen, D., & Strayer, J. (1996). Empathy in conduct-disordered and comparison youth. *Developmental Psychology, 32*, 988–998.

Coie, J. E., Dodge, K. A., & Coppotelli, H. (1982). Dimensions and types of status: A cross-age perspective. *Developmental Psychology, 18*, 557–570.

Coie, J. D., Lochman, J. E., Terry, R., & Hyman, C. (1992). Predicting early adolescent disorder from childhood aggression and peer rejection. *Journal of Consulting and Clinical Psychology, 60*, 783–792.

Colder, C. R., Lochman, J. E., & Wells, K. C. (1997). The moderating effects of children's fear and activity level on relations between parenting practices and childhood symptomatology. *Journal of Abnormal Child Psychology, 25*, 251–263.

Conduct Problems Prevention Research Group. (1992). A developmental and clinical model for the prevention of conduct disorder: The Fast Track Program. *Development and Psychopathology, 4*, 509–527.

Conduct Problems Prevention Research Group. (2004). The effects of the Fast Track program on serious problem outcomes at the end of elementary school. *Journal of Clinical Child and Adolescent Psychology, 33*, 650–661.

Cornell, D. G., Warren, J., Hawk, G., Stafford, E., Oram, G. & Pine, D. (1996). Psychopathy in instrumental and reactive violent offenders. *Journal of Consulting and Clinical Psychology, 64*, 783–790.

Costello, A. J., Edelbrock, C. S., Dulcan, M. K., & Kalas, R. (1984). *Testing of the NIMH Diagnostic Interview Schedule for Children (DISC) in a clinical population* (Contract No. DB-81-0027, final report to the Center for Epidemiological Studies, National Institute for Mental Health). Pittsburgh, PA: University of Pittsburgh.

Crick, N. R., & Dodge, K. A. (1994). A review and reformulation of social information-processing mechanisms in children's social adjustment. *Psychological Bulletin, 115*, 74–101.

Crick, N. R., & Ladd, G. W. (1990). Children's perceptions of the outcomes of aggressive strategies. Do the ends justify the means? *Developmental Psychology, 26*, 612–620.

Dabbs, J. M., Jr., Jurkovic, G. L., & Frady, R. L. (1988). *Saliva testosterone and cortisol among young male prison inmates.* Unpublished manuscript, Georgia State University.

Dishion, T. J., & Andrews, D. W. (1995). Preventing escalation in problem behaviors with high risk young adolescents: Immediate and 1-year outcomes. *Journal of Consulting and Clinical Psychology, 63*, 538–548.

Dishion, T. J., Patterson, G. R., & Griesler, P. C. (1994). Peer adaptations in the development of antisocial behavior: A confluence model. In L. R. Huesmann (Ed.), *Aggressive behavior: Current perspectives* (pp. 61–95). New York: Plenum Press.

Dix, T., & Lochman, J. E. (1990). Social cognition and negative reactions to children: A comparison of mothers of aggressive and nonaggressive boys. *Journal of Social and Clinical Psychology, 9*, 418–438.

Dodge, K. A. (1980). Social cognition and children's aggressive behavior. *Child Development, 51*, 162–170.

Dodge, K. A., Coie, J. D., & Brakke, N. P. (1982). Behavior patterns of socially rejected and neglected preadolescents: The roles of social approach and aggression. *Journal of Abnormal Child Psychology, 10*, 389–410.

Dodge, K. A., & Frame, C. L. (1982), Social cognitive biases and deficits in aggressive boys. *Child Development, 53*, 620–635.

Dodge, K. A., Laird, R., Lochman, J. E., Zelli, A., & the Conduct Problems Prevention Research Group. (2002). Multidimensional latent-construct analysis of children's social information processing patterns: Correlations with aggressive behavior problems. *Psychological Assessment, 14*, 60–73.

Dodge, K. A., Lochman, J. E., Harnish, J. D., Bates, J. E., & Pettit, G. S. (1997). Reactive and proactive aggression in school children and psychiatrically impaired chronically assaultive youth. *Journal of Abnormal Psychology, 106*, 37–51.

Dodge, K. A., & Newman, J. P. (1981). Biased decision-making processes in aggressive boys. *Journal of Abnormal Psychology, 90*, 375–379.

Dodge, K. A., Pettit, G. S., McClaskey, C. L., & Brown, M. M. (1986). Social competence in children. *Monographs of the Society for Research in Child Development, 51*(2, Serial No. 213).

Dodge, K. A., & Somberg, D. R. (1987). Hostile attributional biases among aggressive boys are exacerbated under conditions of threat to the self. *Child Development, 58*, 213–224.

Dubow, E. F., Huesmann, L. R., & Eron, L. D. (1987). Mitigating aggression promoting prosocial behavior in aggressive elementary schoolboys. *Behavior Research and Therapy, 25*, 527–531.

Dunn, S. E., Lochman, J. E., & Colder, C. R. (1997). Social problem-solving skills in boys with conduct and oppositional defiant disorders. *Aggressive Behavior, 23*, 457–469.

Eddy, J. M., Reid, J. B., Stoolmiller, M., & Fetrow, R. A. (2003). Outcomes during middle school for an elementary school-based preventive intervention for conduct problems: Follow-up results from a randomized trial. *Behavior Therapy, 34*, 535–552.

Emery, R., & O'Leary, D. (1982). Children's perceptions of marital discord and behavior of boys and girls. *Journal of Abnormal Child Psychology, 10*, 11–24.

Erdley, C. A. (1990). *An analysis of children's attributions and goals in social situations: Implications of children's friendship outcomes.* Unpublished manuscript, University of Illinois.

Erdley, C. A., & Asher, S. R. (1993, March). *To aggress or not: Social-cognitive mediators of children's responses to ambiguous provocation.* Paper presented at the biennial meeting of the Society for Research in Child Development, New Orleans, LA.

Evans, S. W., & Short, E. J. (1991). A qualitative and serial analysis of social problem-solving in aggressive boys. *Journal of Abnormal Child Psychology, 19*, 331–340.

Eyberg, S. M. (1980). Eyberg Child Behavior Inventory. *Journal of Clinical Child Psychology, 9*, 29–40.

Fiske, S. T., & Taylor, S. W. (1984). *Social cognition.* Reading, MA: Addison-Wesley.

Forman, S. G. (1980). A comparison of cognitive training and response cost procedures in modifying aggressive behavior of elementary school children. *Behavior Therapy, 11*, 94–100.

Gainetdinov, R. R., Wetsel, W. C., Jones, S. R., Levin, E. D., Jaber, M., & Caron, M. G. (1999). Role of serotonin in the paradoxical calming effect of psychostimulants on hyperactivity. *Science, 283*, 397–401.

Garrison, S. R., & Stolberg, A. L. (1983). Modification of anger in children by affect imagery training. *Journal of Abnormal Child Psychology, 11,* 115–130.

Giancola, P. R., Martin, C. S., Tarter, R. E., Pelham, W. E., & Moss, H. B. (1996). Executive cognitive functioning and aggressive behavior in preadolescent boys at high risk for substance abuse/dependence. *Journal of Studies on Alcohol, 57,* 352–359.

Giancola, P. R., Moss, H. B., Martin, C. S., Krisci, L., & Tarter, R. E. (1996). Executive cognitive functioning predicts reactive aggression in boys at high risk for substance abuse: A prospective study. *Alcoholism: Clinical and Experimental Research, 20,* 740–744.

Giancola, P. R., Zeichner, A., Yarnell, J. E., & Dickson, K. E. (1996). Relation between executive cognitive functioning and the adverse consequences of alcohol use in social drinkers. *Alcoholism: Clinical and Experimental Research, 20,* 1094–1098.

Goleman, D. (1995). *Emotional intelligence.* New York: Bantam Books.

Halperin, J. M., Newcorn, J. H., Kopstein, I., McKay, K. E., Schwartz, S. T., Siever, L. J., & Sharma, V. (1997). Serotonin, aggression, and parental psychopathology in children with attention-deficit disorder. *Journal of the American Academy of Child and Adolescent Psychiatry, 36,* 1391–1399.

Hart, C. H., Ladd, G. W., & Burleson, B. R. (1990). Children's expectations of the outcomes of social strategies: Relations with sociometric status and maternal disciplinary style. *Child Development, 61,* 127–137.

Harter, S. (1985). *The Self-Perception Profile for Children: Revision of the Perceived Competence Scale for Children* (manual). Denver, CO: University of Denver.

Hawkins, J. D., Catalano, R. F., Morrison, D. M., O'Donnell, J., Abbott, R. D., & Day, L. E. (1992). The Seattle Social Development Project: Effects of the first four years on protective factors and problem behavior. In J. McCord & R. E. Tremblay (Eds.), *Preventing antisocial behavior: Interventions from birth through adolescence* (pp. 139–161). New York: Guilford Press.

Herrenkohl, I. T., Maguin, E., Hill, K. G., Hawkins, J. D., Abbott, R. D., & Catalano, R. F. (1998). *Developmental predictors of violence in late adolescence.* Unpublished manuscript, University of Washington, Seattle.

Hill, L. G., Coie, J. D., Lochman, J. E., Greenberg, M. T., & the Conduct Problems Prevention Research Group. (2004). Effectiveness of early screening for externalizing problems: Issues of screening accuracy and utility. *Journal of Consulting and Clinical Psychology, 72,* 809–820.

Hodges, V. K. (1987). Assessing children with a clinical research interview: The Child Assessment Schedule. In R. J. Prinz (Ed.), *Advances in behavioral assessment of children and families* (pp. 65–81). Greenwich, CT: JAI Press.

Ingram, R. E., & Kendall, P. C., (1986). Cognitive clinical psychology: Implications of an informational processing perspective. In R. E. Ingram (Ed.), *Information processing approaches to clinical psychology* (pp. 3–21). New York: Academic Press.

Joffe, R. D., Dobson, K. S., Fine, S., Marriage, K., & Haley, G. (1990). Social problem-solving in depressed, conduct disordered and normal adolescents. *Journal of Abnormal Child Psychology, 18,* 565–575.

Johnson, J. H., Jr., & Farrell, W. C., Jr. (1997). *The Durham Scholars Program: An evaluation research proposal.* Chapel Hill: University of North Carolina Department of Geography, Department of Sociology, and the Kenan-Flagler Business School.

Jurkovic, G., & Prentice, N. M. (1977). Relation of moral and cognitive development to dimensions of juvenile delinquency. *Journal of Abnormal Psychology, 86,* 414–420.

Kaufman, A. S., & Kaufman, N. L. (1990). *Kaufman Brief Intelligence Test (K-BIT) manual.* Circle Pines, MN: American Guidance Service.

Kazdin, A. E. (1995). *Conduct disorders in childhood and adolescence* (2nd ed.). Thousand Oaks, CA: Sage.

Kazdin, A. E., Bass, D., Siegel, T., & Thomas, C. (1989). Cognitive-behavioral therapy and relationship therapy in the treatment of children referred for antisocial behavior. *Journal of Consulting and Clinical Psychology, 57,* 522–535.

Kazdin, A. E., & Esveldt-Dawson, K. (1986). The Interview for Antisocial Behavior: Psychometric characteristics and concurrent validity with child psychiatric inpatients. *Journal of Psychopathology and Behavioral Assessment, 8,* 289–303.

Kazdin, A. E., Esveldt-Dawson, K., French, N. H., & Unis, A. S. (1987a). Effects of parent management training and problem-solving skills training combined in the treatment of antisocial child behavior. *Journal of the American Academy of Child and Adolescent Psychiatry, 26,* 416–424.

Kazdin, A. E., Esveldt-Dawson, K., French, N. H., & Unis, A. S. (1987b). Problem-solving skills training and relationship therapy in the treatment of antisocial child behavior. *Journal of Consulting and Clinical Psychology, 55,* 76–85.

Kazdin, A. E., Siegel, T. C., & Bass, D. (1992). Cognitive problem-solving skills training and parent management training in the treatment of antisocial behavior in children. *Journal of Consulting and Clinical Psychology, 60,* 733–747.

Kazdin, A. E., & Weisz, J. R. (2003). *Evidence-based psychotherapies for children and adolescents.* New York: Guilford Press.

Kellam, S. G., & Rebok, G. W. (1992). Building etiological theory through epidemiologically based preventive intervention trials. In J. McCord & R. E. Tremblay (Eds.), *Preventing antisocial behavior: Interventions from birth through adolescence* (pp. 139–161). New York: Guilford Press.

Kendall, P. C. (1998). Empirically-supported psychological therapies. *Journal of Consulting and Clinical Psychology, 66,* 3–6.

Kendall, P. C., & Braswell, L. (1993). *Cognitive-behavioral therapy for impulsive children* (2nd ed.). New York: Guilford Press.

Kendall, P. C., & Choudhury, M. S. (2003). Children and adolescents in cognitive-behavioral therapy: Some past efforts and current advances, and the challenges in our future. *Cognitive Therapy and Research, 27,* 89–104.

Kendall, P. C., & Ingram, R. E. (1989). Cognitive behavioral perspective: Theory and research. In P. C. Kendall & D. Watson (Eds.), *Anxiety and depression: Distinctive and overlapping features.* New York: Academic Press.

Kendall, P. C., & MacDonald, J. P. (1993). Cognition in the psychopathology of youth and implications for treatment. In K. S. Dobson & P. C. Kendall (Eds.), *Psychopathology and cognition* (pp. 387–489). San Diego, CA: Academic Press.

Kendall, P. C., Ronan, K. R., & Epps, J. (1991). Aggression in children-adolescents: Cognitive-behavioral treatment perspectives. In D. Pepler & K. Rubin (Eds.), *Development and treatment of childhood aggression* (pp. 341–360). Toronto, ON, Canada: Erlbaum.

Kettlewell, P. W., & Kausch, D. F. (1983). The generalization of the effects of a cognitive-behavioral treatment program for aggressive children. *Journal of Abnormal Child Psychology, 11,* 101–114.

Larrance, D. T., & Twentyman, C. T. (1983). Maternal attributions and child abuse. *Journal of Abnormal Psychology, 92,* 449–457.

Larson, J., & Lochman, J. E. (2002). *Helping schoolchildren cope with anger: A cognitive behavioral intervention.* New York: Guilford Press.

Lazarus, R. S. (1993). From psychological stress to the emotions: A history of changing outlooks. *Annual Review of Psychology, 44,* 1–21.

Lochman, J. E. (1985). Effects of different treatment lengths in cognitive behavioral interventions with aggressive boys. *Child Psychiatry and Human Development, 16,* 45–56.

Lochman, J. E. (1990). Modification of childhood aggression. In M. Hersen, R. Eisler, & P. M. Miller (Eds.), *Progress in behavior modification* (Vol. 25, pp. 48–86). Newbury Park, CA: Sage.

Lochman, J. E. (1992). Cognitive-behavioral intervention with aggressive boys: Three-year follow-up and preventive effects. *Journal of Consulting and Clinical Psychology, 60*, 426–432.

Lochman, J. E. (2003). Preventive intervention targeting precursors. In Z. Sloboda & W. J. Bukoski (Eds.), *Handbook of drug abuse prevention: Theory, science, and practice.* New York: Plenum.

Lochman, J. E. (2004). Contextual factors in risk and prevention research. *Merrill-Palmer Quarterly, 50*, 311–325.

Lochman, J. E., Burch, P. R., Curry, J. F., & Lampron, L. B. (1984). Treatment and generalization effects of cognitive-behavioral and goal-setting interventions with aggressive boys. *Journal of Consulting and Clinical Psychology, 52*, 915–916.

Lochman, J. E., Coie, J. D., Underwood, M., & Terry, R. (1993). Effectiveness of a social relations intervention program for aggressive and nonaggressive rejected children. *Journal of Consulting and Clinical Psychology, 61*, 1053–1058.

Lochman, J. E., & Curry, J. F. (1986). Effects of social problem-solving training and self-instruction training with aggressive boys. *Journal of Clinical Child Psychology, 15*, 159–164.

Lochman, J. E., & Dodge, K. A. (1994). Social-cognitive processes of severely violent, moderately aggressive and nonaggressive boys. *Journal of Consulting and Clinical Psychology, 62*, 366–374.

Lochman, J. E., & Dodge, K. A. (1998). Distorted perceptions in dyadic interactions of aggressive and nonaggressive boys: Effects of prior expectations, context, and boys' age. *Development and Psychopathology, 10*, 495–512.

Lochman, J. E., Dunn, S. E., & Wagner, E. E. (1997). Anger. In G. Bear, K. Minke, & A. Thomas (Eds.), *Children's needs II* (pp. 149–160). Washington, DC: National Association of School Psychology.

Lochman, J. E., FitzGerald, D., Gage, S., Kanaly, K., Whidby, J., Barry, T. D., et al. (2001). Effects of a social cognitive intervention for aggressive deaf children: The Coping Power Program. *Journal of the American Deafness and Rehabilitation Association, 35*, 38–61.

Lochman, J. E., FitzGerald, D. P., & Whidby, J. M. (1999). Anger management with aggressive children. In C. Schaefer (Ed.), *Short-term psychotherapy groups for children* (pp. 301–349). Northvale, NJ: Aronson.

Lochman, J. E., & Lampron, L. B. (1985). The usefulness of peer ratings of aggression and social acceptance in the identification of behavioral and subjective difficulties in aggressive boys. *Journal of Applied Developmental Psychology, 6*, 187–198.

Lochman, J. E., & Lampron, L. B. (1986). Situational social problem-solving skills and self-esteem of aggressive and nonaggressive boys. *Journal of Abnormal Child Psychology ,14*, 605–617.

Lochman, J. E., & Lampron, L. B. (1988). Cognitive behavioral interventions for aggressive boys: Seven months follow-up effects. *Journal of Child and Adolescent Psychotherapy, 5*, 15–23.

Lochman, J. E., Lampron, L. B., Burch, P. R., & Curry, J. F. (1985). Client characteristics associated with behavior change for treated and untreated boys. *Journal of Abnormal Child Psychology, 13*, 527–538.

Lochman, J. E., Lampron, L. B., Gemmer, T. V., & Harris, R. (1987). In P. A. Keller & S. R. Heyman (Eds.), *Innovations in clinical practice: A source book* (Vol. 6, pp. 339–356). Sarasota, FL: Professional Resource Exchange.

Lochman, J. E., Lampron, L. B., Gemmer, T. C., Harris, R., & Wyckoff, G. M. (1989). Teacher consultation and cognitive-behavioral interventions with aggressive boys. *Psychology in the Schools, 26*, 179–188.

Lochman, J. E., Lampron, L. B., & Rabiner, D. L. (1989). Format and salience effects in the social problem-solving of aggressive and nonaggressive boys. *Journal of Clinical Child Psychology, 18*, 230–236.

Lochman, J. E., Nelson, N. W., III, & Sims, J. P. (1981). A cognitive behavioral program for use with aggressive children. *Journal of Clinical Child Psychology, 13,* 527–538.

Lochman, J. E., & van den Steenhoven, A. (2002). Family-based approaches to substance abuse prevention. *Journal of Primary Prevention, 23,* 49–114.

Lochman, J. E., & Wayland, K. K. (1994). Aggression, social acceptance and race as predictors of negative adolescent outcomes. *Journal of the American Academy of Child and Adolescent Psychiatry, 33,* 1026–1035.

Lochman, J. E., Wayland, K. K., & White, K. J. (1993). Social goals: Relationship to adolescent adjustment and to social problem-solving. *Journal of Abnormal Child Psychology, 21,* 135–151.

Lochman, J. E., & Wells, K. C. (1996). A social-cognitive intervention with aggressive children: Prevention effects and contextual implementation issues. In R. D. Peters & R. J. McMahon (Eds.), *Prevention and early intervention: Childhood disorders, substance use, and delinquency* (pp. 111–143). Thousand Oaks, CA: Sage.

Lochman, J. E., & Wells, K. C. (2002a). Contextual social-cognitive mediators and child outcome: A test of the theoretical model in the Coping Power program. *Development and Psychopathology, 14,* 945–967.

Lochman, J. E., & Wells, K. C. (2002b). The Coping Power program at the middle-school transition: Universal and indicated prevention effects. *Psychology of Addictive Behaviors, 16,* S40–S54.

Lochman, J. E., & Wells, K. C. (2003). Effectiveness of the Coping Power program and of classroom intervention with aggressive children: Outcomes at a 1-year follow-up. *Behavior Therapy, 34,* 493–515.

Lochman, J. E., & Wells, K. C. (2004). The Coping Power Program for preadolescent aggressive boys and their parents: Outcome effects at the 1-year follow-up. *Journal of Consulting and Clinical Psychology, 72,* 571–578.

Lochman, J. E., Wells, K. C., & Murray, M. (in press). The Coping Power program: Preventive intervention at the middle school transition. In P. Tolan, J. Szapocznik, & S. Sambrano (Eds.), *Preventing substance abuse: 3 to 14.* Washington, DC: American Psychological Association.

Lochman, J. E., Whidby, J. M., & FitzGerald, D .P. (2000). Cognitive-behavioral assessment and treatment with aggressive children. In P. C. Kendall (Ed.), *Child and adolescent therapy: Cognitive-behavioral procedures* (2nd ed., pp. 31–87). New York: Guilford Press.

Lochman, J. E., White, K. J., & Wayland, K. K. (1991). Cognitive behavioral assessment and treatment with aggressive children. In P. C. Kendall (Ed.), *Child and adolescent therapy: Cognitive-behavioral procedures* (pp. 25–35). New York: Guilford Press.

Loeber, R. (1990). Development and risk factors of juvenile antisocial behavior and delinquency. *Clinical Psychology Review, 10,* 1–41.

Loeber, R., & Dishion, T. J. (1983). Early predictors of male delinquency: A review. *Psychological Bulletin, 94,* 68–99.

Matthys, W., van Goozen, S. H. M., de Vries, H., Cohen-Kettenis, P .T., & van Engeland, H. (1998). The dominance of behavioural activation over behavioural inhibition in conduct disordered boys with or without Attention Deficit Hyperactivity Disorder. *Journal of Child Psychology and Psychiatry, 39,* 643–651.

McKinnon, C. E., Lamb, M. E., Belsky, J., & Baum, C. (1990). An affective-cognitive model for mother–child aggression. *Development and Psychopathology, 2,* 1–13.

McMahon, R. J., & Estes, A. M. (1997). Conduct problems. In E. J. Mash & L. G. Terdal (Eds.), *Assessment of childhood disorders* (3rd ed., pp. 130–193). New York: Guilford Press.

McMahon, R. J., & Forehand, R. (1988). Conduct disorder. In E. J. Mash & L. G. Terdal (Eds.), *Behavioral assessment of childhood disorders* (2nd ed., pp. 105–153). New York. Guilford Press.

Meichenbaum, D. (1985). *Stress inoculation training.* New York: Pergamon Press.

Meichenbaum, D. H., & Goodman, J. (1971). Training impulsive children to talk to themselves: A means of developing self control. *Journal of Abnormal Psychology, 77,* 115–126.

Milich, R., & Dodge, K. A. (1984). Social information processing in child psychiatric populations. *Journal of Abnormal Child Psychology, 12,* 471–490.

Miller, P. A., & Eisenberg, N. (1988). The relation of empathy to aggressive and externalizing/antisocial behavior. *Psychological Bulletin, 103,* 324–344.

Miller-Johnson, S., Lochman, J. E., Coie, J. D., Terry, R., & Hyman, C. (1998). Comorbidity of conduct and depressive problems at sixth grade: Substance use outcomes across adolescence. *Journal of Abnormal Child Psychology, 26,* 221–232.

Miller-Johnson, S., Winn, D. M., Coie, J., Maumary-Gremaud, A., Hyman, C., Terry, R., & Lochman, J. E. (1999). Motherhood during the teen years: A developmental perspective on risk factors for childbearing. *Development and Psychopathology, 11,* 85–100.

Mirsky, A. F. (1989, August). *The neuropsychology of attention: Developmental neuropsychiatric implications.* Paper presented at the 97th annual convention of the American Psychological Association, New Orleans, LA.

Moffit, T. E. (1993). Adolescence-limited and life-course persistent antisocial behavior: A developmental taxonomy. *Psychological Review, 100,* 674–701.

Novaco, R. W. (1978). Anger and coping with stress: Cognitive-behavioral intervention. In J. P. Foreyet & D. P. Rathjen (Eds.), *Cognitive behavioral therapy: Research and application* (pp. 135–173). New York: Plenum Press.

O'Brien, M., & Chin, C. (1998). The relationship between children's reported exposure to interparental conflict and memory biases in the recognition of aggressive and constructive conflict words. *Social Psychology Bulletin, 24,* 647–657.

Olweus, D. (1979). Stability of aggressive behavior patterns in males: A review. *Psychological Bulletin, 86,* 852–875.

Orobio de Castro, B., Slot, N. W., Bosch, J. D., Koops, W., & Veerman, J. W. (2003). Negative feelings exacerbate hostile attributions of intent in highly aggressive boys. *Journal of Clinical Child and Adolescent Psychology, 32,* 56–65.

Orobio de Castro, B., Veerman, J. W., Koops, W., Bosch, J. D., & Monshouwer, H. J. (2002). Hostile attribution of intent and aggressive behavior: A meta-analysis. *Child Development, 73,* 916–934.

Perry, D. G., Perry, L. C., & Rasmussen, P. (1986). Cognitive social learning mediators of aggression. *Child Development, 57,* 700–711.

Piers, E. V., & Harris, D. B. (1964). Age and other correlates of self-concept in children. *Journal of Educational Psychology, 55,* 91–95.

Porter, B., & O'Leary, K. D. (1980). Marital discord and child behavior problems. *Journal of Abnormal Child Psychology, 8,* 287–295.

Quay, H. C., & Peterson, D. R. (1983). *Interim manual for the Revised Behavior Problem Checklist.* Unpublished manuscript, University of Miami.

Rabiner, D. L., & Gordon, L. V. (1992). The coordination of conflicting goals: Differences between rejected and nonrejected boys. *Child Development, 63,* 1344–1350.

Rabiner, D., Lenhart, L., & Lochman, J. E. (1990). Automatic versus reflective social problem-solving in popular, average, and rejected children. *Developmental Psychology, 26,* 1010–1016.

Raine, A., Venables, P. H., & Williams, M. (1990). Relationships between central and autonomic measures of arousal at age 15 years and criminality at age 24 years. *Archives of General Psychiatry, 47,* 1003–1007.

Reynolds, C. R., & Kamphaus, R. W. (1992). *Behavior Assessment System for Children.* American Guidance Service.

Rose, S. D., & Edleson, J. L. (1987). *Working with children and adolescents in groups.* San Francisco: Jossey-Bass.

Rotter, J. B., Chance, J. E., & Phares, E. J. (1972). *Applications of a social learning theory of personality.* New York: Holt, Rinehart & Winston.

Schwartz, D., Dodge, K. A., Coie, J. D., Hubbard, J. A., Cillessen, A. H., Lemerise, E. A., & Bateman, H. (1998). Social-cognitive and behavioral correlates of aggression and victimization in boys' play groups. *Journal of Abnormal Child Psychology, 26,* 431.

Seguin, J. R., Pihl, R. O., Harden, P.W., Tremblay, R. E., & Boulerice, B. (1995). Cognitive and neuropsychological characteristics of physically aggressive boys. *Journal of Abnormal Psychology, 104,* 614–624.

Shaw, D. S., & Bell, R. Q. (1993). Developmental theories of parental contributions to antisocial behavior. *Journal of Abnormal Child Psychology, 21,* 493–518.

Slaby, R. G., & Guerra, N. G. (1988). Cognitive mediators of aggression in adolescent offenders: 1. Assessment. *Developmental Psychology, 24,* 580–588.

Southam-Gerow, M. A., & Kendall, P. C. (1997). Parent-focused and cognitive-behavioral treatments of antisocial youth. In D. M. Stoff, J. Breiling, & J. D. Maser (Eds.), *Handbook of antisocial behavior* (pp. 384–394). New York: Wiley.

Spanier, G. B. (1976). Measuring dyadic adjustment: New scales for assessing the quality of marriage and similar dyads. *Journal of Marriage and the Family, 38,* 15–28.

Straus, M. A. (1979). Measuring intrafamily conflict and violence: The Conflict Tactics (CT) Scales. *Journal of Marriage and the Family, 41,* 79–88.

Sukhodolsky, D. G., Kassinove, H., & Gorman, B. S. (2004). Cognitive-behavioral therapy for anger in children and adolescents: A meta-analysis. *Aggression and Violent Behavior, 9,* 247–269.

Sulzer, B., & Mayer, G. R. (1972). *Behavior modification procedures for school personnel.* Hinsdale, IL: Dryden.

Thompson, L. L., Riggs, P. D., Mikulich, S. E., & Crowley, T. J. (1996). Contributions of ADHD symptoms to substance problems and delinquency in conduct-disordered adolescents. *Journal of Abnormal Child Psychology, 24,* 325–348.

Tremblay, R. E., Pagani-Kurtz, L., Masse, L. C., Vitaro, F., & Pihl, R. O. (1995). A bi-modal preventive intervention for disruptive kindergarten boys: Its impact through mid-adolescence. *Journal of Consulting and Clinical Psychology, 63,* 560–568.

van de Weil, N. M. H., Matthys, W., Cohen-Kettenis, P., & van Engeland, H. (2003). Application of the Utrecht Coping Power Program and care as usual to children with disruptive behavior disorders in outpatient clinics: A comparative study of cost and course of treatment. *Behavior Therapy, 34,* 421–436.

van Goozen, S. H. M., Matthys, W., Cohen-Kettenis, P. T., Gispen-de Wied, C., Wiegant, V. M., & van Engeland, H. (1998). Salivary cortisol and cardiovascular activity during stress in oppositional-defiant disorder boys and normal controls. *Biological Psychiatry, 43,* 531–539.

van Goozen, S. H. M., Matthys, W., Cohen-Kettenis, P. T., Thijssen, J. H. H., & van Engeland, H. (1998). Adrenal androgens and aggression in Conduct Disorder prepubertal boys and normal controls. *Biological Psychiatry, 43,* 156–158.

van Goozen, S. H. M., Matthys, W., Cohen-Kettenis, P. T., Westenberg, H., & van Engeland, H. (1999). Plasma monoamine metabolites and aggression: Two studies of normal and oppositional defiant disorder children. *European Neuropsychopharmacology, 9,* 141–147.

Waas, G. A., & French, D. C. (1989). Children's social problem solving: Comparison of the open middle interview and children's assertive behavior scale. *Behavioral Assessment, 11,* 219–230.

Wayland, K. K., Schoenwald, S. K., & Lochman, J. E. (1989, August). *Marital adjustment, fam-*

ily conflict and children's perceptions of marital discord. Paper presented at the American Psychological Association annual convention, New Orleans, LA.

Webster-Stratton, C., Reid, J., & Hammond, M. (2001). Social skills and problem-solving training for children with early-onset conduct problems: Who benefits? *Journal of Child Psychology and Psychiatry, 42,* 943–952.

Werry, J. S., Elkind, G. S., & Reeves, J. C. (1987). Attention deficit, conduct, oppositional and anxiety disorders in children: III. Laboratory differences. *Journal of Abnormal Child Psychology, 15,* 409–428.

Williams, S. C., Lochman, J. E., Phillips, N. C., & Barry, T. D. (2003). Aggressive and nonaggressive boys' physiological and cognitive processes in response to peer provocations. *Journal of Clinical Child and Adolescent Psychology, 32,* 568–576.

Wills, T. A., & Filer, M. (1996). Stress-coping model of adolescent substance use. In T. H. Ollendick & R. J. Prinz (Eds.), *Advances in clinical child psychology* (Vol. 18, pp. 91–132). New York: Plenum Press.

Wills, T. A., McNamara, G., Vaccaro, D., & Hirkey, A. E. (1996). Escalated substance use: A longitudinal grouping analysis from early to middle adolescence. *Journal of Abnormal Child Psychology, 105,* 166–180.

Windle, M. (1990). A longitudinal study of antisocial behavior in early adolescence as predictors of late adolescent substance use: Gender and ethnic group differences. *Journal of Abnormal Psychology, 99,* 86–91.

Wootton, J. M., Frick, P. J., Shelton, K. K., & Silverthorn, P. (1997). Ineffective parenting and childhood conduct problems: The moderating role of callous-unemotional traits. *Journal of Consulting and Clinical Psychology, 65,* 301–308.

Zelli, A., Dodge, K. A., Lochman, J. E., Laird, R. D., & the Conduct Problems Prevention Research Group. (1999). The distinction between beliefs legitimizing aggression and deviant processing of social cues: Testing measurement validity and the hypothesis that biased processing mediates the effects of beliefs on aggression. *Journal of Personality and Social Psychology, 77,* 150–166.

CHAPTER 3

Treatment for Children and Adolescents with Attention-Deficit/ Hyperactivity Disorder

STEPHEN P. HINSHAW

For this, the third edition of *Child and Adolescent Therapy: Cognitive-Behavioral Procedures*, one might expect that my primary aim would be to present the latest research on, as well as current treatment procedures related to, cognitive-behavioral treatments for children and adolescents with attention-deficit/hyperactivity disorder (ADHD). Yet, research on such forms of therapy for youth with ADHD has been at a near standstill in recent years. Unlike most of the other disorders, conditions, and problems represented in the companion chapters, children and adolescents with ADHD have typically proved refractory to the types of treatment procedures categorized as cognitive or cognitive-behavioral. Even in terms of more strictly behavioral treatment procedures, for which better evidence regarding ADHD-related efficacy exists, several key investigations completed in recent years indicate the superiority of pharmacological treatments with respect to important domains of outcome (Abikoff et al., 2004; MTA Cooperative Group, 1999a; Pelham, Carlson, Sams, Vallano, & Dixon, 1993).

As a result, many individuals in the field have begun to conclude that medication is the only viable option for treating youngsters with ADHD and that behavioral, much less cognitive-behavioral, intervention strategies are not important for intervening with the core symptoms of the disorder (see Abikoff et al., 2004; Barkley et al., 2000; Goldstein, 2004). One key question for this chapter is thus whether there is, in fact, a role for behavioral and cognitive-behavioral treatments for youth with ADHD. I believe that there is (see also Anastopoulos & Farley, 2003); and in addressing this question further, I cover a number of the core issues discussed in the first two editions of this chapter related to the viability of psychosocial intervention for ADHD (see Hinshaw, 2000; Hinshaw & Erhardt, 1991) I aim to do so with a fresh perspective from the vantage point of accumulated research efforts regarding youth with ADHD over the past decade.

At the outset, I make some evidence-based points and, in the process, attempt to dispel myths that have accumulated regarding treatment for children and adolescents with ADHD.

1. Although "cognitive" interventions for ADHD, based on approaches designed to change self-talk and verbal mediation, may be at least somewhat successful with subclinical cases or school-identified impulsive children and adolescents, these strategies are not viable for yielding meaningful change in clinical samples of youth with ADHD (see review in Abikoff, 1991).

2. On the other hand, despite the relatively stronger short-term effects of medication, psychosocial treatments grounded in behavioral contingencies can yield a positive impact on ADHD-related symptomatology as well as important impairments related to this condition (see review in Hinshaw, Klein, & Abikoff, 2002). Furthermore, for children who show negative or adverse responses to medication, or whose parents oppose medication treatments, such strategies are the only evidence-based interventions for ADHD (Pelham, Wheeler, & Chronis, 1998).

3. Furthermore, medication treatments for ADHD do not yield any kind of curative effect. That is, their benefits, which are strong in many cases, dissipate when medications are discontinued or when monitoring is faded (MTA Cooperative Group, 2004). In addition, such benefits do not extend to the full range of intraindividual, familial, academic, and peer-related contexts in which ADHD and its common impairments exist. Promoting long-term, clinically meaningful change for this disorder is still an unattained objective.

4. Combining medication with viable psychosocial interventions, particularly contingency-based behavioral procedures, has often (but not always) been shown to yield benefits closer to normalization than pharmacologic treatments alone (e.g., Hinshaw et al., 2002; Swanson et al., 2001). Thus, behavioral interventions are key components of the kinds of multimodal interventions that appear to be the treatments of choice for most youth with ADHD.

5. Common comorbidities of ADHD—including learning disorders, aggressive-spectrum disorders, and internalizing conditions such as anxiety disorders or depression—show little evidence of benefit from medication strategies alone, virtually requiring the presence or addition of psychosocial treatments, including

cognitive-behavioral intervention strategies (see Hinshaw, in press). This important point is often overlooked in considering treatments for youth with ADHD.

6. Finally, there is the distinct possibility that adding self-management-based components to traditional behavioral contingencies can help to extend the benefits of the latter strategies over time and across settings. In other words, there may still be a viable role for some forms of cognitive-behavioral procedures in future treatment packages for ADHD, with the objective of extending the benefits of contingency-based interventions. Evidence is mounting that interventions for youth with ADHD need to be continued over a long course in many cases, but the ultimate goal is still to promote self-management and self-control. Hence, cognitive aspects of treatment should not be ignored, so long as they are based on empirically supported behavioral approaches.

With these points in mind, I review the existing behavioral and cognitive-behavioral treatment literature regarding ADHD and provide exemplars of the kinds of self-management procedures that have yielded initial evidence of promise, with the potential for their extension and expansion in future applications. An overarching point for the entire chapter is that the more that is learned about the impairments that attend to children with attentional deficits and hyperactivity (Hinshaw, 2002a) as well as the neurological, neuropsychological, behavioral, familial, and social/interpersonal underpinnings of ADHD (see Nigg, Hinshaw, & Huang-Pollack, in press), the more it is realized that (1) ADHD-related impairments are not limited to childhood; (2) the core deficits lead to lowered self-awareness of problems in functioning and, as a result, decreased motivation to sustain change efforts; and (3) the current arsenal of empirically supported pharmacologic and behavioral treatments is still well below the threshold of providing lasting, clinically meaningful benefits for most children with this disorder. Thus, the ADHD treatment field has few laurels on which to rest, and innovative means of altering the disorganized, impulsive, dysregulated behavior related to this condition, both pharmacologic and psychosocial, are strongly needed.

BEHAVIORAL, COGNITIVE, OR BOTH?

As in the first two editions of this chapter, I initially highlight two key facts. First, traditional contingency-based "behavioral" treatments contain a number of cognitive elements. Specifically, the child or adolescent must, of necessity, be involved in the selection of reinforcers and must be "on board" with the family's and school's implementation of behavioral procedures. The youth's input is clearly required for initiating and maintaining a viable behavioral treatment plan. In addition, reward schedules must be thinned as the youngster makes behavioral, academic, or social gains, with the ultimate goal of fostering self-reinforcement and self-management. Cognitive strategies may be a key means of attaining this goal. Relatedly, effective behavior management programs should emphasize the youth's need for planning and problem solving. As development proceeds, behavioral programs must include negotiated contracts between adults and adolescents (for explication of the need for such mutual contracting work by adolescents, see Robin, 1998), with an emphasis on give-and-take exchanges and enhancement of problem-solving procedures. Thus, as in other applications of cognitive and/or behavioral therapy, the distinction between behavioral and cognitive elements is not clear-cut; an integrated cognitive-behavioral (or, more accurately, cognitive-behavioral-affective) treatment plan is the objective. For example, Anastopoulos and Farley (2003) brand their parent training approach for families of youth with ADHD as cognitive-behavioral, even though it largely contains elements of operant behavioral procedures from earlier versions of the curriculum.

Second, if they are to be at all effective for children with clinical levels of ADHD, cognitive procedures must explicitly include contingency management and other empirically supported behavioral strategies. Self-instructional training alone is simply not a viable treatment strategy for this population, as indicated in more detail below. The road to intrinsic motivation for most children and adolescents with ADHD incorporates skill building and behavior management—involving extrinsic rewards before internal cognitive changes can be expected to appear. This point is essential: Those practitioners promising meaningful clinical change for ADHD through an exclusive focus on altering cognitions or discussing emotions are likely to be met with disappointed, frustrated families along with youth whose problems have persisted if not escalated.

In short, given the pressing need to develop, investigate, and disseminate effective psychosocial and multimodal treatments for the multiple problems related to ADHD, I do not aim to debate what is "behavioral" and what is "cognitive" but rather to focus on an integrated conception of cognitive-behavioral interventions as inclusive of affect, motivation, and family and school contexts, as well as modification of cognitions per se (Braswell & Bloomquist, 1991; Kendall & MacDonald, 1993).

ADHD FUNDAMENTALS

In the interests of space, I present a brief overview of facts and conceptual models related to ADHD (for more thorough reviews, see Barkley, 1998, 2003; Hinshaw, 1999; Nigg et al., in press; Tannock, 1998).

Clinical Features, Prognosis, and Impairments

The diagnostic criteria for ADHD mandate developmentally extreme symptoms in the domains of inattention/disorganization, hyperactivity/impulsivity, or both that are of early onset (before the age of 7 years), long-standing (at least 6 months' duration), pervasive (displayed in multiple situations), and impairing (see American Psychiatric Association, 2000). The ubiquitous nature of difficulties with allocating sustained attention to academic tasks, inhibiting behavior in the face of temptation for immediate gain, and refraining from excess motor behavior in early to middle childhood—particularly in structured educational settings—has prompted critics to contend that ADHD has been overdiagnosed in recent years (e.g., DeGrandpre & Hinshaw, 2000). Yet, substantial evidence supports the validity of ADHD on the basis of such important features as diagnostic reliability, coherence of the syndrome, cross-cultural manifestations, and evidence for clear impairment that emanates from the symptom picture when an appropriate diagnosis is made (Barkley, 2003; Hinshaw, 1999, Lahey & Willcutt, 2002).

Children with extreme levels of inattention (but not hyperactivity/impulsivity) are categorized as the predominantly inattentive type; those with high degrees of hyperactivity/impulsivity (but not inattention) are placed in the predominantly hyperactive/impulsive type; and those with impairing symptoms in both domains constitute the combined type. Although epidemiological studies suggest that, in community samples, the inattentive type is the most prevalent (e.g., Lahey & Willcutt, 2002), the combined type is the most likely to be referred for clinical services. Thus, clinicians who treat ADHD must often contend with multiple problems of sustaining attention, managing impulse control, and regulating excessive motor activity, in addition to the crucial impairments and comorbidities that pertain to this multifaceted symptom presentation (Hinshaw, in press).

Once believed to be a transient disorder limited to childhood, ADHD has been shown to persist through adolescence in a majority of cases and through young adulthood in at least a plurality (Mannuzza & Klein, 2000). Viable intervention during a child's early years thus has the potential of preventing or attenuating a lifetime of accumulating difficulties. The overall prevalence of ADHD appears to be approximately 3–7% of the school-age population (American Psychiatric Association, 2000), with boys more likely than girls to meet diagnostic criteria, particularly for the hyperactive/impulsive and combined types. Girls with ADHD are, in fact, an understudied population (see Hinshaw, 2002c); treatment research with female samples is rare but much needed.

Children and adolescents with ADHD typically have extensive problems in everyday interactions with parents, teachers, friends, and the world at large. The intensity of reactions, the problems in emotion regulation (see Hinshaw, 2003), the poor judgment, the "out-of-sync" quality of social interactions, the problems with keeping organized, and the long-term risk for substance abuse and delinquency—all combine to document the devastating impact of ADHD on children, families, and schools. Indeed, ADHD yields considerable impairment in academic achievement, parent–child interactions, peer relations, independence in functioning, and risk for accidental injury (see review in Hinshaw, 2002a). Nearly all of these impairments are independent of comorbid conditions that may accompany ADHD (e.g., Lahey et al., 1998), meaning that ADHD is specific in its linkage with such major life handicaps. Thus, rather than constituting a set of problems that are merely annoying to parents and teachers, ADHD has real-world consequences in precisely those domains of functioning that are predictive of life success.

Comorbidity

It is a relative rarity to witness a case of ADHD that is unaccompanied by one or more additional disorders (Angold, Costello, & Erkanli, 1999; Jensen, Martin, & Cantwell, 1997). First, over half of ADHD cases display comorbid aggressive-spectrum symptomatology, which, in psychiatric terminology, qualifies for diagnoses of oppositional defiant disorder (ODD) or conduct disorder (CD) (Hinshaw, 1987; Jensen et al., 1997). Children with combinations of ADHD and such disruptive disorders typically display a host of difficulties, including family histories encompassing both ADHD and antisocial-spectrum problems, deficits in verbal skills, serious peer rejection, and a long-term course marked by substantial risk for continuing antisocial behavior patterns (Hinshaw, 1999). Second, ADHD also displays overlap with internalizing disorders, marked by a predominance of anxious, withdrawn, and depressive features. Up to one-third of youth with ADHD show such patterns of comorbidity (Jensen et al., 1997; MTA Cooperative Group, 1999b). This comorbid pattern may have particular implications for differential treatment response, as discussed subsequently. Third, as many as one fourth of youth with ADHD also display learning disorders, defined as clearly subaverage achievement in reading or math. When ADHD is combined with such learning disabilities, stimulant medication facilitates some aspects of achievement but does not alter the underlying processing deficits—for example, phonemic awareness and phonologic processing related to reading—that compromise learning. Thus, psychosocial interventions that directly target academic problems are a priority for this subgroup (Lyon, Fletcher, & Barnes, 2003). Overall, the strong overlap between ADHD and other syndromes/disorders signals both the considerable distance the field must travel to understand the mechanisms responsible for such association and the clear clinical challenges presented by children and adolescents with these multiple-symptom pictures. Cognitive-behavioral treatments are of particular value for some of the aggressive features that often accompany ADHD as well as depressive and anxiety disorders (see Kendall & Suveg, Chapter 7, this volume; Lochman, Powell, Whidby, & FitzGerald, Chapter 2, this volume; and Stark et al., Chapter 5, this volume), and direct academic remediation is indicated for learning disabilities (Lyon et al., 2003).

Assessment and Evaluation

The core point here is that ADHD cannot be accurately evaluated in a brief office examination—which may be all too common in some pediatric practice. For one thing, there are many reasons why children show high levels of inattention or overactivity at school or home—including neurological disorders, reactions to traumatic stressors (including abuse), or family dysfunction—and the process of differential diagnosis cannot be performed casually or quickly. Indeed, one essential aspect of a viable assessment is a thorough history of the child and family, in order to contextualize the symptom picture and rule out a host of alternate conceptualizations. In addition, clinicians cannot typically discern ADHD-related symptomatology on the basis of the child's office behavior. During a clinic visit, a child with markedly disorganized and disruptive behavior patterns at school or home can often hold it together quite well. Information from parents and teachers, who see the child as he or she typically performs in daily life functions, is essential for assessment and diagnosis. Well-normed rating scales, which allow parent and teacher perspectives on typical functioning, are therefore a useful first step in the evaluation process (Hinshaw & Nigg, 1999).

Also crucial are testing for cognitive and learning patterns, evaluation of comorbid disorders, school observations when feasible, and observation of family interaction patterns. As well, obtaining information about peer relations is important, given the crucial nature of this domain for current functioning and for predictive validity regarding future problems (Parker & Asher, 1987). Neurological and medical evaluations may be necessary to the process of differential diagnosis. Laboratory tasks measuring attentional functioning are yielding important empirical findings related to underlying mechanisms (see Nigg et al., in press) but are not, at present, sufficiently sensitive or specific for evaluation of individual children. Thus, despite active investigation into fundamental cognitive, attentional, and information-processing mechanisms pertinent to the underpinnings of ADHD, the diagnosis remains a behavioral one. Finally, evaluation of ADHD and its associated impairments must be ongoing, to monitor the success (or lack thereof) of the chosen intervention strategies (Hinshaw, March, et al., 1997). Such repeated evaluation need not be as time-consuming as the initial workup; brief symptom checklists and ongoing appraisals of functioning can be performed economically.

Risk Factors and Underlying Mechanisms

There is no single etiological sequence or pathway leading to this disorder. ADHD has substantial heritability (Tannock, 1998), meaning that genes largely determine individual differences in the propensity to display the constituent symptomatology. Indeed, the heritability estimates related to ADHD pertain to dimensions of the core symptoms and not to the diagnostic category per se; what tends to be inherited is a vulnerability to the spectrum of ADHD-related behaviors rather than a "disorder" (Levy, Hay, McStephen, Wood, & Waldman, 1997). Other biological risk factors (low birth weight; maternal alcohol or substance use during pregnancy) are related to some cases of ADHD. Yet, it should not be assumed that these psychobiological risk factors rule out the contributions of environmental factors to symptom expression or display of impairments. In fact, maternal negativity and hostility (even controlling for the negativity and noncompliance directed by the child) are relevant to concurrent and longitudinal aspects of disruptive behavior (e.g., Anderson, Hinshaw, & Simmel, 1994; Campbell, 2002; Morrell & Murray, 2003). Adaptive parenting predicts social competence in youth with ADHD as well (Hinshaw, Zupan, Simmel, Nigg, & Melnick, 1997). Thus, despite the biological underpinnings of ADHD, family socialization is critical in shaping aggressive and antisocial comorbidity as well as peer-related competencies.

Substantial debate surrounds the core mechanism or deficit related to ADHD. At a neural level, frontal and frontal–striatal circuits have received the most consistent support in recent years as crucial for symptom display (Castellanos, 1999), with implications for deficits in executive functions. More explicitly psychological theories have also been proffered, but some that were once ascendant (e.g., a fundamental deficit in sustained attention) are highly debated. Is ADHD a problem of oversensitivity to reward (Sagvolden, Aase, Zeiner, & Berger, 1998)? Of poorly regulated arousal or difficulties in mustering cognitive energy (Douglas, 1983, 1999; Sergeant, in press)? Of fundamental problems in motivation or dysregulation of emotional control (Hinshaw, 2003)? Barkley's (1997) unifying theory of ADHD has captured considerable interest; he posits that basic inhibitory processes, such as those related to the need to suspend a previously rewarded or prepotent response or to control "interference," are the core deficit (see also Nigg, 2001).

To the extent that it is accurate, this model implies that the fundamental deficit of ADHD occurs at a basic neuropsychological level of inhibitory processing, which occurs temporally prior to (and, indeed, sets the stage for) such verbal processes as self-directed speech (Berk & Potts, 1991). One implication is that interventions attempting to teach self-regulation through verbal self-control may be occurring too late and too far downstream for clinical success. Indeed, as noted at the outset, treatments emphasizing verbal mediation have proven notoriously unsuccessful with clinical samples of youth with ADHD.

Summary

ADHD is a disorder involving long-standing, developmentally extreme, and pervasive difficulties in attentional deployment, impulse control, and regulation of excessive motor behavior. Its subtypes are focused around the "poles" of inattentive/disorganized versus hyperactive/impulsive domains. Often occurring with comorbid conditions—most notably, antisocial-spectrum disorders, internalizing syndromes, and learning deficits—ADHD yields substantial impairment in key domains (school functioning, home life, peer relations, accidental injuries, adaptive behavior) that are highly related to long-term success. The symptom composite is strongly heritable; yet other biological risks (prenatal insult, low birth weight) exist, and environmental factors clearly play a role in outcome. Among a host of competing explanations, fundamental problems in inhibitory control appear central, at least for the combined and hyperactive/impulsive types. Left untreated, ADHD portends a lifelong pattern of compromised functioning, mandating the development and promotion of effective treatment procedures.

BEHAVIORAL AND COGNITIVE TREATMENTS FOR ADHD: RATIONALE AND EVIDENCE

Linking Deficits to Procedures

Extrapolating from the foregoing material, children with ADHD lack behavioral compliance and control, they fail to display intrinsic motivation for task completion, they do not show adequate levels of rule-governed behavior, and they respond erratically under typical home and classroom conditions of delayed and inconsistent reward (Barkley, 1997, 2003; Hinshaw, 1994; Nigg et al., in press). Thus, ADHD would appear to be tailor-made for intervention programs that feature regular and consistent reinforcers. Such reinforcement could pave the way toward skill building and behavior management, with the gradual development of intrinsic motivation in task performance.

A long-standing issue with respect to contingency-based programs for such children is the extent to which gains will generalize across situations or maintain over time, once such structured extrinsic reinforcement is absent. Several decades ago, a key rationale for adding cognitive components to behavioral contingencies was to foster explicitly just such extensions of treatment gains, by teaching the child to manage his or her own behavior through problem-solving, verbal mediation, and error-coping strategies. Indeed, the 1970s witnessed a surge of interest in the application of cognitive-behavioral treatment procedures to children and adolescents with this disorder. Innovators such as Meichenbaum (1977) contended that the regulatory deficits of what was then termed "hyperactivity" were extremely well matched for the types of self-instructional, problem-solving interventions that were being developed (for empirical evidence, see Bugental, Whalen, & Henker, 1977).

From a different perspective, Kendall and MacDonald (1993) have differentiated two fundamental classes of cognitive disturbance in child psychopathology. First, cognitive *distortions* pertain to certain child disorders: for example, anxiety and depression, in the form of overgeneralization and catastrophizing, and reactive aggression, with its characteristic hostile attributional bias in the face of ambiguous social situations. Many specific cognitive strategies have been developed to modify and redirect such cognitive distortions. Second, cognitive *deficiencies* apply to other conditions, in particular ADHD, which is characterized by deficient problem solving and verbal mediation plus a general cognitive immaturity (Barkley, 1997). It looks to be a far more difficult task to promote or remediate deficient thinking patterns than to modify distortions in cognition. Also, as just noted, it is conceivable that the core deficit of ADHD occurs preverbally, so that approaches based on verbal mediation may not address underlying mechanisms.

Behavioral and Cognitive-Behavioral Approaches for ADHD: Types and Outcomes

The class of behavioral interventions for children and adolescents with ADHD and "externalizing" or disruptive behavior disorders is typically divided into several categories (see Hinshaw et al., 2002; Pelham & Hinshaw, 1992).

Direct Contingency Management

Positive and aversive contingencies are implemented in carefully engineered environments, such as special education, summer camp, or residential settings. Strong effects of reward programs and response–cost contingencies on behavioral and academic targets have been repeatedly demonstrated in such programs, typically through single-case experimental designs (see Pelham et al., 1993). A major issue, however, is the transportability and generalizability of such highly individualized, reinforcement-rich contingency management programs to home, school, and peer settings.

Clinical Behavior Therapy

In this, the most common application of behavioral procedures to youth with disruptive and attentional problems, parents and teachers receive consultation from a behavioral expert in such tactics as measuring behavior, targeting problems for intervention, devising a reinforcement menu and token reward program, utilizing consistent (and nonphysical) punishment procedures, and coordinating programs between home and school. The objective is to make the everyday environment of the child more structured, consistent, and positive. Although such interventions have led to significant gains for children with ADHD (Hinshaw et al., 2002), improvements are not as large as those from direct contingency management per se, and benefits typically fall short of normalization or full clinical significance (Pelham & Hinshaw, 1992). Furthermore, the outcome measures that show improvement usually constitute ratings from the same parents and teachers who conduct the intervention, potentially involving a positive "halo" from satisfaction with the treatment rather than from objectively observed social or academic improvements.

Cognitive-Behavioral Interventions

Here, the intervention is typically conducted directly with the child, either individually or in small-group formats. Common procedures include training in (1) self-instructions, designed to enhance verbal mediation and self-control by fading from adult-directed instruction to child "overt" speech, to child self-directed speech that is "covert"; (2) problem solving, with the aim of providing a scheme for better planning of social and academic behavior; (3) self-reinforcement, so that there is less dependence on adult sources of reward; and (4) error coping, in order that the child redirect him- or herself from mistakes or problematic situations (see Abikoff & Gittelman, 1985; Douglas, Parry, Marton, & Garson, 1976; Meichenbaum, 1977). Application of these procedures to analogue tasks, actual academic work, and social predicaments is performed according to systematic curricula.

Although one might consider ADHD to be an ideally suited diagnostic group for such applications, given its association with poor self-regulation and mediational deficits, when these procedures have been applied in experimental trials with clinical samples of youth with ADHD (e.g., Abikoff & Gittelman, 1985; Abikoff et al., 1988), treatment gains have been found to be almost nonexistent (for reviews, see Abikoff, 1991; Hinshaw & Erhardt, 1991). Children and adolescents with subclinical levels of attentional deficits or impulsivity may benefit from intervention focused on verbal mediation (Braswell & Bloomquist, 1991)—the original focus of cognitive training for ADHD—but youth with diagnostic levels of this disorder have proved to be quite refractory to these kinds of treatment. Exceptions have appeared when behavioral reinforcement programs are explicitly supplemented with cognitive strategies designed to extend benefits or teach social and anger management skills. For example, in Hinshaw, Henker, and Whalen (1984a), cognitive-behavioral training for anger control was shown to be superior to cognitive training in empathy. And Hinshaw, Henker, and Whalen (1984b) demonstrated that the addition of a cognitive self-evaluation procedure enhanced the effects of behavioral reinforcement for promoting improved social behavior in playground settings. The blending of cognitive and behavioral elements was crucial in both instances: Only when cognitive-mediational procedures for anger management and self-evaluation were paired with traditional behavioral contingency management did significant gains emerge. No evidence was found for clinically sufficient benefits of self-instructional training or mediational strategies alone. Note, however, that both of these investigations evaluated only short-term benefits; the long-term viability of such integrated cognitive-behavioral procedures is indeterminate.

Social Skills Training

To the three categories of behavioral intervention just noted, a fourth comprises treatment explicitly designed to teach peer interaction skills. This type of treatment is typically performed in small groups, where clinicians utilize discussions of relevant concepts (e.g., cooperation, validation), repeated behavioral rehearsal, and direct reward of socially skilled behaviors to promote better interpersonal interactions (for an early prototype, see Oden & Asher, 1977). Because the clinical focus is on direct work with children or adolescents rather than application of contingencies in school settings or consultation with adults, social skills intervention is similar in format to cognitive-behavioral treatment. The key distinction is that it deemphasizes verbal self-instructions and training in self-reinforcement and focuses on rehearsal and direct rewards for better approximations of socially competent behavior. Although early manifestations of social skills training produced mixed results, more recent and systematic applications have produced noteworthy benefits (Pfiffner & McBurnett, 1997). Excerpts from the social skills curriculum used in this investigation appear later in the chapter.

Note that both direct contingency management and clinical behavior therapy procedures attempt to shape the environment of the individual with ADHD, by providing clear rewards and punishments, by altering parent and teacher expectations, and by making appropriate accommodations in task demands. Cognitive-mediational and social skills treatments, on the other hand, prioritize changing the inner workings of the child, through the teaching of self-instructional speech, problem-solving strategies, self-evaluation and self-reinforcement skills, and explicit instruction in peer-related competencies. In actual practice, however, this differentiation between outer environmental strategies versus inner cognitive/psychological treatments is more apparent than real (Kendall & MacDonald, 1993). The ultimate goal of environmental modifications for youth with ADHD is to encourage better behavior, academic performance, and social competence in more naturalistic settings—through thinning of reward schedules, fading of prompts and cues, and the addition of cognitive self-evaluation, self-reinforcement, and error-coping strategies to promote generalization and maintenance. In parallel, cognitive procedures expected to be useful for this population cannot be taught in a vacuum, as direct rewarding of self-control procedures, behavioral rehearsal, and promoting environmental encouragement of self-regulation must supplement direct work with the individual. Thus, as noted earlier, partisanship about what is "behavioral" versus what is "cognitive" is likely to be counterproductive.

Comparison and Combination with Stimulant Medication

Any evaluation of psychosocial treatments for youth with ADHD must contend with the high levels of efficacy that have been shown for medications for this population (see Greenhill & Osman, 2000). Indeed, the use of stimulant medications is sufficiently prevalent and effective that no discussion of psychosocial treatment procedures for ADHD can be complete without considering medication as a standard of comparison. In a clear majority of carefully diagnosed youth with ADHD, medications produce clear benefits with respect to core symptomatology, associated impairments in home and school domains, and interactions with parents, teachers, and peers (Greenhill & Osman, 2000; MTA Cooperative Group, 1999a). Individual differences regarding medication response are vast, however, and the role of medications with respect to actual academic progress is less clear. Most important, pharmacologic benefits last only as long as the medication is in the child's system. In this respect, stimulant treatment of ADHD is quite similar to contingency management or clinical behavior therapy, the benefits of which also tend not to persist beyond the life of the contingencies that are put in place. Indeed, a major impetus for the development and promotion of cognitive-behavioral treatments for ADHD three decades ago was the hope that such mediational procedures—"portable coping strategies," in the terminology of Meichenbaum (1977)—could promote generalization and maintenance of contingency-based gains for this population. A continuing challenge for the field is to discover interventions that can produce lasting benefits.

Medications may induce side effects, most of which are manageable but, in some cases, can be prohibitive. Furthermore, medication alone is rarely sufficient to normalize functioning across relevant functional domains, and the benefits of initially successful medication treatment often dissipate over time. Thus, limitations of pharmacological intervention mandate that psychosocial/behavioral treatments continue to be developed and investigated (for discussion, see Klein, Abikoff, Hechtman, & Weiss, 2004).

As reviewed in Hinshaw and colleagues (2002), well-conducted head-to-head comparisons of behavioral versus pharmacological procedures have yielded provocative results. First, even powerful direct-contingency management procedures have been found to produce smaller effect sizes regarding important behavioral outcomes than stimulant medication (Pelham et al., 1993). Thus, even the strongest behavioral treatments may not fare as well as medications in terms of magnitude of effect. Second, in the Multimodal Treatment Study of Children with ADHD (MTA)—a long-term (14-month) comparison of systematic medication management versus an intensive combination of clinical behavior therapy (over 35 parent-training sessions paired with regular teacher consultation) plus direct contingency management (8-week summer treatment program as well as a paraprofessional aide in the child's classroom setting for 3 months), implemented for 7- to 9-year-old youth with ADHD–combined type—the medication procedures proved superior with regard to ADHD symptomatology and associated disruptive behaviors (MTA Cooperative Group, 1999a). Indeed, one-fourth of the participants randomly assigned to the behavior therapy procedures needed to have medication added to their treatment regimen before the end of the treatment period. At the same time, (1) the behavior therapy procedures proved equivalent to medication as practiced in the general community (MTA Cooperative Group, 1999b), and (2) follow-up of the study participants beyond the 14-month period of active intervention showed that those initially assigned to behavioral intervention maintained their gains better than those initially assigned to the medication management condition, as the benefits of the latter faded once the optimal monitoring of this treatment ended (MTA Cooperative Group, 2004).

Another important question concerns the incremental benefit of combining effective behavioral or psychosocial treatments with medication-based interventions. Initial research, reviewed in Pelham and Murphy (1986), revealed that combined treatment regimens yielded greater levels of improvement than single-modality interventions, even if the differences were not always statistically significant. Larger-scale clinical trials have produced mixed evidence: Abikoff and colleagues (2004) found no significant increment from adding systematic behavioral and other psychosocial treatments to individually titrated medication. On the other hand, the MTA Study showed that for the outcomes of (1) clinically significant response, as categorically determined, and (2) a composite outcome measure spanning symptom improvement, decreases in comorbid symptomatology, and improvements in academic, parent-child, and social skills, the combination of medication management plus intensive behavior therapy proved superior to medication only (Conners et al., 2001; Swanson et al., 2001). Furthermore, Hinshaw and colleagues (2000) demonstrated that when families receiving the combination treatment (multimodal combination of medication management plus intensive behavior therapy) showed clinically significant improvements in their discipline style at home—that is, when negative/ineffective discipline was enhanced—the children of such parents showed full normalization of school-based disruptive behavior and important improvements in school-based social skills. In other words, even for a condition as biologically based as ADHD, socialization practices at home were central in explaining major improvements in functioning (see the section on moderators and mediators of treatment outcomes).

Overall, a continuing question is whether combination treatments may be better able to arrest the difficult trajectory traversed by many children with ADHD. Relatedly, it is still an open question whether the right kinds of cognitive extensions of contingency management may help to extend benefits. Finally, for the minority of children with ADHD who either show prohibitive side effects to medication or whose families are not comfortable with a pharmacological approach, psychosocial treatments must be able to stand on their own.

Summary

Regarding behavioral interventions, direct contingency management can yield large effects for youth with this disorder, but usually in highly specialized settings and only so long as the contingencies are in effect. Clinical behavior therapy consultation with parents and teachers also yields significant improvement, but gains are typically smaller and are usually restricted to outcomes comprising ratings from the parents and teachers who are the recipients of the intervention (Hinshaw et al., 2002). Crucially, cognitive treatments designed to enhance mediation and problem solving have not yielded positive effects for children and adolescents with clinical levels of ADHD. Yet, combining cognitive procedures with specific contingencies and extensive behavioral rehearsal (Hinshaw et al., 1984a, 1984b) should still be explored. Social skills training has shown promise when rehearsal, specific contingencies, and coordination with parent-training efforts are combined with cognitive strategies designed to promote social competence. Stimulant medication treatment provides a standard against which psychosocial treatments are typically compared. Medication effects are typically superior to those of behavioral intervention but last only as long as pills are ingested; combining behavioral with pharmacological approaches may yield optimal benefits in several key domains of functioning. Overall, the types of cognitive approaches that have been found effective for other child and adolescent populations are insufficient for children with ADHD, necessitating that the illustrations below combine cognitive strategies with direct contingency management, behavioral rehearsal, and promotion of generalization and maintenance.

CLINICAL ILLUSTRATIONS

An essential aspect of intervening with the population under consideration is coordination and collaboration. That is, because of the multiple problems and impairments displayed by children and adolescents with ADHD across diverse settings (home, school, peer groups, leisure activities) and the typical need for treatments to span educational, family-related, social, and behavioral goals, consistency in service delivery and coordination of efforts is paramount. If educators, medical personnel, psychologists, and paraprofessionals do not coordinate efforts, it is virtually a guarantee that intervention effects will be limited. The disorganization manifested by most individuals with ADHD must be countered by intensive organization and coordination among those attempting to forge more consistent environments and more productive performance.

Intervention for Social Skills

The social skills training (SST) curriculum of Pfiffner and McBurnett (1997, 2004) provides for just such coordination, as in one of their treatment conditions they combined social skills groups for youth with supplemental parent groups, with the goal of teaching parents to support the generalization of child gains to home and play environments. For the child-focused SST program, I excerpt

from the manualized examples of the behavioral and cognitive-behavioral procedures (Pfiffner & McBurnett, 2004).

In this training program, participants (boys and girls with ADHD, with the
group size ranging from six to nine) receive eight weekly 90-minute sessions.
The goals of improving relationships with both peers and adults are addressed
through (1) remediating skills knowledge and skills performance deficits, (2) fostering the child's recognition of verbal and nonverbal social cues, (3) teaching
adaptive responding to new problem situations that arise, and (4) promoting generalization. In the words of Pfiffner and McBurnett (2004):

> The group includes a highly structured, high-density contingency management pro-
> gram. This reward system serves not only to increase the motivation of the children
> to participate but creates a more playful, "game-like" atmosphere for them. Specific
> skills are selected each day from the current skill module being taught. The session
> always begins with a clear introduction of the "skill of the week." These skills are
> presented didactically and through modeling (using enthusiasm and humor!). They
> are then taught to students using prompting, shaping, and rehearsal during "skill
> games" and role plays. Children are actively involved in generating examples, par-
> ticipating in the role plays, and evaluating when, where, and why to use the skill.
> To promote generalization, counselors prompt or suggest role plays for three differ-
> ent situations: (1) with peers, (2) in the classroom, and (3) at home with siblings or
> parents. . . . Feedback, both during training and activities, includes attempts to help
> children self-monitor and self-evaluate their social behavior (e.g., "Did you show
> 'accepting' when you were called 'out' in the game? Did you use your 'ignoring'
> skill to deal with that problem?"). If a child has not grasped a key concept (as
> revealed through lack of participation or inability to succeed at a task), the concept is
> reviewed verbally and practiced. (pp. 3–4)

This excerpt reveals the explicit inclusion of both a high-density reward
program and cognitive elements, exemplifying the prior discussion's emphasis of
integrated cognitive-behavioral intervention for children with ADHD. Indeed,
skills to be taught (e.g., good sportsmanship, accepting consequences, ignoring
provocation, problem solving) are first discussed and modeled, using both pretend (e.g., through the use of puppets) and live modeling. Extensive role playing
next takes place in the context of school, peer, and home applications, as children
evaluate their own and one another's skill performance. Then, during a 30-min-
ute indoor or outdoor free play game, the skills are practiced in more realistic
contexts, with prompting and feedback from the counselors. Tangible reinforcers
(called "good sports bucks") with backup rewards (e.g., a pizza party) are used to
motivate utilization of the social skill. Points can also be earned throughout the
session for following rules, attending, and listening; these are traded for child-
selected activities at the end of the training session. Response–cost is included, as
points can be lost for such behaviors as interrupting, name calling, cursing,
aggressing, and destroying property. In-room time-outs are also in place for

aggressive or disruptive behavior. The following excerpt demonstrates procedures related to the skill of "accepting":

> Announce (with a finger drumroll) that the skill of the week is Accepting. Counselors will hide a piece of paper with the word "Accepting" written on it somewhere in the room. Tell the children that they are going to pretend to be detectives. First, they are assigned the mission to find the piece of paper. . . . Once it is found, they have the mission of figuring out how to show good acceptance by watching the counselors. One counselor will role play being a teacher, and the other, a student. *Role Play Description*: The student is on the playground playing dodgeball, her favorite game, and really wants to win. She ends up getting hit by the ball and must sit out of the game until the next round. She shows the right way to accept (going to the end of the line, "good sport" face and body, etc.). The teacher praises the behavior.
>
> Ask the children what clues they detected that showed good accepting. Encourage them to come up with the following by asking what the counselor looked like, what she did, and what she said. Write the children's ideas on poster board or chalkboard: *staying calm, *following rules, *following directions right away, *good-sport face, *verbalizing compliance (e.g., "OK, I'll do that"), *continuing to get along with others. Announce that "good sport bucks" will be given each time the children show good accepting.
>
> Now, the counselors will role play the wrong way to accept (leaving the game, clenching fists, calling names, etc.). The teacher will give consequences for the non-accepting behavior (benching the student for the rest of recess). As always, the role play should be animated and entertaining. . . . *Role Plays*: Children will volunteer to participate, and each child gets a chance. The children who are not participating will vote on how well the actors showed accepting skills in the role play by thumbs up vote. (Pfiffner & McBurnett, 2004, pp. 11–12)

During the Free Play module, children play small-group board games or outdoor sports, with the opportunity to earn "good sport bucks" for appropriately demonstrating and utilizing the skill of the week. These "bucks" can be traded for credits toward a pizza party. Also, a Good Sport Thermometer is used as a visual aide for goal setting and self-evaluation. At the bottom level (1), the rating is that all of the kids showed poor acceptance; at the top (5), all showed good acceptance (furthermore, if everyone showed "super" acceptance, they "break" the thermometer). The children predict the group's performance before the game and review ratings afterward. Counselors prompt and encourage throughout the game, with a careful review following the game.

Finally, in the treatment condition termed SST-PG (parent-mediated generalization), parents meet in groups at the same time that their children's SST groups occur. They receive similar instruction as the children and observe SST sessions from behind a one-way mirror. The objective is then to learn to prompt and reinforce their children's budding use of the social-cognitive skills at home. They also establish a daily report card with their child's teacher, who rates the target behavior of "getting along with peers" daily. Parents provide the backup reward of "good sports bucks" at home for the child's earning of high teacher ratings on this criterion.

Self-Evaluation Procedures

Following from the previous editions of this volume (Hinshaw & Erhardt, 1991; Hinshaw, 2000), I describe a procedure that provides explicit training in self-monitoring and self-evaluation, two essential skills for the academic, behavioral, and social competence that appear to be quite deficient in most children with ADHD (e.g., Douglas, 1999; Hinshaw, 1992). Indeed, deficient "checking" of task performance and a resultant array of academic errors, behavioral disorganization, and social rejection are hallmarks of ADHD. Children with this disorder appear to pay poor attention not only to adults who give them directions and commands but also to their own behavioral performance. Thus, explicit training in the ability to self-monitor and self-evaluate one's performance in the context of initial goals is crucial. Hinshaw and colleagues (1984a) evaluated these procedures in the context of a summer treatment program.

The procedure in question has been utilized most often in small-group therapy formats, but it can also be applied in individual training sessions. The overall goal of the "Match Game" is to encourage a more self-reflective approach to any academic, behavioral, or social enterprise. It can be used only when behavioral contingencies and token rewards for appropriate behavior are established, exemplifying the type of integrated cognitive-behavioral intervention that is the focus of this chapter. The goal of self-evaluation training is, in fact, to extend the benefits of reward programs for children with ADHD by encouraging them to "take over" the monitoring of progress usually left up to the supervising adults. Thus, self-evaluation exercises such as the Match Game do not stand on their own but need to be paired with a curriculum emphasizing problem solving, to encourage the child's generalization and maintenance of skills learned.

Leaders begin by introducing a salient skill or concept to be learned and practiced. For example, *Cooperation* may be the day's focus (or, in other sessions, *Paying Attention,* or *Helping Others*). This skill is defined by the group leaders and discussed by the group, with key points written on a large chart. Following role plays of both good and poor examples of the criterion behavior, first by the leaders and then by the group members, the group members are periodically rewarded for their display of the criterion behavior while performing academic work or playing a social game. Rewards are given in the form of points, with 5 signaling excellent behavior and 1, no semblance of the criterion (these points are redeemable for subsequent backup reinforcers). The leaders occasionally remind the children to be thinking of how well they are performing with respect to the criterion.

The leaders announce that it is time to play the Match Game. Stopping the activity, they explain that each participant will try to guess or "match" which point on the rating scale the adults have evaluated his or her behavior. The leaders then model a Match Game session. Pretending to be a child, one leader states, "In that work period, I kept following the rules of the game, I shared my materials. . . . Yeah, I was really cooperating. But, oh yeah, I did grab the ball a couple of times, and I got upset when I thought Billy did a better job of playing than I did. Overall, though, I think that I did a pretty good job of cooperating—I'll give myself a 4."

The other adult, modeling the trainer, then might say the following: "Well, Betty, you did start out with good cooperation—I noticed that your hands were to yourself and that you really took turns well. You did share the ball. But you did get quite upset when the other team won a round, and when you grabbed the ball away, Billy could have been hurt. So I gave you a 3—OK for cooperating, with some excellent work but also some examples of poor cooperation." Essential here is the specificity of the leader's "report," which is designed to model and motivate specific recall on the part of the children. During this modeled Match Game, it works best for the trainer role playing the child to overestimate his or her score, as befits the overly generous self-evaluations of many children with ADHD.

At the conclusion of this role-played Match Game, each child then individually completes a rating form while the leaders privately discuss the ratings they will award. The key part of the training now occurs as each child, in sequence, discusses his or her self-ratings—and, crucially, their reasons for the ratings they make—after which the leaders discuss *their* ratings of the child, noting precise examples of good and poor performance. The child receives the number of points awarded by the trainer, but the point total is doubled (or, if preferred, 3 bonus points can be awarded) when there is accurate self-evaluation—that is, when there is a "match." Initially, the bonus can occur for self-ratings that are within a point of the adult rating. Over time, only accurate matches would receive the bonus.

During its initial phases, the Match Game can be played several times within a training session, with emphasis again placed on eliciting the child's reasons for his or her particular self-rating and on the leaders' rewarding the accuracy of the self-evaluation. Gradually, the time span for self-evaluation can be lengthened. In addition, note the following: A wise, if devious, child with ADHD may soon learn that intentional misbehavior (earning a 1 or 2 rating from the adult) can easily be matched—"I completely messed up, so I'll give myself a 1"—earning an easy bonus. Thus, across sessions the criterion should be tightened so that only adult ratings of at least 3 (or even 4) will receive a bonus with accurate self-evaluation. Note also that the behavioral target can shift over sessions in accordance with the curriculum, so that social and behavioral goals, as well as attentional and academic objectives, can be "matched."

The ultimate goal is for the child to require less and less adult reinforcement, as self-evaluation becomes an end unto itself. Still, periodic "checks" by the adult are necessary. Extending the Match Game from the clinic setting to home and school environments, where parents and teachers provide the adult criterion ratings, is important for generalizing the self-evaluation skills. Thus, blending child-focused self-evaluation with parent and teacher training can help to promote generalization.

Anger Management

Anger is a component of certain forms of aggressive behavior (see Lochman et al., Chapter 2, this volume; Nelson, Finch, & Ghee, Chapter 4, this volume). Because children with ADHD—particularly those with comorbid disruptive behavior disorders—tend to emotionally overreact (Melnick & Hinshaw, 2000) and distort interpretations of interpersonal provocations (Milich & Dodge, 1984), they are prone to display retaliatory, reactive aggression, which places them at high risk for interpersonal rejection. In the curriculum highlighted here, procedures that are both behavioral (i.e., repeated rehearsal of the anger-control strategies; explicit reward for successive approximations) and cognitive (i.e., reframing of the interpersonal stimulus, self-monitoring of the attempted plan) are salient. Indeed, as shown in Hinshaw and colleagues (1984a), rehearsal-based cognitive-behavioral intervention for anger control surpassed a treatment emphasizing solely cognitive elements of emotion recognition and empathy enhancement with respect to observed outcome behaviors.

Utilizing elements from Novaco (1979) regarding adult anger management, the curriculum utilizes peers, in a group training format, to facilitate improved self-control. Because the training procedures (and the behavioral provocations that are used to generate outcome assessment data) involve the active use of provocation to provide a realistic environment for the practice of anger control, I highlight at the outset that this is not a curriculum that should be attempted lightly, nor should it constitute material for a one- or two-shot training program. Several initial sessions are mandatory, in which leaders balance clinical sensitivity with a commitment to enhanced self-regulation on the part of the participants.

At the outset, leaders ask the children to disclose those names and phrases used by their peers that really "get under their skin," writing these down on a large chart and explaining that the group will make use of such words to help practice self-control in later sessions. Such open disclosure could lead to embarrassment or even ridicule unless an atmosphere of trust has been modeled in the group and unless there are clear behavioral contingencies in place.

As the actual training begins, leaders raise the topic of name calling and teasing, probing how much of a problem the youngsters perceive this issue to be and asking for suggestions as to how best to cope with this problem. The children's initial plans are carefully written down; after discussion, good versus not-so-good ideas are discussed and sorted through. Next, the pair of leaders engages in a spontaneous (but preplanned) mock argument, with the "victim" initially responding in a verbally retaliatory fashion. The goal is to surprise the children and promote discussion of "what happened" and "what else could the leader who was teased have done better?" Leaders typically need to walk the group through the steps of this provocation afterward, in order to draw out the sequence of events (and ensuring that the group realizes it was a role play). The "argument" can then be repeated, this time incorporating the children's suggestions for greater self-control on the part of the victim.

Anger may develop quite rapidly in individuals with emotional dysregulation, including many children with ADHD. Thus, another phase of training involves prompting the participants to probe how they know when they are becoming upset or angry. For older verbally skilled children and adolescents, knowledge of incipient feeling states may be relatively accessible ("I can feel my blood start to boil"). For younger children or those with little access to internal processes, this exercise is indeed a difficult one.

The active cognitive-behavioral training procedures are then put into place. With ample adult support, each child first generates several specific procedures that he or she will use to counter the developing feelings of anger. Following group discussion and individual consultation, the child selects a specific alternative to anger, rehearsing it while the group provides ever increasing levels of verbal provocation and teasing—using the names initially generated and placed onto each child's list. For children in the early elementary grades, chosen strategies may be quite behavioral in nature (e.g., sitting on one's hands, covering one's ears), whereas children closer to adolescence may be able to utilize more sophisticated cognitive mediational strategies to supplement specific behavioral actions. The repeated practice of the selected strategy under conditions of provocation—with feedback from both the leaders and the group, and incorporation of adjustments based on such feedback—is the key ingredient.

Again, clinical sensitivity and skill are salient. If the provocation exercises are rote and staged, there will not be sufficient affect to motivate any need to employ the newly learned strategies, and the procedure will fall flat. On the other hand, if the leaders fail to enforce rules of "no touching" and "stop the teasing on our cue," the procedures can quickly backfire.

Modifications of these anger-control procedures have been incorporated into the intensive Summer Treatment Program curriculum of Pelham and Hoza (1996) and the social skills curriculum of Pfiffner and McBurnett (1997). Although not clinically sufficient in and of itself, this cognitive-behavioral anger management procedure may be integrated with other programs and skills to help address a fundamental interpersonal problem for many youth with ADHD. Hinshaw, Buhrmester, and Heller (1989) showed that that combining active anger management with relatively high doses of stimulant medication led to optimal self-regulation.

MEDIATORS AND MODERATORS OF TREATMENT OUTCOME

Kazdin and Weisz (1998) highlighted that identification of factors and processes that predict and shape treatment response are of the utmost importance in child therapy research. Moderators are defined as preexisting characteristics that influence treatment response; mediators are those variables occurring during treatment—such as attendance, "dosage" received, relationship with therapist, cognitive changes, family processes—that explain why the treatment works (see Hinshaw, 2002b; Kraemer, Wilson, Fairburn, & Agras, 2002). Despite growing interest in the search for moderator and mediator processes, few existing treatment studies have used appropriate designs or measures or have had sufficient statistical power to examine such essential processes (see Weersing & Weisz, 2002).

With respect to treatments emphasizing cognitive procedures, the child's age or developmental level must certainly be considered as a key moderator (for a lucid discussion, see Holmbeck, Greenley, & Franks, 2003). Specifically, children in the preschool- or early-elementary-school-age range may lack the cognitive sophistication and abstract thinking abilities to demonstrate self-reflective strategies in the service of self-control. Therapeutic strategies for youngsters of this age should probably be quite concrete (e.g., Hinshaw et al., 1984a). As emphasized throughout this chapter, however, even older children with ADHD show a poor response to exclusively cognitive interventions, perhaps validating the contention that ADHD encompasses an overall developmental immaturity (Barkley, 1997). In other words, one potential explanation for the relative lack of efficacy of cognitive strategies with ADHD is that youth with this disorder continue to function, verbally and emotionally, at a level younger than their chronological years.

The comorbidity of ADHD with additional behavioral, emotional, and learning disorders is another prime candidate as a moderator variable. The MTA Study featured a sample size sufficient for moderator analyses, with a total n of 579. Somewhat surprisingly, comorbid oppositional defiant disorder or conduct disorder did not appreciably alter the main findings—that is, children both with and without this comorbidity displayed greater response to medication management than intensive behavior therapy for core symptom outcome measures. Yet, 34% of the sample displayed comorbidity with an anxiety disorder prior to treatment. This subgroup showed a particularly good response to the behavioral intervention: For them, end-of-treatment outcomes were equivalent for medication management versus behavior therapy, with even better response for the combination treatment (MTA Cooperative Group, 1999b). In other words, for the outcome variables of parent-reported ADHD symptomatology and internalizing features, comorbid anxiety disorder status predicted an enhancement of the effectiveness of behavior therapy procedures. Jensen and colleagues (2001) further clarified that double patterns of comorbidity were important to detect: Children with anxiety disorders without concomitant ODD or CD showed a greatly enhanced response to behavior therapy alone, whereas those with both comorbidities (anxiety plus oppositional defiant disorder or conduct disorder) virtually required combination treatment for provide benefits. Mechanisms underlying these effects are not completely understood. For example, the ADHD/anxious group did not have differential symptom severity related to ADHD at baseline, compared to the non-comorbid group. Were such families somehow more motivated for treatment, or does the conjoint presence of ADHD plus anxiety produce superior response to systematic rewards? Overall, clinicians should carefully appraise comorbidity in children with ADHD and consider that highly anxious youth with ADHD may fare relatively better with an exclusively behavioral/psychosocial approach.

With respect to mediator processes that helped to explain how and why the MTA findings emerged as they did, recall the findings from Hinshaw and colleagues (2000), in which it was discovered that changes in family discipline style (specifically, reductions in negative/ineffective discipline) were closely linked to normalization of disruptive behavior at school as well as major improvements in social skills for those families receiving multimodal (combined medication and behavior therapy) treatment. The message here is that family socialization is still important for a condition as psychobiologically based as ADHD. No investigations, however, have examined the potential mediating role of altered (or enhanced) cognitive style in youth with ADHD as related to optimal outcome.

CONCLUSIONS AND KEY ISSUES

Several key themes are apparent from the preceding pages.

- ADHD is an impairing and often chronic disorder, characterized by inhibitory dysregulation and resulting from substantial genetic and prenatal risk operating transactionally with family and school environments. Its impact on multiple life domains mandates intensive intervention in childhood.
- Procedures based on cognitive self-instructional methods are not sufficiently powerful to influence the symptomatology or course of ADHD; their use is not empirically supported.
- More traditional behavioral treatments (direct contingency management; clinical behavior therapy) form the basis of effective psychosocial intervention for this condition, despite their relatively short-term benefits and their relatively weaker effects than those of medication.
- Cognitive enhancements of such contingency-based interventions in the realms of social skills training, intervention for self-evaluation, and promotion of anger management may be valuable for enhancing social competence and promoting maintenance of treatment gains.

- No treatments to date, either pharmacological or psychosocial in nature, are typically sufficient for the multiple problems, impairments, and long-term course related to ADHD; prevention and alteration of the trajectory of ADHD remain elusive goals.

In my limited remaining space, I elaborate on these conclusions and speculate about the directions that future treatment research will need to take for youth with ADHD.

How Well Do Current Approaches Meet the Needs of Children with ADHD?

Core features of behavioral interventions—including a graduated approach to teaching, consistent positive reinforcement, and clear negative consequences for misbehavior—appear well suited to the disorganized style and stimulus-bound nature of children and adolescents with ADHD. At the same time, it is not at all clear that direct contingency management or clinical behavior therapy programs actually remediate any underlying deficit. Rather, they attempt to rework environmental contingencies in the hope of promoting skills learning and reducing problem behavior. Furthermore, behavioral programs take considerable effort to mount and maintain, and there is no automatic transfer of gains once the contingent reinforcers are tapered. Perhaps this is as much as can be expected, given present knowledge of ADHD, but it can certainly be hoped that future advances will yield the promise of greater hopes for lasting change.

The early claims of cognitive-behavioral theorists and practitioners regarding ADHD continue to be conceptually appealing. That is, treatments intended to foster intrinsic motivation and self-regulation would be preferable to operant behavioral approaches, with their focus on extrinsic reinforcement and environmental shaping (e.g., Henker, Whalen, & Hinshaw, 1980; Whalen, Henker, & Hinshaw, 1985). It would also seem logical, to some extent, that self-instructions or other means of enhancing the development of internal speech—which is often lacking, delayed, or nonproductive in children with ADHD (Berk & Potts, 1991)—could foster a more reflective cognitive style, that self-reinforcement could bring internal control of contingencies, and that problem-solving and error-coping procedures could counter behavioral disorganization and impulsivity.

Still, as noted throughout, empirical data do not support the use of these procedures in isolation from strong behavioral contingencies. Explaining this "disconnect" is a difficult challenge. For one thing, the multiple cognitive, motivational, behavioral, and emotional problems that characterize youth with ADHD may simply prevent the conceptually appealing cognitive principles and strategies from ever getting learned (Hinshaw, 2000). In addition, the frequent association of ADHD with clinically significant aggression means that one is often attempting to intervene with youngsters at severe risk for achievement deficits, highly disorganized familial functioning, neuropsychological/executive difficulties, and extreme peer rejection (Hinshaw, 1999). Such severe psychopathology is quite resistant to the field's most intensive treatment efforts. Next, as suggested above, the underlying deficit in ADHD may be closely linked to fundamental problems in inhibitory control that occur prior to the potentially ameliorative effects of verbal self-regulation. Finally, cognitive therapies may be better situated to alter *distortions* in belief systems than to replace or supplement *deficiencies* in cognitive strategies—and the latter appear to be the norm for ADHD (see Kendall & MacDonald, 1993).

For such reasons, if not many others, cognitive approaches have represented an extremely difficult target with respect to children with diagnosable ADHD. Truly integrated cognitive-behavioral treatments, based on contingency management, have yielded documentable benefits. Yet, as just indicated, these treatments may be best considered as rehabilitative rather than truly curative, at least as currently administered.

Assuming that at least part of the underlying deficit of ADHD is linked to inhibitory control mechanisms (Barkley, 1997; Nigg, 2001), how can clinicians influence such primary difficulties? Will sophisticated computer games of the future be able to help a child incorporate more reflective, inhibited responding? Will it be possible, in other words, for repeated trials of successful inhibition of prepotent responses to "reset" inhibitory control mechanisms? Importantly, if such proves to be the case, will gains be imprinted in neural architecture, automatically transferring to the child's home behavior and school performance? This would signal a huge advance over current behavioral, cognitive, or pharmacological treatments, none of which generalizes to periods beyond the active intervention. As for medication, will more specific targeted pharmacological treatments be able to narrow in on receptor subtypes that mediate inhibitory control? Such questions remain unanswered at present.

More fundamentally, can consistent application of more traditional reinforcement programs, which aim to reinforce planful, nonimpulsive actions and developing skills, serve (over time) to help rewire key brain regions and neural tracts toward the end of facilitating inhibitory control? If this optimistic scenario is the case, then perhaps there is a more fundamentally curative role for behavioral contingency management, particularly if it is employed with utter consistency and implemented early in development. Along this line, perhaps the field's efforts have been occurring too late developmentally. In the case of autism, for example, extremely early and intensive behavioral intervention may be beneficial in altering the course of the disorder, at least in relatively mild cases (see McEachin, Smith, & Lovaas, 1993). With early identification, could similar type "immersion" benefit preschool-age youngsters with ADHD? Certainly, intervention during more "plastic" periods of development would be far preferable to performing rehabilitation with a child or adolescent who has undergone many years of failure. Note, however, that the accurate identification of which overactive, impulsive preschoolers truly have ADHD (as opposed to transitory behavior patterns) is far from an exact science at this point (see Campbell, 2002).

Parallels with Other Disorders

Furthermore, I have noted that Barkley's (1997) neuropsychological model of ADHD posits that basic inhibitory deficits occur prior to such executive functions as verbal mediation, implying that cognitive self-instructional training targets a process that follows from rather than precedes inhibitory control. Yet, it is not an automatic assumption that successful interventions must occur at basic levels of mechanism or process. In adult depression, for example, few would argue that depressive cognitions and interpersonal consequences of depression temporally precede affective symptoms. Nonetheless, cognitive therapy and interpersonal therapy have clearly been found to benefit major depression (Craighead, Hart, Craighead, & Ilardi, 2002). Consider further the parallels between ADHD and such severe disorders as schizophrenia and bipolar disorder, for which exclusively psychological/behavioral treatments have proven largely insufficient. In these highly heritable conditions, complex psychobiological causal pathways have been traced, but the core underlying mechanism(s) remain obscure. For bipolar disorder, the beneficial nature of adjunctive individual, group, and family psychoeducational therapies designed to enhance self-awareness and medication adherence cannot be overlooked (Craighead, Miklowitz, Frank, & Vajk, 2002). Thus, there may well be a place for psychosocial therapies in such conditions.

Future Directions

First, intervention efforts directed specifically toward functional impairments should be emphasized. Organizational skills, social competence, and academic remediation are three key target domains for the majority of youth with ADHD. Even if a given treatment fails to normalize the underlying psychopathology of ADHD, successful remediation of impairments in such crucial areas may greatly facilitate adaptive functioning and the long-term course. Along this line, it is tempting to ponder somewhat different targets from the field's traditional treatments. For example, Hinshaw, Zupan, and colleagues (1997) found that authoritative parenting was associated with ADHD boys' peer acceptance and that it also served as a buffer against peer rejection. Thus, it is conceivable that parenting interventions should attempt to promote, more specifically, the warmth, limit setting, and promotion of independence that characterize this child-rearing style. Also, given that parental psychopathology often appears in conjunction with ADHD, it may be quite important to deal with maternal depression, paternal substance use, or extreme marital conflict in addition to focusing on the child's problems.

Second, few research efforts have been directed toward the treatment of children and adolescents with the inattentive type of ADHD. Such youth do not demonstrate the kinds of disruptive, impulsive behaviors that frequently get their counterparts with the hyperactive/impulsive and combined types of ADHD into conflicts with authority and with their peer group, but they show impairment in social, academic, and personal domains (Lahey et al., 1994, 1998). Linda Pfiffner at the University of California, San Francisco, is completing the first randomized trial of behaviorally oriented treatment for children with this variant of ADHD (L. Pfiffner, personal communication, January 2005), with initially promising results.

Third, a great deal more needs to be learned about combining psychosocial treatment strategies with medications for ADHD. Several key questions remain unanswered: What is the optimal temporal patterning of combining these treatment modalities—that is, should the interventions be started simultaneously, or should behavioral approaches be tried first, with medications added only if needed? Alternatively, should medications be considered the treatment of choice, with adjunctive behavioral treatments to be utilized only after pharmacologic control of symptoms occurs? In addition, will the potential benefits of combination treatments appear over longer time periods than the acute effects of either intervention modality alone? In passing, I note that optimal medication treatment may be sufficiently powerful with respect to core symptomatology that further improvements from behavioral approaches are difficult to discern. Incremental gains may be far more apparent, however, in domains of functional impairment (academic achievement, social relationships) that are not measured as easily or readily in most clinical trials.

Finally, throughout the chapter I have emphasized that cognitive-behavioral approaches for ADHD must clearly incorporate explicit reward programs and behavioral contingencies; they must also directly incorporate parent and teacher involvement if optimal and lasting benefits are desired. Altering thinking patterns or teaching problem solving at a cognitive level, in the absence of either clear contingencies or explicit programming for generalization and maintenance, is not likely to show success for youth with ADHD. Yet, a crucial question remains as to how long optimal treatment programs should last for individuals with this disorder—and whether cognitive enhancements of behavioral programs can help to extend benefits. ADHD is increasingly viewed as a condition with lifelong symptoms and impairments, yet most intervention programs are predicated on models of short-term treatments, spanning weeks or at most months. The hope is that the next generation of clinical scientists can persuade parents and families, schools, and those who fund coverage to provide extended treatments for this condition, which explicitly incorporate evidence-based integrated procedures for maintaining and extending important clinical gains.

REFERENCES

Abikoff, H. (1991). Cognitive training in ADHD children: Less to it than meets the eye. *Journal of Learning Disabilities, 24,* 205–209.

Abikoff, H., Ganeles, D., Reiter, G., Blum, C., Foley, C., & Klein, R. G. (1988). Cognitive training in academically deficient ADHD boys receiving stimulant medication. *Journal of Abnormal Child Psychology, 16,* 411–432.

Abikoff, H., & Gittelman, R. (1985). Hyperactive children treated with stimulants: Is cognitive therapy a useful adjunct? *Archives of General Psychiatry, 42,* 953–961.

Abikoff, H., Hechtman, L., Klein, R. G., Weiss, G., Fleiss, K., Etcovitch, J., et al. (2004). Symptomatic improvement in children with ADHD treated with long-term methylphenidate and multimodal psychosocial treatment. *Journal of the American Academy of Child and Adolescent Psychiatry, 43,* 802–811.

American Psychiatric Association. (2000). *Diagnostic and statistical manual of mental disorders* (4th ed., text rev.). Washington, DC: Author.

Anastopoulos, A. D., & Farley, S. E. (2003). A cognitive-behavioral training program for parents of children with attention-deficit/hyperactivity disorder. In A. E. Kazdin & J. R. Weisz (Eds.), *Evidence-based psychotherapies for children and adolescents* (pp. 187–203). New York: Guilford Press.

Anderson, C. A., Hinshaw, S. P., & Simmel, C. (1994). Mother–child interactions in ADHD and comparison boys: Relationships to overt and covert externalizing behavior. *Journal of Abnormal Child Psychology, 22,* 247–265.

Angold A., Costello E.J., & Erkanli, A. (1999). Comorbidity. *Journal of Child Psychology and Psychiatry, 40,* 57–87.

Barkley, R. A. (1997). Behavioral inhibition, sustained attention, and executive functions: Constructing a unifying theory of ADHD. *Psychological Bulletin, 121,* 65–94.

Barkley, R. A. (1998). *Attention-deficit/hyperactivity disorder: A handbook for diagnosis and treatment* (2nd ed.). New York: Guilford Press.

Barkley, R. A. (2003). Attention-deficit/hyperactivity disorder. In E. J. Mash & R. A. Barkley (Eds.), *Child psychopathology* (pp. 75–143). New York: Guilford Press.

Barkley, R. A., Shelton, T. L., Crosswait, C., Moorehouse, M., Fletcher, K., Barrett, S., et al. (2000). Multi-method psycho-educational intervention for preschool children with disruptive behavior. *Journal of Child Psychology and Psychiatry, 41,* 319–322.

Berk, L. E., & Potts, M. (1991). Development and functional significance of private speech among attention-deficit hyperactivity disordered and normal boys. *Journal of Abnormal Child Psychology, 19,* 357–377.

Braswell, L., & Bloomquist, M. L. (1991). *Cognitive-behavioral therapy with ADHD children: Child, family, and school interventions.* New York: Guilford Press.

Bugental, D. B., Whalen, C. K., & Henker, B. (1977). Causal attributions of hyperactive children and motivational assumptions of two behavior change approaches: Evidence for an interactionist position. *Child Development, 48,* 874–884.

Campbell, S. B. (2002). *Behavior problems in preschool children: Clinical and developmental issues* (2nd ed.). New York: Guilford Press.

Castellanos, F. X. (1999). The psychobiology of attention-deficit/hyperactivity disorder. In H. C. Quay & A. E. Hogan (Eds.), *Handbook of disruptive behavior disorders* (pp. 179–190). New York: Kluwer Academic/Plenum.

Conners C. K., Epstein J. N., March, J. S., Angold, A., Wells, K. C., Klaric, J., et al. (2001). Multimodal treatment of ADHD in the MTA: An alternative outcome analysis. *Journal of the American Academy of Child and Adolescent Psychiatry, 40,* 159–167.

Craighead, W. E., Hart, A., B., Craighead, L. W., & Ilardi, S. S. (2002). Psychosocial treat ments for major depressive disorder. In P. E. Nathan & J. M. Gorman (Eds.), *A guide to treatments that work* (2nd ed., pp. 245–261). New York: Oxford University Press.

Craighead, W. E., Miklowitz, D. J., Frank, E., & Vajk, F. C. (2002). Psychosocial treatments for bipolar disorder. In P. E. Nathan & J. M. Gorman (Eds.), *A guide to treatments that work* (2nd ed., pp. 263–275). New York: Oxford University Press.

DeGrandpre, R., & Hinshaw, S. P. (2000). Attention-deficit hyperactivity disorder: Psychiatric problem or American cop-out? *Cerebrum: The Dana Foundation Journal on Brain Sciences, 2,* 12–38.

Douglas, V. I. (1983). Attention and cognitive problems. In M. Rutter (Ed.), *Developmental neuropsychiatry* (pp. 280–329). New York: Guilford Press.

Douglas, V. I. (1999). Cognitive control processes in attention-deficit/hyperactivity disorder. In H. C. Quay & A. E. Hogan (Eds.), *Handbook of disruptive behavior disorders* (pp. 105–138). New York: Kluwer Academic/Plenum.

Douglas, V. I., Parry, P., Marton, P., & Garson, C. (1976). Assessment of a cognitive training program for hyperactive children. *Journal of Abnormal Child Psychology, 4,* 389–410.

Goldstein, S. (2004). Do children with ADHD benefit from psychosocial intervention? *ADHD Report, 12*(6), 1–4.

Greenhill, L. L., & Osman, B. O. (2000). *Ritalin: Theory and patient management* (2nd ed.). Larchmont, NY: Liebert.

Henker, B., Whalen, C. K., & Hinshaw, S. P. (1980). The attributional contexts of cognitive intervention strategies. *Exceptional Education Quarterly, 1,* 17–30.

Hinshaw, S. P. (1987). On the distinction between attentional deficits/hyperactivity and conduct problems/aggression in child psychopathology. *Psychological Bulletin, 101,* 443–463.

Hinshaw, S. P. (1992). Intervention for social skill and social competence. *Child and Adolescent Psychiatric Clinics of North America, 1,* 539–552.

Hinshaw, S. P. (1994). *Attention deficits and hyperactivity in children.* Thousand Oaks, CA: Sage.

Hinshaw, S. P. (1999). Psychosocial intervention for childhood ADHD: Etiologic and developmental themes, comorbidity, and integration with pharmacotherapy. In D. Cicchetti & S. L. Toth (Eds.), *Rochester Symposium on Developmental Psychopathology: Vol. 9: Developmental approaches to prevention and intervention* (pp. 221–270). Rochester, NY: University of Rochester Press.

Hinshaw, S. P. (2000). Attention-deficit hyperactivity disorder: The search for viable treatments. In P. C. Kendall (Ed.), *Child and adolescent therapy: Cognitive-behavioral procedures* (2nd ed., pp. 88–128). New York: Guilford Press.

Hinshaw, S. P. (2002a). Is ADHD an impairing condition in childhood and adolescence? In P. S. Jensen & J. R. Cooper (Eds.), *Attention-deficit hyperactivity disorder: State of the science, best practices* (pp. 5-1–5-21). Kingston, NJ: Civic Research Institute.

Hinshaw, S. P. (2002b). Intervention research, theoretical mechanisms, and causal processes related to externalizing behavior patterns. *Development and Psychopathology, 14,* 789–818.

Hinshaw, S. P. (2002c). Preadolescent girls with attention-deficit/hyperactivity disorder: I. Background characteristics, comorbidity, cognitive and social functioning, and parenting practices. *Journal of Consulting and Clinical Psychology, 70,* 1086–1098.

Hinshaw, S. P. (2003). Impulsivity, emotion regulation, and developmental psychopathology: Specificity vs. generality of linkages. *Annals of the New York Academy of Sciences, 1008,* 149–159.

Hinshaw, S. P. (in press). Psychosocial interventions for attention-deficit disorders and comorbidities. In T. E. Brown (Ed.), *Attention-deficit disorders and comorbidities in children, adolescents, and adults* (2nd ed.). Washington, DC: American Psychiatric Press.

Hinshaw, S. P., Buhrmester, D., & Heller, T. (1989). Anger control in response to verbal provocation: Effects of methylphenidate for boys with ADHD. *Journal of Abnormal Child Psychology, 17,* 393–407.

Hinshaw, S. P., & Erhardt, D. (1991). Attention-deficit/hyperactivity disorder. In P. C. Kendall (Ed.), *Child and adolescent therapy: Cognitive-behavioral procedures* (pp. 98–128). New York: Guilford Press.

Hinshaw, S. P., Henker, B., & Whalen, C. K. (1984a). Cognitive-behavioral and pharmacologic interventions for hyperactive boys: Comparative and combined effects. *Journal of Consulting and Clinical Psychology, 52,* 739–749.

Hinshaw, S. P., Henker, B., & Whalen, C. K. (1984b). Self-control in hyperactive boys in anger-inducing situations: Effects of cognitive-behavioral training and of methylphenidate. *Journal of Abnormal Child Psychology, 12,* 55–77.

Hinshaw, S. P., Klein, R. G., & Abikoff, H. (2002). Nonpharmacologic treatments and their combination with medication. In P. E. Nathan & J. M. Gorman (Eds.), *A guide to treatments that work* (2nd ed., pp. 3–23). New York: Oxford University Press.

Hinshaw, S. P., March, J. S., Abikoff, H., Arnold, L. E., Cantwell, D. P., Conners, C. K., et al. (1997). Comprehensive assessment of childhood attention-deficit hyperactivity disorder in the context of a multisite, multimodal clinical trial. *Journal of Attention Disorders, 1,* 217–234.

Hinshaw, S. P., & Nigg, J. T. (1999). Behavior rating scales in the assessment of disruptive behavior problems in childhood. In D. Shaffer, C. P. Lucas, & J. E. Richters (Eds.), *Diagnostic assessment in child and adolescent psychopathology* (pp. 91–126). New York: Guilford Press.

Hinshaw, S. P., Owens, E. B., Wells, K. C., Kraemer, H. C., Abikoff, H. B., Arnold, L. E., et al. (2000). Family processes and treatment outcome in the MTA: Negative/ineffective parenting practices in relation to multimodal treatment. *Journal of Abnormal Child Psychology, 28,* 555–568.

Hinshaw, S. P., Zupan, B. A., Simmel, C., Nigg, J. T., & Melnick, S. M. (1997). Peer status in boys with and without attention-deficit hyperactivity disorder: Predictions from overt and covert antisocial behavior, social isolation, and authoritative parenting beliefs. *Child Development, 64,* 880–896.

Holmbeck, G. N., Greenley, R. N., & Franks, E. A. (2003). Developmental issues and considerations in research and practice. In A. E. Kazdin & J. R. Weisz (Eds.), *Evidence-based psychotherapies for children and adolescents* (pp. 21–41). New York: Guilford Press.

Jensen, P. S., Hinshaw, S. P., Kraemer, H. C., Lenora, N., Abikoff, H. B., Conners, C. K., et al. (2001). ADHD comorbidity findings from the MTA study: Comparing comorbid subgroups. *Journal of the American Academy of Child and Adolescent Psychiatry, 40,* 147–158.

Jensen, P. S., Martin, D., & Cantwell, D. P. (1997). Comorbidity in ADHD: Implications for research, practice, and DSM-V. *Journal of the American Academy of Child and Adolescent Psychiatry, 36,* 1065–1079.

Kazdin, A. E., & Weisz, J. R. (1998). Identifying and developing empirically supported child and adolescent treatments. *Journal of Consulting and Clinical Psychology, 66,* 19–36.

Kendall, P. C., & MacDonald, J. P. (1993). Cognition in the psychopathology of youth and implications for treatment. In K. S. Dobson & P. C. Kendall (Eds.), *Psychopathology and cognition* (pp. 387–427). San Diego, CA: Academic Press.

Klein, R. G., Abikoff, H., Hechtman, L., & Weiss, G. (2004). Design and rationale of controlled study of long-term methylphenidate and multimodal psychosocial treatment in children with ADHD. *Journal of the American Academy of Child and Adolescent Psychiatry, 43,* 792–801.

Kraemer, H. C., Wilson G. T., Fairburn C. G., & Agras, W. S. (2002). Mediators and moderators of treatment effects in randomized clinical trials. *Archives of General Psychiatry, 59,* 877–884.

Lahey, B. B., Applegate, B., McBurnett, K., Biederman, J., Greenhill, L., Hynd, G., et al.

(1994). DSM-IV Field Trials for attention deficit hyperactivity disorder in children and adolescents. *American Journal of Psychiatry, 151,* 1673–1685.

Lahey, B. B., Pelham, W. E., Stein, M. A., Loney, J., Trapani, C., Nugent, K., et al. (1998). Validity of DSM-IV attention-deficit/hyperactivity disorder for younger children. *Journal of the American Academy of Child and Adolescent Psychiatry, 37,* 695–702.

Lahey, B. B., & Willcutt, E. (2002). Validity of the diagnosis and dimensions of attention-deficit hyperactivity disorder. In P. S. Jenson & J. R. Cooper (Eds.), *Diagnosis and treatment of attention-deficit/hyperactivity disorder: An evidence-based approach* (pp. 1-1–1-23). Kingston, NJ: Civic Research Institute.

Levy, F., Hay, D. A., McStephen, M., Wood, C., & Waldman, I. (1997). Attention-deficit hyperactivity disorder: A category or a continuum? Genetic analysis of a large-scale twin study. *Journal of the American Academy of Child and Adolescent Psychiatry, 36,* 737–744.

Lyon, G. R., Fletcher, J. M., & Barnes, M. C. (2003). Learning disabilities. In E. J. Mash & R. A. Barkley (Eds.), *Child psychopathology* (2nd ed., pp. 520–586). New York: Guilford Press.

Mannuzza, S., & Klein, R. G. (2000). Long-term prognosis in attention-deficit/hyperactivity disorder. *Child and Adolescent Psychiatric Clinics of North America, 9,* 711–726.

McEachin, J. J., Smith, T., & Lovaas, O. I. (1993). Long-term outcome of children with autism who received early intensive behavior therapy. *American Journal of Mental Retardation, 97,* 359–372.

Meichenbaum, D. H. (1977). *Cognitive-behavior modification: An integrative approach.* New York: Plenum Press.

Melnick, S. M., & Hinshaw, S. P. (2000). Emotion regulation and parenting in AD/HD and comparison boys: Linkages with social behaviors and peer preference. *Journal of Abnormal Child Psychology, 28,* 73–86.

Milich, R., & Dodge, K. A. (1984). Social information processing in child psychiatry populations. *Journal of Abnormal Child Psychology, 12,* 471–489.

Morrell, J., & Murray, L. (2003). Parenting and the development of conduct disorder and hyperactive symptoms in childhood: A prospective longitudinal study from 2 months to 8 years. *Journal of Child Psychology and Psychiatry, 44,* 489–508.

MTA Cooperative Group. (1999a). Fourteen-month randomized clinical trial of treatment strategies for attention-deficit hyperactivity disorder. *Archives of General Psychiatry, 56,* 1073–1086.

MTA Cooperative Group. (1999b). Moderators and mediators of treatment response for children with ADHD: The MTA Study. *Archives of General Psychiatry, 56,* 1088–1096.

MTA Cooperative Group. (2004). The National Institute of Mental Health MTA follow-up: 24-month outcomes of treatment strategies for attention-deficit hyperactivity disorder. *Pediatrics, 113,* 754–761.

Nigg, J. T. (2001). Is ADHD an inhibitory disorder? *Psychological Bulletin, 127,* 571–598.

Nigg, J. T., Hinshaw, S. P., & Huang-Pollack, C. (in press). Disorders of attention and impulse regulation. In D. Cicchetti & D. Cohen (Eds.), *Developmental psychopathology* (2nd ed.). New York: Wiley.

Novaco, R. W. (1979). The cognitive regulation of anger and stress. In P. C. Kendall & S. D. Hollon (Eds.), *Cognitive-behavioral interventions: Theory, research, and procedures* (pp. 241–283). New York: Academic Press.

Oden, S., & Asher, S. R. (1977). Coaching children in social skills for friendship making. *Child Development, 48,* 495–506.

Parker, J. G., & Asher, S. R. (1987). Peer relations and later personal adjustment: Are low-accepted children at risk? *Psychological Bulletin, 102,* 357–389.

Pelham, W. E., Carlson, C. L., Sams, S. E., Vallano, G., & Dixon, M. J. (1993). Separate and combined effects of methylphenidate and behavior modification on boys with attention-deficit hyperactivity disorder in the classroom. *Journal of Consulting and Clinical Psychology, 61*, 506–515.

Pelham, W. E., & Hinshaw, S. P. (1992). Behavioral intervention for attention-deficit hyperactivity disorder. In S. M. Turner, K. S. Calhoun, & H. E. Adams (Eds.), *Handbook of clinical behavior therapy* (2nd ed., pp. 259–283). New York: Wiley.

Pelham, W. E., & Hoza, B. (1996). Intensive treatment: A summer treatment program for children with ADHD. In E. D. Hibbs & P. S. Jensen (Eds.), *Psychosocial treatments for child and adolescent disorders: Empirically based strategies for clinical practice* (pp. 311–340). Washington, DC: American Psychological Association.

Pelham, W. E., & Murphy, H. A. (1986). Behavioral and pharmacological treatment of hyperactivity and attention-deficit disorders. In M. Hersen & S. E. Breuning (Eds.), *Pharmacological and behavioral treatment: An integrative approach* (pp. 108–147). New York: Wiley.

Pelham, W. E., Wheeler, T., & Chronis, A. (1998). Empirically supported psychosocial treatments for attention deficit hyperactivity disorder. *Journal of Clinical Child Psychology, 27*, 190–205.

Pfiffner, L., & McBurnett, K. (1997). Social skills training with parent generalization: Treatment effects for children with attention deficit disorder. *Journal of Consulting and Clinical Psychology, 65*, 749–757.

Pfiffner, L. & McBurnett, K. (2004). *Social skills training for children with ADHD.* Unpublished manual, University of California, San Francisco.

Robin, A. L. (1998). Training families with ADHD adolescents. In R. A. Barkley (Ed.), *Attention deficit hyperactivity disorder: A handbook for diagnosis and treatment* (2nd ed., pp. 413–457). New York: Guilford Press.

Sagvolden, T., Aase, H., Zeiner, P., & Berger, D.F. (1998). Altered reinforcement mechanisms in attention deficit/hyperactivity disorder. *Behavioral Brain Research, 94*, 61–71.

Sergeant, J. A. (in press). The cognitive energetic model and ADHD. *Biological Psychiatry.*

Stein, M. A., Szumowski, E., Blondis, T. A., & Roizen, N. J. (1995). Adaptive skills dysfunction in ADD and ADHD children. *Journal of Child Psychology and Psychiatry, 36*, 663–670.

Swanson, J. M., Kraemer, H. C., Hinshaw, S. P., Arnold, L. E., Conners, C. K., Abikoff, H. B., et al. (2001). Clinical relevance of the primary findings of the MTA: Success rates based on severity of ADHD and ODD symptoms at the end of treatment. *Journal of the American Academy of Child and Adolescent Psychiatry, 40*, 168–179.

Tannock, R. (1998). Attention deficit hyperactivity disorder: Advances in cognitive, neurobiological, and genetic research. *Journal of Child Psychology and Psychiatry, 39*, 65–99.

Weersing, V. R., & Weisz, J. R. (2002). Mechanisms of action in youth psychotherapy. *Journal of Child Psychology and Psychiatry, 43*, 2–29.

Whalen, C. K., Henker, B., & Hinshaw, S. P. (1985). Cognitive-behavioral therapies for hyperactive children: Premises, problems, and prospects. *Journal of Abnormal Child Psychology, 13*, 289–308.

CHAPTER 4

Anger Management with Children and Adolescents

Cognitive-Behavioral Therapy

W. MICHAEL NELSON III, A. J. FINCH, Jr.,
and A. CASH GHEE

When he said that to me, I just saw red and felt like I was going to explode! My fists just balled up and I thought, "I'm gonna hurt him bad!" The next thing I knew, I was in the principal's office and she was calling my parents to come and get me.

  —11-year-old boy described as being a "hot-headed problem child"

Although official rates of aggression and violence in children, adolescents, and adults in the United States have shown some leveling off or slight decline during the 1990s (e.g., Fagan, Zimring, & Kim, 1998; Fingerhut & Kleinman, 1990; Snyder & Sickmund, 1995), few would argue that anger and aggression still remain among the most salient and difficult problems faced by our society. The United States continues to surpass other industrialized nations in terms of levels of violence (e.g., Loeber & Hay, 1997; Rutter, Giller, & Hagell, 1998). Anger, aggression, severe acting out, and disruptive behavior patterns have continued to rank among the most common reasons for referral for mental health services from the 1960s to the present (Achenbach & Howell, 1993). More specifically, the adverse impact this has on our society is reflected in several facts:

- Prevalence rates for conduct disorder range from 2 to 6%, or approximately 1.4–4.2 million children in the United States.
- Thirty-three to 50% of such severe acting-out youth are referred for outpatient treatment. In fact, disruptive, aggressive, and delinquent child and adolescent behavior accounts for almost 25% of all special services in school and almost half of all juvenile referrals to community mental health agencies (e.g., Stewart, deBlois, Meardon, & Cummings, 1980; Stouthamer-Loeber, Loeber, & Thomas, 1992).
- These youngsters are "at risk" in that approximately 80% are likely to meet the criteria for some type of psychiatric disorder in the future, particularly other externalizing or disruptive disorders (e.g., oppositional defiant disorder, conduct disorder, attention deficit/hyperactivity disorder), but also, to a lesser extent, internalizing disorders (e.g., anxiety disorders, mood disorders).
- Numerous adverse consequences follow for others, including parents, siblings, peers, and teachers, as well as strangers, who are the targets of such aggressive and antisocial behavior. Those youth with a history of severe aggressive and antisocial behavior are generally more likely to continue such acts as they grow up, oftentimes leaving many victims of murder, rape, robbery, spouse and child abuse, arson, and drunk driving (Farrington, Loeber, & Van Kammen, 1990; Kazdin, 1995). Such youth have also been shown to be at high risk for adult crime, alcoholism, drug abuse, unemployment, divorce, and mental illness (e.g., Farrington, 1995; Horne & Sayger, 1990; McCord & McCord, 1960; Robins, 1966).
- Enormous societal monetary costs also accrue, as these youth often are placed in special education classes, receive mental health services, are caught up in the juvenile justice system, and receive various social services over the course of their lives. In fact, the staggering costs borne by such systems in our country make this disorder the most costly mental health problem in North America (Cohen, Miller, & Rossman, 1994; Lipsey, 1992). In commenting on the social and economic costs related to severe acting out, Donna E. Shalala noted that "the world remains a threatening, often dangerous place for children and youths. And in our country today, the greatest threat to the lives of children and adolescents is not disease or starvation or abandonment, but the terrible reality of violence" (U.S. Department of Health and Human Services, 2001).

Although rural and small-town communities continue to be alarmed by the aggressive, violent acts of these children, the typical adolescent homicide still involves inner-city ethnic minority males and occurs six times each day in the United States (National Institute of Mental Health, 2000). Externalized anger and aggression within African American boys has been linked to high levels of socioecological stress (e.g., joblessness, alienation, racism) (Nyborg & Curry, 2003). Violence has disproportionate consequences for African American youth: African American girls are 4 times and boys 11 times more likely to be murdered;

and these youth constitute 67% of the incarcerated juveniles (Commission for the Prevention of Youth Violence, 2000). Boys, in general, are far more likely to engage in physically aggressive behaviors and other antisocial behaviors as compared to girls, whose infrequent violent behaviors are often related to abuse and violence in their homes and relationships (Chesney-Lind & Brown, 1999). Although only a small percentage of youth are classified as *life-course-persistent* offenders (NIMH, 2000), early aggression seems to foreshadow problems in adulthood (Kazdin, 1987; Mash & Wolfe, 2005; Sanford et al., 1999), with such aggression predicting later violence, including frequent fighting by late adolescence, partner assault, and conviction for violent offenses by the early 30s (Farrington, 1991, 1994; Stattin & Magnusson, 1989). The National Institute of Mental Health (2000) advises against using a violent child profile; instead, several factors must be considered, including mental health and cognitive deficits, exposure to abuse and violence, stressful neighborhood, home conditions that support violence, and ineffective parenting.

Among nations, the United States ranks first in its rates of interpersonal violence (American Psychological Association, 1993). Although there has been a 61% increase in arrest for violent offenses between 1988 and 1994, the juvenile arrest rate for homicide increased a staggering 90% from 1987 to 1991, and it remained fairly constant thereafter (Snyder & Sickmund, 1995). Although the patterns and consequences of aggression and violence may vary according to the gender and race of the perpetrator, the impact of youth aggression/violence on communities and societies is penetrating. Boys tend to engage in direct physical aggression, whereas girls tend to use more indirect relational or social methods of aggression (e.g., verbal rejection, social exclusion, slander) typically resulting in emotional harm and social damage to other girls (Xie, Cairns, & Cairns, 2002). Children who are victimized physically or overtly tend to experience internalized distress, which may lead to difficulties in controlling their anger and possible oppositional behavior directed against their aggressors (Crick & Bigbee, 1998; Crick, Grotpeter, & Rockhill, 1999). Individuals and communities suffer in both situations, whether social aggression is used to ostracize, defame, and control, or physical aggression is used to abuse and terrorize. Climates of fear, intimidation, and deprivation in many communities result from the threat or reality of violence (Richters & Martinez, 1993).

Even though such behavior decreases with age, children who exhibit these behaviors maintain their relative standing in terms of aggressive behavior with peers over time (Broidy et al., 2003). In fact, longitudinal studies find severe aggressive acting out (e.g., persistent physical fighting) to be highly stable (with an average correlation of approximately .70 for measures of these behaviors taken at different times) (Loeber, Green, Lahey, & Kalb, 2000), which makes aggressive behavior about as stable as some reports of IQ.

Although there appears to be stability of aggression over time, this does not mean that such behavior in children and adolescents is immutable. In fact, there is some evidence that physical altercations and aggressive acting out generally decrease from childhood to adulthood (e.g., Loeber & Stouthamer-Loeber, 1998). There appear to be three developmental types of aggressive, violent youngsters: (1) life-course-persistent, (2) limited-duration, and (3) late-onset (Loeber & Stouthamer-Loeber, 1998; Moffit, 1993; Moffit, Caspi, Dickson, Silva, & Stanton, 1996). The life-course-persistent (LCP) path describes youngsters who engage in aggressive social behavior at an earlier age and continue to do so into adulthood. Such severe acting out with these children begins early, likely due to subtle neuropsychological deficits that may interfere with their language and self-control, resulting in cognitive delays and temperamental difficulties that are evident by the age of 3 or younger. Such deficits heighten the child's vulnerability to environmental deficits such as poor parenting or abuse, which fuels oppositional and conduct problems (Lansford et al., 2002; Moffit, 1993). Such children account for the largest proportion of highly aggressive persons emerging in later life. The adolescent-limited (AL) path involves youngsters whose aggressive acting out begins around puberty and continues into adolescence, although they outgrow their aggression during young adulthood (Farrington, 1986). This acting out is more limited to their teenage years, and they display less extreme aggression and acting out than those on the LCP path. Such youngsters appear to have stronger family ties and are less likely to drop out of school. Their aggression and acting out are generally not as consistent across situations, as with their LCP counterparts. It should be noted, however, that some youngsters on the AL path continue to exhibit aggressive and antisocial behavior well into their 20s before such behavior diminishes. Still others do not desist in their 20s but continue to exhibit such severe acting out, impulsivity, substance abuse, property crimes, and mental health problems (Moffitt, Caspi, Harrington, & Milne, 2002). In identifying these LCP and AL path youngsters, it should be remembered that most adolescents do not go on to become antisocial adults (Robins, 1978). At the crossroads of early adulthood, they differentiate, diverge, and go different ways—aggression and antisocial behavior being stable for LCP youth as they continue on the same road, but discontinuation characterizing the AL path. Finally, violent behavior in a smaller subset, the late-onset type, emerges only during adulthood and may be a function of overcontrol, which diminishes as inhibitions against anger abate.

Overall, aggressive behavior is susceptible to change with systematic interventions (e.g., Southam-Gerow & Kendall, 1997; Tate, Reppucci, & Mulvey, 1995; Wasserman & Miller, 1998). Thus, the notion that early onset and stable forms of aggression during childhood and adolescence develop into stable personality traits is not entirely accurate. There is evidence and subsequent hope that, when exposed to effective interventions, at-risk youth not only can learn to deal with problems in other ways than aggression and violence but also can lead productive lives. The clinical picture is not all doom and gloom.

A variety of intervention strategies have been evaluated for more seriously acting-out, conduct-disordered children, such as psychotherapeutic medication interventions and home, school, and community-based programs, as well as hospital and residential treatment (for reviews, see Brandt & Zlotnick, 1988; Dumas, 1989; Eyberg, Boggs, & Algina, 1995; Kazdin, 2003; Miller, 1994; Nelson, Finch, & Hart, in press; Pepler & Rubin, 1991; Stoff, Breiling, & Maser, 1997; U.S. Congress, 1991). In fact, Kazdin (1993) described several criteria in evaluating the promise of intervention programs, including (1) a theoretical conceptualization of the disorder that guides treatment, (2) a conceptualization of how it is supported by research, (3) a characterization of how outcome research supports the treatment's efficacy, and (4) explication of how the outcome is related to processes identified in the conceptualization of the disorder. Currently, there are no treatments that adequately meet all of these criteria, although two interventions seem more promising for severely acting-out children—the family-/parent-focused therapies derived from social learning theory and the child-focused cognitive-behavioral interventions (Kazdin, 2003; Miller & Prinz, 1990; Southam-Gerow & Kendall, 1997). This chapter focuses primarily on the cognitive-behavioral interventions.

THEORIES, CONCEPTS, CENTRAL FEATURES, AND THE CATEGORIZATION OF ANGER AND AGGRESSION

The value of any psychological theory is measured, at least in part, by its usefulness in improving assessment and therapeutic intervention procedures. Interest in several traditional theories of aggression has diminished, particularly as deficiencies in their conceptional and derived therapeutic techniques have become apparent. Among these are theories that view aggressive behavior, like virtually all other social behavior, as under instinctual control (instinctual theory: McDougall, 1931); the view that aggression is an expression of a death instinct (psychoanalytic theory: Freud, 1920); the notion that aggressive behavior consists of clearly organized response patterns released in each species by specific external or "sign" stimuli (ethological theory: Lorenz, 1966); and the view that aggression is a frustration-produced drive (frustration–aggression hypotheses: Dollard, Doob, Miller, Mowrer, & Sears, 1939). In addition, some of the more behaviorally oriented theories suggest that aggressive behavior is a result of poor role models, reinforcement, and/or deficits in social cognition. There is no single-cause theory about the etiology of anger, aggression, and conduct problems, although each may highlight a potentially important factor or determinant. Aggressive behavior and conduct problems result from an interplay among predisposing/mediating factors—child-level factors (e.g., genetic influences, prenatal factors, birth complications, neurobiological factors, poor social-cognitive and problem-solving skills, poor self-regulation and perceived peer context, as well as deficits in resisting peer pressure) (e.g., Trembley, 2000); contextual factors—family influences such as poor parental models, caregiving, and discipline of the child (Wasserman & Seracini, 2001); more indirect factors such as the community (e.g., parents' workplace and social networks, local government); and cultural factors (e.g., broader culture, historical events) (Bronfenbrenner, 1989; Hill, 2002; Lahey, Moffitt, & Caspi, 2003; Raine, 2002). In considering such multiple factors, also remember that (Mash & Wolfe, 2005) note that:

- Genetic influences account for about 50% of the variance in aggressive/antisocial behavior.
- Aggression and antisocial behavior may be a function of the behavioral activation system (BAS) that stimulates behavior and responses to signals of reward or nonpunishment, coupled with deficits in the behavioral inhibition system (BIS), responsible for anxiety and inhibiting ongoing behavior.
- Several family factors, such as intense marital conflict, family isolation, negative/inconsistent and coercive disciplinary practices, violence in the home, lack of parental supervision, and deficits in attachment, may also play a role.
- Parental criminality and antisocial personality, family instability, divorce, antisocial family values, and unemployment may also contribute to the problem.
- Community factors such as poverty, neighborhood crime, family disruption, residential mobility, and low socioeconomic status may provide a "fertile ground" for the emergence of aggression and severe acting out.
- School, peer, and media influences also seem to be potential risk factors, as well as minority-group status and ethnicity, as minority status has been associated with aggressive/antisocial behavior in the United States. Such findings, however, are likely related to economic hardship, limited employment opportunities, residence in high-risk urban neighborhoods, and membership in gangs.

With such multiple causes what is a therapist to do? Of the psychological theories, it is the social learning theory (Bandura, 1986) and cognitive-behavioral theories (Novaco, 1978, 1979) that have emerged and been sustained as the most widely held theories of aggressive behavior in children and adolescents (Nelson, Finch, & Hart, in press; Nelson, Hart, & Finch, 1993). Social learning theory holds that aggressive behaviors are learned through either direct experience or observation. The cognitive-behavioral model expands this position and views *anger* as an intense emotional response to frustration or provocation characterized by heightened automatic arousal, changes in central nervous system activity, and cognitive labeling of the physiological arousal as anger. Thus, aggression is viewed as only one of the potential overt expressions of the subjective experience of anger.

The first step in the therapeutic process is to recognize that there are a variety of terms used to describe acting-out behavior in children and adolescents, with the result being confusion and lack of precision. Our difficulties in understanding acting out in youth comes not only as a function of the entanglement of terms used to describe such behavior but also from the differing conceptional models employed in understanding such emotion and behavior. Thus, it is important to clarify the terms used to describe acting–out behavior in children and adolescents. *Anger* is the internal experience of a private, subjective event (i.e., emotion) that has cognitive (e.g., thoughts, self statements, private speech, images, attributions) and physiological components. *Aggression* involves behavioral acts that inflict bodily or mental harm on others (Loeber & Hay, 1997). Aggression causes less serious harm than *violence*, which denotes aggressive acts that cause serious harm (e.g., aggravated assault, rape, robbery, homicide; Loeber & Stouthamer-Loeber, 1998). There are two primary classification approaches in describing aggressive acting out in youth. The first is the empirically derived multivariate statistical approach that distinguishes between externalized (typified by impulsive, overactive, aggressive, antisocial actions) and internalized (characterized by dysphoric, withdrawn, anxious, somaticizing features) conflict (Achenbach, 1991; Quay, 1986). The second is the more clinically derived DSM-IV-TR approach to labeling (American Psychiatric Association, 2000). The diagnostic categories of conduct disorder (CD) and oppositional defiant disorder (ODD) are the two primary classification categories for youth in DSM-IV-TR, while antisocial personality disorder is reserved for adults. Despite the wide acceptance of these classification systems, they do not necessarily provide better understanding of the problem for the practicing clinician. There are more clinically useful ways of categorizing the levels of aggressive behavior of children and adolescents.

Distinctions among various levels of anger and aggression are an important first step in not only multimethod clinical assessment but also in setting the stage for cognitive-behavioral interventions. Such clinically useful diagnostic distinctions, as opposed to the clinically derived DSM-IV-TR and empirically derived (e.g., Achenbach Child Behavior Checklist) classification systems, not only assist the therapist in planning appropriate interventions but also help the family of the youngster accurately assess the severity and dangerousness of the aggressive behavior. This distinction is particularly important in dealing with clients whose primary problems are anger and aggression in that their behavior frequently elicits strong emotional responses not only in family members and significant individuals around them, but also in the therapist. Such emotional reactions may result in immediately assuming that the youngster is "bad" or more seriously dangerous than is actually the case.

In general, therapists tend to err in the direction of assuming greater danger than is warranted (Buchanan, 1997; Limandri & Sheridan, 1995; Monahan & Walker, 1990). As such, a therapist's assessment in evaluating a problem may be skewed because of the level of fear a parent or teacher may have in being able to manage the youngster who seems out of control. Therefore, it is important to distinguish among anger, threats of violence against others, and actually carrying those threats out. In such a diagnostic process, parents and significant others need to be sensitized to and recognize the differences among anger, verbal aggression, and different levels of physical aggression in the sense that such behaviors may cover a wide range, from being merely obnoxious and inflammatory to being seriously harmful or violent. In addition, universal diagnostic formulations should not be generally assumed for cross-cultural clients, despite the therapist's temptation to view expressions of anger and aggression as race- or culture-free. For example, higher diagnostic rates of conduct disorder within African American youth (Spencer & Oatts, 1999; Steiner, 1997) may be influenced by racial insensitivity, in view of the findings that African American youth who receive a conduct disorder diagnosis are less likely to have chart documentation supporting their diagnoses (Jerrell, 2003). A similar concern is the higher frequency of a schizophrenia diagnosis and the less frequent occurrence of an affective disorder diagnosis among African American adults (Chen, Swann, & Burt, 1996). The problems of incorrectly diagnosing and overdiagnosing clients from multicultural populations are reduced through cultural competency training and consultation, which assumes that cultural differences are of major importance when assessing human behavior (Dana, 2000). Given the tendency to assume greater danger, it is helpful to differentiate anger and aggression in a more clinically useful fashion, such that a clearer and more realistic picture of the seriousness of the problem can be ascertained. The relevant dimensions of anger, aggression, and violence in the clinically useful classification system (adapted from Price, 1996) are depicted in Table 4.1 and explained below.

TABLE 4.1. Relevant Dimensions in a Clinically Useful Classification System

Anger	Verbal aggression directed at self	Verbal aggression directed at others	Physical aggression against inanimate objects	Physical aggression against others	Violence

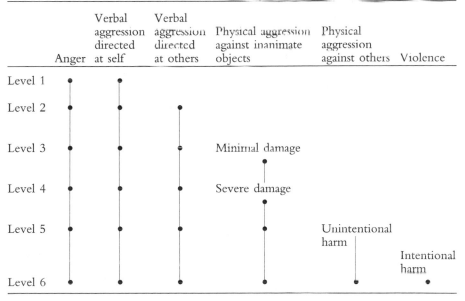

Level 1: The Impatient/Annoying/Irritating Child

Youngsters at Level 1 whine, complain, and become enraged whenever they are told "no," do not get their way, or are challenged. They raise their voices, hold their breath, and their faces become red. Such anger is "controlled," and they may even turn such anger against themselves and say, "I hate myself; I'm always doing the wrong thing; I'm stupid [etc.]."

Level 2: The Stubborn/Dramatic Child

Children and adolescents at Level 2 stubbornly refuse to follow directions or comply with requests. They become enraged and exhibit verbal aggression in the sense of swearing, calling others names, hurling insults, and so on. Such verbally assaultive behavior may be interpreted by parents as indicating that their child is on the verge of violence. Children's dramatic behavior often is sufficient (in terms of intensity and/or frequency) to convince adults that their children are "out of control" when, in fact, they are angry and expressing this feeling only verbally. A fifteen-year-old who takes a few steps toward his mother and calls her a "bitch" demonstrates Level 2 behavior.

Level 3: The Threatening Child and the Beginning of Damage

At level 3, children become increasingly angry (in terms of frequency and/or intensity), and the range of their verbal aggression includes threats to injure or kill parents, siblings, peers, and/or animals. It should be noted that at Level 3 the youngster has never really injured any human being or living thing. He or she is still primarily engaged in verbal aggression and threats, although the child may have caused minimal damage to nonvaluable inanimate objects. A 10-year-old kicks his chair and it puts a good-sized dent in the plaster wall, but the fact that he avoids throwing knives, glasses, or objects at the TV demonstrates he is still cognizant of how serious more severe forms of aggression against inanimate objects might be. Thus, he is clearly thinking about how far he is going, even though parents (or the therapist) may interpret this behavior as clearly "out of control."

Level 4: The "Taking It Up a Notch" Child

Children at Level 4 are purposely and intentionally venting their anger against inanimate objects by seriously damaging or destroying things. They become so enraged and exhibit aggressive behavior such as punching a hole in the wall, throwing an object through a window, and breaking increasingly valuable objects. Youngsters may threaten to actually hit the family member with an object or weapon such as a baseball bat, hammer, or knife. However, the most important distinction to make at this level is the fact that there is no actual physical contact or harming of another. These teenagers, when they become enraged, may threaten others but keep a distance between the person they view as the antagonist and themselves. They usually retreat or storm out of the room, however, when approached. Most parents believe that their child is very dangerous at this time and can become quite intimidated by him or her. Nevertheless, these youngsters are exhibiting some cognitive and behavioral control in the sense that their verbal aggression against others and their physical aggression against inanimate objects is not escalating into actual physical violence against others.

Level 5: The Assaultive Child

At Level 5 the child has moved well beyond expressions of verbal anger and physical aggression exhibited against inanimate objects to physical aggression involving acts that inflict bodily harm on others. Thus, actual physical aggression often accompanies verbal threats. At this level, however, the aggression does not involve violence or serious bodily injury. Such behavior includes pushing, shoving, shouldering, hitting, and throwing objects at others that would not result in serious harm (e.g., tennis ball, pencil, plastic cup, stuffed animal). Actual physical injuries at this level are minor, and such injuries tend to be more incidental rather than directly intentional. For example, a 12-year-old boy might throw a tennis ball across the room and accidentally hit his sister. Even though she may have fallen down and bruised her arm, this injury is basically unintentional inasmuch as he did not anticipate the outcome. Although it may be difficult, it is important to assess whether or not the adolescent has actually made a choice to physically injure someone or whether the injury was an unintentional outcome of an angry or aggressive outburst. At this point the parents are usually very frightened and are legitimately fearful that their child might truly lose control and physically harm someone in a violent fashion.

Level 6: The Violent Child

Adolescents or children at Level 6 are exhibiting violent behavior that causes serious harm to others and are dangerous to others. They deliberately throw dangerous objects at others or attack others with their fists with the intention of injuring them. Weapons may be more deliberately used, such as when a 15-year-old girl deliberately struck her 9-year-old brother with a tree limb because he would not give her a ball. The important dimension in Level 6 is actual violent behavior where physical harm is intended and occurs. At this stage, parents feel intimidated, hopeless, and even abused. They may seem "shell-shocked" or "burned out" because of the humiliation and abusiveness they have suffered over the years. They may even feel resigned to the violence that has escalated from verbal expressions of anger to aggression against inanimate objects, to aggression unintentionally resulting in minor bodily harm, to actual violence toward others. Parents often view their situation as being so terrible that they no longer have any control over the situation whatsoever, and feel lost, abandoned, and hopeless. Price (1996) refers to these parents as being "emotionally and physically abused" by their children.

THE COGNITIVE-BEHAVIORAL TREATMENT OF ANGER AND AGGRESSION IN YOUTH

Cognitive-behavioral treatment draws upon the rich traditions of behavior modification, rational-emotive, and cognitive therapy and integrates knowledge about social cognition (Dodge, 1991). As such cognitive-behavioral treatment interventions do not involve a single therapeutic technique, but rather consist of multiple intervention components: (1) problem solving and social skills education, (2) coping models, (3) role playing, (4) *in vivo* experiences and assignments, (5) affective education, (6) homework assignments, and (7) operant conditioning, most typically response cost (Kendall & Braswell, 1993; see Kendall, Chapter 1, this volume). In addition, therapeutic interventions include a variety of self-control strategies that not only teach the child to inhibit aggressive behavior through the use of cognitive processing (in other words, to put thought between the environmental stimulus or "trigger" and the overt aggressive response) but also teach alternative skills to inhibit acting in an aggressive fashion. The cognitive-behavioral approach is unified by the principles of learning theory and information processing, and therefore is not simply a loose technical eclecticism.

To date, there have been only two meta-analysis anger management studies (Beck & Fernandez, 1998; Tafrate, 1995). However, Tafrate's survey was confined to adult samples. On the other hand, Beck and Fernandez's study not only involved adults and children but also incorporated unpublished studies. Their final sample consisted of 50 nomothetic studies that included 1,640 participants and provided at least one anger-related measure of change. They included only cognitive-behavioral interventions for anger that typically involved multiple intervention techniques. Their results indicated that cognitive-behavioral interventions were suggestive of moderate treatment gains in that the average treatment participant improved more than 76% of the control participants. Twenty-five of the 35 studies (two articles reported results of two different studies) used in their meta-analytic calculations had different samples of children and/or adolescents. These 25 studies were examined as to the number of participants, sex, age, intervention techniques, outcome measures, and results.[1] There were multiple cognitive-behavioral interventions employed in these studies (e.g., self-monitoring, self-instruction, problem solving, relaxation, assertion training, goal setting, perspective taking). In addition, samples included youth ranging in age from 8 to 21 years. Seventeen involved males only and eight involved males and females. Outcome measures also varied, but typically self-reported anger was utilized as the dependent variable for these younger populations. When self-reported anger was not feasible, behavioral ratings of aggression and/or ratings by significant others were often employed as dependent variables.

THE COGNITIVE-BEHAVIORAL MODEL OF ANGER

Guided by the cognitive-behavioral model of anger (see Figure 4.1), such therapy includes a set of general therapeutic interventions that are individually tailored to fit the child's specific circumstances in terms of dealing with the external/environmental and/or internal stimuli and the specific aggressive responses to these. Any model of anger needs to be comprehensive enough to guide the clinician in effectively utilizing therapy interventions but also simple enough for the child or adolescent as well as his or her family and others to understand (at least with the assistance of the therapist) the nature of his or her anger and subsequent aggressive behavior. Thus, the cognitive-behavioral model provides the framework not only for the therapist to understand the child but also for the child to understand his or her problems that have necessitated therapy.

The cognitive-behavioral model is based on the rationale that children's emotions and subsequent actions are regulated by the way they perceive, process, and/or mediate environmental events. The problems or environmental events themselves do not directly determine how a person feels or what he or she actu-

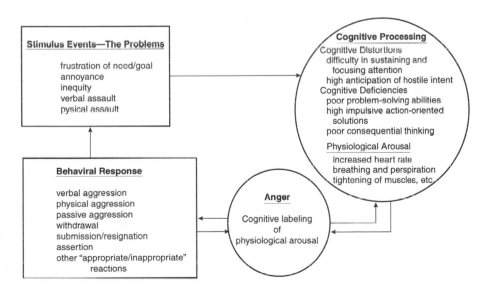

FIGURE 4.1. Cognitive-behavioral model of anger and aggression.

ally does in any given circumstance. Anger is a subjective reaction to day-to-day problems, or "triggers." The experience of the emotion of anger reflects one's integration of cognitive processing of physiological events (the cognitive arousal theory of emotion; Mandler, 1984; Schachter, 1964; Schachter & Singer, 1962). It is assumed that aggressive youngsters lack the necessary psychological resources for coping with problems and are, therefore, prone to reacting in an aggressive fashion when encountering a provoking situation. Thus, the cognitive-behavioral model is a skills-deficit one. In order to cope with problems or stressors, the child needs to develop the necessary skills to effectively manage the subjective state of anger, which then results in more adaptive behavioral reactions. Specific cognitive-behavioral intervention techniques involve both direct-action procedures (e.g., assertion training, relaxation techniques) and/or cognitive interventions (e.g., self-talk, problem solving, humor). In the former procedures, the focus is on teaching the child alternative ways of responding to problems or stress. In the latter cognitive techniques, the focus is on changing the child's cognition concerning anger-provoking situations or the processing of such situations. In both cases the desired outcome is a more adaptive change in subsequent behavior.

THE THERAPEUTIC RELATIONSHIP AND THE STRESS INOCULATION PARADIGM FOR AGGRESSIVE YOUTH

It is essential for the clinician to have not only a conceptual model of anger and aggression to understand such emotions and behavior but also a model in which a variety of intervention techniques can be conceptualized and integrated into an effective therapeutic intervention treatment plan (Finch, Nelson, & Ott, 1993; Meichenbaum, 1977; Novaco, 1979). The stress inoculation model provides such a framework and can be seen in Table 4.2.

Before discussing specific stress inoculation strategies, it is important to consider the type of therapeutic relationship a cognitive-behavioral therapist attempts to establish with aggressive youth. Such clients provide a variety of challenges in therapy because of their dysfunctional beliefs, self-statements, and ways of interacting with others. Aggressive youngsters may believe that no one understands them, especially because they frequently believe that it is others who pro-

---

TABLE 4.2. Four Phases in the Stress Inoculation Training Model

1. Assessment
2. Educational Phase (cognitive preparation)
3. Skills Acquisition Phase (rehearsal)
4. Application Training (practice, practice, and more practice . . .)

voke them into aggressive responses. They may believe that "others will get me if I don't get them first" or "if I don't push other people, I will get pushed around." Not only do aggressive youngsters frequently not want to come to therapy but also when forced to do so by parents or others in authority, they often view the therapist in the same negative light they perceive adults outside of therapy. Thus, therapists "have their work cut out for them" in trying to establish a positive therapeutic relationship with aggressive children and adolescents.

Cognitive-behavioral interventions are best grounded in a "collaborative empiricism" (Beck, Rush, Shaw, & Emery, 1979). In other words, a collaborative relationship (see Kendall, Chapter 1, this volume) is established with the child so that the "therapist–client team" works against the common opponent, anger/aggression. It is essential to form such a collaborative relationship with acting-out youngsters, who frequently view adults or authority figures as "the enemy." Such relationships are forged by aligning or "joining" with children to assist them in developing better skills to avoid suffering aversive consequences after behaving in a maladaptive, aggressive fashion. Most acting-out children are acutely aware of the fact that it is they who "end up in hot water" or "get the short end of the stick" in many situations, even though they frequently minimize or deny their own responsibility in the aggressive cycle or chain of events. Thus, they view themselves as victims in most situations. Attempts to convince them otherwise, especially in the initial phases of therapy, frequently lead to a rift in the therapist–client relationship. Consequently, it is recommended that therapists "side-step" such a power struggle and form a strategic alliance with the youngster against what can be conceptualized as "the enemy"—unbridled anger and subsequent maladaptive aggression or violence.

In terms of more formal evaluation, multimethod assessment over the course of treatment is useful in order to ascertain any therapeutic gains. This may not always be feasible for practicing clinicians who frequently rely more on self- or parent-report devices. For experimental studies, in assessing anger management interventions it is important to assess during at least two time periods, once initially for selection for treatment/therapy and once immediately before intervention is to begin. In this way, the actual status of the client immediately preceding treatment can be ascertained, as well as the issue of stability of self-report measures (Kendall & Flannery-Schroeder, 1995; Kendall, Hollon, Beck, Hammen, & Ingram, 1987).

For the practicing clinician, it is also important to note that there are gender-related differences in forms of overt aggression. Girls tend to be nominated more by their peers as relationally aggressive, while boys are described more frequently as overtly aggressive (e.g., Cairns, Cairns, Neckerman, Ferguson, & Gariepy, 1989; Crick & Grotpeter, 1995; Lagerspetz, Bjorkqvist, & Peltonen, 1988). Overt aggression involves both direct verbal and physical aggression that can be harmful to others, whereas relational aggression tends to be more harmful to others indirectly, causing damage to peer relationships by way of manipulation and control (Crick, Casas, & Mosher, 1997). Examples of such aggression include creating false rumors to end existing friendships or intimate relationships, publicly displaying demoralizing or sexually degrading accusations, and persuading the group to collaborate in assigning an individual to an outcast status. This is an important factor to remember when developing anger hierarchies during the initial assessment and treatment.

The first stage of treatment, the Assessment Phase, involves a thorough multimethod process to identify the external environmental stimuli and/or internal "triggers"—through such means as behavioral interviews and observations, rating forms from parents, teachers, and peers, and self-reports. Assessment techniques not only help the clinician understand the interconnections between cognition, emotion, and behavior but also can be utilized to "join" with and develop the collaborative alliance with the child. The second stage, the Educational Phase, involves teaching the child about the nature of his or her feelings of anger and how subsequent aggressive behavior can be self-defeating and "get them into trouble." Thus, the Educational Phase sets the stage for the youngster to become more aware of how the anger experience (involving cognitions and physiological events) can lead to maladaptive acting out. This increased awareness involves a self-observation or self-monitoring of autonomic and physiological processes so that the child can better understand the two components of anger (physiological feelings and cognitions) and how these can be utilized in stage three, the Skills Acquisition Phase, to better manage anger and subsequent aggression. Thus, these self-observations are utilized not only to increase the child's awareness of the environmental "triggers" for anger and aggressive acting out but also to help him or her recognize the maladaptive cognitive-physiological-behavioral chain. In the Application Training Phase, children are exposed in a hierarchical fashion to progressively more problematic situations in order to practice their newly learned anger management skills. Finally, relapse prevention and actual termination need to be planned for and addressed to ensure maximum generalization and maintenance of treatment effects.

Nelson and Finch (1996) developed a treatment workbook, *Keeping Your Cool*, that integrates five of the most often utilized cognitive-behavioral intervention techniques for use with acting-out children into a structured yet flexible intervention regimen. There is also an accompanying video, *"Keeping Your Cool": The Anger Management Video* (Nelson, 1998), that can be directly employed in therapy sessions where models educate the client (and parents) about the nature of anger and teach the client the specific anger management skills. Such a prevention program can be utilized as a primary or secondary intervention strategy in groups or individually. In fact, the *Summary Report of the American Psychological Association Commission on Violence and Youth* (American Psychological Association, 1993) indicated that "primary prevention programs that promote social and cognitive skills seem to have the greatest impact on attitudes about violent behavior among children and youth" (p. 56) and "secondary prevention programs that focus on improving individual affective, cognitive, and behavioral skills . . . offer promise of interrupting the path toward violence for high-risk or predelinquent youth" (p 56). The *Keeping Your Cool* workbook has integrated a number of these empirically supported procedures into a psychoeducational workbook format—verbal self-instructions, relaxation training, problem solving, assertion training, and humor. These particular procedures were selected because of their individually demonstrated usefulness and their theoretical consistency within the cognitive-behavior model of anger management. The use of verbal self-instructions as a treatment approach grew out of the theories of Vygotsky (1962, 1987) and Luria (1959, 1961). These two Soviet psychologists suggested that verbal commands need to be internalized in order for a child to gain voluntary control over overt behavior. A potential model for this development of control was presented by Luria and later utilized by Meichenbaum and Goodman (1971) in modifying an impulsive cognitive style in normal children.

Relaxation training usually follows a set of procedures first introduced by Jacobsen (1938). Various muscle groups are isolated, and the feeling of relaxation is enhanced by comparison with tension. These procedures have been modified for children by Koeppen (1974). Relaxation training has been found to be useful in children not only for the reduction of anxiety (Eisen & Silverman, 1993), depression (Dujovne, Barnard, & Rapoff, 1995; Reynolds & Coats, 1986), and anger (Deffenbacher, Lynch, Oetting, & Kemper, 1996) but also for the increase of positive psychological attitudes (Benson, Kornhaber, Kornhaber, & LeChanu, 1994). In addition, there is some suggestion that relaxation training may be more effective with physical symptoms than cognitive ones (Eisen & Silverman, 1993). We have found this to be consistent with our clinical work with angry children. Most children and adolescents who have anger management problems tense their muscles as their anger increases. This increase in tension seems to be a signal that is often interpreted by the individual as a preparation for some aggressive act. Through relaxation training, the child is taught to reinterpret these signals as a call to relax.

The third treatment strategy in the *Keeping Your Cool* workbook is problem solving. Problem-solving skills have been identified as deficit in a variety of disorders. For example, training in problem solving has been employed in the treatment of depression (Clarke, Lewinsohn, & Hops, 1990; Stark et al., 1996) and anger (Larson & Lochman, 2002; Lochman, 1992). Clinically, aggressive children and adolescents appear markedly deficient in solving their interpersonal problems. Their first response to a wide range of problem situations is anger and they seem to lack other skills in seeking alternative solutions.

Assertiveness training has been a widely used and popular intervention, as indicated by the publication of the seventh edition of Alberti and Emmons's self-help book, *Your Perfect Right*, in 2001. Within the anger management area, the rationale for the use of assertiveness training is that individuals have difficulty standing up for themselves and/or making their needs known to others in an appropriately assertive manner. As a result of these skill deficits, they respond in an aggressive or angry manner. With children and adolescents, assertiveness training has been found to be effective in improving self-concept (Waksman, 1981), improving self-esteem in minority females (Stewart & Lewis, 1986), increasing appropriate interaction with teachers (Pentz, 1980), and decreasing self-reported aggressiveness (Dong, Hallberg, & Hassard, 1979).

Humor, by design, is comical or amusing and therefore to elicit an emotional response incompatible with anger. Its use in psychotherapy (Buckman, 1994; Chapman & Chapman-Santana, 1995; Fry & Salameh, 1993) and assessment (Bernet, 1993; Dana, 1994) has been widely discussed. Specific guidelines for its use with children and adolescents have been published (Ventis & Ventis, 1988). Despite all the discussion about the use of humor, there is a dearth of research on the effectiveness of its use. It has been our clinical impression that humor not only can be an effective tool in the reduction of tension and anger with children and adolescents but also can serve to improve the collaborative therapeutic relationship between the therapist and the client.

Although the use of psychotherapy training manuals has been hotly debated (e.g., Beutler, 2004; Levant, 2004), we hope that the manual and workbook provide clinicians with concrete descriptions and procedures of intervention techniques, as well as a theoretical framework to guide or augment treatment. The workbook format is not meant to be a mechanical set of rules but rather a way of structuring interventions for therapists wanting to use a cognitive-behavioral approach. In addition, such workbooks may become increasingly useful for clients, as increasing pressure from third-party reimbursers and policymakers frequently caps the number of therapy sessions available to clients. Workbooks can expand the therapeutic armaments of the clinician by providing a way to offer more structured interventions outside of the typical therapy hour.

Thus, the *Keeping Your Cool* workbook offers a sequential stepwise program to teach cognitive-behaviorally based anger management skills to acting-out youth. The five specific interventions strategies or "plays" presented in the workbook help children identify potentially problematic situations early on, process the environmental cues of which they become more accurately aware, and provide a variety of anger management skills they can draw upon in dealing with day-to-day problems or anger-provoking situations. These basic strategies in the workbook are also augmented by other cognitive-behavioral techniques found to have some empirical support in the cognitive-behavioral literature—goal setting, self-monitoring, perspective taking, and changing irrational beliefs.

Phase I: Assessment

The assessment of anger in children is a multidimensional process and one that is likely to be shaped by the nature of the anger management problems presented. However, certain core components should be considered. The initial decision concerns with whom should the therapist meet for the initial interview. Some therapists suggest that parents should be seen initially to determine the nature of the problem; others suggest meeting with the child alone initially, and still others suggest meeting with the entire family during this initial session. We recommend that the entire family be seen during the initial session, if at all possible. One reason for this approach is to avoid the perception by the child that anything secretive is being planned. Children with anger management problems generally have a history of conflict with authority figures and are quick to believe that they are in trouble again. Having their parents meet with another authority figure, without personally hearing what is said, has the potential to result in a negative perception by the child. Additional concern may exist for youth in single-parent homes; they may be worried that the outside authority will build a threatening alliance with their parent, which puts their tenuous parent–child relationship at further risk. Many of these children have fears about what will be said, and their misconceptions are generally worse than what is actually conveyed.

When working cross-culturally, the effective therapist is familiar with family structures, gender roles, and protocols specific to the racial ethnic or cultural group. For example, in view of their cultural value of *respeto* (respect), Latino families can be deeply insulted when adults and elders are addressed without titles, such as Mr. and Mrs. (Santiago-Rivera, Arredondo, & Gallardo-Cooper, 2002). Similarly, use of certain verbal communications such as the minimal encourager "umm-hmm" is considered an effective psychotherapy skill, though this expression is often regarded as a disrespectful (and condescending) term when spoken to a middle-class African American elder. Moreover, this term would have no reference for a Chinese client who is unfamiliar with the nuances of the English language, because "umm-hmm" does not exist in many languages (Helms & Cook, 1999).

Another advantage of meeting with the entire family at once is to observe the interactions of the family members. Considerable information about interactions, respect, lines of communication, alliances, and roles can be learned quickly by observing interactions firsthand. Estimations of how best to deal with issues of compliance and sabotage can be assessed quickly. In addition, the clinician can obtain some indication of how angry the parents are with the child, and with each other, about the problem. Such information can be very useful once treatment begins.

After the initial session with the entire family, the next session can be divided between meeting with the parents alone and/or with the child. During these meetings, more detailed information is obtained about the specific behaviors, including a description of general and specific incidences of problems in dealing with anger. Care should be taken to ensure that the child is not made to feel defensive. Often, the natural response is to withdraw and remain silent. Minimization is to be expected, and the therapist is likely to need a "warm-up" period with the child in which other issues are discussed rather than the specific problems which brought the child to the office. This "warm-up" period is essential for ethnic minorities, especially when the client and therapist differ in race or ethnicity. African American male teenagers, for example, require additional time to build trust in view of their potential to generalize expectations of legal or police injustice to the therapeutic relationship. Similarly, Latino youth may resist a therapeutic alliance, particularly if family members have previously been subjected to fear of immigration authorities, as well as the disillusionment of discrimination. The therapist must form an alliance with the child against a "common enemy," anger or aggression. However, this alliance may have to be developed slowly and indirectly.

Interviewing children can take a variety of directions. Children with anger management problems frequently answer even open-ended questions with one- or two-word answers or simply shrugs. Given that many of the factors that the cognitive-behavioral therapist wants to explore are private (e.g., negative self-statements), the therapist must be patient and supportive of the child while not undermining parental authority. Frequently children will minimize or present themselves in the "best light." We have found that confrontation does not help, but only increases the child's defensiveness.

A more indirect approach may be necessary. The following case material with 11-year-old Josh illustrates this point.

Inside the Therapist's Office

THERAPIST: Tell me about the last time you were angry with your sister.

JOSH: I was running late getting ready for school . . .

THERAPIST: Tell me a little more about your "running late." What happened?

JOSH: She called me a "slug."

THERAPIST: When she called you a slug, what did you do?

JOSH: I told her that it made me mad when she called me a slug, and she said she was sorry.

[*Comments*: The therapist knew that Josh actually threw his books at his sister and a physical fight followed, in which Josh was so angry/aggressive that his mother had to seek assistance in controlling him. However, the therapist also believed that Josh was attempting to place himself in the best light. The therapist believed that, if confronted, Josh would simply react in a more defensive manner. The therapist responds with a "side step."]

THERAPIST: I wonder if you would tell me about another time your sister made you mad and you did not handle it so well. Tell me about a time you kind of lost it with her.

[*Comments*: Here, the therapist is giving Josh permission to share freely an incident that is selected because he did not handle his anger very well. By definition, there is no need for Josh to present himself in the best light.]

As a number of interview techniques for use with children with anger management problems have previously been presented (Finch, Nelson, & Moss, 1993), only a brief discussion is included here. We have found it very useful to have the child "run a movie" of an incident. Children are familiar with VCR/DVD terms such as "pausing," "reversing," and "rerunning" from their home videos/DVDs and seem to have little difficulty with engaging in this activity. The therapist simply asks the child to close his or her eyes and visualize the event. Next, the child is asked to "play" the scene and provide the therapist with a verbal description of what is being played. The therapist can help the child focus attention by asking specific questions about internal dialogue, visual images, physiological sensations, and other potentially important details. While the child is providing this description, the therapist needs to "record" the scene (take detailed notes) for later "playback" and "editing" during future sessions. Remember, during this early phase while the collaborative alliance is still being formed, the therapist seeks to understand, rather than challenge, judge, or correct, the adolescent's behavior.

Younger children (below about 10 years of age) frequently have difficulty with "running a movie." Their attention typically drifts and they appear to need a more concrete approach. With this age group we have attempted a variety of other approaches. One of the most useful has been "action figure drawings." In this task, the child is asked to describe the scene and the therapist makes a stick figure drawing of the described scene. The therapist can ask questions to help "make the drawing" while actually obtaining information about the desired feelings, thoughts, and physical sensations. Internal dialogue can be noted with bubbles (as utilized in cartoons), while external speech is denoted by drawing a continuous line. Children tend to enjoy this task, and it can help to develop a sense of collaboration that becomes useful later in therapy.

Other procedures for assessing anger with children include self-report measures. Because anger is an internal feeling and not an external behavior, self-report measures provide the most direct means of assessing it. As has been pointed out by Quay and La Greca (1986), internal self-statements and emotions are difficult for parents and teachers to identify accurately. There are serious questions that have to be realized when self-report measures are being used. As Finch and Politano (1994) have pointed out, self-report measures assume that the child is willing and able to report his or her internal feelings. This fact makes the development of a trusting and collaborative relationship even more important in the assessment of anger.

One of the most useful measures that we have found in the self-report of anger is the Children's Inventory of Anger (ChIA; Nelson & Finch, 2000). The ChIA consists of 48 items that require children to rate how the items apply to them on a 4-point scale ranging from "I don't care. That situation doesn't even bother me. I don't know why that would make anyone mad (angry)" to "I can't stand that! I'm furious! I feel like really hurting or killing that person or destroying that thing!" The items are written on a fourth-grade reading level and involve a variety of situations that might occur at home, at school, in peer interactions, and in other potentially anger-provoking situations. A number of other self-report measures have also been found to be useful. The Children's Action Tendency Scale (CATS) is a self-report inventory developed to evaluate levels of assertiveness in children (Deluty, 1979). One of the various potential responses to conflict situations is anger and aggression. The CATS has been found to be useful in a variety of situations and has acceptable levels of reliability. Self-report measures should be interpreted within the context of the child's racial and ethnic background as well as the standards of his or her youth subgroup. For example, an African American girl is likely to communicate emotions through hyperbole, so interpreting words such as "kill" requires additional interviewing.

Information about the child's anger management may be obtained from parents and teachers as well as other individuals who have the opportunity to observe the problem. A "multisystems" therapy model recognizes that, based on socioeconomic, cultural, and racial circumstances, varied key authority figures should be included in children's intervention, especially for African-American children and economically disadvantaged families (Boyd-Franklin, 2003). Some examples are a nonrelated godmother who has unofficial custody, a caseworker who is involved in a family reunification plan, or a mentor in a mandated rites-of-passage program. These individuals can provide important information for the therapist about the circumstances of the child's behavior, precipitating events, and the subsequent outcomes. In addition, other family members should be consulted, especially when the therapist's background is different than the family's. Corroborating information and collaborative support from one's extended family often proves highly useful in individually tailoring the treatment program for the particular child. In addition, children are not always the best reporters of their own behavior. Sometimes they are unaware of their own behaviors, while at other times they deny or minimize their role in the situation (Finch & Politano, 1994).

As was discussed by Finch, Nelson, and Moss (1993), the therapist focuses the interview with significant others on obtaining information on (1) the informant's view of the child's complaint, symptoms, and stressors; (2) the informant's view of the child's current environment (home, school, peers); (3) the informant's view of the child's development and history; and (4) the informant's expectations about the child's future.

More general measures of behavior can be obtained from behavioral checklists. Popular rating scales frequently employed include the Behavioral Assessment System for Children (BASC; Reynolds & Kamphaus, 1992) and the Child Behavior Checklist (Achenbach & Edelbrock, 1983). Both of these scales provide different forms to be completed by parents, teachers, and older children. These different perspectives can be very useful in evaluating the effectiveness of treatment as well as planning it.

Another useful anger scale is the Children's Hostility Inventory (Kazdin, Rodgers, Colbus, & Siegel, 1987). This scale consists of 38 items related to hostility and aggression and can be completed by parents. It is clinically useful to ask the children themselves to respond to these items and then to compare their responses to those of their parents. Frequently, the clinician can gain some understanding of the differences in perspective between parents and their children. However, there are no data available on the psychometric properties of this scale when completed by children.

On a more informal basis, we have found it useful to use behavioral role playing of anger-provoking situations. In these role-playing situations, anger-provoking interactions are staged and the child is asked to respond to them. Selective behavioral role modeling is an adaptation in which the adolescent identifies and role-plays a popular person from a movie, music video, video game, and so on, who reminds him or her of his or her own situation. This method allows adolescents to work within the framework of their own subculture, acknowledging their gender, race, or ethnic differences, and it facilitates disclosure for those who find that difficult to do. An example is the "Incredible Hulk," an iconic cartoon character who experiences destructive rage and superhuman strength when frustrated, offended, or perturbed. Youth with anger problems easily identify with the Incredible Hulk. His green color and unfavorable circumstances seem to strike a chord with angry youth while transcending race, ethnicity, and social class. After a few minutes of "warm-up," most children are able to become comfortable with these situations and fall into the same behaviors that have led to their being referred. We have been surprised at the number of times children have become angry in these artificial situations. It is important to establish the "ground rules" before these role-playing situations are initiated in order to have clearly defined limits and signals to "stop the action." Parents, siblings, and peers can be used successfully when clearly defined escape plans are established. The amount of information that can be obtained by using such "staged" interactions is very impressive.

Phase II: Educational Phase

Although an extension of the Assessment Phase rather than a discrete shift in therapy, the Educational Phase has four main purposes: (1) to continue forming a collaborative alliance with the child to work against the common "enemy," anger; (2) to help the child further understand the nature of his or her anger and subsequent aggressive behavior; (3) to quickly recognize the cognitive–affective–behavioral links early in the anger-arousing response chain; and (4) to continue to identify and recognize the specific environmental stimuli or problems that "trigger" the anger–aggression response pattern. First, the strategy of joining with the child to form a "team" works better with aggressive youngsters because it helps avoid the aversive consequences that typically follow maladaptive aggressive acting out; the goal of collaborative empiricism is facilitated. Second, in a collaborative attempt to teach the child the two components of anger (cognitions and physiological processes) that precede aggressive behavior, the child is given the clear message that he or she can control and better manage his or her own thoughts/images and feelings and is not a helpless victim solely at the mercy of anger-engendering stressors. Clients are taught that they are not at the mercy of, or a "puppet" of, "the problem" (person or situation) but have a choice in behaving aggressively or not (see Figure 4.2). They are educated in "short-circuiting" their anger by "cutting" their fuse with their mind (cognitive anger management strategies such as anger-reducing self-talk) before they "blow" (or react in a self-defeating aggressive fashion (see Figure 4.3).

The workbook provides specific psychoeducational tasks to augment the therapist's skillful persuasive efforts aimed not only at teaching the child about his or her own experience of anger but also at setting the stage for how the intervention strategies in the skills acquisition phase can be utilized to short-circuit the maladaptive cognitive–affective–behavioral reaction. The "Keeping Your Cool" video (Nelson, 1998) can also be particularly useful in this stage of awareness training, as it provides a model describing the basic components of anger and how to better manage such emotions.

The understanding of anger and aggression is integrated into the cognitive-behavioral framework of personality and presented as the "ABCs of personality." In other words, an individual's personality and the experience of anger is determined by how one thinks (A), feels (B), and acts (C). This ABC paradigm is derived from the rational–emotive model (Ellis, 1970; Ellis & Bernard, 1985). A, the activating experience, refers to the external event, problem, or "trigger" to

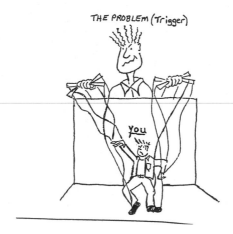

FIGURE 4.2. Illustration used to discuss the control that the client can have over anger.

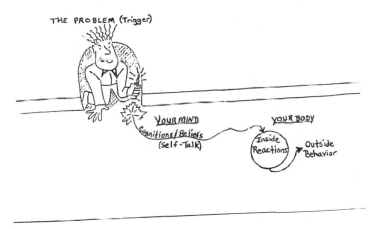

FIGURE 4.3. Illustration used to discuss potential of gaining control over anger.

which the child is exposed. B, the belief, refers to the chain of thoughts, images, or specific self-verbalizations that result in internal feelings and subsequent actions (behaviors) the adolescent goes through in response to A. Thus, B symbolizes the cognitive processes that occur within the adolescent in response to external events. Such processes include the child's appraisal of the situation, anticipated reactions of others, and self-statements in response to activating events. Finally, C, the consequences, refers to the environmental reactions that result from others reacting to the behavior of the adolescent.

Inside the Therapist's Office

The following is a brief interaction between the therapist and Dante, a 14-year-old African American referred for his anger management problems by his grandmother, who has custody of him. Dante's mother voluntarily gave custody of him to his grandmother 6 months earlier so that he could attend a better high school than the one in her neighborhood.

THERAPIST: I understand that you and your grandmother had a big problem Saturday.

DANTE: Yeah.

THERAPIST: Would you tell me a little more about it?

DANTE: (*Silence*) She's trying to treat me like a baby or something (*very angry tone*).

THERAPIST: You're 14 years old? A freshman, right? So, tell me about your grandmother treating you like a baby on Saturday.

DANTE: She kept getting in my face and told me I was grounded (*angry tone*).

[*Comments*: This is a fairly typical exchange with an adolescent; he is not forthcoming initially and is focusing blame on someone else. The therapist finds him- or herself in the middle of the interaction. It seems likely that grounding Dante is an event that happened as part of a more complex interaction but was not the start of it.]

THERAPIST: Let's start at the beginning. What time did you get up Saturday morning?

[*Comments*: This is a closed-ended question that the therapist hopes will help Dante begin discussing the interaction at the beginning and at a less emotionally charged part of the interaction.]

DANTE: I don't know (*resistant*).

THERAPIST: That's okay. It's a Saturday morning—tell me how you began your day?

DANTE: She came in my room and told me to get up and clean my room while she was cooking breakfast. I started to clean my room and I watched a little TV too, this one cartoon that I like.

THERAPIST: A typical Saturday morning? Cartoons and your grandmother cooks breakfast?

DANTE: Yeah, on weekends, Grandma cooks a big breakfast and I have to sit at the table and eat with her.

THERAPIST: During the week I guess mornings are pretty rushed with you getting ready for school and your grandmother getting ready for work. But on Saturday it sounds like it is a little more relaxed.

DANTE: Relaxed, right (*sarcastically*).

THERAPIST: So you *had* to eat breakfast with her. Then what happened?

DANTE: She was yelling at me, saying that I was supposed to clean my room since Friday, and that she was going to take my videogames and TV.

THERAPIST: So you didn't get around to cleaning your room on Friday?

DANTE: No, my friend came over so we could finish our championship game.

THERAPIST: Championship game?

DANTE: Yeah, John Madden Football. We had tied three games and he had to give the game back to his cousin the next day. Then I was too tired to clean up when we finished playing.

THERAPIST: So you put off cleaning your room until Saturday. It's Saturday and here is the room still waiting to be cleaned. What happened after breakfast?

DANTE: Well, after breakfast I started to clean it. My room was all messed up, and I knew it was going to take forever to clean it.

THERAPIST: (*Laughs*) Yeah, even I feel that way sometimes. Then what happens?

DANTE: I felt like I was going to be inside a long time, so I turned the TV on again.

THERAPIST: Umm-hmm, and what happened next?

DANTE: I heard Grandma saying that she was going to choir practice.

THERAPIST: So, you were now home alone?

DANTE: Yeah.

THERAPIST: What happens with the room?

DANTE: I noticed that the Madden game was left on the table. I decided to work on my football Playstation skills before my friend came to get it. Then, before I knew it, Grandma was back from choir practice. She was standing at my door!

THERAPIST: About how long was she gone?

DANTE: I don't know; probably the usual 2 hours.

THERAPIST: Then what happened?

DANTE: She comes in and unplugs my game and says that I need to clean my room now.

THERAPIST: She wanted you to start back cleaning your room.

DANTE: Yeah, she said I couldn't do anything else until my room was clean.

THERAPIST: What did you say?

DANTE: I told her I was getting ready to clean it, but she didn't have to disrespect my videogame system. I bought it with my own money!

THERAPIST: How were you feeling?

DANTE: I was cool—no, I was pissed! I'm tired of being treated like a baby. I don't have no privacy, not even with my own stuff!

THERAPIST: You were pissed. Then what happened?

DANTE: I started to make up my bed, but my friend knocked at the door to get his game. I heard her tell him that I couldn't come to the door because my room was a mess!

THERAPIST: Umm-hmm, so what happened?

DANTE: I went and opened the door and gave him the game. She was embarrassing me and stuff, so I went back to my room and slammed the door.

THERAPIST: Is that when you punched through the door?

DANTE: I guess so.

THERAPIST: Sounds like you were really angry then.

DANTE: Yeah. Who wouldn't be! I can't do anything! Nothing, without my grandmother all in my business! She didn't have to act like that, in front of my boy.

THERAPIST: Is this when you got grounded?

DANTE: First she took all my stuff! She didn't buy any of it. I'm the one who had to go out and cut all those lawns.

THERAPIST: And then you trashed your room?

DANTE: Yeah, I guess. It just happened; I was just throwing everything.

From a cognitive-behavioral model the above interaction is replete with a series of escalating interactions that can be conceptualized as a string of ABCs. This scenario depicts a fairly typical situation for a single parent or caretaker who is dealing with a variety of demands and stressors. There is a 14-year-old who is self-focused (not atypical) and believes that *all* things should go his way. In addition, as an urban African American male teenager, he may be particularly sensitive to being "controlled," particularly by a woman, since his environment requires him to be "tough." Furthermore, Dante is especially vulnerable to feeling disempowered—often a reaction to discrimination in society at large. However, his negative feelings are intensified because he is engaging in all-or-nothing thinking in which he is either a "baby" or a grown-up. A series of interactions leads to an escalating series of emotionally charged reactions.

In this interaction we can assume that the grandmother is already being pushed by Dante, who has not done what he was expected to do—clean his room on Friday. Dante finds himself faced with a boring task that he really does not want to do. In the ABC conceptualization, first there is the loss of his video game and his privacy—both are very important to him. This is an activating event (A) for Dante. He is frustrated and believes that things must go his way and according to his own schedule. In addition, Dante believes that he is being treated like a "baby" (a previously mentioned concern). He is fearful of being viewed by his friends as weak and unable to determine even the most ordinary decisions within his grandmother's house. A prized requirement within Dante's black urban adolescent peer group is to "act like a man," so being perceived as "a child" could be disastrous to his image. Yet, in Dante's catastrophic way of thinking, he believes that the worst outcome is the only possibility for him. This type of belief (B) leads to angry feelings and a subsequent aggressive outburst that is very frightening to his grandmother. She grounds him and contacts their social worker (C) in reaction to his inappropriate behavior.

Later in the session, the therapist attempts to help Dante understand how his negative self-talk and expectations and dysfunctional thinking served to escalate his anger and resulted in an even more undesirable outcome. Dante must first be invested. Therefore, it is crucial that the therapist help Dante regard his angry, aggressive behavior as the "enemy" that he wants to defeat before it defeats him. The therapist must be careful not to invalidate Dante's specific socioenvironmental experiences while exploring his irrational belief system.

Phase III: Skills Acquisition

The third phase within the training stress inoculation model is designed to provide the child with specific techniques, both cognitive and behavioral, to use during the coping process. During this phase, self-management strategies are targeted at the cognitive, affective, and behavioral levels, as anger-reducing self-talk, relaxation techniques, problem-solving skills, assertion training, and humor are introduced and taught. By having the "stage set" during the educational phase, children are further presented with the notion that what they ultimately do in any situation (behavior) is a choice and basically a function of how they feel (feelings), which, in turn, is more a function of how they think about a situation and what they say to themselves (e.g., explicit self-talk and thoughts). Thus, aggression is not triggered merely by environmental events but rather by the way in which these events are perceived and processed. Children with anger-control problems have been found to exhibit egocentric and distorted perceptions of social situations (Crick & Dodge, 1994; Lochman & Dodge, 1998; Lochman & Wells, 2002). In general, aggressive children typically attend to and remember hostile cues selectively in their interactions with others (Dodge, Price, Bachorowski, & Newman, 1990). Children with anger-control problems exhibit tendencies to overrecall hostile cues and may even remember situations in hostile terms, even if they were originally positive or neutral (Milich & Dodge, 1984). Perspective taking is a key cognitive element in adolescents' understanding of relationships (e.g., Chandler & Boyes, 1982). Aggressive children and adolescents overattribute hostility on the part of others (e.g., Dodge, Lochman, Harnish, Bates, & Petit, 1997; Lochman, Meyer, Rabiner, & White, 1991) in that aggressive adolescents quickly assume hostile intent on the part of others and subsequently are more likely to respond in an aggressive fashion based on inaccurately perceived threats. This distorted "viewpoint" of aggressive youth understandably makes them particularly prone to impulsively react aggressively in a wide range of problem situations.

One's ability to take the perspective of others and make inferences about their thoughts and attentions is called cognitive perspective taking. One's understanding of the feelings and internal emotions of others is called affective perceptive taking. Both are clearly influenced by developmental factors (e.g., Kimball, Nelson, & Politano, 1993). Such maladaptive interpersonal processing exacerbates the difficulties aggressive children have in interpersonal situations. Thus, aggressive youngsters seem to quickly assume that others will behave in a hostile fashion toward them and are more likely to respond in an aggressive fashion based on inaccurately perceived threats. The "Perspective Check" exercises in the workbook provide therapists with opportunities to deal with such distorted perspective taking and helps the youngster infer more accurately others' thoughts and intentions (cognitive perspective taking) and to subsequently enhance their understanding of others' feelings and emotional states (affective perspective taking). Workbook tasks assist adolescents in accurately identifying similarities and differences among individuals by considering alternative interpretations of social cues and considering alternatives inferences about what others may be thinking or feeling. For example, using the "Perspective Check" cartoon, the child is asked, "How does the boy feel about the mess?", "How does the mother feel?", and "How do their perspectives differ?" (see Figure 4.4).

The basic educational purpose in these tasks is to help adolescents better understand the idea that individuals (including themselves) have different perspectives and frequently misinterpret the intent, thoughts, and/or feelings of others. This idea may also be presented by having the therapist ask how the class bully or someone with a "chip on their shoulder" might respond to someone asking "Where'd you get that?" (in a gruff voice) and how his or her response would be different from someone else who did not have a "chip on their shoulder." In this way, adolescents learn to evaluate more accurately the intent of others by considering additional alternatives to hostile intent. Again, they are empowered in the sense that it is clarified how their hostile perceptions and appraisals in interpersonal situations, and their subsequent interpretation of others as threatening, can be altered, and they can engage in other cognitive or behavioral activities directed at developing more effective behavioral responses to their problems.

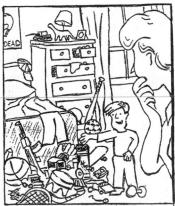

"But it looks better this way!"

FIGURE 4.4. Cartoon used to conduct a "perspective check."

Anger-reducing self-verbalizations and humor are employed in a systematic fashion that involves overt cognitive modeling, overt external guidance, overt self-guidance, faded overt modeling, faded overt self-guidance, covert guidance modeling, and covert self-guidance. The basic strategy is to have individuals engage in anger-reducing self-talk or to think of something funny to "short-circuit" the cognitive–affective–behavioral aggression chain.

Interventions at the cognitive level involve four of the five anger management skills in the stress inoculation model—self-talk, problem solving, assertion training, and humor. The following are brief descriptions of how these intervention techniques are presented in the *Keeping Your Cool* workbook. For each anger management skill, the technique is outlined in a "Playbook" that is employed in sessions and for homework. In this way the skill to be learned is taught in a step-by-step simplified fashion. Thus, we hope the reader can better understand how these "Plays" are run for individual children and adolescents. Play 1 (Self-Talk) fundamentally involves teaching the child to engage in anger-reducing self-talk rather than their well-learned anger-increasing self-talk in response to problem situations (see Figure 4.5). Anger-increasing self-talk has been popularized, and many youth, especially Latino, African American, and urban teenagers, may consider it to be beneficial in terms of peer group popularity, as being tough is a requisite of survival within the urban "street culture." Shaped by youth-oriented music, such as "gangsta rap" (Ghee, 1994; Rich, Woods, Goodman, Emans, & DuRant, 1998) and the violent themes in movies and video games (American Academy of Pediatrics, 2001), a youth subculture that glorifies aggression and anger has been propagated. Therefore, shifting from angry self-talk is unlikely to occur if it is to be replaced with what adolescents perceive as seemingly impotent or cowardly expressions. An effective strategy toward a positive cognitive shift for these youth is to tap into the potency of their media and challenge them to analyze and rewrite negative messages as prosocial ones while maintaining the empowering, vigorous self-images—but stripped of the violence (Ghee, Walker, & Younger, 1997). The "rap" music genre offers an opportune framework for these cognitive shifts because of its angry themes bolstered by rhythmic beats that intensify the lyrics. An exercise with a teenager referred for oppositional behavior demonstrates the effectiveness of this strategy. During therapy sessions, first this young man acknowledges that the lyrics of a popular and controversial rap musician (Eminem, in his song entitled "I Never Knew") represent his own situation. In this song, a violent but lyrical solution is presented in response to the question, "What, you want me to watch my mouth?".

Subsequently, the therapist discusses with the client the dysfunctional thoughts and negative consequences of the violent reactions prescribed in the lyrics. The therapist then works with the client to rewrite the lyrics, opting for a nonviolent solution:

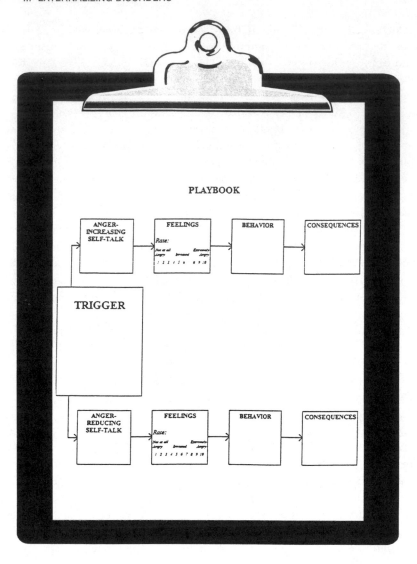

FIGURE 4.5. The Self-Talk Playbook.

> What, you want me to watch my mouth?
> How? If you look at my eyeballs for long,
> You'll know that I am strong.
> I don't need you telling me right from wrong,
> I need someone to understand my song.

A change in one's self-talk hopefully results in different feelings, behaviors, and consequences in response to problems that aggressive youngsters frequently encounter. A similar playbook is employed for Play 5 (Humor) (see Figure 4.6). Again, the basic strategy is to insert different cognitive processes between the anger-provoking situation and subsequent behavior.

Problem-solving and assertion training are more complex skills that involve systematic training. Play 3 (Problem Solving) basically teaches the adolescent the problem-solving process. The Problem Solving Playbook is depicted in Figure 4.7. As can be seen, the problem-solving sequence involves the following steps:

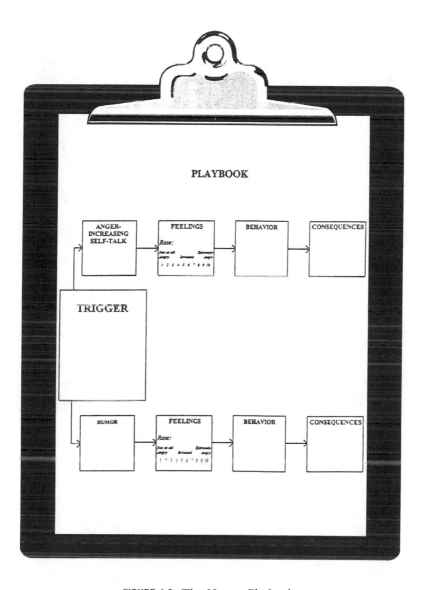

FIGURE 4.6. The Humor Playbook.

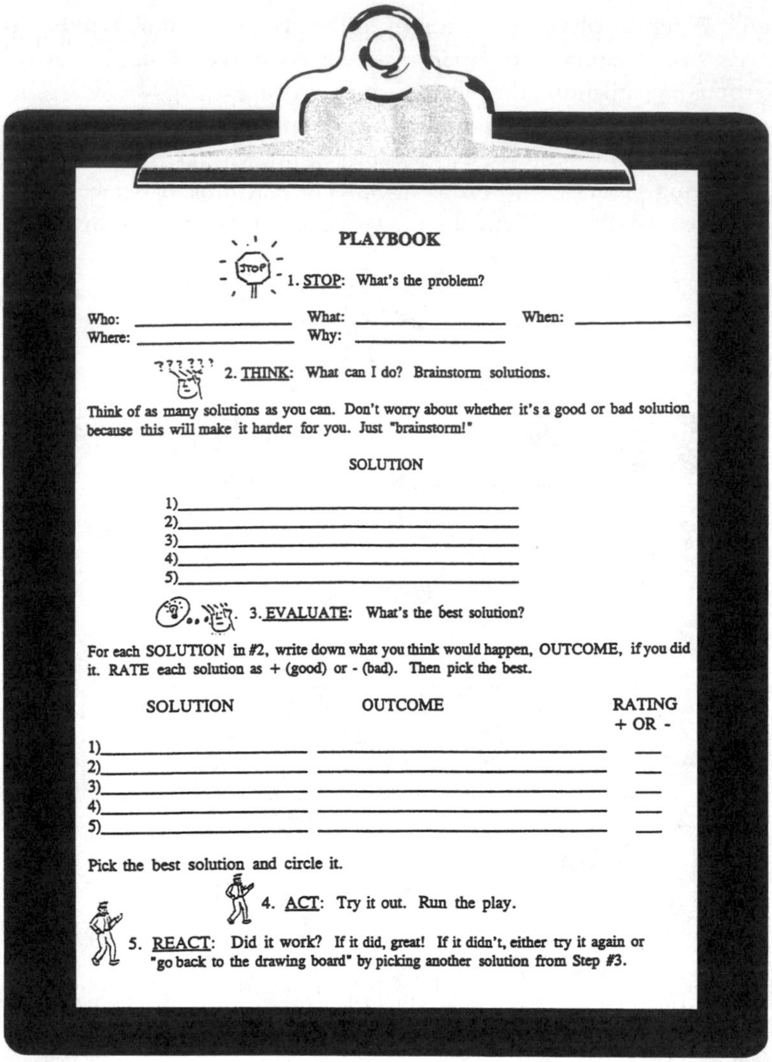

PLAYBOOK

1. STOP: What's the problem?

Who: ______ What: ______ When: ______
Where: ______ Why: ______

2. THINK: What can I do? Brainstorm solutions.

Think of as many solutions as you can. Don't worry about whether it's a good or bad solution because this will make it harder for you. Just "brainstorm!"

SOLUTION

1)______
2)______
3)______
4)______
5)______

3. EVALUATE: What's the best solution?

For each SOLUTION in #2, write down what you think would happen, OUTCOME, if you did it. RATE each solution as + (good) or - (bad). Then pick the best.

SOLUTION	OUTCOME	RATING + OR -
1)______	______	___
2)______	______	___
3)______	______	___
4)______	______	___
5)______	______	___

Pick the best solution and circle it.

4. ACT: Try it out. Run the play.

5. REACT: Did it work? If it did, great! If it didn't, either try it again or "go back to the drawing board" by picking another solution from Step #3.

FIGURE 4.7. The Problem-Solving Playbook.

1. *Stop*: What's the problem?
2. *Think*: What can I do? Brainstorm solutions.
3. *Evaluate:* What's the best solution?
4. *Act:* Try it out.
5. *React*: Did it work?

Play 4 (Assertion Training) is a more complex set of skills that are beyond the scope of this chapter to review. Nevertheless, the basic strategy is to teach aggressive adolescents alternative responses to situations that typically evoke anger and aggression. The basic format of assertion training involves assisting youth (1) to distinguish among aggressive, passive–aggressive, and assertive responses; (2) to identify their personal rights in various situations, (3) to identify and change irrational thoughts supporting nonassertive behavior; and (4) to practice assertive responses to various anger-arousing situations. The first step involves sharpening the children's ability to recognize the various ways of responding to different problems and to help identify their "Personal Rights" (see Figure 4.8). The Assertion Playbook is depicted in Figure 4.9.

YOUR BILL OF RIGHTS

1. You have the right to experience and express your feelings.

2. You have the right to voice your opinion about things.

3. You have the right to be treated with respect.

4. You have the right to say "no" to others and not feel guilty.

5. You have the right to take time to slow down and think.

6. You have the right to change your mind.

7. You have the right to be different or "your own person."

8. You have the right to ask for things you want.

9. You have the right to make mistakes.

10. You have the right to feel good about yourself.

Can you think of any others?

11. _____

12. _____

13. _____

FIGURE 4.8. Your Bill of Rights.

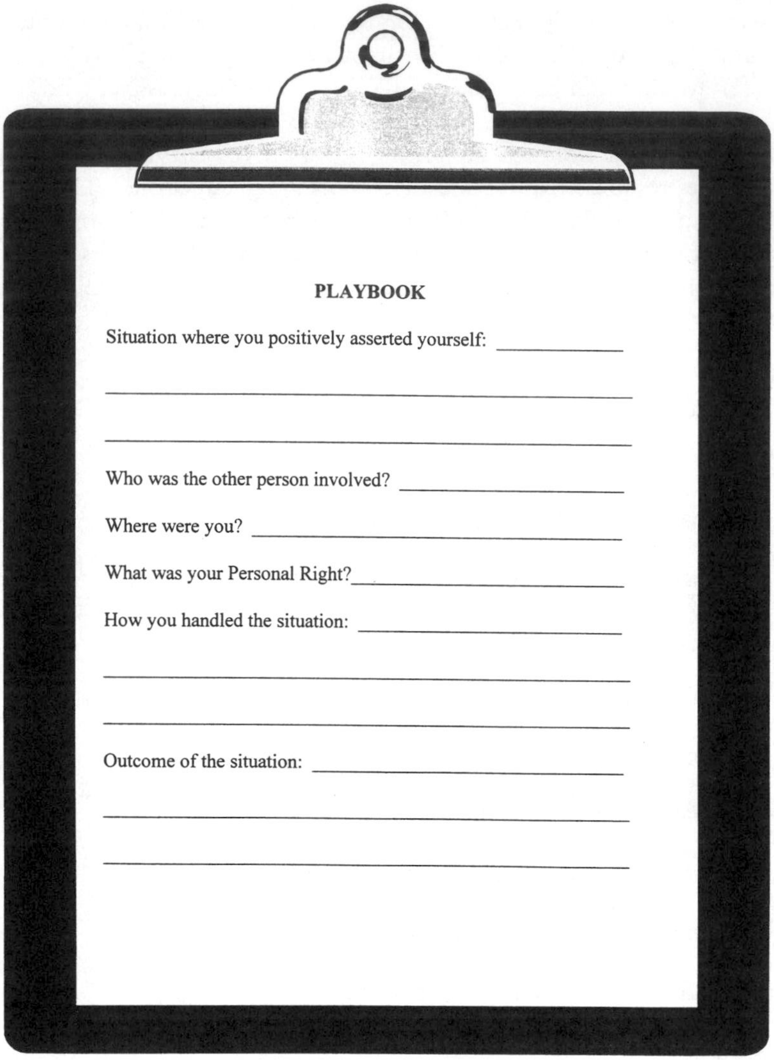

PLAYBOOK

Situation where you positively asserted yourself: _____

_____

_____

Who was the other person involved? _____

Where were you? _____

What was your Personal Right?_____

How you handled the situation: _____

_____

_____

Outcome of the situation: _____

_____

_____

FIGURE 4.9. The Assertion Playbook.

Play 2 (Relaxation) involves teaching youngsters deep breathing and relaxation techniques to use as an anger-reducing coping skill. The intervention takes place at the affective level and not the cognitive level, as do self-talk, humor, problem solving, and assertion training. Again, it is beyond the scope of this chapter to detail the specifics of relaxation training, although children are encouraged to rate their ability to use this by using the Relax-O-Meter (see Figure 4.10).

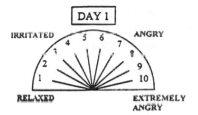

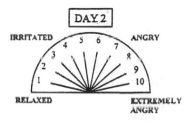

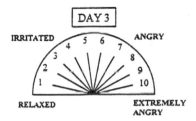

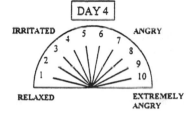

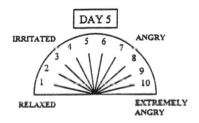

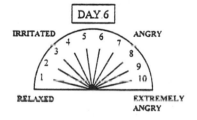

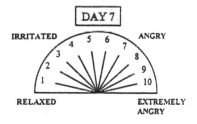

FIGURE 4.10. The Relax-O-Meter.

Overall, the goal is to help the child recognize the cognitive–physiological elements of anger, to decide whether or not expression of anger is appropriate, and then either to communicate feelings (anger) in a nonhostile, more adaptive manner or to engage in some form of problem-solving action that may include direct expressing of feelings.

Inside the Therapist's Office

In the following transcript the therapist works with the child to see the potential benefits of learning how to manage her anger. Although many youngsters we see with anger management problems do not admit they have a problem, they do recognize that they are not obtaining what they want in life. They are the ones who frequently find themselves in trouble and are losing various privileges. In the following exchange, the therapist attempts to form a "partnership" with the 12-year-old youngster, Megan, in managing her anger and thus prevent experiencing negative consequences.

THERAPIST: We've been talking about aggression and the various problems that people have with anger management. Do you have any ideas about your aggression and how you can better manage it, so you won't keep getting into trouble?

MEGAN: Yeah, I have lots of ideas, but I wouldn't be in trouble if people like Laura would just get a life and stop wishing she could live mine.

THERAPIST: Perhaps that is true. Anyway, you feel like her reporting you to the principal, who then suspended you, was an injustice because you didn't physically hurt anyone.

MEGAN: Damn right. There are some kids who deserve to be suspended; this is so unfair!

THERAPIST: I understand that you've had two detentions and now this suspension?

MEGAN: Does that file of yours say that I'm an honor student, the best forward on the soccer team, and I was the first student nominated for homecoming court?

THERAPIST: Thanks for giving me the bigger picture; some things are going really well for you. What I think we should do is to try to stop the detentions and suspensions, and aim for a very impressive record, not one that is marred. What do you think?

MEGAN: If it keeps me from competing for homecoming court, OK—but it's still not fair.

THERAPIST: OK. From what your mom and teacher said, it seems that you've been named for bullying other girls this year—but never before this year?

MEGAN: Yeah, it wasn't important before. Now, my school is full of those nerdy kids from that other school who think we're supposed to feel sorry for them because their school closed.

[*Comments*: Megan is an only child living in a two-parent household. Although both of her parents work outside the home, she lives near older relatives, being the third generation to live in their upper-middle-class neighborhood. Recently, Megan's school merged with another school since both had a low enrollment. However, there was a lengthy protest from the adults in the community. Megan's once familiar environment has changed significantly: Half of the students are new, and students now have to compete for membership in extracurricular programs. Megan has repeatedly been identified as the leader of a group of girls who have been intimidating and humiliating some of the new students using indirect relational aggression (e.g., sending cruel notes, telling nasty lies, spreading rumors, designating seats in the cafeteria to ostracize them, and pressuring other students to join together and chant insults at the new students). Initially, her parents ignored the complaints, assured that Megan had not physically endangered anyone; now that the school has suspended Megan, they are very concerned.

THERAPIST: It seems like you would be much better off if you did not have to deal with any more detentions or suspensions.

MEGAN: Just send all those nerds like Laura to another school!

THERAPIST: That's an idea, but I don't think that is something you and I are going to make happen.

MEGAN: Whatever (*sarcastically*). You think I don't already know that?

THERAPIST: But you and I can work together in getting you back into school next week. And I understand that they will clear your record if there are not any more problems for the rest of the school year.

MEGAN: I can't let this hurt my chances of winning homecoming court.

THERAPIST: OK, we have a goal. And it seems that you agree that it would be good if I could help you return to school and stay out of the principal's office.

MEGAN: OK.

THERAPIST: Good! Now let's look at what aggression is and see where we can break the chain of events that leads to your getting into trouble.

The therapist has formed an agreement with Megan to help her attain a desirable and mutually agreed-upon goal—eliminating referrals to the principal's office and subsequent discipline. This goal is likely to meet both Megan's needs (a more acceptable school record and a chance at winning homecoming court) and to decrease the relationally aggressive behaviors that resulted in the referral for psychological treatment. All of Megan's school problems are related to aggressive manipulation of other girls. Although she believes her behavior is justified, she escalates her aggressiveness when she is angry and concerned that a student will report her to the principal. Megan sees the "problem" as being the fault of other students but now is willing to work to develop skills that will stop her detentions and suspensions.

Phase IV: Application Training

After the youngster has become proficient in one or more of the skills taught during Phase III, the therapist provides the opportunity to test these skills in controlled situations. Note that proficiency in all five anger management skills is not necessary. It is better to work on only several of these, learn them well, and then practice these newly learned anger management skills. Thus, the workbook allows the gradual build-up to the more difficult interactions in an anger hierarchy. The workbook is designed to ensure that the child understands and has learned the anger management strategies before having to apply them in emotionally arousing anger situations, thus optimizing successful outcomes. This is accomplished by having the therapist and child engage in structured role-play scenarios in therapy sessions to "test" their newly learned skills. This practice is done in both imaginal and direct-action role-play scenarios, employing a number of anger situations the child is likely to encounter in real life. Once the child is proficient, the therapist can use "barbs" (Kaufmann & Wagner, 1972). A "barb" is a provocative statement that is applied in situations other than in the training/ therapy situation. The rationale and procedure are explained to the child, whom the therapist then warns, "I'm going to barb you" (e.g., "Don't look at me like that! You're grounded tomorrow!"). Parents, teachers, staff members, and other significant individuals deliver the barbs and record the child's responses for review and discussion in subsequent therapy sessions. Overall, homework assignments are very familiar to children and play a pivotal role in cognitive-behavioral interventions. It is the main mechanism to foster generalization of treatment effects into the real world by providing a structure in which the child practices anger management skills. The implication also is that children (as well as parents) are taught that improvement in their situation is a product of their own efforts rather than those of the therapist.

The workbook also includes a series of bookmarks and other ways of providing prompts or external cues to utilize the newly learned anger management skills in real-life situations. Finally, the workbook encourages youngsters to "make a commercial" (e.g., produce a commercial; write a poem, poster, or sign; draw a picture) to show others how they learned to defeat the opponent, anger. Such "peer teaching" not only facilitates the learning of anger management strategies but also helps prepare the client for termination that is celebrated with a Certificate of Achievement that announces that the child has now learned to better manage his or her anger. The process of termination from a cognitive-behavioral perspective is part of the planned intervention process (see Nelson & Politano, 1993, for further discussion).

INTEGRATION OF INDIVIDUAL AND FAMILY INTERVENTIONS: FUTURE DIRECTIONS

There is an increasing awareness of the benefits of involving parents in the treatment of children and adolescents. Such involvement has ranged from an exclusive focus on parent training treatments (e.g., Patterson, 1982, 1986) to parents' indirect supporting roles in cognitive interventions (e.g., Kendall & MacDonald, 1993). Within the child-focused cognitive-behavioral treatments, broadening these to include parent training seems to facilitate treatment efficacy. Although several treatment programs have combined some type of parent training with individual cognitive-behavioral approaches (e.g., Horne & Sayger, 1990; Kazdin, 2003; Webster-Stratton & Hammond, 1997), more research on the implications of active involvement of parents in these more individually tailored treatment programs is needed. For example, Kazdin (1993) found problem-solving training combined with parent management training to be superior in children and adolescents (ages 7–23 years) referred for severe antisocial/aggressive behavior. In addition, Brestan and Eyberg (1998) reviewed 82 controlled studies involving psychosocial interventions for child and adolescent conduct problems and found videotape modeling parent-training programs and those based on Patterson and Gullion's (1971) manual, *Living with Children*, to be effective. Reviews (Chamberlain & Rosicky, 1995; Estrada & Pinsof, 1995) found that family interventions consistently improved child and parent functioning in their analyses of the scientific evidence for the effectiveness of family-based approaches in the treatment of aggressive children with conduct disorders. Thus, the involvement of parents in treatment programs seems like a good idea, as the family plays a critical role in a child's development. Nevertheless, there can be difficulties with parental participation in a child's treatment. Involving more than one person in a treatment program can make it more complex for the therapist to manage. Furthermore, therapists using parent-based child interventions for youth with conduct disorders have found that it is often difficult to persuade parents to participate (e.g., Hawkins, von-Cleve, & Catalano, 1991) and attrition rates are high (Forehand, Middlebrook, Rogers, & Steffe, 1983). In addition, parents of highly aggressive children can be as difficult to work with as the children themselves, because the parents of acting-out children have shown a higher frequency of deviant behavior, exhibit less mature moral judgment, and have been found to be more rejecting, to use harsh power-assertive punishment, to model aggressive criminal behavior, and to be erratically permissive and inconsistent in enforcing rules. Also they are simply "worn-out" in dealing with their children and although they may love them, they may not like them at the beginning of therapy. Despite these difficulties, the potential benefits for involving parents are notable insofar as treatment gains not only need to be generalized to the home, school, and elsewhere, but also maintained over time. Because the parents, in large part, contribute to the environment in which a child develops over time, they can contribute to the generalization and treatment gains over time and prevent relapse. Although it is beyond the scope of this chapter, Kazdin and Kendall (1998) outlined a blueprint for progress in treatment research that recommends expanded assessment, addressing a broad range of treatment questions, evaluating "clinical significance," replicating findings, and exploring how to make use of research findings for practicing clinicians.

Key issues still remain as to what types of interventions are most effective for what specific children, how to best integrate the various parent-training components with individual interventions, and how to determine the conditions under which therapeutic interventions are maximally effective (e.g., school-/community-based programs). In this endeavor, any intervention components need to be fundamentally based on social learning, cognitive-behavioral, and behavioral principles. Parents of acting-out youngsters need to be taught to carefully observe the child and to clearly identify positive and maladaptive behaviors. Most parent training focuses on how to reinforce children's attempts at better managing their anger and to effectively deal with incidents when their children do not manage their anger. Consistency, negotiation, and behavioral contracting are all elements of parent training that have been employed for years, and for which manuals for parents and therapist are available (e.g., McMahon, Forehand, & Guest, 1981; Patterson & Forgatch, 1987; Patterson & Gullion, 1971; Patterson, Reid, Jones, & Conger, 1975). These and other techniques, especially from strategic family therapists, also offer the potential to augment individual child/adolescent treatment interventions (e.g., Price, 1996; Sells, 1998). Remember that cognitive-behavioral treatments are also "behavioral" in nature, in the sense that the use of clear, effective consequences for severe acting should be integrated with the more "cognitive" approaches. For example, in employing the *Keeping Your Cool* workbook (Nelson & Finch, 1996), one of the authors (Nelson) has had some success in teaching anger management skills to angry/aggressive parents who have problems with managing their own anger, requiring that they immediately teach these same self-control techniques to their acting-out child. In this way, both the adult (typically the father in two-parent homes) and child are treated, and the parent is "hooked" into treatment himself by having him help his child. Such a task alters the father–son relationship and places the father more in the role of educator than disciplinarian. Not only does this therapeutic intervention provide the father with needed anger management skills, but it also aims at shifting and ultimately improving the father–son relationship. Coupled with such an approach is also the "behavioral" side, where parents are coached in developing consequences that are effective in stopping extreme aggressive acting out without being abusive. Notwithstanding, specific parent interventions should be designed to meet the needs of the increasing number of single-parent homes, the majority of which are headed by women. Because these women tend to be younger, poorer, and less educated (Amato, 2000), providing the single mother with anger management skills while improving child–mother relationships promises to enhance the child's supervision and guidance.

The use of manuals in providing psychological treatments for children and adolescents has been a source of controversy over the past 15 years. Heated discussions of politics and religion, as well as the usefulness of projective testing among psychologists, attest to the emotionally charged conflicting opinions surrounding the use of empirically supported treatments. Before "jumping into the fray" in such heated discussions, it is important to know the difference between treatments that have been labeled as "empirically validated," "empirically supported," and "empirically evaluated" (e.g., Chambless et al., 1996). The first term suggests that treatments that are already validated assume a state of completeness or finality. In point of fact, it may be argued that there are no treatments for children and adolescents that are so validated that the use of them is a closed question. Validation is never completed and closed, and some have argued that the notion that therapy provides a "cure" is a misleading belief (Kendall, 1989). Those therapies that purport to be "empirically supported" suggest that treatment has been supported by acceptable empirical studies. The implication, however, is that there is some empirically based evidence to label therapy as such. Finally, the third type, "empirically evaluated" therapies, simply suggests that treatments have been empirically evaluated and that, at least to some degree they have been supported, but such a statement does not prematurely close the process of evaluation (see Kendall, 1998, for further discussion).

Labeling treatments as described has become such an emotionally charged topic because of the potential for use and abuse of such connotations. Such questions as "Would it be ethical to provide an as-yet-unevaluated treatment when there are already some data supporting other therapies and other theoretical orientations?" have been raised. Will empirically supported treatments lead to a restrictive list of treatments taught in graduate schools and clinics (and reimbursed by third parties)? Will such treatments be viewed as simply being "mandated"? To what degree should flexibility be allowed in using treatment manuals, or in adhering to a manual that does not guarantee quality therapy? Certainly we know about some efficacy for some treatments for some disorders, but the effectiveness or clinical utility of such interventions certainly requires more work (see Christopherson & Mortweet, 2003; Kazdin, 2003). These issues hit upon the age-old tension between scientists and practitioners and how interventions found to be efficacious can be transported into service provider settings.

It is with such issues in mind that *"Keeping Your Cool": The Anger Management Workbook* (Nelson & Finch, 1996) was developed. Such a workbook is empirically supported because it was developed by carefully surveying cognitive-behavioral procedures that were found to have some empirical support within the literature (Beck & Fernandez, 1998; Digiuseppe & Tafrate, 2003; Wilson, Gottfredson, & Najaka, 2001; Wilson, Lipsey, & Derzon, 2003). This workbook was also designed to facilitate "transportability" (see Kendall, 1998; Stirman, Crits-Christoph, & De Rubeis, 2004), in the sense that it makes cognitive-behavioral interventions "user-friendly" for both therapists and clients by providing a structured manual-based format for working with clients. It provides an overall framework that outlines treatment sessions and goals, supplies strategies that aid the therapist from different theoretical orientations in achieving their goals, and guides the therapist as he or she tries to tailor interventions to the particular client over the course of treatment. It provides a blueprint for practitioners who need to "breathe life into the manual" (Kendall et al., 1998). Despite the proliferation of a variety of empirically evaluated treatment programs and manuals, the impact of these interventions on actual clinical practice has been modest, at best (e.g., Addis & Krasnow, 2000; Chorpita & Nakamura, 2004). A major challenge still lies ahead of us—just how not only to increase the availability of the latest knowledge about psychological treatments to deliverers and consumers of mental-health services, but also to actively facilitate the actual use of such treatments in actual practice (e.g., Stirman et al., 2004).

In sum, considerable progress toward refining theoretical models, making meaningful differential diagnoses, and formulating adequate treatments for aggressive youth has been made (Nelson et al., in press). Nevertheless, much more remains to be done. Being equipped with the best possible therapeutic approaches and the continued empirical evaluation of these interventions will hopefully lead us to being able to even better assist acting-out, aggressive children and adolescents in developing into adults who are healthy, productive members of society.

NOTE

1. A copy of a summary table of the child/adolescent studies cited in the Beck and Fernandez (1998) study is available from W. Michael Nelson, III, Department of Psychology, Xavier University, Cincinnati, OH 45207-6411.

REFERENCES

Achenbach, T. M. (1991). *Manual for the Child Behavior Checklist/4–18 and 1991 profile.* Burlington: University of Vermont, Department of Psychiatry.

Achenbach, T., & Edelbrock, C. (1983). *Manual for the Child Behavior Checklist and Revised Behavior Profile.* Burlington: University Associates in Psychiatry.

Achenbach, T., & Howell, C. (1993). Are American children's problems getting worse? A 13-year comparison. *Journal of the American Academy of Child and Adolescent Psychiatry, 32*(6), 1145–1154.

Addis, M. E., & Krasnow, A. D. (2000). A rational survey of practicing psychologists' attitudestoward psychotherapy treatment manuals. *Journal of Consulting and Clinical Psychology, 68*, 331–339.

Alberti, R., & Emmons, M. (2001. *Your perfect right* (8th ed.). San Luis Obispo, CA: Impact

Amato, P. R. (2000). Diversity within single-parent families. In D. H. Demo, K. R. Allen, & M. Fine (Eds.), *Handbook of family diversity* (pp. 149–172). New York: Oxford University Press.

American Academy of Pediatrics. (2001). Media violence. *Pediatrics, 108*(5), 1222–1226.

American Psychiatric Association. (2000). *Diagnostic and statistical manual of mental Disorders* (4th ed., text rev.). Washington, DC: Author.

American Psychological Association. (1993). *Summary report of the American Psychological Association Commission on violence and youth: Vol. 1. Psychology's response.* Washington, DC: Author.

Bandura, A. (1986). *Social functions of thought and action: A social cognitive theory.* Englewood Cliffs, NJ: Prentice-Hall.

Beck, R., & Fernandez, E. (1998). Cognitive behavioral therapy in the treatment of anger: A meta-analysis. *Cognitive Therapy and Research, 22*, 63–74.

Beck, A. T., Rush, A. J., Shaw, B. F., & Emery, G. (1979). *Cognitive therapy of depression.* New York: Guilford Press.

Benson, H., Kornhaber, A., Kornhaber, C., & LeChanu, M. (1994). Increases in positive psychological characteristics with a new relaxation-response curriculum in high school students. *Journal of Research and Development in Education 27*, 226–231.

Beutler, L. E. (2004). The empirically supported treatments movement: A scientist-practitioner's response. *Clinical Psychology: Service and Practice, 11*, 225–229.

Boyd-Franklin, N. (2003). *Black families in therapy: Understanding the African American experience* (2nd ed.). New York: Guilford Press.

Brandt, E. E., & Zlotnick, S. J. (1988). *The psychology and treatment of the youthful offender.* Springfield, IL: Thomas.

Brestan, E. V., & Eyberg, S. M. (1998). Effective psychological treatments of conduct-disordered children and adolescents: 29 years, 82 studies, 5,272 kids. *Journal of Clinical Child Psychology, 27*, 180–189.

Broidy, L. M., Nagin, D. S., Tremblay, R. E., Bates, J. E., Brame, B., Dodge, K. A., et al. (2003). Developmental trajectories of childhood disruptive behaviors and adolescent delinquency: A six-site, cross-national study. *Developmental Psychology, 39*, 222–245.

Bronfenbrenner, U. (1989). Ecological systems theory. In R. Vasta (Ed.), *Analysis of child development* (Vol. 6, pp. 187–250). Greenwich, CT: JAI Press.

Buchanan, A. (1997). The investigation of acting on delusions as a tool for risk assessment in the mentally disordered. *British Journal of Psychiatry, 170*(Suppl. 32), 12–14.

Buckman, E. (Ed.). (1994). *The handbook of humor: Clinical applications in psychotherapy.* Malabar, FL: Krieger.

Cairns, R. B., Cairns, B. D., Neckerman, H. J., Ferguson, L. L., & Gariepy, J. L. (1989). Growth and Aggression 1: Childhood to early adolescence. *Developmental Psychology, 25*, 320–330.

Chamberlain, P., & Rosicky, J. G. (1995). The effectiveness of family therapy in the treatment of adolescents with conduct disorders and delinquency. *Journal of Marital and Family Therapy, 21*, 441–459.

Chambless, D. L., Sanderson, W. C., Shohan, V., Johnson, S. B., Pope, K. S., Crits-Christoph, P., et al. (1996). An update on clinically validated therapies. *Clinical Psychologist, 49*, 5–18.

Chandler, M., & Boyes, M. (1982). Social cognitive development. In B. Wolman (Ed.), *Handbook of developmental psychology* (pp. 387–402). New York: Wiley.

Chapman, A. & Chapman-Santana, M. (1995). *The use of humor in psychotherapy. Arquivos de Neuro-Psiquiatria, 53*, 153–156.

Chen, Y., Swann, A., & Burt, D. (1996). Stability of diagnosis in schizophrenia. *American Journal of Psychiatry, 153*(5), 682–686.

Chesney-Lind, M., & Brown. M. (1999). Girls and violence: An overview. In D. J. Flannery & C. R. Huff (Eds.), *Youth violence: Prevention, intervention, and social policy* (pp. 171–199). Washington, DC: American Psychiatric Press.

Chorpita, B. F., & Nakamura, B. J. (2004). Four considerations for dissemination of intervention innovations. *Clinical Psychology: Science and Practice, 11*, 364–367.

Christopherson, E. R., & Mortweet, S. L. (2003). "Treatments that work with children: Empirically suggested strategies for managing problems. Washington, DC: American Psychological Association.

Clarke, G., Lewinsohn, P., & Hops, H. (1990). *Adolescent coping with depression course.* Eugene, OR: Castalia Press.

Cohen, M., Miller, T., & Rossman, S. (1994). The costs and consequences of violent behavior in the United States. In A. J. Reiss & J. A. Roth (Eds.), *Understanding and preventing violence: Vol. 4. Consequences and control* (pp. 67–167). Washington, DC: National Academic Press.

Commission for the Prevention of Youth Violence. (2000). *Youth and violence: Medicine, nursing, and public health: Connecting the dots to prevent violence.* Retrieved on November 7, 2004, from www.ama-assn.org/upload/mm/386/fullreport.pdf.

Crick, N. R., & Bigbee, M. A. (1998). Relational and overt forms of peer victimization: A multi-informant approach. *Journal of Consulting and Clinical Psychology, 66*(2), 337–347.

Crick, N. R., Casas, J. F., & Mosher, M. (1997). Relational and overt aggression in preschool. *Developmental Psychology, 33*, 579–588.

Crick, N. R., & Dodge, K. A. (1994). A review and reformulization of social-information processing mechanisms in children's social adjustment. *Psychological Bulletin, 115*, 74–101.

Crick, N. R., & Grotpeter, J. K. (1995). Relational aggression, gender, and social-psychological adjustment. *Child Development, 66*, 710–722.

Crick, N. R., Grotpeter, J. K., & Rockhill, C. M. (1999). A social information-processing approach to children's loneliness. In K. J. Rothenberg & S. Hymel (Eds.), *Loneliness in childhood and adolescence* (pp. 153–175). New York: Cambridge University Press.

Dana, R. (1994). Humor as a diagnostic tool in child and adolescent groups. In E. Buckman (Ed.), *The handbook of humor: Clinical applications in psychotherapy* (pp. 41–51). Malabar, FL: Kriegar Publishing.

Dana, R. H. (2000). An assessment-intervention model for research and practice with multicultural populations. In R.H. Dana (Ed.), *Handbook of cross-cultural and multicultural personality assessment* (pp. 5–16). Mahwah, NJ: Erlbaum.

Deffenbacher, J., Lynch, R., Oetting, E., & Kemper, C. (1996). Anger reduction in early adolescents. *Journal of Counseling Psychology, 43*, 149–157.

Deluty, R. H. (1979). Children's Action Tendency Scale: A self-report measure of aggressiveness, assertiveness, and submissiveness in children. *Journal of Consulting and Clinical Psychology, 47*, 1061–1071.

DiGiuseppe, R., & Tafrate, R. C. (2003). Anger treatment for adults: A meta-analytic review. *Clinical Psychology: Science and Practice, 10*, 70–84.

Dodge, K. A. (1991). The structure and function of reactive and protective aggression. In D. J. Pepper & K. H. Rubin (Eds.), *The development and treatment of childhood aggression* (pp. 210–218). Hillsdale, NJ: Erlbaum.

Dodge, K. A., Lochman, J. E., Harnish, J. D., Bates, J. E., & Petit, G. (1997). Reactive and proactive aggression in school children and psychiatrically impaired chronically assaultive youth. *Journal of Abnormal Psychology, 106*, 37–51.

Dodge, K. A., Price, J. M., Bachorowski, J., & Newman, J. P. (1990). Hostile attributional biases in severely aggressive adolescents. *Journal of Abnormal Psychology, 99*, 385–392.

Dollard, J., Doob, L. W., Miller, N. E., Mowrer, O. H., & Sears, R. R. (1939). *Frustration and aggression.* New Haven, CT: Yale University Press.

Dong, Y., Hallberg, E., & Hassard, H. (1979). Effects of assertion training on aggressive behavior of adolescents. *Journal of Counseling Psychology, 26*, 459–461.

Dujovne, V., Barnard, M., & Rapoff, M. (1995). Pharmacological and cognitive behavioral approaches in the treatment of childhood depression: A review and critique. *Clinical Psychology Review, 15*, 589–611.

Dumas, J. E. (1989). Treating antisocial behavior in children: Child and family approaches. *Clinical Psychology Review, 9*, 197–222.

Eisen, A., & Silverman, W. (1993). Should I relax or change my thoughts? A preliminary examination of cognitive therapy, relaxation training, and their combination with overanxious children. *Journal of Cognitive Psychotherapy, 7*, 265–279.

Ellis, A. (1970). *The essence of rational psychotherapy: A comprehensive approach to treatment.* New York: Institute for Rational Living.

Ellis, A., & Bernard, M. E. (1985). *Rational-emotive approaches to the problems of childhood.* New York: Plenum Press.

Estrada, A. U., & Pinsof, W. M. (1995). The effectiveness of family therapies for selected behavioral disorders of childhood. *Journal of Marital and Family Therapy, 21*, 403–440.

Eyberg, S. M., Boggs, J. P., & Algina, J. (1995). New developments in psychosocial, pharmacological, and combined treatments of conduct disorders in aggressive children. *Psychopharmacology Bulletin, 31*, 83–91.

Fagan, J., Zimring, F. E., & Kim, J. (1998). Declining homicide in New York City: A tale of two trends. *Journal of Criminal Law and Criminology, 88*(4), 1277–1323.

Farrington, D. P. (1991). Childhood aggression and adult violence: Early precursors and life outcomes. In D. J. Pepler & K. H. Rubin (Eds.), *The development and treatment of childhood aggression* (pp. 5–29). Hillsdale, NJ: Erlbaum.

Farrington, D. P. (1995). The development of offending and antisocial behavior from childhood: Key findings from the Cambridge Study in Delinquent Development. *Journal of Child Psychology and Psychiatry, 36*, 929–964.

Farrington, D. P. (1994). Childhood, adolescent, and adult features of violent males. In L. R. Huesmann (Ed.), *Aggressive behavior: Current perspectives* (pp. 215–240). New York: Plenum Press.

Farrington, D. P. (1986). The application of stress theory to the study of family violence: Principles, problems, and prospects. *Journal of Family Violence, 1*(2), 131–147.

Farrington, D. P., Loeber, R., & Van Kammen, W. B. (1990). Long-term clinical outcomes of hyperactivity-impulsivity-attention deficit and conduct problems in childhood. In L. N. Robins & M. Rutter (Eds.), *Straight and devious pathways from childhood to adulthood* (pp. 62–81). Cambridge, UK: Cambridge University Press.

Finch, A. J., Jr., Nelson, W. M., III, & Moss, J. H. (1993). Childhood aggression: Cognitive-behavioral therapy strategies and interventions. In A. J. Finch, Jr., W. M. Nelson, III, & E. S. Ott (Eds.), *Cognitive-behavioral procedures with children and adolescents: A practical guide* (pp. 148–205). Boston: Allyn & Bacon.

Finch, A. J., Jr., Nelson, W. M., III, & Ott, E. S. (1993). *Cognitive-behavioral procedures with children and adolescents: A practical guide.* Boston: Allyn & Bacon.

Finch, A. J., Jr., & Politano, P. M. (1994). Projective techniques. In T. H. Ollendick, N. J. King, & W. Yule (Eds.), *International handbook of phobic and anxiety disorders in children and adolescents* (pp. 381–393). New York: Plenum Press.

Fingerhut, L. A., & Kleinman, J. C. (1990). International and interstate comparisons of homicide among young males. *Journal of the American Medical Association, 263*, 3292–3295.

Forehand, R., Middlebrook, J., Rogers, T., & Steffe, M. (1983). Dropping out of parent training. *Behaviour Research and Therapy, 21,* 663–668.

Freud, S. A. (1920). *A general introduction to psycho-analysis.* New York: Boni & Liveright.

Fry, W., & Salameh, W. (Eds.). (1993). *Advances in humor and psychotherapy.* Sarasota, FL: Professional Resources Press.

Ghee, K. L. (1994). Edu-Culture: An innovative strategy for promoting identity and scholarship in young African American males. In B. A Jones & K. M. Borman (Eds.), *Investing in U.S. schools: Directions for educational policy* (pp. 102–125). Norwood, NJ: Ablex.

Ghee, K. L., Walker, J., Younger, A. (1997). The RAAMUS Academy: Evaluation of an educultural after-school intervention for young African American males. *Journal of Prevention and Intervention in the Community, 16*(1/2), 87–102.

Hawkins, J. D., von Cleve, E., & Catalano, R. F. (1991). Reducing early childhood aggression: Results of a primary prevention program. *Journal of the American Academy of Child and Adolescent Psychiatry, 30,* 208–217.

Helms, J., & Cook, D. (1999). *Using race and culture in counseling and psychotherapy: Theory and practice.* Boston: Allyn & Bacon.

Hill, J. (2002). Biological, psychological and social processes of conduct disorders. *Journal of Child Psychology and Psychiatry, 43,* 133–164.

Horne, A. M., & Sayger, T. V. (1990). *Treating conduct and oppositional defiant disorders in children.* Elmsford, NY: Pergamon.

Jacobsen, R. (1938). *Progressive relaxation.* Chicago: University of Chicago Press.

Jerrell, J. (2003). Are assessment and treatment influenced by ethnicity and gender? *Psychiatric Times, 20*(10), 71–74.

Kaufman, L., & Wagner, B. (1972). Barb: A systematic treatment technology for temper control disorders. *Behavior Therapy, 3,* 84–90.

Kazdin, A. E. (1987). Treatment of antisocial behavior in children: Current status and future directions. *Psychological Bulletin, 102,* 187–203.

Kazdin, A. E. (1993). Treatment of conduct disorder: Progress and directions in psychotherapy research. *Development and Psychopathology, 5,* 277–310.

Kazdin, A. E. (1995). *Conduct disorder in childhood and adolescence* (2nd ed.). Thousand Oaks, CA: Sage.

Kazdin, A. E. (2003). Problem-solving skills training and parent management training for conduct disorder. In A. E. Kazdin & J. R. Weisz (Eds.), *Evidence-based psychotherapies for children and adolescents* (pp. 241–262). New York: Guilford Press.

Kazdin, A. E., & Kendall, P. C. (1998). Current progress and future plans for developing effective treatments: Comments and perspectives. *Journal of Clinical Child Psychology, 27,* 217–226.

Kazdin, A. E., Rodgers, A., Colbus, D., & Siegel, T. (1987). Children's Hostility Inventory: Measurement of aggression and hostility in psychiatric inpatient children. *Journal of Clinical Child Psychology, 16,* 320–328.

Kendall, P. C. (1998). Empirically supported psychological therapies. *Journal of Consulting and Clinical Psychology, 66,* 3–6.

Kendall, P. C., Chu, B., Gifford, A. Hayes, C., & Nauta, M. (1998). Breathing life into a manual: Flexibility and creativity with manual-based treatments. *Cognitive and Behavioral Practice, 5*(2), 177–198.

Kendall, P. C., & Flannery-Schroeder, E. C. (1995). Rigor, but not rigor mortis, in depression research. *Journal of Personality and Social Psychology, 69,* 892–894.

Kendall, P. C., Hollon, S. D., Beck, A. T., Hammen, C. H., & Ingram, R. E. (1987). Issues and recommendations regarding use of the Beck Depression Inventory. *Cognitive Therapy and Research, 11,* 289–299.

Kendall, P. C., & MacDonald, J. P. (1993). Cognition in the psychopathology of youth and complications for treatment. In K. S. Dobson & P. C. Kendall (Eds), *Psychopathology and cognition* (pp. 387–432). San Diego, CA: Academic Press.

Kimball, W., Nelson, W. M., III, & Politano, P. M. (1993). The role of developmental variables in cognitive-behavioral interventions with children. In A. J. Finch, Jr., W. M. Nelson, III, & E. S. Ott (Eds.), *Cognitive-behavioral procedures with children and adolescents* (pp. 25–66). Boston: Allyn & Bacon.

Koeppen, A. (1974, October). Relaxation training for children. *Elementary School Guidance and Counseling*, pp. 14–21.

Lagerspetz, K. M., Bjorkqvist, K., & Peltonen, T. (1988). Is indirect aggression more typical of females? Gender differences in 11- to 12-year-old children. *Aggressive Behavior, 14*, 403–414.

Lahey, B. B., Moffitt, T. E., & Caspi, A. (Eds.). (2003). *Causes of conduct disorder and juvenile delinquency*. New York: Guilford Press.

Lansford, J. E., Dodge, K. A., Petit, G. S., Bates, J. E., Crozier, J., & Kaplow, J. (2002). Long-term effects of early child physical maltreatment on psychologinormalities. *Journal of Autism and Developmental Disorders, 26*, 205–209.

Larson, J., & Lochman, J. E. (2002). *Helping schoolchildren cope with anger: A cognitive-behavioral intervention*. New York: Guilford Press.

Levant, R. F. (2004). The empirically validated treatments movement: A practitioner's perspective. *Clinical Psychology: Service Practice, 11*, 219–224.

Limandri, B., & Sheridan, D. (1995). Prediction of intentional interpersonal violence. An introduction. In J. C. Campbell (Ed.), *Assessing dangerousness: Violence by sexual offenders, batterers, and child abusers* (pp. 1–19). Thousand Oaks, CA: Sage.

Lipsey, M. W. (1992). Juvenile delinquency treatment: A meta-analytic inquiry into the variability of effects. In T. D. Cook, H. Cooper, D. S. Cordray, H. Hartmann, L. V. Hedges, R. J. Light, et al. (Eds.), *Meta-analysis for explanation: A casebook* (pp. 83–126). New York: Russell Sage Foundation.

Lochman, J. E. (1992). Cognitive-behavioral interventions with aggressive boys: Three-year follow-up and preventive effects. *Journal of Consulting and Clinical Psychology, 60*, 426–432.

Lochman, J. E., & Dodge, K. A. (1998). Distorted perceptions in dyadic interactions of aggressive and nonaggressive boys: Effects of prior expectations, context, and boys' age. *Development and Psychopathology, 10*, 495–512.

Lochman, J. E., Meyer, B., Rabiner, D., & White, K. (1991). Parameters influencing social problem solving of aggressive children. In R. Prinz (Ed.), *Advances in behavioral assessment of children and families* (Vol. 5, pp. 31–63). Greenwich, CT: JAI Press.

Lochman, J. E., & Wells, K. C. (2002). Countertextual social-cognitive mediators and child outcome: A test of the theoretical model in the Coping Power Program. *Development and Psychopathology, 14*, 971–993.

Loeber, R., Green, S. M., Lahey, B. B., & Kalb, L. (2000). Physical fighting in childhood as a risk factor for later mental health problems. *Journal of the American Academy of Child and Adolescent Psychiatry, 39*, 121–128.

Loeber, R., & Hay, D. F. (1997). Key issues in the development of aggression and violence from childhood to early adulthood. *Annual Review of Psychology, 48*, 371–410.

Loeber, R., & Stouthamer-Loeber, M. (1998). Development of juvenile aggression and violence: Some common misperceptions and controversies. *American Psychologist, 53*, 242–259.

Lorenz, K. (1966). *On aggression*. New York: Harcourt Brace Jovanovich.

Luria, A. (1959). The directive function of speech in development and dissolution. *Word, 15*, 341–352.

Luria, A. (1961). *The role of speech in the regulation of normal and abnormal behaviors*. New York: Liveright.

Mandler, G. (1984). *Mind and body: Psychology of emotion and stress.* New York: Norton.

Mash, E. J., Wolfe, D. A. (2005). *Abnormal child psychology* (3rd ed.) Belmont, CA: Thomson Wadsworth.

McCord, W., & McCord, J. (1960). *Origins of alcoholism.* Stanford, CA: Stanford University Press.

McDougall, W. (1931). *An introduction to social psychology.* London: Methuen.

McMahon, R. J., Forehand, R., & Guest, D. L. (1981). Effects of knowledge of social learning principles on enhancing treatment outcome and generalization in a parent training program. *Journal of Consulting and Clinical Psychology, 49,* 526–532.

Meichenbaum, D., & Goodman, J. (1971). Training impulsive children to talk to themselves: A means of developing self-control. *Journal of Abnormal Psychology, 77,* 115–126.

Milich, R., & Dodge, K. A. (1984). Social information processing in child psychiatric populations. *Journal of Abnormal Child Psychology, 12,* 471–490.

Miller, L. S. (1994). Preventive interventions for conduct disorders: A review. *Child and Adolescent Psychiatric Clinics of North America, 3,* 405–420.

Miller, G. E., & Prinz, R. J. (1990). Enhancement of social learning family intervention for childhood conduct disorder. *Psychological Bulletin, 108,* 291–307.

Moffitt, T. E. (1993). Adolescence-limited and life-course-persistent antisocial behavior: A developmental taxonomy. *Psychology Review, 100,* 674–701.

Moffitt, T. E., Caspi, A., Dickson, N., Silva, P., & Stanton, W. (1996). Childhood-onset versus adolescent-onset antisocial conduct problems in males: Natural history from ages 3 to 18 years. *Development and Psychopathology, 8,* 399–424.

Moffitt, T. E., Caspi, A., Harrington, H., & Milne, B. J. (2002). Males on the life-course-persistent and adolescence-limited antisocial pathways: Follow-up at age 26 years. *Development and Psychopathology, 14,* 179–207.

Monahan, J., & Walker, L. (Eds.). (1990). *Social science in law: Cases and materials* (2nd ed.). Westbury, NJ: Foundation Press.

National Institute of Mental Health. (2000). *Child an Adolescent Violence Research at the NIMH* (NIH Publication No. 00-4706). Washington DC: U.S. Government Printing Office.

Nelson, W. M., III. (1998). *"Keeping your cool": The anger management video.* Ardmore, PA: Workbook Publishing.

Nelson, W. M., III, & Finch, A. J., Jr. (1996). *"Keeping your cool": The anger management workbook* (Parts 1 and 2). Ardmore, PA: Workbook Publishing.

Nelson, W. M., III, & Finch, A. J., Jr. (2000). *Children's Inventory of Anger (CHIA) manual.* Los Angeles: Western Psychological Services.

Nelson, W. M., III, Finch, A. J., Jr., & Hart, K. J. (in press). *Comparative treatments for conduct disorder.* New York: Springer.

Nelson, W. M., III, Hart, K. J., & Finch, A. J., Jr. (1993). Anger in children: A cognitive-behavioral view of the assessment–therapy connection. *Journal of Rational-Emotive and Cognitive-Behavior Therapy, 11,* 135–150.

Nelson, W. M., III, & Politano, P. M. (1993). The goal is to say "good-bye" and have the treatment effects generalize and maintain: A cognitive-behavioral view of termination. *Journal of Cognitive Psychology, 7,* 249–261.

Novaco, R. W. (1978). Anger and coping with stress. In J. P. Foreyt & D. P. Rathjen (Eds.), *Cognitive behavior therapy: Research and application* (pp. 241–286). New York: Plenum Press.

Novaco, R. W. (1979). The cognitive regulation of anger and stress. In P. C. Kendall & S. D. Hollan (Eds.), *Cognitive-behavioral interventions: Theory, research, and procedures* (pp. 241–285). New York: Academic Press.

Nyborg, V. M., & Curry, J. F. (2003). The impact of perceived racism: Psychological symptoms among African American boys. *Journal of Clinical Child and Adolescent Psychology, 32*(2), 258–266.

Patterson, G. R. (1982). *Coercive family process*. Eugene, OR: Castalia Press.

Patterson, G. R. (1986). Performance models for antisocial boys. *American Psychologist, 41*, 432–444.

Patterson, G. R., & Forgatch, M. (1987). *Parents and adolescents living together: Part 1. The basics*. Eugene, OR: Castalia Press.

Patterson, G. R., & Gullion, M. E. (1971). *Living with children: New methods for parents and teachers*. Champagne, IL: Research Press.

Patterson, G. R., Reid, J. B., Jones, R. R., & Conger, R. W. (1975). *A social learning approach to family intervention* (Vol. 1). Eugene, OR: Castalia Press.

Pentz, M. (1980). Assertion training and trainer effects on unassertive and aggressive adolescents. *Journal of Counseling Psychology, 27*, 76–83.

Pepler, D. J., & Rubin, K. H. (Eds.). (1991). *The development and treatment of childhood aggression*. Hillsdale, NJ: Erlbaum.

Price, J. A. (1996). *Power and compassion: Working with difficult adolescents and abused parents*. New York: Guilford Press.

Quay, H. C. (1986). Conduct disorders. In H. C. Quay & J. S. Werry (Eds.), *Psychopathological disorders of childhood* (3rd ed., pp. 35–72). New York: Wiley.

Quay, H. C., & La Greca, A. M. (1986). Disorders of anxiety, withdrawal, and dysphoria. In H. C. Quay & J. S. Werry (Eds.), *Psychopathological disorders of children* (3rd ed., pp. 73–110). New York: Wiley.

Reynolds, W., & Coats, K. (1986). A comparison of cognitive-behavioral therapy and relaxation training for the treatment of depression. *Journal of Consulting and Clinical Psychology, 54*, 653–660.

Reynolds, C., & Kamphaus, R. (1992). *Behavior Assessment System for Children: Manual*. Circle Pines, MN: American Guidance Services.

Rich, M., Woods, E. R., Goodman, E., Emans, S. J., & DuRant, R. H. (1998). Aggressors or victims: Gender and race in music video violence. *Pediatrics, 101*(4), 669–674.

Richters, J. E., & Martinez, P. E. (1993). Violent communities, family choices, and children's chances: An algorithm for improving the odds. *Development and Psychopathology, 5*, 609–627.

Robins, L. N. (1966). *Deviant children grown up: A sociological and psychiatric study of sociopathic personality*. Baltimore: Williams & Wilkins.

Robins, L. N. (1978). Sturdy childhood predictors of adult antisocial behavior: Replications from longitudinal studies. *Psychological Medicine, 8*(4), 611–622.

Rutter, M., Giller, H., & Hagell, A. (1998). *Antisocial behavior by young people*. New York: Cambridge University Press.

Sanford, M., Boyles, M. H., Szatmari, P., Offord, D. R., Jamieson, E., & Spinner, M. (1999). Age-of-onset classification of Conduct Disorder: Reliability and validity in a prospective cohort study. *Journal of the American Academy of Child and Adolescent Psychiatry, 38*, 992–999.

Santiago Rivera, A. L., Arredondo, P., & Gallardo-Cooper, M. (2002). *Counseling Latinos and la familia*. Thousand Oaks, CA: Sage.

Schachter, S. (1964). The interaction of cognitive and physiological determents of emotional state. In L. Berkowitz (Ed.), *Advances in experimental social psychology* (pp. 49–80). New York: Academic Press.

Schachter, S., & Singer, J. (1962). Cognitive, social and physiological determinants of emotional state. *Psychological Review, 69*, 379–399.

Sells, S. P. (1998). *Treating the tough adolescent: A family-based, step-by-step guide*. New York: Guilford Press.

Snyder, H. N., & Sickmund, M. (1995). *Juvenile offenders and victims: A national report* (Document No. NCJ-153569). Washington, DC: U.S. Department of Justice, Office of Juvenile Justice and Delinquency Prevention.

Southam-Gerow, M. A., & Kendall, P. C. (1997). In D. M. Stoff, J. Breiling, & J. D. Moser (Eds.), *Handbook of antisocial behavior* (pp. 384–394). New York: Wiley.

Spencer, L., & Oatts, T. (1999). Conduct disorder vs. attention-deficit hyperactivity disorder: Diagnostic implications for African-American adolescent males. *Education, 119*(3), 514–518.

Stark, K., Kendall, P. C., McCarthy, M., Stafford, M., Barron, R., & Thomeer, M. (1996). *Taking action: A workbook for overcoming depression.* Ardmore, PA: Workbook Publishing.

Stattin, H., & Magnusson, D. (1989). The role of early aggressive behavior in the frequency, seriousness, and types of later crime. *Journal of Consulting and Clinical Psychology, 57,* 710–718.

Steiner, H. (1997). Practice parameters for the assessment and treatment of children and adolescents with conduct disorder. *Journal of American Academy of Child and Adolescent Psychiatry, 36,* 1225–1395.

Stewart, C., & Lewis, W. (1986). Effects of assertiveness training on the self-esteem of Black high school students. *Journal of Counseling and Development, 64,* 638–641.

Stewart, M. A., deBlois, S., Meardon, J., & Cummings, C. (1980). Aggressive conduct disorder of children: The clinical picture. *Journal of Nervous and Mental Disease, 168,* 604–615.

Stirman, S. W., Crits-Christoph, P., & De Rubeis, R. J. (2004). Achieving successful dissemination of empirically-supported psychotherapies: A synthesis of dissemination theory. *Clinical Psychology: Science and Practice, 11,* 343–359.

Stoff, D. M., Breiling, J., & Maser, J. D. (Eds.). (1997). *Handbook of antisocial behavior.* New York: Wiley.

Stouthamer-Loeber, M., Loeber, R., & Thomas, C. (1992). Caretakers seeking help for boys with disruptive and delinquent behavior. *Comprehensive Mental Health Care, 2,* 159–178.

Tafrate, R. C. (1995). Evaluation of treatment strategies for adult anger disorders. In H. Kassinove (Ed.), *Anger disorders: Definition, diagnoses, and treatment* (pp. 109–130). Washington, DC: Taylor & Francis.

Tate, D. C., Reppucci, N. D., & Mulvey, E. P. (1995). Violent juvenile delinquents: Treatment effectiveness and implications for future action. *American Psychologist, 50,* 777–781.

Tremblay, R. E. (2000). The development of aggressive behaviour during childhood: What have we learned in the past century? *International Journal of Behavioural Development, 24,* 129–141.

U.S. Congress, Office of Technology Assessment. (1991). *Adolescent health* (OTA-H-468). Washington, DC: U.S. Government Printing Office.

U. S. Department of Health and Human Services. (2001). *Youth violence: A report of the Surgeon General.* Retrieved December 13, 2004, from http://www.surgeongeneral. gov/library/ youthviolence/sgsummary/summary.htm

Ventis, W., & Ventis, D. (1988). Guidelines for using humor in therapy with children and young adolescents. *Journal of Children in Contemporary Society, 20,* 179–197.

Vygotsky, L. (1962). *Thought and language.* New York: Wiley.

Vygotsky, L. (1987). Thinking and speech. In *The collected works of L. S. Vygotsky: Vol. 1. Problems of general psychology* (N. Minick, Trans.) (pp. 43–243). New York: Plenum Press. (Original work published 1934)

Waksman, S. (1981). A controlled evaluation of assertion training with adolescents. *Adolescence, 19,* 277–282.

Wasserman, G. A., & Miller, L. S. (1998). The prevention of serious and violent juvenile offending. In R. Loeber & D. P. Farrington (Eds.), *Serious and violent juvenile offenders: Risk factors and successful interventions* (pp. 197–247). Thousand Oaks, CA: Sage.

Wasserman, G. A., & Seracini, A. G. (2001). Family risk factors and family treatments for early-onset offending. In R. Loeber & D. P. Farrington (Eds.), *Child delinquents: Development, intervention, and service needs* (pp. 165–190). Thousand Oaks, CA: Sage.

Webster-Stratton, C., & Hammond, M. (1997). Treating children with early onset conduct problems: A comparison of child and parent training interventions. *Journal of Consulting and Clinical Psychology, 65*, 93–109.

Wilson, D. B., Gottfredson, D.C., & Najaka, S. (2001). School-based prevention of problem behaviors: A meta-analysis. *Journal of Quantitative Criminology, 17*(3), 247 272.

Wilson, S. J., Lipsey, M. W., & Derzon, J. (2003). The effects of school-based intervention programs on aggressive behavior: A meta-analysis. *Journal of Consulting and Clinical Psychology, 71*(1), 136–149.

Xie, H., Cairns, R. B., & Cairns, B. D. (2002). The development of social aggression and physical aggression: A narrative analysis of interpersonal conflicts. *Aggressive Behavior, 28*, 341–355.

PART III
INTERNALIZING DISORDERS

CHAPTER 5

Treatment of Childhood Depression
The ACTION Treatment Program

KEVIN D. STARK, JENNIFER HARGRAVE,
JANAY SANDER, GILBERT CUSTER,
SARAH SCHNOEBELEN, JANE SIMPSON,
and JOHANNA MOLNAR

Cognitive-behavioral therapy (CBT) continues to be a preferred and highly investigated intervention for depressive disorders in youth. One feature of CBT that is not often discussed in the literature is the role of case conceptualization as a road map to treatment. The ACTION program is a manual-based treatment, but it is designed so that it is guided by a case conceptualization for each participant. The program and the measures that contribute to conceptualizing each case are described. The ACTION program presented here is a cognitive-behavioral intervention for depressed girls; in addition, there is a parent training component and a teacher consultation component. Thus, in the ideal situation, the participating girls learn the coping, problem-solving, and cognitive restructuring skills at the same time that their environments are being changed to support the changes and other people in the girls' environments are working with the therapist to support application of the skills. The program is modified to address the needs of youth with comorbid conditions. Before describing the details of the program, we first review recent outcome research.

PSYCHOSOCIAL TREATMENT OUTCOME RESEARCH

Treatment in the Community

Most depressed youth do not receive treatment and those that do, do not receive evidence-based treatments (Olfson, Gameroff, Marcus, & Waslick, 2003). Among those depressed youth who do receive treatment, 79% complete one or more sessions of psychotherapy and 59.8% are treated with medication. Twenty-one percent are treated solely with medication, and almost half of treated youth receive a combination of therapy and medication. Among youth who receive psychotherapy, 75% complete less than eight sessions per year (Olfson et al., 2003), which is less than a minimally acceptable dose of psychotherapy (Howard, Kopta, Krause, & Orlinsky, 1986). Most depressed youth are treated by a physician (76.7%), a third are treated by a psychologist, and the remainder are treated by another type of provider (Olfson et al., 2003).

The majority of depressed youth receive treatment through a community mental health center (CMHC), private practitioner, or therapist in another setting. Few receive state-of-the-art evidence-based interventions. In general, child psychotherapists in the community use an eclectic mix of treatments (Addis & Krasnow, 2000) that lack an evidence base (Weisz, 2000). There is no evidence to support the efficacy of this approach to psychotherapy with children (Bickman, Noser, & Summerfelt, 1999). Furthermore, this form of child psychotherapy is said to be no more effective than no treatment (Andrade, Lambert, & Bickman, 2000). Consistent with these findings for children in general seeking psychotherapy, Weersing and Weisz (2002) reported that the standard of care for depressed youth who received services through a CMHC is an eclectic mix of primarily psychodynamic procedures with some cognitive and behavioral techniques delivered in a median of 11 sessions. A substantial percentage of these youth (35.8%) completed fewer than eight sessions (Weersing & Weisz, 2002).

Treatment as usual in the community does not appear to be as effective as treatment delivered within a research protocol (Weersing & Weisz, 2002). The median number of sessions in a research protocol for depressed youth is 12, and depressed youth who received treatment through a research protocol relative to those that received treatment in a CMHC improved very quickly and their scores were significantly better than those for the CMHC sample following treatment. Depressed youth who received CBT reported enough improvement in depressive symptoms that their scores fell near those of a normative sample. This significant difference between the youth who received CBT and those that received treatment through the CMHC held at 3-month follow-up. Youth who received treatment through the CMHC showed a trajectory of change that was similar to participants that had not received treatment—change occurred at a slow rate. Treatment as usual produced no more improvement in depressive symptoms than that which occurs due to the natural passing of time.

It could be argued that the failure of treatment as usual is due to the limited number of sessions that the youngsters received and to a failure to assess change that accrues over longer periods of time. Weiss, Harris, and Han (2003) addressed this issue in an open-ended treatment protocol that allowed the therapists to work with children for up to 18 months and did not place any limits on the type of treatment or number of meetings. In addition, internalizing and externalizing symptoms were tracked over a 2-year follow-up period. Results provided little to no support for the effectiveness of traditional child psychotherapy: Symptom severity did not approach a normal level of functioning following treatment. Overall, there is no evidence to support the effectiveness of traditional child therapy for youth with depressive disorders. How do these disappointing results compare to the results of interventions that are delivered as part of a research protocol?

Protocol-Based Treatments

Concerns about the State of the Art

Results of protocol-based treatments for depressed youth are more encouraging and suggest that CBT can be effective. However, the conclusions that can be drawn from the literature have to be tempered by the limitations of existing outcome research. An agenda for improving the state of treatment outcome research with children was outlined (see Kazdin, 2000; Kendall, 2000; Weisz, 2000). Limitations in existing outcome research with children in general also concern investigations with depressed youth. According to Kazdin (2000), children in most outcome studies may be less seriously depressed, experience less comorbidity, be exposed to less parental psychopathology, and are less disadvantaged in general. With the exception of the Treatment for Adolescents with Depression Study (TADS; March, 2004), these criticisms may be true of the existing studies of depressed youth. Given these issues, it is not clear whether or not the results of studies that included youth with mild depression can be applied to youth who present at clinics with more severe depression.

Although the primary objective of a treatment for depressed youth is symptom reduction, an effective intervention also produces improvements in functional impairment, academic functioning, parent and family functioning, and social functioning. To date, this broader set of outcome variables has not been assessed in the treatment outcome research with depressed youth.

Weisz (2000) believes that a very basic issue is that, although effective interventions have been found, virtually none of the empirically supported treatments has made its way into regular practice. One method for promoting transportability is to manualize treatments. However, manuals need to recognize the individuality of each child and therapist (Kendall, 2000), and some manuals do not achieve this goal. In reality, there is great variability in the training, theoretical orientation, experience, skills, interpersonal abilities, and other personal differences that challenge one to truly "even the playing field" among the therapists (Kendall, 2000). Children vary too, and this requires that the application of a manualized treatment be implemented by a trained therapist. To flexibly and realistically implement a manualized treatment the therapist benefits from an ability to conceptualize the youngster's problems from a consistent theoretical perspective. In addition, the therapist must understand the "big picture" of the manual, a skill that permits the therapist to be able to recognize opportunities to spontaneously apply treatment strategies. Without a basic understanding of treatment, a manual will be implemented in a stilted fashion that is not adapted to the specific needs of the child.

Research-Based Interventions

Psychosocial Interventions. Since the prior edition of this text, a modest amount of additional treatment outcome research has been conducted with depressed youth. CBT has been labeled "possibly efficacious" for depressed children and "probably efficacious for depressed adolescents" (Kazdin & Weisz, 1998), according to the criteria for empirically supported treatments (Chambless & Hollon, 1998). Although several different research teams have reported that CBT was effective in producing significant improvements in depressive symptoms and an average of 60% of the youngsters are no longer depressed following treatment, the label of "well-established" has not been applied to CBT for depressive disorders in youth.

Lewinsohn, Clarke, and colleagues have adapted and tested their Coping with Depression Course as both a prevention and treatment program for depressed adolescents (Clarke et al., 1995, 2001; Clarke, Rohde, Lewinsohn, Hops, & Seeley, 1999; Lewinsohn, Clarke, Hops, & Andrews, 1990), which included standard delivery of intervention plus booster sessions. The course was effective in treating depression when used with adolescents alone or with their parents (Clarke et al., 1999; Lewinsohn et al., 1990). Booster sessions did not prevent recurrence of depressive episodes. However, adolescents who were depressed at posttreatment assessment had quicker recovery rates if they received booster sessions (Clarke et al., 1999). Other researchers have also indicated that continuation of CBT is effective in preventing relapse (Kroll, Harrington, Jayson, Fraser, & Gowers, 1996).

Brent and colleagues (Birmaher et al., 2000; Brent, Holder, & Kolko, 1997) compared CBT, systematic behavior family therapy, and nondirective supportive therapy for the treatment of depressed adolescents. At posttreatment, participants who completed CBT reported more change than participants in the other treatment conditions. However, the mean differences between conditions on those variables at long-term follow-up were not significantly different.

What variables predict improvement through completion of a trial of CBT? It appears as though a less severe depressive disorder prior to initiation of treatment, lower rates of parent child conflict, lower levels of cognitive distortion, lower hopelessness, and greater general functioning predict a better treatment outcome (Birmaher et al., 2000). Kendall (2000) and Kazdin (2000) emphasize the importance of determining whether interventions produce changes in the targets of treatment (e.g. depressive cognition) and whether changes in these variables predict improvement in depression. There is some evidence that CBT produces changes in depressive cognition, such as changes in negative self-talk (Kaufman, Rohde, Seeley, Clarke, & Stice, 2005; see also Treadwell & Kendall, 1996). However, there also were some changes in family functioning that were not targeted by the CBT (Kolko, Brent, Baugher, Bridge, Birmaher, 2000). In a meta-analysis of CBT interventions for children with a variety of disturbances including depression, the effectiveness of CBT was reported to be moderated by cognitive developmental level, a finding that suggests that CBT is impacting child functioning through changes in cognition (Durlak, Fuhrman, & Lampman, 1991). However, these same investigators did not find that changes in cognitive processes were related to improvements in behavior. Is there a dosage effect for psychosocial treatments of depression in youth? In other words, do children who complete more treatment sessions report greater improvement than those who complete fewer sessions? A dosage effect for CBT was found in one study (Weersing & Weisz, 2002).

In the adult treatment literature there is a phenomenon referred to as "sudden gains" in which a participant reports significant improvement between one session and the next session. This change can occur at any time during treatment. Gaynor and colleagues (Gaynor et al., 2003) evaluated this phenomenon with depressed youth. Sudden gains were found for depressed adolescents who participated in individual treatment with either CBT or nonspecific supportive therapy, but they were not found among participants who received systematic family therapy. It is thought that sudden gains stem from some kind of cognitive click that occurs during treatment. However, this hypothesis remains untested.

In a rigorous study with a large sample of clinically depressed youths, referred to as the TADS study (March, 2004), the efficacy of CBT as a stand-alone intervention for depressed adolescents is brought into question. March (2004) evaluated the relative efficacy of fluoxetine, CBT, the combination of fluoxetine and CBT, and placebo for the treatment of 351 adolescents who received primary diagnoses of moderate to severe major depressive disorder (MDD). Participants received 12 weeks of treatment. The CBT had both "required" skill-building sessions and optional or "modular sessions" that allowed flexible, developmentally sensitive, and individual tailoring of the treatment to address the adolescent's needs. The required skill-building sessions were completed over the first six meetings and included psychoeducation about depression, goal setting, mood monitoring, increasing engagement in pleasant activities, social problem solving, and cognitive restructuring. In the subsequent optional modules (meetings 7 to 12), the child and therapist collaboratively chose the relevant social skills deficits of the teenager and worked on the development of these skills (e.g. social engagement, communication, negotiation, compromise, or assertion). Additional family sessions could be completed that included psychoeducation for parents about depression and conjoint sessions that focus on addressing identified parent–adolescent concerns. Although the specific CBT that was evaluated was not a program that had been previously found to be efficacious, participants in the program did complete a mean of 11 sessions that contained sets of features of CBT.

Results indicated that the combination of fluoxetine and CBT produced the greatest improvement in symptoms of MDD. Fluoxetine alone was effective, but not as effective as its combination with CBT. CBT alone was less effective than fluoxetine and not significantly more effective than placebo. Results of the clinical significance of the improvements indicates that a positive response to treatment was reported for 71% of the participants in the combined treatment, 60.6% of the youngsters who received fluoxetine, 43.2% of the youngsters who received CBT, and 34.8% of the youngsters who received a placebo.

The lower rate of effectiveness of CBT in the TADS cannot solely be based on differences in the severity of depression experienced by participants in the majority of studies relative to the TADS. Participants in both of the Brent and colleagues (1997) and March (2004) studies were clinic-referred youth who were experiencing MDD and a multiplicity of comorbid conditions. Despite the similarity of samples with respect to severity of their depressive disorders, the results for the two forms of CBT used in these investigations are very different despite the fact that they were similar in terms of the number of sessions that participants completed in each study. In the Brendt and colleagues investigation a treatment that was more true to cognitive therapy (Beck, Rush, Shaw, & Emery, 1979) was used, and it emphasized collaborative empiricism, socialization to the cognitive therapy model, and monitoring and modification of automatic thoughts, assumptions, and beliefs. Participants also acquired problem-solving, affect regulation, and social skills. Therapists in TADS did not use cognitive therapy; rather, participants learned six cognitive and behavioral skills in the first six meetings, followed by six sessions of social skills training. Perhaps it is this difference in the two treatments that causes the difference in rates of clinical improvement. Brent and colleagues reported that the depressive episodes of 60% of youth were in remission at posttreatment versus 43% of youth in the TADS study.

A major issue in the medication treatment of depressed youth is the concern about increases in suicidal ideation and behavior that have been said to be associated with taking a selective serotonin reuptake inhibitor (SSRI). In a later section of this chapter, this issue is discussed in greater depth. A trend toward more suicidal behavior but not suicidal ideation was found in the fluoxetine-only group in the TADS (March, 2004). Of greatest relevance to this chapter is that CBT appeared to have a protective effect on suicidal ideation and behavior.

Pharmacological Treatments. As noted earlier, the most common practice in the community is to provide depressed youth with a combination of antidepressant medication and psychotherapy. The results of studies of the efficacy of antidepressant medications will be described briefly. Several SSRIs have been reported to be superior to placebo in treating MDD in youth, with fluoxetine being the most widely studied of the SSRIs. Emslie and colleagues (1997) randomized youth ages 7–17 years with MDD to an 8-week trial of 20 mg of fluoxetine or placebo. A significantly larger percentage of participants receiving fluoxetine (56%) relative to those receiving placebo (33%) were rated "much" or "very much" improved at the end of the study. Complete symptom remission was reported by 31% of fluoxetine-treated and 23% of the placebo-treated participants. Response rates were comparable across age and gender.

In a larger multicenter study, Emslie and colleagues (2002) compared fluoxetine to placebo for the treatment of children and adolescents with MDD. Fluoxetine-treated patients received 10 mg/day for 1 week, followed by 20 mg/day for 8 weeks. Fluoxetine treated participants relative to placebo-treated participants reported a significantly greater decrease in severity of depressive symptoms on a semistructured interview at endpoint. Remission of the depressive episode was reported by 41.3% of the participants who were treated with fluoxetine, whereas only 19.8% of the participants in the placebo group reported that their depressive episode was in remission. A clinical response was reported by 65% of the fluoxetine-treated and 53% of the placebo-treated participants.

Wagner and Ambrosini (2003) evaluated the efficacy and safety of sertraline relative to placebo in the treatment of MDD in children and adolescents ages 6–17. Participants were randomized to receive a flexible dosage of (50–200 mg/day) of sertraline or matching placebo tablets for 10 weeks. Sertraline-treated participants relative to participants who received the placebo experienced significantly greater improvement in severity of depressive symptoms, and 69% of sertraline-treated participants compared with 59% of placebo-treated participants were considered responders.

Wagner and colleagues (2004) randomized 7–17-year-olds with MDD to a placebo-controlled 8-week trial of citalopram. Participants were treated initially with placebo or 20 mg/day of citalopram, with an option to increase the dose to 40 mg/day at week 4. The overall mean citalopram dose was approximately 24 mg/day. Clinical response was better in the citalopram-treated group relative to the placebo-treated group (36% vs. 24%). The change from baseline in symptom severity was significantly better in the citalopram-treated group relative to the placebo group.

Depressed youth who are treated with an SSRI experience a 2–3% higher rate of suicidal behavior, and they are at heightened risk for developing a manic or hypomanic episode during treatment (*Physician Desk Reference*, 2004). Family history of suicide and bipolar disorder may be associated with increased suicidal ideation and manic reactions when a child or adolescent with MDD is treated with an SSRI. Patients treated with antidepressants should be closely observed, especially during the early phase of treatment, for worsening of depression, increased suicidal ideation and impulses, manic reactions, anxiety, agitation, irritability, hostility, and impulsivity.

NEUROBIOLOGICAL CORRELATES OF SYMPTOM REMISSION

What might be happening in the brain during treatment for depression? Just as neuroplasticity is argued to be a mechanism through which early life stress induces functional neural change, creating depressive vulnerability (Penza, Heim, & Nemeroff, 2003), adaptive functional changes have also been observed upon remission of depression. Research has pointed to normalization of brain activation in some areas upon successful treatment with antidepressant medications and psychotherapy, although there have been very few studies evaluating the latter. The majority of literature to date has focused on brain changes following successful psychopharmacological treatment, with much of the research suggesting changes in brain abnormalities (e.g. Baxter et al., 1989; Bench, Frackowiak, & Dolan, 1995; Kennedy et al., 2001; Mayberg et al., 1999), although symptom remission has also been associated with additional, non-normalizing patterns of neural activation (Mayberg, 2003). Although few studies have utilized psychotherapy to study brain changes, there is early indication that psychotherapy can mediate recovery through effecting change in neural regions slightly different than those observed for medication (Brody et al., 2001; Martin, Martin, Rai, Richardson, & Royall, 2001) and that perhaps various forms of therapy result in brain changes (Goldapple et al., 2004).

It is of interest to consider the psychological processes that may be represented by the neurofunctional changes occurring after symptom remission from either medication or psychotherapy. Although the studies beginning to address this question are exploratory and suffer from small sample size, they are interesting to consider. Healthy adults who receive a single dose of either the noradrenergic reboxetine (Harmer, Hill, Taylor, Cowen, & Goodwin, 2003) or an SSRI (Harmer, Bhagwager, et al., 2003) demonstrated an information processing bias toward positive emotional information when compared to participants receiving a placebo. The investigators highlight the similarity of psychological and biological mechanisms in the treatment of depression. CBT seeks to aid the client in shifting processing biases away from negative information to more positive and realistic information. Although the above-cited studies indicate the potential of a common neural pathway leading to remission, other studies suggest the picture may be more complex. Depressed patients who have been treated with SSRIs tend to show a reduction in mood during tryptophan–depletion challenge (Delgado et al., 1990, 1999). However, in a recent study comparing previously depressed individuals who had been successfully treated with either an SSRI or cognitive therapy, it was found that the group that received cognitive therapy did not exhibit the worsening of mood noted in the SSRI-treated group during tryptohan depletion (O'Reardon et al., 2004). The authors hypothesize that remission induced by cognitive therapy is not necessarily mediated by a normally functioning serotonin system. Thus, it may impact a different system. If CBT and SSRIs impact different systems, this could explain the beneficial impact of combined treatment.

OUTCOME MEASURES

Due to space limitations, the present focus will be on selected outcome measures and the way that they are used to inform intervention. When treating depression with CBT, it is believed that symptom reduction occurs as a result of changes in explanatory style and cognitive processing. Social skills and the family environment also may be targets and mechanisms of treatment change. Thus, it is important to include measures of these constructs.

Assessment of Depression

Best practices for assessing depression in youth include multiple measures and multiple methods completed by multiple raters. Measures of symptom severity including self-report questionnaires such as the Children's Depression Inventory (CDI; Kovacs, 1981), interviews such as the Schedule for Affective Disorders and Schizophrenia for School-Age Children (K-SADS; Ambrosini & Dixon, 2000), and parent report measures such as the Child Behavior Checklist (Achenbach & Rescorla, 2001) serve as a means of assessing the presence and severity of depressive symptoms. The K-SADS can also be used to diagnose depressive disorders and comorbid conditions. The K-SADS is independently administered to the child and primary caregiver. The severity of each symptom is determined through combining information about frequency, duration, and phenomenological experience. The severity of the depressive disorder is determined by combining severity ratings across all of the symptoms that constitute the disorder. While the K-SADS is cumbersome upon initial use, requires extensive training, and is designed for use in research, its format is flexible enough that it can be adapted by the skilled interviewer for clinical practice.

A self-report measure such as the CDI or the depression section of the Beck Youth Inventory (BYI; Beck, Beck, & Jolly, 2003) can be used as a means of further quantifying the severity of depressive symptoms. Although the interview provides the clinician with an opportunity to establish rapport and inquire about each symptom, a self-report questionnaire often results in additional information about subjective distress. The youngsters' responses to the BYI items can be compared to the same symptoms on the interview, and differences can be discussed through a follow-up interview.

Results of the interview and BYI provide a measure of severity of the episode, and since research suggests that more severe episodes have a more protracted course (McCauley et al., 1993), the therapist may use this information to plan for a more intense or protracted intervention. Intensity can be increased through scheduling more frequent meetings and by coordinating adjunctive interventions or a referral for hospitalization. The diagnostic interview also guides treatment through the identification of comorbid conditions, as the overall intervention would have to be altered to address comorbid disorders.

Information from the depression measures regarding the presence of specific depressive symptoms also guides treatment. For example, if a child reports sleep disturbance, then sleep hygiene behaviors are integrated into the intervention along with an emphasis on soothing and relaxing coping skills. If the child reports the presence of a number of very severe vegetative symptoms along with anhedonia, then pharmacological intervention may be initiated. Another example would be the child who reports a mood disturbance, excessive fatigue, or hypersomnia, but does not have the associated cognitive symptoms of depression. This youngster would be referred for an assessment of hypothalamic functioning and possibly related medical treatment.

Another important concern is assessment of suicidal risk. The K-SADS includes a section that assesses the severity of suicidal risk and risk of self-damaging behaviors. While this section of the interview is useful, it represents only a start to a thorough risk assessment. Consequently, we supplement this section of the interview with a set of questions that allows for a more thorough assessment. Similarly, we have trained our interviewers to ask additional questions about self-damaging behaviors such as cutting. Thus, while the K-SADS includes relevant items, it does not include an adequate interview in these areas. If the youngster is at risk for suicidal behavior, steps are immediately taken to ensure the youngster's safety, and an emergency referral is made to a psychiatrist.

In addition to assessing the presence of a depressive disorder, the measures of symptom severity can be used as a means of assessing the effectiveness of treatment over time. The K-SADS is an excellent outcome measure because of the sensitivity and range of the severity ratings. A self-report measure such as the BYI can be used to assess progress of treatment over time. For example, we ask the children to complete the depressive disorders section of the BYI at the beginning of every other treatment meeting. We have used both the CDI and the depressive disorders section of the BYI for this purpose, and children prefer the BYI due to its simpler format, Likert-scaled response choices, and shorter duration of time to complete.

Assessment of Related Constructs

Additional measures can be used to assess variables that are theoretically related to depression. A few paper and-pencil measures have been developed for assessing important cognitive variables. The Automatic Thoughts Questionnaire for Children (ATQ-C; Stark, Humphrey, Laurent, Livingston, & Christopher, 1993), a version of the ATQ (Hollon & Kendall, 1980), consists of 30 depressive self-statements. The child rates the frequency of occurrence of each thought. The youngster's ratings can be reviewed and used to guide cognitive interventions. Another useful questionnaire is the Cognitive Triad Inventory for Children, which assesses the youngster's beliefs about the self, world, and future (CTI-C; Kaslow, Stark, Printz, Livingston, & Tsai, 1992). The CTI-C consists of 36 items that are equally distributed across the three scales. The youngster's scores on the three scales and on the specific items that each scale comprises guide treatment. For example, a child who reports a negative view of the self would have this as a target of treatment. The therapist would continually help the youngster to identify evidence that contradicts the negative self-view and supports a more positive self-view. The Children's Cognitive Style Questionnaire (CCSQ; Mezulis, Hyde, Abramson, Stark, & Simpson, 2004) consists of six scenarios, including four negative scenarios and two positive scenarios. Accompanying each scenario are statements regarding the internality, stability, and globality of attributions (three items per scenario); self-inferences (one item); and anticipated consequences (one item). Each scenario contains one attribution emphasizing internality, one emphasizing stability, and one emphasizing globality. Children indicate agreement with each item on a 5 point scale. The 12 items specifically related to attributional style are summed for a negative attributional style score. The four items assessing negative self-inferences are summed to create a negative self-inferences score, and the four items assessing negative consequences are summed to create a negative consequences score. If the child has the depressive attributional style (internal, global, stable attributions for negative events), then cognitive restructuring and planned learning experiences would be used to help the youngster to make more adaptive attributions for negative events.

The assessment of interpersonal behaviors can be accomplished using therapist observations and through using a paper-and-pencil self-report measure such as the Matson Evaluation of Social Skills in Youths (Matson, Rotatori, & Helsel, 1983). When a disturbance in interpersonal skills or functioning is identified, then the therapist determines whether this disturbance is due to a maladaptive belief such as "If I get close to someone they will hurt me" or due to a skills deficit such as a failure to engage in age–appropriate behaviors. If a cognitive disturbance produces a performance deficit, then cognitive restructuring procedures, especially behavioral homework assignments, would be used to build new more adaptive beliefs. When a maladaptive pattern of behavior is recognized, the therapist shares his or her observations with the child and helps the youngster identify his or her thoughts surrounding it. Subsequently, they develop a plan for preventing the maladaptive behavior from reoccurring and for replacing it with a behavior that is more adaptive and yet serves the same function (assuming that the function is a healthy one).

Guiding the assessment of family functioning is the belief that the family represents the context in which the child develops essential cognitive and interpersonal skills. As such, the therapist observes and assesses the family with the goal of identifying interaction patterns that could produce and maintain maladaptive beliefs, information processing errors, and maladaptive interpersonal behaviors. Perhaps the most effective method for accomplishing this is to join the family and observe their interactions in times of stress. In addition, we have developed a few measures that are designed to aid in the assessment of family functioning and interaction patterns that could contribute to the development of a depressive style of thinking. To assess characteristics of the family milieu that are associated with depressive disorders, we have developed a children's version of the Self-Report Measure of Family Functioning (Stark, Humphrey, Crook, & Lewis, 1990). This measure has undergone extensive revision and currently consists of 65 items and 10 scales that reliably assess important characteristics of the family environment including cohesion, expression, conflict, organization, democratic family style, authoritarian family style, laissez faire family style, sociability, active recreational orientation, and intellectual/cultural orientation. Another measure that has proven to be very useful and to differentiate depressed youth from youth with other disorders (Schmidt, Stark, Carlson, & Anthony, 1998) is the Family Messages Measure (Stark et al., 1996). This 36-item self-report questionnaire assesses messages about the self, world, and future that the child perceives receiving from each parent. The child's responses to these questionnaires serve as hypotheses that are tested during observation of family interactions.

THE ACTION TREATMENT PROGRAM: AN EXAMPLE OF COGNITIVE-BEHAVIORAL THERAPY FOR DEPRESSION

Overview

The intervention for depressed girls that we describe is one that we are evaluating as part of an NIMH-funded investigation. The intervention is prototypical of CBT for depressed youths and consistent with previously developed and reported CBT programs (e.g., Stark, Schnoebelen, et al., 2005; Stark, Simpson, et al., 2005). Preliminary results with the first 60 participants suggest that the intervention is effective and is producing greater than 70% recovery rates. The primary components are appropriate for males and females, and for children and adolescents. However, by design, the delivery format, treatment activities, specific coping skills, emphasis on interpersonal relationships, and the illustrations in the treatment materials are specific to girls ages 9–13 years. In addition, the treatment manual is designed so that the examples used within the meetings and the material that the girls bring to the meetings is specific to this age range. Thus, the examples used to illustrate the application of the treatment are based on our experiences with girls that have completed treatment.

Overview of Child Treatment

Girls who are experiencing a depressive disorder are identified through a multiple-gate assessment procedure (e.g. Kendall, Cantwell, & Kazdin, 1989). After parental consent and child assent are secured, girls complete the CDI in large groups. As girls complete their questionnaire, research staff members check the suicidal ideation item (no. 9) and immediately interview any child who endorses "I want to kill myself." The questionnaires are scored immediately after they are completed. Girls who score in excess of one standard deviation above the mean are interviewed with a DSM symptom interview that assesses the presence of depressive symptoms. This 10- to 15-minute interview is used to eliminate the relatively large number of false positives. If a girl reports the presence of depressive symptoms during the DSM interview, her parent receives a phone call from the interviewer inviting the child and parent to complete a diagnostic interview, and a permission letter is sent home. If parental consent and child assent are received, she passes through the screening gates and is interviewed with the K-SADS. In addition, her primary caregiver is interviewed with the K-SADS. If the youngster receives a diagnosis of MDD or dysthymic disorder (DD), she is invited to participate in the evaluation of the treatment program. The participants are moderately to severely depressed, as 71% are experiencing MDD as their primary disorder and over 60% are experiencing additional comorbid conditions.

The ACTION treatment is a gender-specific, developmentally sensitive group treatment program for depressed girls that follows a structured therapist's manual (Stark, Simpson et al., 2005) and workbook (Stark, Schnoebelen et al., 2005). The treatment is conducted in the schools in groups of two to five girls. Each of the 20 group and 2 individual meetings lasts approximately 60 minutes and is conducted twice a week for 11 weeks. The child treatment is designed to be fun and engaging while teaching the youngsters a variety of skills that are applied to their depressive symptoms, interpersonal difficulties, and other stressors. The skills are taught to the children through didactic presentations and activities, they are rehearsed during in-session activities, and they are applied through therapeutic homework. Skills application is monitored and recorded through completion of workbook activities, and completion of the therapeutic home-work is encouraged through an in-session reward system.

The treatment program is based on a self-control model in which youngsters use skills to achieve and maintain a pleasant mood, or they use a change in mood, negative thoughts, or another depressive symptom as a sign that they need to engage in the coping, problem-solving, and/or cognitive restructuring strategies taught within the program. By paying attention to their experiences in these three realms, the youngsters are better aware of their own emotions and thus can use progressively smaller changes as a cue to engage in coping, problem solving, or cognitive restructuring. A variety of activities completed within the meetings and as homework help the participants to become more aware of their personal experiences.

Participants are taught coping skills for managing their unpleasant emotions and other depressive symptoms. The skills are taught to the youngsters within the sessions through activities that demonstrate the impact of the coping skills on their unpleasant moods. Depressed youth often experience undesirable situations that are not within their control and thus cannot be changed by the youngsters. In such situations, the children can take action to improve their mood and other depressive symptoms through using the coping skills that are taught and applied during the first nine meetings.

Problem solving is taught to depressed youth to help them change undesir-able situations that are within their control and can be changed. The youth are taught a five-step problem-solving process. The steps include (1) problem defini-tion, (2) goal definition, (3) solution generation, (4) consequential thinking, and (5) self-evaluation. The steps are defined in a developmentally sensitive way. The steps are modeled by the therapist and then applied to hypothetical situations. Once again, activities are used to illustrate the meaning and purpose of each step. Over time, the therapist helps the youngsters to apply problem solving to their own real-life problems. The workbook has problem-solving worksheets that guide the youngsters through the process as they apply it outside of meetings. By the middle of treatment, the youngsters typically are proficient at using coping and problem-solving skills. Use of these skills provides them with symptom relief, including an improvement in mood. This improvement allows them to enter the next phase of treatment that focuses on identifying, self-monitoring, evaluating, and changing negative thoughts.

Depressed youths commonly view themselves, their daily experiences, and the future in an unrealistically negative way. To counter this, depressed youths are taught to recognize their negative thoughts. Oftentimes, they have a very dif-ficult time pulling themselves out of the quagmire of negative thinking. We refer to this as getting "stuck in the negative muck." The youngsters are taught to rec-ognize their negative thoughts and then to evaluate them using a number of cog-nitive restructuring strategies. Once again, a variety of within-session activities and therapeutic homework exercises are used to teach youngsters to be "thought judges" who evaluate the validity of their negative thoughts using two questions: What is another way of looking at it? What is the evidence? If their negative thought is realistic and reflects a situation that can be changed, then the youngster is encouraged to use problem solving to develop and follow a plan that produces improvement. If the situation is real but cannot be changed, then the youngster is taught to use a coping strategy to manage his or her reaction to the situation.

A more complete description of each treatment component appears in the following sections. In general, the first nine sessions focus primarily on affective education and teaching coping and problem-solving skills. Sessions 10–19 focus primarily on learning and applying cognitive restructuring as well as continued use of previously learned strategies. Beginning with the 11th meeting and continuing through the 20th meeting, children work to improve their sense of self. Prior to describing the intervention strategies, the format, group size, duration, spacing of meetings, and structure of meetings are described. These are less obvious but important ingredients in the treatment program.

Therapist Issues

For CBT to be effective, the therapist needs to be able to develop a conceptualization of the child's depressive disorder and then have a map in her mind of where she needs to take the child in order for her to effectively manage depressive symptoms and to change the core beliefs that underlie the depressive disorder. In addition, the therapist must have an understanding of cognitive behavioral therapy so that she can artistically apply CBT to the conceptualization of the child's depressive disorder. This ability to use the big picture to guide treatment is necessary for effective treatment. The ACTION treatment program, like any other manualized intervention, cannot be effectively applied in a cookbook fashion. Rather, it can only be effectively employed when the therapist has an understanding of depressive disorders and of cognitive therapy for depression. Since CBT for depression is driven by both an idiosyncratic case conceptualization and research with depressed children, the therapist is trying to evaluate the validity of the conceptualization for each child during the interactions within the meeting. Then the therapist has to integrate the conceptualization with the meeting from the manual. The conceptualization typically evolves over the course of treatment.

Within any given treatment session, the therapist is confronted with numerous statements made by multiple participants, so she has to decide what to attend to and what to try to address. Thus, the therapist has to know if the time is right—in other words, whether the child is ready to accept the intervention—and whether the material to be addressed is the most important material from a therapeutic perspective. Guiding this decision making is the cognitive behavioral case conceptualization. The therapist asks herself if the statement the child has made, or the situation that she has described, represents (1) an opportunity to help her see how the evidence from her life is contradictory to her depressive schema or consistent with a new, more adaptive, schema; (2) an opportunity to help her see how using a coping strategy has helped her to alleviate depressive symptoms or how a coping skill could be used to alleviate depressive symptoms; or (3) an opportunity to use problem solving or a situation where problem solving could have been used.

Group CBT can be very taxing on the therapist, as she has to be cognizant of so many things at once. For example, the therapist has an agenda. Each agenda item may or may not be appropriate for the children's current concerns. Thus, a judgment about how to proceed has to be made. The therapist has to determine whether the participants are engaged in the activity or procedure that is being used to help them acquire the therapeutic skills. The therapist has to watch for opportunities to make the skill real for the children. In other words, the therapist has to watch for opportunities to show the children how they can apply that skill to a real-life situation. The therapist has to be alert for negative thoughts and schema-consistent thoughts, and then make a decision about whether to restructure them or to note them for future meetings. The therapist has to watch for and encourage prosocial behavior, and she has to try to manage group behavior.

Implementation

Format of Treatment

In the majority of treatment outcome studies, the treatment is delivered using a group format, while most youth seen on an outpatient basis receive individual therapy. For research purposes, we have used a group format due to the need to treat a large number of girls in a relatively short period of time. However, an important question has not been addressed in the literature, namely, is one format more effective than the other? Based on clinical experience, there are some advantages for each format, and at times a hybrid model that includes both has appeared to be ideal, though impractical. Some of the advantages and disadvantages of the group format for CBT with depressed youth are reported in Table 5.1. For a discussion regarding this issue, see Stark and colleagues (in press).

Group Size

Although groups enable the therapist to see multiple children at once, there is a point at which a group becomes too large to be of therapeutic value. We suggest that four is a good size for a group of depressed 9- to 13-year-old girls. With four participants, it feels and works like a group but is small enough that there is enough time to attend to each participant. In a group that is working well (e.g. no interpersonal conflicts, participants are actively engaged in treatment, etc.),

TABLE 5.1. Advantages and Disadvantages of Group CBT

Advantages of group CBT	Disadvantages of group CBT
• Economy of therapist's time. • Recognition that other same-age girls experience depression. • Group members provide social and emotional support. • Group members are a source of encouragement. • Facilitates acquisition of social skills. • Provides evidence that counters negative beliefs. • Group members give each other therapeutically relevant feedback. • Peer restructuring of beliefs. • Peer-generated solutions to problems. • Peer-generated coping behaviors. • Begin recognizing depressive thoughts in others. • Begin restructuring negative thoughts in others. • Counters the negative thought "No one likes me." • Facilitates building of friendships. • Participants may know more about other group members. • Peers have a more powerful impact on one another.	• Less intense for any given group member. • Less attention for any given group member. • Less time focused on any given group member. • Participants lose focus and get bored. • Participants disengage. • Interpersonal conflict between group members. • Greater complexity for the therapist. • Very taxing on the therapist. • Child who is the focus of restructuring may become self-conscious. • Too much process information for one therapist. • More process factors to recognize and work with. • Participants may be reluctant to self-disclose in the presence of their peers.

the maximum number of children appears to be five. The primary problem of having more participants is that there isn't enough time to attend to each youngster's concerns. The more children in the group, the less time there is for each person to talk about the topic of the day or their individual concerns. At the simplest level, a larger number of participants would slow treatment down and reduce the time spent directly focused on each individual.

Duration and Spacing of Meetings

How many meetings are necessary and sufficient for treatment to be maximally effective? This question is yet to be empirically addressed in the literature. The answer is not simple, as it is idiosyncratic to each client. Currently, our treatment groups are completing 20 meetings plus two individual meetings over 11 weeks. Additional individual meetings are completed during this period on an as-needed basis. The duration of each meeting is developmentally dependent. The meetings are scheduled for more time for older youth and for less time with younger children. We prefer 1-hour meetings with groups of 9- and 10-year-olds and 75-

TABLE 5.2. Advantages to Meeting Twice a Week

- Builds group cohesion more quickly.
- Builds the therapeutic relationship more quickly.
- Participants remember more from one meeting to the next.
- Need less time to review the previous meeting.
- More likely to remember and complete therapeutic homework.
- Can thread meetings together more effectively.
- Consciousness of participants is filled with the therapeutic dialogue.
- Meeting is closer in time to occurrence of critical events.
- More likely to remember thoughts and feelings associated with critical events.
- Less time between destructive between-session events, and the outcome of therapeutic homework is processed closer in time to the event.
- Participants can be reinforced closer in time to the use of therapeutic skills.
- Minimizes the impact of destructive between-session events.
- Participants receive social reinforcement for the use of skills closer in time to the event.

minute meetings with children 11 and older. A possible developmental difference between the treatment of depressed adults and children is that children benefit from meeting twice a week rather than once a week. There are numerous advantages to twice-weekly meetings (see Table 5.2).

Structure of Meetings

The therapy sessions in CBT for depression are structured, and each meeting follows a sequence of events (J. Beck, 1995). We have modified the sequence that has been outlined by Judith Beck (1995) to be developmentally appropriate (see Table 5.3). Following a consistent sequence provides participants with a sense of security, as they know what to expect and it helps to focus the meeting on therapeutically relevant material. Beck has described the structure as it applies to treating depressed adults, and the authors have described this structure for depressed

TABLE 5.3. Structure of Meetings

- Rapport building
- Set agenda
- Goal attainment check-in
- Review of previous meeting and homework
- Coping skills activity
- Skill building
- Review
- Positive behavior review
- Assignment of therapeutic homework

children and adolescents (Stark et al., in press). In the following paragraphs, the segments of treatment that are unique to youths will be briefly described.

Rapport Building. Meetings begin with 5 minutes of unstructured "chat time" to reestablish rapport and to ease participants into more personal discussions. This "chat time" appears to be important to young teens, as they have a greater need to get to know their peers and the therapist as a means of gaining trust. Youth like to use this time to talk about what happened between meetings as a means of getting to know one another. These discussions may be completely irrelevant to treatment, or they may be relevant and allow the therapist to identify possible agenda items. If the discussion becomes therapeutically relevant, then the therapist may decide to move into skill building and use the discussion to teach skills or concepts. When the situation is therapeutically relevant, but doesn't fit with the skill that was scheduled to be taught, the therapist has the flexibility to teach the situation-relevant skill instead.

Goal Attainment Check-In. During every meeting the therapist asks the participants whether they have made any progress toward goal attainment. If they have made progress, then the participant is asked to describe the progress and the therapeutic skills used. The group celebrates the progress through a round of applause or some other form of recognition. In some cases, children have difficulty making progress toward goal attainment. The group may problem-solve to help the youngster develop new plans, or the therapist might meet individually with the child to see if the primary roadblock is negative thinking or something that she doesn't want to discuss in group. If it is due to negatively distorted thoughts, the therapist will restructure the negative thoughts. In some cases, the child may need additional encouragement through an in-session or home reward system. Sometimes, the goals are too ambitious and have to be broken down into subgoals, and plans have to be revised.

Coping Skills Activity. One of the developmental considerations in the design of the treatment manual is that it is believed that children and adolescents have to experience the benefits of a coping skill before they will believe that it works and consider using it. Experiencing the benefits of using a coping skill also helps to restructure the belief that "there isn't anything I can do to help myself feel better." Thus, a powerful way to teach youngsters coping skills is to demonstrate their effectiveness within the meeting. Typically, this can be accomplished using a brief 5- to 10-minute activity. These activities and the specific skills are described in a later section of this chapter. The activity can be enacted at any point during the meeting, and the therapist is free to choose the coping skill that she thinks would be most beneficial for the group at the moment. For example, if the group seems especially flat or depressed, an activity that is energizing would be used. There is one requirement: All five categories of coping strategies (see later section of the chapter) have to be demonstrated by the ninth meeting—thus ensuring that participants experience and know how to use each strategy by the midpoint of treatment. This gives them a number of additional weeks to practice using the skills and prove to themselves that they help improve mood.

Positive Interpersonal Behavior Review. This segment of the meeting is referred to as the "Catch the Positive Activity." It represents an opportunity for the therapist to use praise to shape the behavior of the participants and to help them build a new, positive self-schema. Child clients do not know how to derive the most out of therapy. Thus, it is important to teach them how to be effective clients. The therapist provides each child with a compliment that specifically tells her what she did that would help her derive maximum benefits from the group. In other words, the therapist socially reinforces the participants for behaviors that maximize their therapy experiences (e.g., listening, contributing to the discussion, discussing how something applies to themselves, being supportive of other group members, etc.). As the therapist compliments each child, she tosses a soft, spongy, smiley-faced ball to the child who is the recipient of the compliment— for example, "Kate, you did a great job of helping Melissa see the evidence that she has friends." For some participants it is important to reinforce desirable interpersonal behaviors to prevent conflict or to help a participant to be accepted by other group members. As treatment progresses, participants are assigned by the therapist to compliment one another—for example, "Lindsey, you will compliment Sarah today and Sarah you will compliment Heather," and so on. During each of the last six meetings, the children are asked to notice what they have done well during the meeting and to give themselves compliments. The youngsters enjoy this part of the meeting and seem to internalize the compliments. In addition, they learn how to compliment others who are their age, which is a powerful social skill that they can use outside of group meetings.

Core Therapeutic Components

Affective Education

Affective education is the educational component of treatment that teaches participants about depression and how to manage it. It helps participants to become more aware of their own experiences of depression, including their thoughts, emotions, and behavior, and the relationships between thoughts, emotions, and behavior. In essence, the girls are taught the CBT model of depression, how to personalize the model, and how to manage depression. In addition, it helps them to become more self-aware, particularly of therapeutically relevant experiences such as their depressive thoughts, unpleasant emotions, and other depressive symptoms. Participants are then taught to use these experiences as cues to engage cognitive strategies and problem-solving or coping skills as a means of managing the unpleasant emotions. Affective education is threaded throughout the treatment program and is especially evident during the first few meetings.

Due to developmental limitations, children are taught a simplified model of depression in which sadness is caused by negative thoughts and undesirable outcomes. To manage depression, participants learn three core strategies: (1) if the undesirable situation can't be changed, use a coping strategy; (2) if the undesirable situation can be changed, use problem solving to improve it; and (3) catch negative thoughts and change them to more realistic and positive thoughts. In order to use these three broad strategies, the youngsters have to recognize their unpleasant emotions, that they are experiencing a problem, and that they are experiencing negative thoughts. We help the youngsters to identify their emotions by acting like "emotion detectives" who investigate their own experience of the "three B's": Body, Brain, and Behavior. Participants are taught greater awareness of their emotional experiences by tuning into how their body is reacting, what they are thinking, and how they are acting. During the meetings, when a child states that she is experiencing a particular emotion, the therapist asks her to describe what is happening in her body, what she is thinking, and how she is behaving. Simultaneously, the therapist may use a simple cookie cutout drawing of a girl (Figure 5.1) to illustrate what is happening in her body, brain, and behavior. As treatment progresses and the girls become more proficient at the process, they complete the drawings themselves. The girls also complete therapeutic homework assignments in which they catch their emotional experiences and independently create a drawing using the three B's.

A critical component of the treatment program is teaching the youngsters the relationship between negative thoughts and undesirable emotions and behav-

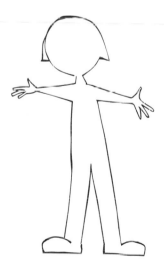

FIGURE 5.1. Drawing used to identify the 3 B's.

iors. To help children understand this relationship, the therapist links thoughts to emotions by asking questions such as "What were you thinking when . . .?" or "What was going through your head when. . .?" Similarly, the therapist might help participants to see the link between thinking and feeling by using an example such as: "A girl thinks, 'No one likes me, I can't do anything right, and I'll always have these problems.' How will she feel? If she thinks, 'I have a couple of really good friends, I do most things well, and I can make things better,' then how would she feel?" Perhaps the most effective way to teach the link between thoughts and emotions is to catch the girls' own examples when they spontaneously verbalize them during the meeting. "I thought that my mom was mad at me, so I felt really down." "Oh, you mean that the way that you thought about the situation caused you to feel down? The thought that your mom was mad at you caused you to feel down?" Such statements also lead to the opportunity to gain an understanding of the *meaning* of the thoughts for the child, thus opening a window to the child's schema or beliefs. The therapist can help the child to become aware of the deeper meaning of events and thus help her to become aware of the schema that is guiding her constructions of situations. This then leads to more elegant and powerful opportunities to restructure the child's core schema. As we will note in a later section, this component is missing from most interventions that are described by investigators as "CBT" and may represent the difference between CBT and cognitive therapy.

Activities and homework assignments also are used to help children become aware of the link between their thoughts and emotions. For example, participants may take turns pulling the name of an emotion out of a bag and then they describe the thoughts that would lead to that emotion. Or they may pull a thought bubble out of a bag and then have to state the emotion that would result from that thought. As treatment progresses, the participants engage in a number of activities that help them become proficient at identifying their negative thoughts.

It is critical to the overall effectiveness of the intervention that the participants be helped to become aware of the link between their thoughts and emotions and that they begin to tune into and verbalize their thoughts early in treatment. This enables them to see that these thoughts cause their upset and maladaptive behaviors, and that these thoughts are not true—that it is the "Muck Monster" (see section on cognitive restructuring) lying to them and that they shouldn't believe what it says.

Goal Setting

CBT is a collaborative approach to psychological treatment in which the child is fully informed of the treatment objectives and the methods that are going to be employed to achieve these objectives. Central to this collaborative process is helping the participant to identify her goals for therapy. In the case of treating children, it may also involve helping the child's parents to identify their goals for their child's treatment as well as their goals for changing their family or parenting practices. In the ACTION program, the therapist begins the goal-setting process by reviewing the plethora of assessment information that each youngster completes prior to treatment. This information is used to complete an initial case conceptualization. The conceptualization is then translated into treatment goals—positively worded statements about desired outcomes. From the CBT perspective, case conceptualization is a fluid process that changes as more is learned about the child (e.g., J. Beck, 1995). The initial conceptualization evolves as new information is gleaned from the group meetings.

The therapist meets individually with each girl between the third and fourth group meetings and collaboratively identifies her greatest concerns and three or four related goals for treatment. Thus, the therapist merges the goals that she has generated during case conceptualization with the child's goals and concerns to develop a set of mutually agreed-upon treatment goals. In addition, the therapist describes treatment procedures that will be used to help her achieve her goals. Before the end of the goals meeting, the therapist asks the child if she would be willing to share her goals with the group. If the child prefers to keep a goal confidential, then this request is respected. During the fourth group meeting, participants share goals with one another and brainstorm how each group member can help the others to attain their goals, a step that can further the sense of cohesion and support within the group. The strategies for helping one another are recorded on their goals sheets so that they can refer to them as needed.

As noted in an earlier section, at the beginning of every subsequent meeting, there is a "goals check-in" time to report progress toward goal attainment and to celebrate progress. As goals are achieved, the therapist helps the participants identify new goals.

Recognizing Progress toward Goals. Progress toward goal attainment can be documented visually for each child. Individual charts are used because a group chart might create competition and reinforce negative thoughts about the self when other group members make more progress toward goal attainment. Problem solving is used to generate new plans if original plans fail. Stickers (for younger children) or check marks (for older children and adolescents) are used to recognize and reinforce progress. Seeing progress toward goal attainment contributes to building a sense of self-efficacy that helps the depressed child feel better about herself and her ability to overcome stressors.

Coping Skills Training

There are a number of underlying assumptions of the ACTION treatment that are rooted in research (for a review see Stark, Sander, Yancy, Bronik, & Hoke, 2000). Thus, coping skills represent a foundational component of the intervention. Depressed youth appear to experience greater mood lability than depressed adults. This may be a developmental phenomenon that is related to their greater exposure to mood-enhancing events and other distractions that naturally occur throughout their day. Even more severely depressed youth experience some temporary reduction in their dysphoria over the course of the day. The greater likelihood of experiencing an improvement in mood may be due to children being less capable of withdrawing and isolating themselves from others and the outside world. It may be due to their exposure to many nondepressed peers who engage them in various social, recreational, and academic activities.

Due to the central role of coping skills in CBT for depressive disorders and the greater reactivity of depressed youth to internal and environmental events, coping skills are included in the ACTION treatment program. A pilot study was conducted to identify developmentally appropriate coping strategies. Five general categories of coping strategies emerged from this research (see Table 5.4).

Coping skills are taught both as a general strategy for enhancing mood and more specifically as a strategy that can be used to enhance mood when a child is experiencing an unfortunate or stressful situation that she cannot change. Thus, clients are taught emotion-focused coping. Coping skills are specifically taught to participants and practiced during meetings 2–9 (see also Kendall & Suveg, Chapter 7, this volume). Coping-skills training is emphasized at the beginning of treatment because these skills help youngsters produce an immediate improvement in mood. This improvement in mood makes it easier for them to learn and benefit from the problem solving and cognitive restructuring that are taught later. There is some flexibility built into the program, as the therapist chooses the coping skills to be taught and applied during each meeting with the constraint that examples from all five of the categories have to be taught within the first nine meetings. Besides this constraint, the therapist chooses the coping skills that she believes are most needed by the group during each meeting. It is important to note that the therapist may include coping skills training at any point during treatment when it would be helpful to the group. For example, students have to complete "high-stakes testing" that determines whether they pass to the next grade. This is a stressful time for the entire school, as funding and individuals' jobs are dependent on the results. This testing occurs over 3 days. The testing was completed during the latter part of treatment for some groups and during the meetings that focused

TABLE 5.4. Five Core Coping Strategies Taught to Participants of the ACTION Program

1. Do something fun and distracting.
2. Do something soothing and relaxing.
3. Do something that expends energy.
4. Talk to someone.
5. Change the way you think about it.

on coping-skills training for other groups. Regardless, the therapists incorporated the testing and the associated negative thoughts and accompanying anxiety into the treatment meetings planned for those days. Soothing and relaxing coping skills were taught and applied to the stress the girls were feeling about the tests. In addition, problem solving was used to help the children develop plans for reducing stress and preparing for anxiety during testing.

Talking about coping skills and how they work is not adequate, as it becomes nothing more than an intellectual exercise. Depressed children, and perhaps children with other disorders, have to experience the benefits of coping skills before they will actually try to use them. When one of the five coping strategies is first taught to the participants, the therapist may notice that the group appears to be flat or down and asks the girls to rate their moods at the moment. If the group is more animated, they may be asked to complete a brief imagery activity in which they imagine experiencing a personally relevant stressful event (e.g., being teased by peers). Then they are asked to rate their mood. After the mood rating, the therapist asks the girls to participate in an activity in which they use a coping skill. For example, the girls may play with hula hoops for 5 minutes along with the therapist (fun and distracting), or they may play freeze tag (exerting energy), wiggle their toes in sand while imaging a relaxing beach scene (soothing and relaxing), they may talk with one another about a stressor (talk to someone), or they may be asked to talk back to their negative thoughts (change your thinking). After completing the activity that takes a few minutes, they stop and rerate their moods. Inevitably, their moods dramatically improve. The therapist asks them what they learned from the experience: "We can help ourselves feel better by doing something fun." "So, what do you think that you can do the next time that you feel down?" The group generates a list of examples of things they can do from this general category of coping strategies. In addition, they discuss the mechanism that makes the coping strategy work. The girls then brainstorm situations where they could use the coping strategy, and they are instructed to try to use one of these coping skills the next time they experience a similar situation.

In addition to teaching girls the coping strategies, the therapist helps the girls to identify situations where it is most advantageous to use particular coping skills. For example, doing something fun and distracting can help lift mood, reduce anger, or reduce anxiety. Soothing and relaxing coping skills are emphasized as a method for reducing anger, irritability, and stress in general. In addition, they can be used to create a calm, pleasant emotional state. Expending energy is useful for generating more energy in general, reducing stress, elevating mood, and fostering better sleep hygiene. Talking to someone can be used as a way to calm down, distract oneself from something that is upsetting, a means of gaining perspective, and a way to feel more connected. Early in treatment, participants are taught to use simple coping statements as a means of managing mood. Coping statements are used by participants during the time that they are acquiring more complex cognitive restructuring strategies. For example, a child may be taught to remind herself that "There are people who love and care about me—what she says isn't true." These statements are designed to help a child to at least temporarily combat depressive thinking. They are not to be confused with the more elegant cognitive restructuring procedures described in a later section.

It is apparent that the youngsters can learn and benefit from using coping skills, but therapeutic improvement is dependent on applying skills outside of group meetings. To facilitate this, therapeutic homework is assigned. This homework progresses from identifying changes in emotion and accompanying thoughts to noting a change in emotions, the context of the emotional change, and the coping skill used to improve mood. In general, participants have a relatively easy time learning coping skills and applying them to their depressive symptoms. By the midpoint in treatment, they give examples of how they use coping skills to improve their moods. In fact, they like the skills so much that it is difficult to get them to use other skills.

Initially, participants are taught to use coping skills as a general strategy for improving mood. Engagement in pleasant activities is used as a method for elevating the participants' overall mood. To accomplish this, the group is asked to generate a list of "fun activities" that are within their control. Each participant is asked to identify activities that give her the most pleasure and to use the list to create a pleasant events schedule ("Take Action List"). These lists consist of mood-enhancing activities and events and a space for indicating their occurrence or nonoccurrence each day. At the bottom of the page is a mood meter where a child rates her mood for the day. The child is instructed to engage in as many pleasant activities as possible and to indicate her involvement by placing a check mark in the appropriate box. Mood is enhanced through increased engagement in pleasant activities and through restructuring the youngster's belief that nothing good ever happens in her life.

Problem-Solving Training

As participants acquire a better understanding of their emotions, accurately identify them, recognize their impact on behavior and thinking, and understand that they can take action to moderate the intensity and impact of their emotions, we teach the girls that some of the undesirable situations that lead to unpleasant affect can be changed. Problem solving is the strategy that they can use to develop a plan for changing undesirable situations. The five-step problem-solving sequence is formally introduced during the fifth meeting. During this meeting, the group also creates a comprehensive list of the problems that girls their age typically face. Without identifying any child, the therapist also contributes examples of problems that the girls experience or have experienced. Then the group goes through the list and determines whether each problem can be changed or whether it is a problem that they can't change. If they can't change the problem, then the therapist queries them about which coping skill they would use to moderate the impact of the event.

The problem-solving procedure that is used is a modification of the one described by Kendall (e.g., Kendall & Braswell, 1993). Children are taught to break problem solving down into five component steps through education, modeling, coaching, rehearsal, and feedback. To simplify the process and to help the girls remember the steps, the therapist refers to the steps as the "five P's" (see Table 5.5). Since the steps have been described elsewhere, only the unique aspects of teaching the steps to depressed youth will be discussed here.

The first step in the process is problem identification and definition. Children refer to this step as "Problem." This may be the most difficult step for depressed children to learn, as they often view a problem as a personal threat. To a depressed child, the existence of a problem means that there is something wrong with herself—or the problem represents an impending loss. In addition, depressed children feel overwhelmed by problems and as if they cannot solve them, and that even if they did solve an existing problem, it would immediately be replaced by another one. Thus, their sense of hopelessness has to be combated through concrete evidence in their life experiences that demonstrates that they can in fact overcome problems. The key to helping depressed youth with identifying their goal for problem solving is helping them to choose constructive goals and to avoid destructive goals. Generating alternative solutions is difficult for depressed youngsters since they typically come up with more reasons for why a plan *won't* work than why it *will* work. Even when they can't identify specific reasons for its not working, they base their prediction on how they are feeling (emotional reasoning). Thus, participants are taught to use coping skills to improve their mood before attempting problem solving as well as during problem solving as they become frustrated or upset. As depressed youth try to use consequential thinking when faced with real-life problems, the therapist often has to help them recognize the potential positive outcomes as well as the limitations and self-defeating consequences of other possibilities. Once again, it is necessary at this step to combat the youngster's pessimism. When the girls first start using problem solving, it is important for the therapist to process the outcome, as depressed youngsters are likely to minimize their successes and magnify the sig-

---

TABLE 5.5. The Five Problem-Solving Steps That Correspond to the Five P's

- Problem—Problem definition
- Purpose—Goal of problem solving
- Plans—Brainstorming solution generation
- Predict and pick—Consequential thinking
- Pat on the back—Self-evaluation of progress toward the goal and self-reinforcement for effort

nificance of their failed attempts and attribute failures to themselves. The girls are taught to use coping statements for unsuccessful plans as well as other coping skills to help themselves deal with the unpleasant affect associated with a failed plan.

Teaching children the problem-solving steps is the easy part of the training. The difficult part is getting them to *use* problem solving to change the situations that cause stress and distress. The participants are formally taught the five steps during meetings 5–9. To facilitate applications of problem solving they are instructed to use problem solving at least once between each of the following meetings and to record their experience with it on one of the problem-solving homework forms. At first, the homework assignments facilitate recognition of problems. Then, the homework forms guide the participants through the application of the steps to their real-life problems.

A secondary issue with the application of problem solving is that the negative thinking of depressed youth gets in the way of their trying to use it. "Why bother? Nothing is going to change, anyway. I'll just mess it up anyway. Nothing is going to work. Even if they change, they'll go back to their old ways again." Thus, cognitive restructuring strategies may have to be used to get participants over the cognitive roadblocks that prevent them from trying problem solving. It often takes the girls a while to build enough of a new-learning history to begin to believe that they can use problem solving to produce significant changes in their lives. Another useful strategy is to teach the girls to combine coping skills with problem solving. They are taught to use the coping skills to elevate their mood or to overcome their pessimism, and then they engage in problem solving when they have more emotional distance and can think more realistically about the problem.

Cognitive Restructuring

A primary objective of the ACTION treatment for depressed children is to change their negatively distorted thinking to more positive and realistic thinking. To accomplish this objective, the therapist has to identify the core beliefs that underlie the youngster's depressive thoughts and then develop a plan for providing the child with corrective learning experiences that help her to evaluate and change dysfunctional beliefs. As noted earlier, the therapist uses assessment information to develop a conceptualization before treatment meetings begin. This conceptualization includes hypotheses about possible core beliefs. As noted by Aaron Beck, the most common core beliefs or schemas underlying depression include "I'm unlovable," "I'm worthless," and "I'm helpless" (e.g. Beck et al., 1979). A depressed child may be experiencing one or more of these beliefs. To determine which belief or beliefs are operating for each child, the therapist listens to the child's self-references and the meanings that she draws from daily experiences. The beliefs are reflected in the themes and consistencies found in each child's thoughts. The meanings of events can be deduced from the discussions and by asking "What does it mean about you if . . . ?" and by following up with additional similar questions until the most basic meaning is uncovered. Judith Beck (1995) refers to this procedure as the downward-arrow technique.

Negative thoughts are restructured directly and indirectly throughout treatment. During the first nine meetings, the therapist identifies negative thoughts and asks the questions that lead to cognitive restructuring. Consequently, the girls don't have to do a lot of self-reflection outside of meetings. Direct restructuring of negative thoughts is completed through teaching youngsters to identify, evaluate, and then replace their own negative thoughts with more realistic and positive thoughts. Girls are taught cognitive restructuring later in treatment (meetings 10–20) because it requires them to become more self-focused and to focus on negative thoughts that can exacerbate depressive symptoms. By providing the girls with coping and problem-solving skills earlier in treatment, they can manage the upset that comes with an increased self-focus. In addition, the cognitive restructuring that the therapist completes helps to start the shift in thinking, and it serves as a model for how to do it. It also appears as though the improvement in mood and symptoms that results from other treatment components and the therapist-led cognitive restructuring provide youngsters with some cognitive distance from their depressive thoughts and beliefs that seems to open them to restructuring their own thoughts.

In order to independently restructure negative thoughts and the beliefs that underlie them, the girls must become aware of their thoughts. It is easier to recognize when someone else expresses negative thoughts, so we begin by asking the girls to do this as a bridge to recognizing and identifying their own negative thoughts. To accomplish this, the therapist and girls discuss how to recognize negative thoughts and then they play a game of catching each other's negative thoughts. The girls are instructed to call out "negative thought" whenever someone expresses one through their in-group statements. The therapist purposely makes many negative statements to give the girls practice at doing this and to normalize being the recipient of the "negative thought" comment. Subsequently, the girls are asked to catch and record their own negative thoughts on homework forms that they bring to the group for help restructuring.

Once a negative thought has been identified, the child asks one of the two "what questions" as a means of evaluating its validity and for developing adaptive thoughts to replace the negative ones. The two "what questions" are (1) What's another way to think about it? and (2) What's the evidence? First, the girls learn the question that is best suited for transforming negative thoughts. "What's another way to think about it?" is the easiest cognitive restructuring question for children to learn. They use this question to generate alternative, plausible, and *positive* thoughts for a distressing situation. So, this is a good question to use when the girls draw a conclusion from a situation that has many other viable conclusions that could be drawn from it. "What's the evidence?" is used when the objective facts do not support the child's negative thought.

The standard cognitive restructuring procedure can be difficult to teach children to use—once again reflecting a developmental difference between children and adults. A powerful tool that is part of the ACTION program is an activity that the girls refer to as "talking back to the Muck Monster." When the participants are having difficulty changing, or letting go of, negative thinking, we refer to this as being stuck in the negative muck. The girls like and understand this metaphor. When they are stuck in the negative muck, it is the "Muck Monster" that is filling them with negative thoughts and holding them back from extricating themselves from the muck. Somewhat surprisingly, the girls consistently report having an image of their muck monster. They are eager to describe it, and they are asked to draw it in preparation for the activity. Therapists encourage this, as it depersonalizes the negative thinking, creates emotional distance between the child and her depressive thinking, and creates a concrete opponent to defeat. Talking back to the muck monster is completed as many times as needed to help the girls learn how to restructure their negative thoughts between the 10th meeting and termination.

Preparation for this activity begins prior to treatment during the assessment process and continues throughout treatment. The therapist maintains a list of each girl's negative thoughts. The list includes thoughts that were endorsed on the pretreatment assessment measures, verbalized during treatment meetings, and recorded on homework forms. This list represents the content of each girl's "muck monster." During an individual meeting that occurs between group meetings 10 and 11, the therapist discusses each girl's list with her in order to confirm that it "rings true" and to make her aware of these thoughts and beliefs as well as their impact on emotions, behavior, and interpersonal relationships. The beliefs are written inside the girls' drawings of their muck monsters, and the thoughts that stem from the beliefs are written in thought bubbles around the muck monster.

To help the girls learn how to independently apply cognitive restructuring, they are asked to talk back to the muck monster by using the two "what questions" during meetings. To accomplish this, an extra chair is brought to the group meetings. The chair is for the muck monster. The therapist moves to the empty chair and holds the child's picture of the muck monster while she states one of the child's negative thoughts. The girl forcefully uses the two "what questions" to guide her talking back to the muck monster. Group members help her to do this by providing additional evidence or alternative interpretations. The girls may be encouraged to very forcefully talk back to the muck monster by yelling at it. Other group members assist and cheer her on as she forcefully evaluates negative thoughts and then replaces them with more realistic positive ones. Sometimes it is helpful to have the girl play the role of the muck monster and have her hold the drawing of the muck monster while she verbalizes her own negative thoughts and while the therapist forcefully talks back to the muck monster by using the two "what questions." The girls enjoy this activity, and it helps them learn how to use cognitive restructuring. To provide the girls with additional help in applying cognitive restructuring outside of the meetings, the workbook has forms that guide the girls through the process of catching, evaluating, and replacing negative thoughts.

Restructuring of negative thoughts also is completed indirectly through guided learning experiences that are incorporated into treatment. These learning experiences are chosen based on the case conceptualization that was initially developed before treatment meetings began and is further refined over the ensuing treatment meetings. Thus, at the same time that the therapist is refining the case conceptualizations she is watching for opportunities to use the child's own experiences to help her process evidence that contradicts her negative beliefs and supports new, more adaptive, beliefs. For example, a girl whose underlying core belief is "I'm unlovable," which results in the intermediate belief "No one likes me," states that the following events happened between meetings. She talked with a friend on the Internet. She had a friend sleep over during the weekend. She was invited to a birthday party. She and her mom baked Christmas cookies together. Her mom tucks her into bed and says prayers with her every night. Through Socratic questioning each of these events can be used to help her see that she is liked by others and that she is loved by significant others. Of course, this would only be done if she truly is liked and loved by others. The therapist also gives the child specific homework assignments that provide her with learning experiences that contradict existing negative beliefs and build new, more adaptive, beliefs. The girls are instructed to complete a diary that guides their attention to events that facilitate cognitive restructuring. The diary is referred to as the "Catch the Positive" Diary (CPD). For example, the girl who believes that she is unlovable would be asked to develop a list of parental behaviors that demonstrate that she is loved. This list would become part of her CPD, and she would be instructed to monitor the occurrence of these behaviors using the CPD between meetings. As they occur, she checks them off in her diary, and the outcome of the assignment is processed during the next meeting. This assignment restructures the child's belief only if it is a reflection of a distortion in her thinking—that is, peers really do like her and significant others really do love her. It would not work so well if the parents did not express their love for her in demonstrable ways.

Building a Positive Sense of Self

The primary objective of cognitive restructuring is to help girls build a positive self-schema. During the last eight meetings additional activities are used to support this positive sense of self. This treatment component appears last because all of the other skills are used during the process of working toward self-improvement and recognizing positive aspects of the self. Depressed children evaluate their performances, possessions, and personal qualities more negatively than nondepressed youth, and their self-evaluations tend to be negatively distorted (Kendall, Stark, & Adam, 1990). In other words, they tend to be unrealistically and unreasonably negative in their self-evaluations. Children can be taught to evaluate themselves more reasonably and positively when it is realistic to do so. During this process they learn to recognize their positive attributes, outcomes, and possessions.

One of the tools used to help youngsters develop a more positive sense of themselves is the "self-map" (see Figure 5.2). Each circle within the figure represents an area of the child's life and an aspect of self-definition. Overall, the "self-map" helps the girls to broaden their self-definition and to recognize more strengths than they were previously aware of. Participants are asked to fill in each bubble with relevant strengths. In addition, parents and teachers are interviewed by the therapist to identify their perceptions of the child's strengths in each of the domains. This information is provided to the girls by the therapist. We have found that this information can be very powerful, as the children enjoy receiving the compliments. In addition, group members provide one another with positive feedback for each circle. Once again, receiving this information from peers appears to be very powerful and believable.

The CPD is used as the children are asked to self-monitor evidence that supports the positive self-description that is outlined on the self-map. For exam-

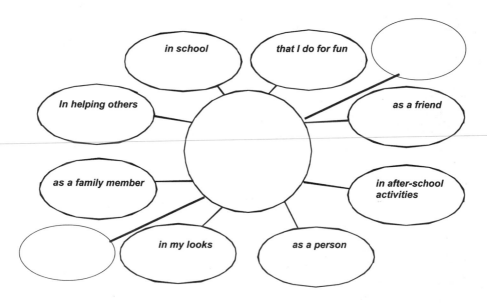

FIGURE 5.2. Self-map.

ple, a child might place a lot of self worth into her musical talent. She would be instructed to self-monitor her successes during class, individual instruction, practice, and concerts. In addition, emphasis would be placed on her effort toward becoming a better musician rather than on comparing herself to others. Furthermore, the *personal* pleasure she derives from playing her instrument would be emphasized.

In some instances, the children's negative self-evaluations are accurate, and they can benefit from change. In such instances, the goal of treatment is to help the youngsters to translate personal standards into realistic goals and then to develop and carry out plans for attaining their goals. Following the translation process, children prioritize the areas where they are working toward self-improvement. Initially a plan is formulated for producing improvement in an area where success is probable. The long-term goal is broken down into subgoals, and problem solving is used to develop plans that will lead to subgoal and eventually goal attainment. Prior to enacting plans, children try to identify possible impediments to carrying out the plans. Once again, problem solving is used to develop contingency plans for overcoming the impediments. Once the plans, including contingency plans, have been developed, children self-monitor their progress toward change. Alterations in plans are made along the way.

ACTION Kits

One of the developmental differences between conducting CBT with depressed children versus depressed adults is that children are less likely to remember what they have discussed in the meetings. To help them remember the central therapeutic concepts, we have constructed "ACTION Kits." The kits consist of a set of five color-coded cards, including (1) a simple schematic depicting when to use coping skills, problem solving, and cognitive restructuring, (2) a visual depiction of how to use the three B's to identify emotions; (3) a visual depiction of the five categories of coping skills; (4) the five problem-solving steps ("five P's"); and (5) the two "what questions" that guide cognitive restructuring. In addition, each kit includes one of the smiley-faced catch-the-positive balls and a personalized goals form including plans for achieving goals. These kits are given to the girls between the sixth and seventh meetings, after all of the major treatment strategies have been introduced. The therapist uses her own kit during group meetings to model its use. For example, when a participant's homework reveals that she was feeling angry between meetings, the therapist pulls out the card that depicts when to use each of the three primary treatment strategies. Since it was a situation with a classmate that could be changed, the group decides to use problem solving, and the therapist uses the problem-solving card to guide the development of a plan. However, the therapist notes that it can be difficult to develop constructive plans when feeling angry, so she also pulls out the coping-skills card and the child chooses coping skills that would help her reduce anger so that she could think more clearly. Thus, the therapist introduces the idea that it is helpful to combine the three primary treatment strategies. For example, a child may have to apply coping skills to improve dysphoric mood before she can effectively restructure a negative thought. It is common for children to have to use multiple skills simultaneously in order to improve their mood and other depressive symptoms. The therapist uses the group members' therapeutic homework and concerns that they bring to group to help them learn how to do this.

Therapeutic Homework

Therapeutic homework is an integral part of treatment. Homework assignments are designed to help children *apply* skills that they have learned within meetings to real-life situations that occur outside of treatment. The workbook (Stark, Schnoebelen, et al., 2005) structures therapeutic homework. Each assignment is designed to support application of the skill that was taught during that meeting. An example of a coping skills, problem-solving, and cognitive restructuring homework form are provided in Figures 5.3, 5.4, and 5.5, respectively.

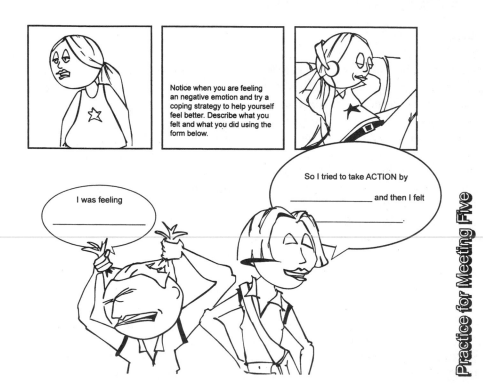

FIGURE 5.3. Coping skills homework form.

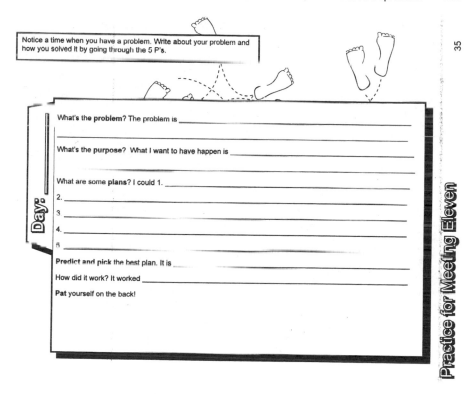

FIGURE 5.4. Problem-solving homework form.

Many children don't like to complete therapeutic homework. To encourage them to do it, we include a within-session reward system. Children who complete the assignment can choose a reward from the preferred prize bag, and children who do not complete the assignment are given the opportunity to choose from the less desirable bag for attending the meeting. The therapists may use additional rewards for the successful completion of homework.

When a child fails to complete a homework assignment, she is asked to complete it to the best of her recollection at the start of the meeting. If a child consistently has problems completing homework, the therapist will meet individually with her, and they will problem-solve to help her develop a plan for completing it. If a participant continues to have difficulty in completing her homework, we have used a number of additional strategies, including e-mail and telephone call reminders as well as having the girl stop by the school counselor's office prior to school each morning. Ideally, with younger children, we like their primary caregiver to encourage them to complete it. With older children and adolescents, parental involvement in homework is less desirable.

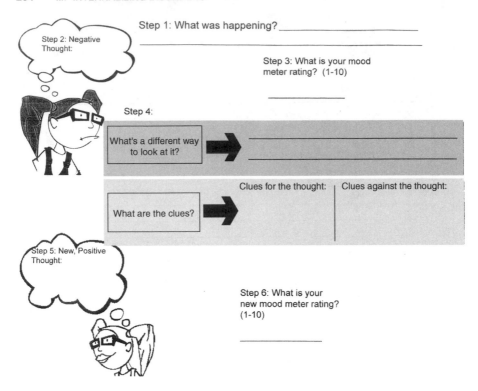

FIGURE 5.5. Cognitive restructuring form.

Parent Training

Currently the efficacy of the ACTION treatment program is being evaluated with and without a parent-training component. Parent training (Stark, Schnoebelen, et al., 2005; Stark, Simpson, et al., 2005) is designed to support the child treatment component and to teach the parents (1) how to support their child's efforts to learn and apply the therapeutic skills, (2) indirectly teach the parents the same skills, and (3) teach the parents skills for improving their behavior management, improving communication, reducing conflict, and helping the girls to identify and change their negative thoughts. The parent training meetings are completed in groups at their daughter's school after school hours. The meetings are conducted by the child's therapist and a co-therapist, and the meetings last approximately 90 minutes. There are eight group parent meetings and two individual family meetings completed over the 11 weeks that their daughters are receiving their group treatment. The individual family meetings occur between the third and fourth group meetings and again between the seventh and eighth group meetings. The daughters are present during the even-numbered group meetings and both individual family meetings. The meetings are structured similarly to the child meetings. However, there is an addition: Prior to reviewing the main points from the previous parent meeting, the therapists, or the therapists and the girls, provide the parents with a description of the skills the girls have learned, and they try to teach the parents how to use the skills.

Skills Taught to the Parents

A number of core therapeutic skills are taught to the parents, based on the literature regarding the impact of the family on depressive disorders in youths. Prior to teaching the parents specific skills, they are provided with information about depression in children and young teens, our model of depressive disorders, and how to successfully treat depression. To create a more positive environment, parents are taught to manage their daughters' behavior through the use of reinforcement for desirable behavior. At the same time, they are instructed to decrease their use of punitive and coercive strategies. Teaching parents this more positive approach to managing their daughters' behavior creates a home environment that has a positive affective valence, and it sends the girls a positive message about themselves (I am a good person) and about their parents (they pay attention to me). Parents learn how to effectively use positive reinforcement and details about the impact of positive reinforcement on their daughters during the first two meetings, and they practice applying it during all of the following meetings that their daughters are present. Subsequently, they are instructed to monitor their use of reinforcement at home. During the second meeting the girls help their parents develop a reward menu, and they identify areas where they think they could benefit from some more parental encouragement. In addition, during this meeting, parents experience the power of doing fun things with their daughters as they play a game together. Parents are encouraged to help their daughters do more fun things as a coping strategy, and they are encouraged to do more recreational things as a family. During the third meeting, the parents are taught the deleterious effects of excessive use of punishment to manage their daughters' behavior. They are helped to identify all of the forms of punishment that they use, and they are encouraged to decrease their use of punishment and replace it with positive reinforcement.

During the same week that the girls set their goals for treatment and collaboratively work with the therapist to identify plans for attaining their goals, the therapist conducts individual family meetings and collaborates with the parents to identify their goals for their daughter and family. In addition, with the girl's permission, the therapist and girl go over her goals for treatment and the plan for realizing the goals. Parents are encouraged to support these goals, and the things that they can do to help their daughter achieve her goals are discussed.

Parents are taught a variety of communication skills. Initially, they are taught how to listen empathically. This skill is taught because it communicates to the child that she is being listened to and understood, which leads to a sense of being loved and worthy. In addition, it is a cornerstone of good communication between the girls and their parents. Whenever they are feeling upset or experiencing a problem, the girls are taught to immediately ask their parents if it is a good time to talk. Similarly, the parents are taught to initiate a conversation with their daughters whenever they sense that she is upset. Once the conversation is initiated, the parent clears his or her mind of distractions and then listens to the daughter without providing her with any quick comforts or solutions to problems. The parent listens for the emotion or message that underlies the girl's statements. This is very difficult for the parents to do. They have a hard time just listening and an even harder time identifying the underlying emotions or broader meaning. It takes a good deal of role playing and coaching for the parents to be able to listen empathically. In some cases, it seems like the best that can be done is to teach the parent to become an active listener. In addition, parents are taught the following communication skills: (1) Keep it brief, (2) don't blame, (3) be specific, (4) listen empathically, (5) make feeling statements, and (6) give options if possible. These skills are modeled by the therapists, role-played by the therapists and parents, and practiced during sessions by the parents and their daughters. The training begins with discussions about easy topics and then progresses to more emotionally laden topics.

Parents are taught the same five-step problem-solving procedure that the girls learn. Parents are taught to view misbehavior and problems that the family faces as problems to be solved. The girls teach their parents the steps, and then they play a game with their parents as a procedure for demonstrating the meaning of each step as well as how to apply each step to a simple situation—the game. Once the parents have been exposed to the steps and understand the process, the therapist breaks the parents and daughters into family units and provides the families with a hypothetical family problem to be solved.

Elevated levels of conflict are commonly reported in families with depressed children (Stark et al., 1990), and the conflict is related to the duration of time that it takes for a depressive episode to naturally remit. Thus, parents are taught conflict resolution skills. More specifically, they are taught how to structure and use family meetings as a tool for reducing conflict. The first step in the family meeting is to say something positive about each family member. Then, the person who calls the meeting sets the agenda. The person who calls the meeting states the issue and gives examples of the personal impact of the point of conflict. Next, this person initiates a discussion about alternative behaviors that would solve the problem, and the family discusses potential outcomes for each alternative. Finally, a plan is chosen and initiated. The families role-play the meeting process with coaching from the therapists. Emphasis is placed on catching the conflict early before the upset gets so bad that it can't be constructively managed. Over the course of the next few meetings, the therapist works with the parents to eliminate barriers to resolving conflict, such as parents' beliefs.

Parents can play a meaningful role in helping their daughters to catch, evaluate, and restructure their negative thoughts and beliefs. During the second individual family meeting and during the seventh and eighth group parent meetings, the parents learn about the impact of negative thinking on their daughters' emotional well-being. During the group meetings, parents learn about the impact of negative thoughts and beliefs on their daughters' emotional functioning, and they are taught to look at the messages that they inadvertently send to their daughters through their own actions and the things that they say. During the individual family meeting and while the families are broken up into their own constellations within the larger group meeting, the girls describe the impact that their specific negative thoughts have on their emotions, and then the parents help their daughters to talk back to the thoughts. Parents are encouraged to identify their own negative thoughts and to restructure them, using the same procedures as their daughters use.

Teacher Consultation

The classroom environment and the relationship that a student has with her teacher and peers have an impact on a child's emotional adjustment. Teacher support and perceived classroom belonging play a role in academic motivation, self-esteem, and depressive symptoms for females (Goodenow, 1993; Midgley, Feldlaufer, & Eccles, 1989). Positive teacher–student relationships promote positive school-related emotions, perceived sense of belonging, and positive self-esteem across age levels (Hoge, Smith, & Hanson, 1990; Murray & Greenberg, 2000; Pianta, 1994; Roeser, Midgley, & Urdan, 1996). Students with low perceptions of belongingness are more likely to experience depression, social rejection, and school problems (Anderman, 2002). Increases in teacher support are related to increases in self-esteem and decreases in depression (Reddy, Rhodes, & Mulhall, 2003). An objective of the ACTION program is to provide teacher consultation as a means of impacting depression.

The ACTION program is implemented in the schools during school hours. Thus, entry has been secured at the highest level of administration (the superintendent of schools) and at the site level through the principal. The administration has communicated its support to the teachers, which makes consultation easier. Teachers are an excellent source of information about the child and more specifically about academic and interpersonal functioning. Interviewing the teacher can provide the therapist with information about the child's academic performance, general mood, frustration tolerance, negative self-statements ("I can't do this!" "Nobody likes me."), frequency of visits to the nurse's office, absences, and interpersonal relationships. If the child is performing well, this can be useful information for cognitive restructuring, and if the child is struggling, the teacher may be able to modify the curriculum or provide tutoring or other assistance to help ensure that the child is successful.

Since students meet in their treatment groups 2 hours per week, and many students, especially those in elementary school, spend more time with their teachers than with their parents, it is important to use teacher consultation to encourage the girls to apply the therapeutic skills. Teachers can provide the girls with additional opportunities to practice their new strategies for relieving depressive symptoms. For example, a teacher might see that a child is frustrated by an assignment. She might discreetly cue the child to use one of her coping strategies to reduce the emotional upset. A child might verbalize a negative thought, and the teacher can discreetly cue her to use her "what questions" and cognitive restructuring worksheets to evaluate and restructure the thought. Optimally the therapist meets with the child's teachers throughout treatment. The therapist introduces the treatment skills to the teacher as the group progresses, and asks the teacher to praise the child for using a skill in the classroom.

Another objective of teacher consultation is to collaboratively design ways that the teachers can facilitate cognitive restructuring. The goal of this consultation is not for teachers to become therapists; rather, it is to collaboratively develop ways that they can provide the girls with new learning experiences that restructure maladaptive beliefs. For example, a child who believes that no one likes her may in fact be approached by many other students during the school day, but she minimizes or in some other way distorts these experiences. The teacher can help her see that other students approached her to initiate social interaction by pointing it out at the moment or by providing the girl with specific examples throughout the day.

Examples of Student-Specific Interventions in the Classroom

Positive Peer Interaction Self-Monitoring—"No one likes me." This intervention restructures the belief "No one likes me." The purpose of this intervention is to provide the child with evidence that restructures this belief by helping the child to become aware of positive interactions with her peers. The child is instructed to tell the teacher about three positive peer interactions. A specific time is established to discreetly discuss these interactions. The teacher can help the student recognize and not minimize simple interactions such as "Lindsey smiled at me" or "said 'Hello' " as well as more extensive interactions such as talking or playing with a classmate. The teacher reinforces self-monitoring and engagement in these positive interactions. If the student has difficulty remembering positive events, the teacher can provide examples that he or she observed. The teacher shares this information with the therapist by recording the outcome of the child's self-monitoring and any comments or concerns.

Positive Teacher Attention Time—"My teacher doesn't like me." A student may believe that a teacher does not like her. When this occurs, it may be due to a core belief of unlovability. Providing evidence that the teacher likes her can help to restructure this belief. The therapist and teacher brainstorm a list of positive characteristics about the child. The teacher uses material from this list to initiate positive interactions or discussions with the student for a few minutes a day. The child and the teacher keep logs of the interactions.

Encouraging Approach-Related Behaviors—"They don't like me/They don't want to hang out with me." Children who believe that their peers do not like them often use withdrawal as a compensatory strategy. Unfortunately this strategy indirectly provides the student with further evidence that peers do not want to spend time with her. This intervention would *not* be used with students who are victims of teasing or bullying, but is appropriate for students who have an unfounded belief that others do not like them. The therapist meets with the student and teacher to discuss some experiments to be conducted with classmates. Examples of approach behaviors would be discussed, and students who are likely to be open to such initiations would be identified. The student is encouraged to try this behavior once a day and report her attempts to the teacher, and the teacher would verbally reinforce her efforts. If she is not successful, the teacher or therapist can help the student problem-solve prior to her next attempt.

Self-Monitoring Negative Predictions—"Things will never be good." Some students possess the belief that "Nothing will ever work out the way I want." After the student has stated her worries to the therapist, they discuss how this belief can be objectively evaluated and observed in school. The therapist develops a self-monitoring form with three columns, marked "Prediction," "More helpful thought," and "Actual event." The student is responsible for writing down two negative predictions each day as well as more helpful thoughts or problem-solving ideas. Then, the participant must note what really happens. Examples of negative predictions could be "I'm going to fail this test," "No one will sit next to me at lunch," or "My teacher will be mad that I forgot my homework." If the child doesn't have any negative predictions on a particular day, she is instructed to list three positive events that worked out the way she hoped. The student can show the teacher her worksheet each day, and the teacher can either help her to see the positive outcomes or to identify desirable events that the girl didn't notice.

Self-Monitoring Success—"I can't do anything right!" Many girls have the core belief that they can't do anything right. Teachers can help children restructure this belief by helping them to become aware of the things they do well and the things that demonstrate that they do things correctly. The student may be asked to tell the teacher or write down three tasks she completed or things she did right. Examples include: "I got to school on time. I followed the rules during a game. I was quiet in the hallways. I raised my hand to ask a question." The goal of this strategy is to help the student recognize that she does many things right many days. Therefore, if she gets in trouble or makes a mistake, it doesn't mean she does everything wrong or can't do anything right.

Self-Monitoring Problem-Solving and Coping Skills. Some students have difficulty noticing when to use problem-solving and coping skills. The therapist can meet with the child and teacher to develop a system that enables the teacher to cue the child to use problem-solving and/or coping skills. The therapist gives the child extra copies of the problem-solving forms from the ACTION workbook. The child is responsible for noticing one problem each day (it can be anything from a small annoyance to a significant problem) and to use problem solving to develop and implement a plan for changing the situation. If she notices a problem that is out of her control, the teacher reminds her to use one of the five coping strategies to manage the emotional upset. Some students are not comfortable with the teacher reading their entries—thus, just showing the teacher that it was completed is sufficient for these results.

SUMMARY AND CONCLUSIONS

Most depressed youth do not receive treatment, and those that do, receive treatment from a provider that typically uses an eclectic mix of dynamic, behavioral, and cognitive procedures (Weersing & Weisz, 2002). Unfortunately, this form of treatment has been found to be no more effective than the changes that occur due to the passage of time (Andrade et al., 2000), and it is less effective than other (research-based) treatments (Weersing & Weisz, 2002). Although the majority of outcome studies that were conducted since the second edition of this book suggest that CBT remains an effective intervention for depressive disorders among youth, the status of CBT as a stand-alone treatment for depressive disorders has been questioned by the results of the TADS, but recall that the TADS CBT was not identical to the other evaluated CBT programs. Perhaps the TADS study raises more questions than it answers, and additional research is necessary to answer them. Are the less-than-typical results due to the specific treatment components included, or perhaps not included? Was the intervention too short? The CBT intervention in TADS consisted of psychoeducation about depression and training in five therapeutic skills in the first six meetings followed by social skills training for the next six meetings. Clinical experience with severely depressed youth suggests that the limited amount of time spent training in the use of each of the therapeutic skills (one meeting per skill) amounts to a very limited psychoeducation. CBT is effective when the participant learns, applies, and experiences the benefits of the skills being taught. It is necessary to demonstrate within the sessions that the skills actually help to break through the hopelessness and other negative thoughts of depressed youth that prevent them from applying the skills in their daily lives. It is not apparent from the TADS manual that this was part of the treatment.

The program has resulted in positive outcomes. If the positive results with the ACTION treatment program hold up for the entire sample being studied, the model can be said to have been effective with girls between the ages of 9 and 13. Are the results due to the gender specificity of the treatment? Are they due to a greater number of treatment sessions (20 group and 2 individual meetings)? Are they due to the specific components included in the treatment or the number of meetings dedicated to certain targets of change? Are they due to the treatment being individualized for each youth based on a cognitive case conceptualization? Are they due to the younger age of the participants? Are they due to the delivery format (group vs. individual)? Once again, additional research is needed to answer these and other related questions.

The ACTION program is designed to teach girls to use unpleasant affect and other depressive symptoms as cues to employ coping, problem-solving, and cognitive restructuring skills to manage their depressive symptoms. Psychoeducation is used to teach the girls to tune into their emotional experiences. Initially, treatment efforts are focused on pleasant emotions and positive experiences as a means of creating an improvement in mood. Subsequently, the girls are taught to use coping strategies when their upset stems from a situation that they can't change, problem solving when their upset stems from a situation that they can change, and cognitive restructuring when their upset stems from negatively distorted thinking. Consistent with principles of cognitive therapy, the treatment sessions are highly structured, with each segment of the meeting being designed to have therapeutic value. Thus, unproductive time is minimized. In addition, the therapist develops a cognitive case conceptualization before treatment begins, and this conceptualization changes as it is informed by experiences during treatment meetings. This conceptualization provides the therapist with a schema for watching for experiences in the child's life that provide contradictory evidence for existing depressive schemas and help build more realistic and positive schemas. In addition, the therapist tries to develop learning experiences for the child that will tear down the negative schemas and build new more adaptive core schemas.

Another objective of the ACTION treatment program is to change the family environment through parent training. The parent training program is designed to teach the parents to use positive reinforcement as the primary means of managing behavior. Simultaneous to increasing the use of positive reinforcement is a decrease of punitive and coercive behavior management procedures. Parents are taught empathic listening as well as other communication skills. This appears to be important to girls who want significant others in their environments to listen to them and understand them. Empathic listening communicates both. Parents are taught family problem-solving and conflict resolution skills as a means of reducing stress, and more specifically the stress due to conflict within the family. Parents are also taught how to identify their daughters' negative thoughts and methods for helping them to restructure these thoughts. Another important aspect of the parent training component is to help parents understand how they can support their daughters in the application of the ACTION skills in the home environment. Finally, parents are encouraged to apply the skills that their daughters are learning to their own lives.

School-age youth spend more time in school interacting with their teachers and peers than they do at home interacting with their parents. Consequently, the ACTION program includes a teacher consultation component. Teacher consultation is designed to help teachers encourage girls to apply the ACTION skills to the classroom and other school environments. In addition, teachers may be asked to assist the girls in their homework activities that are designed to produce cognitive restructuring.

Each depressed youth represents a complex and unique case. To be effective, the therapist has to be facile in the use of CBT for depressive disorders, and he or she has to be able to blend this treatment with treatments for the other comorbid conditions that the youngster is likely to be experiencing. This is an exciting time in the study of interventions for depressed youth, as a great deal of research is underway. It is expected that many of the questions raised by current outcome research will be answered by the printing of the fourth edition of this text.

REFERENCES

Addis, M. E., & Krasnow, A. D. (2000). A national survey of practicing psychologists' attitudes toward psychotherapy treatment manuals. *Journal of Consulting and Clinical Psychology, 68,* 331–339.

Ambrosini, P. J., & Dixon, J. F. (Eds.). (2000). *Schedule for Affective Disorders and Schizophrenia for School Age Children (6–18 yrs.) KIDDIE-SADS (K-SADS) Present State and Lifetime Version. K-SADS-IVR (Revision of K-SADS).* Unpublished manuscript.

Anderman, E. M. (2002). School effects on psychological outcomes during adolescence. *Journal of Educational Psychology, 94,* 795–809.

Andrade, A., Lambert, W., & Bickman, L. (2000). Dose effect in child psychotherapy: Outcomes associated with negligible treatment. *Journal of the American Academy of Child and Adolescent Psychiatry, 39,* 161–168.

Baxter, L. R., Schwartz, J. M., Phelps, M. E., Mazziotta, J. C., Guze, B. H., Selin, C. E., et al. (1989). Reduction of prefrontal cortex glucose metabolism common to three types of depression. *Archives of General Psychiatry, 46,* 243–250.

Beck, A. T., Rush, J., Shaw, B. F., & Emery, G. (1979). *Cognitive therapy of depression.* New York: Guilford Press.

Beck, J. S. (1995). *Cognitive therapy: Basics and beyond.* New York: Guilford Press.

Beck, J. S., Beck, A. T., & Jolly, J. B. (2001). *Beck Youth Inventories.* San Antonio, TX: Psychological Corporation.

Bench, C. J., Frackowiak, R. S. J., & Dolan, R. J. (1995). Changes in regional cerebral blood flow on recovery from depression. *Psychological Medicine, 25,* 247–251.

Bickman, L., Noser, K., & Summerfelt, W. T. (1999). Long-term effects of a system of care on children and adolescents. *Journal of Behavioral Health Services Research, 26,* 185–202.

Birmaher, B., Brent, D. A., Kolko, D., Baugher, M., Bridge, J., Holder, D., et al. (2000).

Clinical outcome after short-term psychotherapy for adolescents with Major Depressive Disorder. *Archives of General Psychiatry, 57*, 29–36.

Brent, D. A., Holder, D., & Kolko, D. (1997). A clinical psychotherapy trial for adolescent depression comparing cognitive, family, and supportive therapy. *Archives of General Psychiatry, 54*, 877 885.

Brody, A. L., Saxena, S., Mandelkern, M. A., Fairbanks, L. A., Ho, M. L., & Baxter, L. R. (2001). Brain metabolic change associated with symptom factor improvement in Major Depressive Disorder. *Biological Psychiatry, 50*, 171–178.

Chambless, D. L., & Hollon, S. D. (1998). Defining empirically supported therapies. *Journal of Consulting and Clinical Psychology, 66*, 7–18

Clarke, G. N., Hawkins, W., Murphy, M., Sheeber, L. B., Lewinsohn, P. M., & Seeley, J. R. (1995). Targeted prevention of unipolar depressive disorder in an at-risk sample of high school adolescents: A randomized trial of group cognitive intervention. *Journal of Child and Adolescent Psychiatry, 32*, 312–321.

Clarke, G. N., Hornbrook, M., Lynch, F., Plen, M., Gale, J., Beardslee, W., et al. (2001). A randomized trial of a group cognitive intervention for preventing depression in adolescent offspring of depressed parents. *Archives of General Psychiatry, 58*, 1127–1134.

Clarke, G. N., Rohde, P., Lewinsohn, P. M., Hops, H., & Seeley, J. R. (1999) Cognitive-behavioral treatment of adolescent depression: Efficacy of acute group treatment and booster sessions. *Journal of the American Academy of Child and Adolescent Psychiatry, 38*, 272–279.

Delgado, P. L., Charney, D. S., Price, L. H., Aghajanian, G. K., Landis, H., & Heninger, G. R. (1990). Serotonin function and the mechanism of antidepressant action: Reversal of antidepressant-induced remission by rapid depletion of plasma tryptophan. *Archives of General Psychiatry, 47*, 411–418.

Delgado, P. L., Miller, H. L., Salomon, R. M., Licinio, J., Krystal, J. H., Moreno, F. A., et al. (1999). Tryptophan-depletion challenge in depressed patients treated with desipramine or fluoxetine: Implications for the role of serotonin in the mechanism of antidepressant action. *Biological Psychiatry, 46*, 212–220.

Durlak, J. A., Fuhrman, T., & Lampman, C. (1991). Effectiveness of cognitive-behavior therapy for maladapting children: A meta-analysis. *Psychological Bulletin, 110*, 204–214.

Emslie, G. J., Rush, A. J., Weinberrg, W. A., Gullion, C. M., Rintelmann, J., & Hughes, C. W. (1997). Recurrence of major depressive disorder in hospitalized children and adolescents *Journal of the American Academy of Child and Adolescent Psychiatry, 36*, 785–792.

Emslie, G. J., Heiligenstein, J. H., Wagner, K. D., Hoog, S. L., Ernest, D. E., Brown, E., et al. (2002). Fluoxetine for acute treatment of depression in children and adolescents: A placebo-controlled, randomized clinical trial. *Journal of the American Academy of Child and Adolescent Psychiatry, 41*, 1205–1215.

Goldapple, K., Segal, Z., Garson, C., Lau, M., Bieling, P., Kennedy, S., & Mayberg, H. (2004). Modulation of cortical-limbic pathways in major depression. *Archives of General Psychiatry, 61*, 34–41.

Goodenow, C. (1993). Classroom belonging among early adolescent students: Relationships to motivation and achievement. *Journal of Early Adolescence, 13*, 21–43.

Harmer, C. J., Hill, S. A., Taylor, M. J., Cowen, P. J., & Goodwin, G. M. (2003). Toward a neuropsychological theory of antidepressant drug action: Increase in positive emotional bias after potentiation of norepinephrine activity. *American Journal of Psychiatry, 160*, 990–992.

Hoge, D. R., Smith, E. K., & Hanson, S. L. (1990). School experiences predicting changes in self-esteem of sixth- and seventh-grade students. *Journal of Educational Psychology, 82*, 117–127.

Hollon, S. D., & Kendall, P. C. (1980). Cognitive self-statements in depression: Development of an Automatic Thoughts Questionnaire. *Cognitive Therapy and Research, 4*, 384–395.

Howard, K. I., Kopta, S. M., Krause, M. S., & Orlinsky, D. E. (1986). The dose–effect relationship in psychotherapy. *American Psychologist, 41,* 159–164.

Kaslow, N. J., Stark, K. D., Printz, B., Livingston, R., & Tsai, S. (1992). Cognitive Triad Inventory for Children: Development and relationship to depression and anxiety. *Journal of Clinical Child Psychology, 21,* 339–347.

Kaufman, N. K., Rohde, P., Seeley, J. R., Clarke, G. N., & Stice, E. (2005). Potential mediators of cognitive-behavioral therapy for adolescents with comorbid major depression and conduct disorder. *Journal of Consulting and Clinical Psychology, 73,* 38–46.

Kazdin, A. (2000). Developing a research agenda for child and adolescent psychotherapy. *Archives of General Psychiatry, 57,* 829 835.

Kazdin, A. E., & Weisz, J. R. (1998). Identifying and developing empirically supported child and adolescent treatments. *Journal of Consulting and Clinical Psychology, 66,* 19–36.

Kendall, P. C. (2000). Round of applause for an agenda and regular report cards for child and adolescent psychotherapy research. *Archives of General Psychiatry, 57,* 839–840.

Kendall, P. C., & Braswell, L. (1993). *Cognitive-behavioral therapy for impulsive children* (2nd ed.). New York: Guilford Press.

Kendall, P. C., Cantwell, D. P., & Kazdin, A. E. (1989). Depression in children and adolescents: Assessment issues and recommendations. *Cognitive Therapy and Research, 13,* 109–146.

Kendall, P. C., Stark, K. D., & Adam, T. (1990). Cognitive deficit or cognitive distortion in childhood depression. *Journal of Abnormal Child Psychology, 18,* 255–270.

Kennedy, S. H., Evans, K. R., Kruger, S., Mayberg, H. S., Meyer, J. H., McCann, S., et al. (2001). Changes in regional brain glucose metabolism measured with positron emission tomography after paroxetine treatment of Major Depression. *American Journal of Psychiatry, 158,* 899–905.

Kolko, D. J., Brent, D. A., Baugher, M., Bridge, J., & Birmaher, B. (2000). Cognitive and family therapies for adolescent depression: Treatment specificity, mediation, and moderation. *Journal of Consulting and Clinical Psychology, 68,* 603–614.

Kovacs, M. (1981). Rating scales to assess depression in school aged children. *Acta Paedopsychiatrica, 46,* 305–315.

Kroll, L., Harrington, R., Jayson, D., Fraser, J., & Gowers, S. (1996). Pilot study of continuation cognitive-behavioral therapy for major depression in adolescent psychiatric patients. *Journal of the American Academy of Child and Adolescent Psychiatry, 35,* 1156–1161.

Lewinsohn, P. M., Clarke, G. N., Hops, H., & Andrews, J. (1990). Cognitive-behavioral treatment for depressed adolescents. *Behavior Therapy, 21,* 385–401.

March, J. (2004). The treatment for adolescents with depression study (TADS): Short-term effectiveness and safety outcomes. *Journal of the American Medical Association, 292,* 807–820.

Martin, S. D., Martin, E., Rai, S. S., Richardson, M. A., & Royall, R. (2001). Brain blood flow changes in depressed patients treated with interpersonal psychotherapy or venlafaxine hydrochloride. *Archives of General Psychiatry, 58,* 641–651.

Matson, J. L., Rotatori, A. F., & Helsel, W. J. (1983). Development of a rating scale to measure social skills in children: The Matson Evaluation of Social Skills with Youngsters (MESSY). *Behavioral Research and Therapy, 41,* 335–340.

Mayberg, H. S. (2003). Modulating dysfunctional limbic-cortical circuits in depression: Towards development of brain-based algorithms for diagnosis and optimized treatment. *British Medical Bulletin, 54,* 193–207.

Mayberg, H. S., Liotti, M., Brannan, S. K., McGinnis, S., Mahurin, R. K., Jerabek, P. A., et al. (1999). Reciprocal limbic-cortical function and negative mood: Converging PET findings in depression and normal sadness. *American Journal of Psychiatry, 156,* 675–682.

McCauley, E., Myers, K., Mitchell, J., Calderon, R., Schloredt, K., & Treder, R. (1993). Depression in young people: Initial presentation and clinical course. *Journal of the American Academy of Child and Adolescent Psychiatry, 29*, 611–619.

Mezulis, A. H., Hyde, J. S., Abramson, L. Y., Stark, K., & Simpson, J. P. (2004). *Measuring cognitive vulnerability to depression in children.* Unpublished manuscript, University of Wisconsin.

Midgley, C., Feldlaufer, H., & Eccles, J.S. (1989). Student/teacher relations and attitudes toward mathematics before and after the transition to junior high school. *Child Development, 60*, 981–992.

Murray, C., & Greenberg, M. T. (2000). Children's relationship with teachers and bonds with school. An investigation of patterns and correlates in middle childhood. *Journal of School Psychology, 38*, 423–445.

Olfson, M., Gameroff, M. J., Marcus, S. C., & Waslick, B. D. (2003). Outpatient treatment of child and adolescent depression in the United States. *Archives of General Psychiatry, 60*, 1236–1242.

O'Reardon, J. P., Chopra, M. P., Bergan, A., Gallop, R., DeRubeis, R. J., & Crits-Christoph, P. (2004). Response to tryptophan depletion in major depression treated with either cognitive therapy or selective serotonin reuptake inhibitor antidepressants. *Biological Psychiatry, 55*, 957–959.

Orvaschel, H., & Puig-Antich, J. H. (1994). *Schedule for Affective Disorders and Schizophrenia for School-Age Children* (Epidemiologic version, 5th ed.). Pittsburgh, PA: Western Psychiatric Institute and Clinic.

Penza, K. M., Heim, C., & Nemeroff, C. B. (2003). Neurobiological effects of childhood abuse: Implications for the pathophysiology of depression and anxiety. *Archives of Women's Mental Health, 6*, 15–22.

Physician Desk Reference. (2004). Upper Saddle River, NJ: Thompson PDR.

Pianta, R. C. (1994). Patterns of relationships between children and kindergarten teachers. *Journal of School Psychology, 32*, 15–31.

Reddy, R., Rhodes, J. E., & Mulhall, P. (2003). The influence of teacher support on student adjustment in the middle school years: A latent growth curve study. *Development and Psychopathology, 15*, 119–138.

Roeser, R. W., Midgley, C., & Urdan, T. C. (1996). Perceptions of the school psychological environment and early adolescents' psychological and behavioral functioning in school: The mediating role of goals and belonging. *Journal of Educational Psychology, 88*, 408–422.

Schmidt, K. L., Stark, K. D., Carlson, C. L., & Anthony, B. J. (1998). Cognitive factors differentiating attention-deficit-hyperactivity disorder with and without a co-morbid mood disorder. *Journal of Counsulting and Clinical Psychology, 66*, 673–679.

Stark, K. D., Humphrey, L. L., Crook, K., & Lewis, K. (1990). Perceived family environments of depressed and anxious children: Child's and maternal figure's perspectives. *Journal of Abnormal Child Psychology, 18*, 527–547.

Stark, K. D., Humphrey, L. L., Laurent, J., Livingston, R., & Christopher, J. (1993). Cognitive, behavioral, and family factors in the differentiation of depressive and anxiety disorders during childhood. *Journal of Consulting and Clinical Psychology, 61*, 878–886.

Stark, K. D., Sander, J., Hauser, M., Simpson, J., Schnoebelen, S., Glenn R., & Molnar, J. (in press). Depressive disorders during childhood and adolescence. In E. J. Mash & R. A. Barkley (Eds.), *Treatment of childhood disorders* (3rd ed.). New York: Guilford Press.

Stark, K. D., Schnoebelen, S., Simpson, J., Hargrave, J., Molnar, J., & Glenn R. (2005). *Treating depressed children: Therapist manual for ACTION.* Ardmore, PA: Workbook Publishing.

Stark, K. D., Simpson, J., Schnoebelen, S., Glenn, R., Hargrave, J., & Molnar, J. (2005). *ACTION workbook*. Ardmore, PA: Workbook Publishing.

Treadwell, K. R. H., & Kendall, P. C. (1996). Self-talk in anxiety-disordered youth: States-of-mind, content specificity, and treatment outcome. *Journal of Consulting and Clinical Psychology, 64*, 941–950.

Wagner, K. D., Robb, A. S., Findling, R. L., Gutierrez, M. M., & Heydom, W. E. (2004). A randomized, placebo-controlled trial of citalopram for the treatment of major depression in children and adolescents. *American Journal of Psychiatry, 161*, 1079–1083.

Wagner, K. D., & Ambrosini, P. (2003) Efficacy of sertraline in the treatment of children and adolescents with major depressive disorder: Two randomized controlled trials. *Journal of the American Medical Association, 290*, 1033–1041.

Weersing, V. R., & Weisz, J. R. (2002). Community clinic treatment of depressed youth: Benchmarking usual care against CBT clinical trials. *Journal of Consulting and Clinical Psychology, 43*, 3–29.

Weiss, B., Harris, V., Catron, T., & Han, S. S. (2003). Efficacy of the RECAP intervention program for children with concurrent internalizing and externalizing problems. *Journal of Consulting and Clinical Psychology, 71*, 364–374.

Weisz, J. R. (2000). Agenda for child and adolescent psychotherapy research: On the need to put science into practice. *Archives of General Psychiatry, 57*, 837–838.

CHAPTER 6

Addressing Adolescent Suicidal Behavior

Cognitive-Behavioral Strategies

ANTHONY SPIRITO
and CHRISTIANNE ESPOSITO-SMYTHERS

It is quite sad but true: Rates of attempted and completed suicide rise precipitously during adolescence (Kessler, Borges, & Walters, 1999). Within a 12-month period, approximately 19% of adolescents in the United States seriously consider attempting suicide, 15% develop a suicide plan, 9% attempt suicide, and 2.6% of adolescents attempt suicide in a manner requiring emergency medical treatment (Department of Health and Human Services, 2002). These rates translate into approximately 2 million attempts per year, of which about 700,000 receive emergency medical treatment (Shaffer & Pfeffer, 2001). Borst, Noam, and Bartok (1991) postulate that, with the advent of puberty, social-cognitive reorganization leads to more internal attribution of unhappiness from previous external attributions. This shift in attributional style leads to more self-blame in response to interpersonal stressors and, in some adolescents, results in increased risk for suicidal behavior.

Although there are important differences between those adolescents who attempt and those who complete suicide, a previous suicide attempt is one of the best predictive risk factors for eventual completed suicide by an adolescent. In one study (LeComte & Fornes, 1998), one-third of youth who died by suicide had previously attempted suicide at least once. Thus, it is clear that effective treatment of adolescents who attempt suicide, the focus of this chapter, is an important facet of addressing the public health problem of youth suicide.

COGNITIVE-BEHAVIORAL MODEL OF SUICIDAL BEHAVIOR

From a cognitive–behavioral model (social–cognitive learning theory) perspective, suicidal behavior is similar to other forms of psychopathology in that it results from faulty learning experiences that are reflected in maladaptive cognition, behavior, and feelings. Drawing in part from a model of suicidal behavior for adults (Rudd, Joiner, & Rajeb, 2001), as well as research and clinical experience with suicidal adolescents, a model of suicidal behavior among adolescents (see Figure 6.1) is presented. Suicidal behavior emerges from reciprocal relations among learned maladaptive cognition, behavior, and affective responses to stressors in adolescents with predisposing vulnerabilities. Predisposing vulnerabilities, derived from poor early learning histories, among others may include exposure to childhood trauma such as abuse or neglect (e.g., Beautrais, Joyce, & Mulder, 1996; Brent et al., 1994) and parental psychopathology, including suicidal behavior (Brent et al., 1994). Peer factors, such as exposure to peer violence, victimization, and suicidal behavior, may also play a role. A genetic predisposition toward psychopathology also serves as a vulnerability factor.

Stress resulting from interpersonal conflict, other negative life events, or worsening of psychiatric symptoms may initially trigger the suicidal crisis in a vulnerable adolescent. In attempting to cognitively process this trigger, distorted thinking may occur and result in cognitive errors (e.g., catastrophizing, personalization) and negative views of self and the future. Indeed, Brent, Kolko, Allan, and Brown (1990) found suicide attempting and ideating adolescent inpatients with a mood disorder to have higher catastrophizing, personalization, selective abstraction, overgeneralization, and total cognitive errors than nonsuicidal adolescents with a mood disorder. Adolescent suicide ideators and attempters also exhibit more hopelessness and lower self-esteem than nonsuicidal controls (e.g., Marciano & Kazdin, 1994; Spirito, Williams, Stark, & Hart, 1988).

Depending upon the degree of distortion and repetitiveness of the trigger, the adolescent may attempt to generate solutions to the trigger, but may be unsuccessful. Studies employing self-report measures have consistently revealed suicidal adolescents to report greater difficulty generating alternatives to problems and choosing/implementing effective alternatives as compared to nonsuicidal adolescents (Adams & Adams, 1996; Sadowski & Kelley, 1993). Often, solutions generated by adolescents are ineffective and cause more problems, or they may be effective but the adolescent does not believe that they can be successfully implemented. This, in turn, results in more distorted thinking as well as affective distress that may include physiological arousal, anger, and/or worsening of the

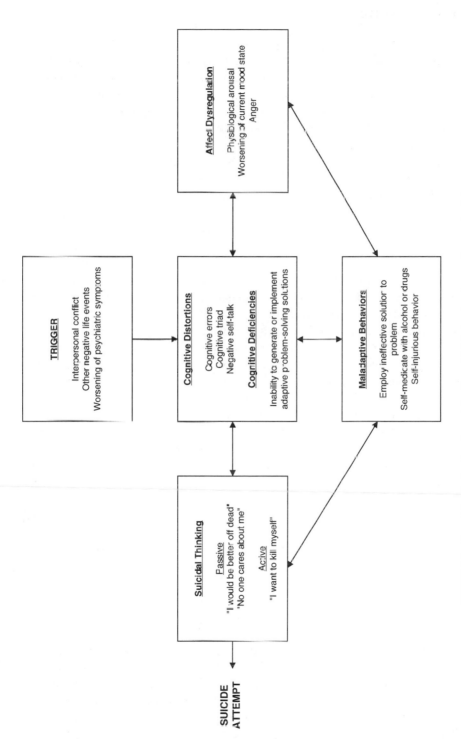

FIGURE 6.1. Cognitive–behavioral model of suicidal behavior in predisposed adolescents.

current mood state. Suicidal adolescents have been shown to have a reduced capacity to regulate their internal states and may use affect regulation skills less frequently relative to nonsymptomatic adolescents (Fritsch, Donaldson, Spirito, & Plummer, 2000). Related research has also shown anger to be associated with adolescent suicidal thoughts and behavior (Boergers, Spirito, & Donaldson, 1998).

The adolescent may then engage in maladaptive behavior in response to cognitive distortions, deficiencies, and affective arousal. This may include the use of passive and/or aggressive communication styles and behavior to deal with interpersonal conflict with peers (Prinstein, Boergers, Spirito, & Little, 2000) and family members (Wagner, 1997). Other adolescents may attempt to self-medicate with alcohol or drugs (Esposito-Smythers & Spirito, 2004). Alternatively, the adolescent may choose to engage in a less lethal self-injurious behavior as a means to temporarily dissociate from the situation, such as superficially cutting or burning oneself (Guertin, Lloyd-Richardson, Spirito, Donaldson, & Boergers, 2001). The behavior chosen is often based on behavior that has been modeled by parents, peers, or other important figures in the adolescent's life.

After a short period of time, if the problem remains unresolved or the adolescent's behavior has generated even more problems, cognitive processes and affect may become increasingly negative. Concurrent with affect dysregulation, the adolescent may also begin to experience passive suicidal thoughts such as "I would be better off dead." Over time these thoughts may switch to active suicidal thoughts such as "I might as well kill myself," and a suicide plan is then developed. Depending upon such factors as the adolescent's affective threshold, level of impulsivity, availability of method, presence of intoxication, degree of isolation, and presence of support, the adolescent may act on his or her suicidal thoughts at that time and make a suicide attempt. Alternatively, the adolescent may cycle through this cognitive, affective, and behavioral process numerous times, with each rotation leading to greater cognitive, affective, and behavioral dysfunction. This may take place over a few days, weeks, or even months. Either way, the end result of this cycle, if not interrupted, is the perception that a solution is hopeless, the affective state intolerable, and suicide is the only means of escape.

Once suicidal behavior occurs, it may sensitize the adolescent to future suicide-related thoughts and behavior (Beck, 1996). Beck conceptualizes these thoughts and behaviors as an orienting schema. Suicidal behavior makes the suicidal schema more easily accessible and easily triggered in future stressful situations. Once the taboo against suicide has been broken, it becomes easier to view suicide as a viable solution to life's problems. Thus, the importance of effective treatment for adolescents following a suicide attempt cannot be underestimated.

Given this model of suicidality, cognitive-behavioral therapy (CBT) may be effective with suicidal adolescents, because it is based on the premise that maladaptive cognition, behavior, and affective responses can be corrected. With such a complex symptom presentation, clinical work with suicidal adolescents may require multiple modes of intervention, including individual, family, and group therapy. Treatments must address not only suicidality but also the underlying disorder(s) and contextual factors. In this chapter, we will limit our discussion to the treatment of suicidal behavior.

ASSESSMENT OF SUICIDALITY FOR TREATMENT PLANNING

When interviewing an adolescent shortly after a suicide attempt, it is important to understand five related aspects of the attempt: suicidal ideation, the method of attempt, suicidal intent, and the attempt precipitant(s), as well as reasons for the attempt. Based on this assessment, considerations regarding the best way to address the suicidality can be made.

Suicidal Ideation

Suicidal ideation can be assumed to underlie almost all suicidal acts. However, the duration and complexity of the suicidal ideation can vary across adolescents. Some adolescents attempt suicide after lengthy thought and detailed plans, whereas others act more impulsively. The assessment of suicidal ideation in adolescents has been conducted with several different instruments. A comprehensive description of assessment tools for suicidal behavior and risk in children and adolescents has been published by Goldston (2003). Instruments such as the Suicide Ideation Questionnaire (SIQ; Reynolds, 1988) and the Beck Scale for Suicide Ideation (BSS; Beck & Steer, 1991) are widely used.

If an assessment instrument is not available, the therapist can ask questions that tap the frequency of suicidal thought (How frequent are your current suicidal thoughts—once a week, a few days a week, daily? How long do they last—a few minutes, a few hours, most of the day?), disclosure (Have you told anyone about your suicidal thoughts? Who did you tell? When?), duration (How long ago did you first start to have these thoughts?), and specificity of any suicidal plans (Did you make a suicide plan? How and when did you plan to attempt suicide? Have you made any preparations such as a suicide note or giving away belongings?).

Method and Lethality of the Suicide Attempt

Among adolescents, the choice of method for attempting suicide seems to be largely dictated by opportunity and availability. Most adolescents attempt suicide by an overdose of over-the-counter medications. Attempts other than by overdose or superficial cutting may be predictive of a higher likelihood of repeat suicide attempts and ultimately completed suicide (Shaffer & Pfeffer, 2001). It is important to assess the availability of means for a future suicide attempt (e.g., pills, firearms, knives) and steps taken to remove them from the home until the episode of suicidality resolves.

Suicidal Intent

When evaluating an attempt of low lethality, it is important to consider other aspects of the attempt, particularly intentionality, and not be misled by the low-risk nature of an attempt method. It is important to ask the adolescent about at least two major aspects of suicidal intent: expected outcome and planning of the attempt (Spirito, Sterling, Donaldson, & Arrigan, 1996). The measure of suicidal intent with the most empirical support with adolescents is the Suicide Intent Scale (SIS; Beck, Schuyler, & Herman, 1974).

Questions that can be asked to tap suicidal intent include: Did you make a suicide plan prior to your attempt? How long did you think about this plan prior to attempting suicide? Did you tell anyone about your plan? Did you make any preparations for your suicide attempt such as a suicide note or giving away belongings? Did you think that your suicide attempt would kill you? If not, what did you think would happen? Did you think anyone would find you in time to keep you from dying? Did you actually want to die? Or, is it that you didn't really want to die but do want to escape an intolerable situation? Do you still feel this way? Do you think that things will get better with time, or is this situation hopeless? If the adolescent remains suicidal after the attempt, specifics about a future plan (how, when, and where) should be asked.

Attempt Precipitants and Reasons for the Attempt

The precipitants to adolescent suicide attempts are typically everyday stressors, particularly interpersonal conflict. Among adolescents who made a medically serious suicide attempt, the most common precipitants included the termination of a relationship (24%) or other interpersonal problems (26%) such as arguments with friends or family members (Beautrais, Joyce, & Mulder, 1997). These apparently minor stressors are often perceived as "the last straw" for individuals who are struggling with other risk factors. The seriousness of an adolescent's suicide attempt should not be underestimated based on the nature of the suicide precipitant.

It is also important to determine whether the precipitating stressor has been resolved and to evaluate whether conflictual interpersonal relationships may have been altered by the suicidal act. Questions that might be asked include: What triggered your suicide attempt? Does that problem still exist? Can you avoid this problem in the future? Do you intend to avoid this problem?

More detailed questioning about the reasons for an attempt can be helpful in clarifying current stressors and the adolescent's motive. In one study (Boergers et al., 1998) the most frequently endorsed motives for suicide attempts were a desire to die (28%), to escape (13%), and to obtain relief (18%). Adolescents who cited a desire to die as a reason for their suicide attempt reported more hopelessness, depression, tendencies for perfectionism, and difficulties with anger expression.

An understanding of the adolescent's own cognition about the attempt is critical for establishing a trusting therapeutic alliance and for tailoring the type of treatment that is offered. For example, therapists and families often view adolescent suicide attempts as a cry for help. However, relatively few adolescents (9%) in the Boergers and colleagues (1998) study acknowledged help seeking as a motivation for their attempt. This suggests that many adolescent suicide attempters might engage in treatment more readily if emphasis were placed on helping them to obtain some sense of relief from an unbearable situation. Thus, if the treatment is focused on the situational problems rather than the suicidal person, engagement in the treatment process may be facilitated.

TREATMENT FOR SUICIDAL BEHAVIOR: CURRENT STATUS OF THE RESEARCH

Empirical studies of psychosocial treatments for adolescents who attempt suicide are few in number. All randomized and selected nonrandomized trials are reviewed below.

Individual Psychotherapy

Rathus and Miller (2002) adapted Linehan's (1993) dialectical behavior therapy (DBT) for use with suicidal adolescents. The focus of DBT is on improving distress tolerance, emotional regulation, and interpersonal effectiveness. Using a quasi-experimental design, they compared treatment efficacy of DBT ($n = 29$) to treatment as usual (TAU) for 82 suicidal adolescents (one-third were attempters) with borderline features. Adolescents in both groups attended approximately 24 sessions over 3 months. The DBT group, which had more severe baseline symptomatology than the TAU group, had fewer psychiatric hospitalizations and higher rates of treatment completion than the TAU group. No differences in repeat suicide attempts were found: About 40% reattempted over the course of treatment.

Donaldson, Spirito, and Esposito-Smythers (2005) conducted the only randomized trial to date of individual therapy. In this trial, CBT was compared to a problem-oriented supportive therapy designed to mimic standard care with adolescent suicide attempters. Both treatments were delivered in an individual format with conjoint parent adolescent sessions. Adolescents were randomized to either 10 sessions of CBT ($n = 18$) or the problem-oriented supportive treatment ($n = 17$). Seven different therapists provided both treatments (to control for therapist effects). The groups were equivalent across baseline variables as well as the percentage of participants placed on medication during the study. More than half of the sample had made multiple suicide attempts. Participants in both conditions reported significant reductions in suicidal ideation and depression at 3-month follow-up, but there were no between-groups differences. At 6 months, both groups retained improvement over baseline; however, levels of suicide ideation and depression were slightly higher than at 3-month follow-up.

Family Therapy

Three nonrandomized interventions and one randomized family-focused intervention have been described in the literature. In a highly structured six-session outpatient family therapy program called "SNAP" (Successful Negotiation/ Acting Positively), problem-solving skills were taught and practiced, using role playing, modeling, and feedback. Negotiating, active listening skills, and strategies for managing affective arousal were also taught. Although a randomized trial was not conducted, SNAP reduced overall symptom levels among 140 female minority-group adolescent suicide attempters (Rotheram-Borus, Piacentini, Miller, Graae, & Castro-Blanco, 1994).

Harrington and colleagues (1998) provided treatment to 162 adolescents (10–16 years old) who had attempted suicide by overdose. Patients were randomly assigned to either routine care ($M = 3.6$ sessions) or routine care plus a four-session home-based family intervention ($M = 3.2$ sessions). The family sessions focused on discussion of the suicide attempt, communication skills, problem solving, and psychoeducation on adolescent development. The additional home-based family intervention resulted in reduced suicidal ideation at 6-month follow-up, but only for adolescents without major depression. There were no differences in rate of suicide reattempts.

Group Therapy

Wood, Trainor, Rothwell, Moore, and Harrington (2001) randomized 63 adolescents, ages 12–16, who had deliberately harmed themselves on at least two occasions within a year, to group therapy plus routine care or routine care alone. The group therapy approach utilized techniques from a variety of theoretical orientations, including CBT techniques previously used with depressed or suicidal adolescents and their families (Harrington et al., 1998) and DBT techniques. Adolescents randomized to the group intervention attended six structured "acute" group sessions, followed by weekly process-oriented long-term group therapy that could continue until the patient felt ready to terminate sessions. Those randomized to this condition attended a median of 8 group sessions (range = 0–25). They were also permitted to attend individual sessions as needed with the group therapist (median of 3, range = 0–10). Adolescents in routine care alone attended a median of 4 sessions (range = 0–30). Adolescents who received group therapy plus routine care, compared to routine care alone, were less likely to make more than one repeat suicide attempt (2 of 32, vs. 10 of 31), had better school attendance, and a lower rate of behavior problems. The interventions did not differ in their effects on depression or global outcome. Interestingly, more sessions of routine care were associated with a worse outcome.

Day Treatment/Multisystemic Therapy

Rudd and colleagues (1996) conducted a randomized trial comparing an experimental problem-solving-based day treatment program to standard care in the community for older adolescents and young adults (42% ideators, 58% attempters). Those in the experimental program received group therapy that primarily focused on psychoeducation, problem solving, and experiential-affective techniques over the course of 2 weeks. The experimental program resulted in improvements in suicidal ideation and behavior, but the comparison group had comparable improvement. However, further analyses revealed that patients with comorbid symptomatology experienced the most improvement with the problem-solving-based experimental day treatment program (Joiner, Voelz, & Rudd, 2001).

Huey and colleagues (2004) randomized adolescents presenting with psychiatric emergencies to either psychiatric hospitalization or multisystemic therapy (MST). MST is a family-focused home-based intervention that addresses home, school, and community factors related to youth difficulties, with a particular emphasis on parenting skills. A variety of behavioral interventions are typically delivered in MST based on a set of nine treatment principles and ongoing supervision. Caseloads are low for each therapist, and treatment ranges from 3 to 6 months, with daily sessions when necessary. At 1-year follow-up, the MST group had significantly lower rates of suicide attempts than the hospitalized adolescents. Depressed mood, hopelessness, and suicidal ideation improved for both groups over follow-up, but there were no differences between the two groups on these variables.

TREATMENT ISSUES WITH ADOLESCENT SUICIDE ATTEMPTERS

Before discussing our CBT program for suicidal adolescents, we must review a few issues pertinent to treatment of suicidal adolescents. First, adolescents who attempt suicide vary greatly in terms of treatment attendance. Follow-up studies of these adolescents have typically found poor adherence with outpatient treatment (Boergers & Spirito, 2003). Therapy dropout among adolescent suicide attempters occurs earlier and at a higher rate, compared to adolescents in therapy for other problems (median session attendance = 3 sessions vs. 11 sessions;

Trautman, Stewart, & Morishima, 1993). One factor that undoubtedly affects treatment attendance is that families who enter into treatment often have multiple sources of stress and adverse conditions in their lives that make participation in treatment a burden, consistent with the "burden of treatment model" (Kazdin, 1996). Thus, efforts must be made early on to problem-solve through obstacles to treatment participation and to build a strong therapeutic alliance with both the adolescent and family. Indeed, a strong therapeutic alliance has been shown to have a positive effect on youth treatment retention and treatment outcome (Chatoor & Krupnick, 2001).

Second, suicidal behavior rarely occurs in the absence of psychopathology (Shaffer et al., 1996). Furthermore, adolescent suicide attempters possess great diagnostic heterogeneity. A diagnosis of a mood disorder has consistently been identified as the most powerful diagnostic predictor of suicide completions, attempts, and ideation in adolescents (Beautrais et al., 1996; Brent et al., 1993; Shaffer et al., 1996). The odds of completing suicide are approximately 27 times greater in adolescents with major depressive disorder as compared to those without major depressive disorder (Beautrais et al., 1996). Anxiety, disruptive behavior, and substance use disorders, which are covered in other chapters of this book, have also been linked with adolescent suicidal behavior (Brent et al., 1993; Shaffer et al., 1996). Comorbid psychiatric disorders further increase risk for suicidality. Rates of suicide attempts in depressed adolescents increase when they are diagnosed with a comorbid anxiety, disruptive behavior (oppositional defiant or conduct disorder), and/or substance use disorder (Brent et al., 1993; Shaffer et al., 1996).

Third, there exists evidence for two distinct types of suicide attempters based on (1) degree of premeditation prior to the suicide attempt and (2) patterns of co-occurring psychopathology. The two types are impulsive suicide attempters with predominant externalizing symptoms and nonimpulsive suicide attempters with predominant internalizing symptoms. Relative to impulsive attempters, nonimpulsive attempters were found to have higher levels of depression and hopelessness and a proclivity toward greater suicidal ideation (Brown, Overholser, Spirito, & Fritz, 1991). Furthermore, anger turned inward was associated with hopelessness only in the nonimpulsive group.

TREATMENT OF ADOLESCENT SUICIDAL BEHAVIOR

Our CBT protocol integrates existing cognitive-behavioral techniques to remediate maladaptive cognition and behavior that underlie suicidality. The treatment protocol includes individual and family sessions. In the individual protocol, sessions include instruction in problem-solving, cognitive restructuring, and affect regulation skills to remediate coping skill deficits, cognitive distortions, affect regulation deficits, and problematic social behavior exhibited by suicidal adolescents. Moreover, these treatment techniques target many of the same cognitive distortions and skill deficits commonly found to underlie other forms of co-occurring psychopathology exhibited by suicidal adolescents (e.g., depression, substance abuse). Our treatment is designed to accommodate rather than exclude adolescents with comorbid mental disorders to increase its transportability.

Here we discuss modules for teaching problem-solving, cognitive restructuring, and affect regulation skills with respect to suicidal episodes. These are the primary skills taught to specifically address suicidality in individual therapy sessions. We also include other skills in our treatment program that are reviewed in other chapters of this book. These include relaxation training (deep breathing, progressive muscle relaxation, guided imagery), increasing pleasant events, and assertiveness training.

All individual sessions in our treatment protocol follow the same format. They begin with a medication adherence check, if applicable, followed by an assessment of suicidal thoughts or behavior experienced since the last session. If the adolescent does appear to be at significant risk for suicidal behavior, we conduct an assessment of current suicidality, using the questions presented above. A no-suicide contract is also negotiated with all adolescents. The adolescent is asked whether he or she can promise, with 100% certainty, to keep him- or herself safe until the next treatment session. Additional safety considerations include how effective the adolescent's home environment is in keeping the adolescent safe. For example, questions that should be considered include whether a parent can safely monitor the adolescent, whether parental mental illness or substance abuse is present that would affect parenting, whether the relationship between the parent and adolescent is at least somewhat positive, and whether there is any abuse or neglect present in the home.

The subsequent portion of the session follows the typical cognitive-behavioral format. First, the adolescent is asked to identify an agenda item for the session, homework from the prior session is reviewed, a new skill is introduced or a previously taught skill reviewed, the skill is practiced, the agenda item is discussed with efforts directed toward incorporating the use of skills learned previously in treatment, and a personalized homework assignment is created. Worksheets and handouts for each skill taught are used in every session. The adolescent is provided with a binder in which to keep all worksheets and assignments completed throughout the course of treatment. He or she is asked to bring this binder to each session. All individual sessions also include a parent check-in at the end.

Overview Session

The first session includes time devoted to rapport building, an overview of the treatment methods, treatment compliance procedures, a review of safety procedures, an overview of CBT, and initial goal setting. The latter two elements will not be discussed here, because they are generic to most cognitive-behavioral protocols. To begin the session, the therapist meets alone with the adolescent to engage in rapport building and conduct safety assessments. Upon completion, the therapist works with the adolescent to create a "personal reasons to live" list and a coping card. For the reasons-to-live list, the adolescent is asked to generate at least five reasons to live (e.g., "to have a family of my own and to see my little brother grow up") and write them on a worksheet. For the coping card, the adolescent generates a list of strategies that he or she can use in coping with difficult situations, as well as numbers to contact in an emergency. The adolescent is asked to place a copy of the reasons-to-live list and coping card in his or her CBT binder. A copy of the coping card is also given to the adolescent to place in his or her wallet for immediate access. The therapist then asks the parent to join the session to introduce the treatment.

Treatment Methods

When parents enter the session, they are provided with an overview of the treatment methods so that they know exactly what to expect in treatment. This description includes anticipated length of treatment, number and schedule of treatment sessions, what can be expected in treatment sessions, goals of the treatment program, and degree of parent involvement. We also share our willingness to advocate for and help families effectively navigate social systems outside the family causing any undue stress (e.g., school, juvenile courts). In addition, we discuss the importance of taking any prescribed medications regularly for optimal treatment outcome.

Compliance Enhancement

Given the high rates of treatment dropout among adolescent suicide attempters, as described above, we employ a brief compliance enhancement protocol that has been previously tested by our group (Spirito, Boergers, Donaldson, Bishop, & Lewander, 2001). As part of this procedure, we provide psychoeducation on adolescent suicidal behavior.

> "It is important for you to know that if nothing changes in your child's life when you leave here, your child is at risk for hurting him- or herself in the future. This is based on years of experience working with teenagers and families who have been in the same situation as yours. In fact, teenagers who attempt suicide are 18 times more likely to make a repeat suicide attempt than those who don't consider attempting suicide. Of those teenagers who are hospitalized for a suicide attempt, approximately 1 in 10 teenagers try to hurt themselves within 3 months of being in the hospital."

We then encourage families to come to counseling regularly and complete the full treatment program. We provide the rationale that it takes time for the family to know the therapist and feel comfortable sharing information. It also takes time for the therapist to get to know the child and family. Furthermore, families have usually struggled for a few years, so it takes time for therapy to produce desired changes. Terminating treatment early can also lead to a relapse of suicidal behavior. We emphasize the importance of completing the full course of treatment to obtain the best treatment outcomes.

Next, we discuss expectations for treatment, factors that may impede compliance with treatment, and then problem-solve through potential obstacles. In discussing expectations for treatment, we ask the adolescent what he or she thinks about coming to counseling, what he or she thinks happens in counseling, and how many visits he or she believes that it will take to get better. We then inquire about obstacles that might get in the way of coming to counseling regularly. It is important for the therapist to be prepared to discuss various factors that may impede adolescent treatment compliance (e.g., stigma, concerns that the therapist will side with parents against the teen or that parents might get upset if the teen discusses family problems, etc.). When obstacles are brought up, we share that these are things that other teenagers have also mentioned, to normalize the experience, and then ask the adolescent to generate all of the things that he or she can think of to prevent the obstacle(s) from getting in the way. The parent is also invited to participate in this conversation. Obstacles introduced by the parent are also discussed in session.

Pragmatic Safety Information

We then review with parents how important it is to provide adult supervision, obtain needed services in case of an emergency, and keep their home safe, which includes the removal of medications and objects that could be used in a suicidal act (e.g., *all* medications, firearms, razors, etc.). The disinhibiting effects of drugs and alcohol are also discussed, along with steps needed to secure or remove drugs and alcohol from the home. We note that these are not permanent changes, but need to be in place as long as the high-risk period lasts. We also emphasize that the parent, not the adolescent, must be responsible for giving the child his or her medications. Parents are instructed to take their teenager to a local emergency room in an emergency. We reemphasize the importance of the safety procedures. It is not uncommon for families to dismiss these procedures—so they are strongly encouraged.

"This may sound excessive but we know that suicide attempts are often impulsive acts. If your child becomes very upset and the means for a suicide attempt are readily available, such as medication, he or she is much more likely to act on suicidal impulses. However, if the means are not available, the suicidal impulse may pass without injury. We cannot stress how important it is to follow these recommendations."

Problem Solving

Deficits in problem solving include limited flexibility, difficulty generating alternative solutions, and limited ability to identify positive consequences of potential solutions. Although there are several approaches to problem-solving training, we developed the "SOLVE" system (Donaldson, Spirito, & Overholser, 2003), which covers the basic steps and has been easily implemented with adolescent suicide attempters. We begin with the generation of a list of triggers for suicidality. After a list has been generated by the adolescent, which tends to range from two to five events, the therapist teaches the adolescent the SOLVE system as follows:

"Today, we are going to talk about a very important skill that you can use to work through problems—a special problem-solving system. We call it the 'S-O-L-V-E system.' Each letter in the word SOLVE stands for a different step of problem-solving. 'S' stands for 'Select a problem.' The first step in solving a problem is to figure out what the problem is. The second step is 'O,' or 'Options.' After you figure out what the problem is, you make a list of ALL possible options to deal with the problem, not just the ones you think would work. The bigger the list you make, the better the chance you have of solving the problem! The next step in problem solving starts with an 'L' and stands for 'Likely Outcomes.' You take the list you made up and decide what might happen when you try each of your 'Options.' Think about whether things would get better or worse with each 'Option' and then rate each option as positive, negative, or even both. Then, you can narrow down your list to one 'Option' by picking the 'very best one' to use. After that, it is time to try it out. And last, after you give the 'Option' a try, you can 'Evaluate' the 'Option' and decide whether or not it worked. If it worked, then your problem is solved! If it did not work, then you go back to your 'Options,' weigh them out, and pick the next 'very best one' to try. You keep doing this until your problem is solved. Let's give it a try."

After the problem-solving system is taught, the subsequent part of the session can be used to address the problem that precipitated the suicide attempt. We have developed a worksheet to assist in the SOLVE process. Often, the adolescent will have initial difficulties generating "Options." The therapist may need to model the skills to help the adolescent accept and use these new behaviors. The adolescent is also encouraged to list a suicide attempt as an option. This demonstrates that it is safe to talk about suicidal thoughts and behavior in session and acknowledges that a suicide attempt is always an option. It also helps to open lines of communication around the suicide attempt and provides the therapist with the opportunity to begin to address any cognitive distortions surrounding this behavior. After the exercise is completed, the therapist can then reframe the suicide attempt as a *failure* in problem solving. This helps provide the adolescent with an adaptive way to understand the suicide attempt and a better sense of control over future problems that may arise.

THERAPIST: What would happen if you only had one Option listed and you tried it but it didn't work?

TEEN: I wouldn't have any other options?

THERAPIST: Yes. That's right. You would be stuck. That's kind of like what happened when you hurt yourself. You didn't feel like you had many Options, you felt pretty stuck, so you picked the only "Option" you thought you had, which was to hurt yourself. That's why we've found "SOLVE" to be helpful to teenagers who have been in that situation. The more you practice coming up with a big list of "Options" and the more "Options" you have to choose from when you have a problem, the less likely you'll feel stuck or like the only thing left to do is to hurt yourself.

Cognitive Restructuring

As with those exhibiting other forms of psychopathology, suicidal adolescents also exhibit cognitive distortion. Much of the distortion stems from co-occurring psychiatric disorders such as mood, anxiety, and conduct disorders. We use a modified version of rational emotive therapy (Bernard & Joyce, 1984) created by McClung (2000) in teaching cognitive restructuring. We call it the ABCDE method to help adolescents better remember the steps in cognitive restructuring. We introduce this method as a skill that helps adolescents deal with negative beliefs or thoughts that they may experience when problems arise. The experience of negative thoughts in and of themselves is normalized for the adolescent, but such thoughts become problematic when they occur too frequently. This is typically what happens when suicidal thoughts emerge. Adolescents are guided to address and change irrational thoughts through the "ABCDE method."

THERAPIST: Each letter of the ABCDE method stands for a different step of thought changing. "A" stands for "Activating Event." The first step in changing negative thoughts is to identify the "Activating Event" associated with the negative thoughts. "Activating Events" can be positive or negative. An example of a positive "Activating Event" may be going to a movie. An example of a negative "Activating Event" may be failing a test. Can you think of one?

TEEN: Getting in a fight with my mom?

THERAPIST: That is a good example of a negative activating event. Now let's skip the second step for a minute and go to the third step. The third step is to identify "Consequences or Feelings" related to the "Activating Event." For example, going to a movie might make people feel "very good or excited." However, after failing a test, they might feel "disappointed or depressed."

Many people believe that negative "Activating Events" cause us to feel badly. For example, people believe that "failing a test *causes* you to feel depressed." But that is not true. It is what occurs between the negative "Activating Event" and our feelings that causes us to feel bad. These things are called "Beliefs," and they occur between steps 1 and 3. These beliefs are typically negative and occur so quickly that we don't even know that we have them. Many of these beliefs are "irrational or untrue."

For example, after failing a test, some people might think things like "If I can't pass this test, then I am going to fail this course." So, it is our negative beliefs, which are often untrue, that make us feel bad. To feel better we must "argue" against these beliefs, or "dispute" them. Disputing is the fourth step, and perhaps the most important step, of thought changing.

Now, say that I was your good friend and I called you up and said, "I failed a test. I am a failure. I am never going to pass this course." What would you tell me to make me feel better?

TEEN: It is only one test. You can get help and pass the next one.

THERAPIST: Great job! That is exactly how you dispute. You just argued against, or "disputed," my negative beliefs. Most people don't dispute their negative beliefs and are left feeling very upset, and that is when they make unsafe decisions, such as hurting themselves.

Finally, the last step begins with an "E" and stands for "Effect." If you have an Effect on something, change will occur. We may not be able to change the fact that a negative activating event happened to us, but we can change our negative beliefs about it. And if we change our negative beliefs about it, we will feel better, and make better and safer decisions.

The therapist practices the ABCDE method using the suicide attempt precipitant as the Activating Event. When teaching the adolescent to dispute, we ask the adolescent to begin by asking him- or herself two simple questions in regard to beliefs surrounding a negative activating event: (1) Is this belief true? And if it is true, (2) Is this belief helpful? If the answer is "no" to either of these questions, then disputing is employed. When adolescents begin to use this method, the therapist will need to provide much guidance in disputing through Socratic questioning. Questions that we commonly use include: What evidence do you have for that belief? (which is followed by the generation of an "Evidence For Belief/ Evidence Against Belief" list). What would your friend say if he or she heard this belief? Does this belief help get you what you want? Does this belief help you feel the way you want? Does this belief help you avoid conflicts? Is there another explanation for why the event occurred?

We also present the adolescent with a list of cognitive distortions (e.g., black/white thinking, predicting the worst, missing the positive, feelings as facts, jumping to conclusions, expecting perfection, see Beck, Rush, Shaw, & Emery, 1979), which we have adapted to include simpler language and call "Thinking Mistakes." We ask the adolescent if he or she can identify any thinking mistakes in his or her beliefs. At the end of session, the therapist then helps the adolescent further reframe the suicide attempt.

THERAPIST: Now, what would happen if you only came up with negative beliefs and did not dispute any of them?

TEEN: I would feel really bad?

THERAPIST: That's right! You would only have negative thoughts running through your head and feel really bad. So, in addition to not seeing any other "options" to suicide, you had all of these negative beliefs running through your head and did not dispute any of them, which left you feeling suicidal. Now, the more you practice disputing negative beliefs, the more positive beliefs you will have running through your head. This will help you to feel better and make better and, most importantly, *safer* decisions. But, it is important to remember that it takes practice to get really good at this. So we will continue to practice this skill together during our sessions.

There are a number of other cognitive techniques specifically useful for suicidal persons that can be integrated into the cognitive restructuring module (Freeman & Reinecke, 1993). Decastrophizing involves having the therapist help the adolescent decide whether he or she is overestimating the catastrophic nature of the suicide attempt precipitant through such questions as: "What would be the worst thing that will arise if _____ occurs again? If _____ does occur, how will it affect your life in 3 months, 6 months? What is the most likely thing to happen? How will you handle it?" Scaling the severity of stressful events involves having the adolescent scale the suicidal precipitant, or anticipated future stressful event (e.g., on a scale from 0 to 100). Scaling helps the adolescent view events on a continuum rather than in a dichotomous (black/white) fashion.

Affect Regulation

Affect regulation techniques that are used include training adolescents to recognize stimuli that provoke negative emotions and learning to reduce physiological arousal via self-talk and relaxation. The following script is used in the initial affect management session.

"Today we are going to talk about some more things that you can do to help yourself feel better when problems come up. As we talked about earlier, when a negative activating event occurs, it triggers negative or untrue beliefs. These beliefs then cause negative feelings such as anger or sadness. In addition to negative feelings, these negative beliefs can also cause our body to start feeling out of control. You might experience muscle tightness, a faster heart rate, sweating, or shortness of breath and not even realize it. The more your body feels out of control, the harder it is to do problem solving or dispute negative beliefs. If you are not able to do these things, then you are more likely to make unsafe decisions. So, today we are going to learn ways to keep your body from spiraling out of control so that you can use your problem-solving and disputing skills to work through your problems."

The therapist then shows the adolescent a series of feelings cards and asks him or her to choose the card that best describes how he or she was feeling when the event that triggered the suicide attempt occurred. Next, the therapist presents the adolescent with a list of physiological and behavioral symptoms associated with negative affect, referred to as "body talk," and asks him or her to circle those symptoms he or she experienced when feeling the way described on the selected feeling card. The therapist notes that these "body talk" symptoms do not occur all at once but successively, like a set of dominos. The adolescent is then introduced to the concept of a "feelings thermometer" (e.g., see Rotheram-Borus et al., 1994). The bottom of the thermometer has a rating of "1" and stands for "calm and cool," and the top is "10" and stands for "extremely upset" or whatever the predominant feeling was for the adolescent at the time of the suicide trigger. The adolescent is then asked to fill in lines by each rating on the thermometer with the "body talk" endorsed on their worksheet. After that is complete, the adolescent's specific negative beliefs are inserted at the appropriate level. Next, the adolescent is asked to indicate his or her personal "danger zone" on the thermometer, or the point where his or her body spirals so far out of control that he or she is at risk for unsafe or suicidal behavior. The importance of recognizing "early" body talk and working on decreasing it before it escalates to the "danger zone" is discussed. Finally, the adolescent is asked to create a "stay cool" plan to use when he or she begins to notice early "body talk" and negative beliefs. This includes various self-soothing behaviors and positive self-statements. Finally, before the adolescent leaves the session, the parents are briefed on the session content so that they are aware of the child's coping plan and can provide their support.

When an adolescent reports instances of suicidal or self-injurious behavior during the course of treatment, we conduct a functional analysis of this behavior with the adolescent. This functional analysis combines the use of problem solving, cognitive restructuring, and other affect regulation techniques and is adapted from Linehan (1993). This technique is called a "chain analysis" and is introduced to the adolescent in the following manner:

"It sounds like you had a pretty rough time dealing with [*cite the specific trigger for suicidal behavior*]. It also sounds like your body spiraled out of control, which made it hard for you to use your problem-solving and disputing skills. Let's try to figure out what went wrong and how you can keep the same thing from happening again. To do this we need to take a look at your behavior, thoughts, feelings, and body symptoms leading up to your suicide attempt. We can do this using what we call a "chain analysis." We call this exercise a chain analysis because it takes a number of links, or a chain of related thoughts, behavior, feelings, and body sensations, to lead to a suicide attempt. The chain analysis helps us figure out what triggered your suicide attempt and each of the negative links that followed so that we can better understand what went wrong. After we figure out what wrong, we can then rebuild the chain with positive or helpful links so that you have a better plan to deal with problems."

The adolescent is first asked a series of questions about his or her intrapersonal behavior within close proximity to the suicide attempt that made him or her particularly vulnerable. This may include questions regarding medication adherence, eating patterns, sleeping patterns, exercise, and the use of alcohol or drugs, as well as various behavior patterns that are specific to the adolescent, such as isolating him- or herself when upset. Next, the adolescent is presented with a worksheet with a series of blank lines representing links and is asked to record the behavior, thoughts, body talk, and feelings (with a severity rating of from 1 to 10) associated with each link. The therapist asks the adolescent to begin the chain with a behavior that occurred earlier in the day that served as the initial trigger for a more negative mood, not the actual suicide attempt. It is not uncommon for adolescents to indicate that they woke up in a bad mood that day, in which case the chain is started with getting out of bed that morning (noting that lack of sleep likely precipitated the bad mood). These links are then completed up to the point of the suicide attempt.

Upon completion of all of the links, the therapist asks the adolescent to identify the "weak links" in the chain by circling the negative behavior and beliefs associated with any negative body talk and feelings. Next, the adolescent is asked to identify and record alternative adaptive behavior, or "strong links" that could be used to replace the "weak links."

THERAPIST: Let's look at the fifth link in your chain. You called your friend (behavior), who told you she was on another call and asked if you could talk tomorrow. You thought to yourself, "She does not want to talk to me (thought)," noticed tension in your body (body talk), and felt rejected (feeling).

You did not identify your behavior in this situation as negative. Good call. Talking to friends when you are sad is a behavior that often helps you to feel better. However, let's take a look at your thought that followed. Can you see a thinking mistake?

TEEN: Jumping to conclusions?

THERAPIST: Right. You assumed that she did not want to talk to you. What skill could you use to work on that thought?

TEEN: Disputing.

THERAPIST: Good. Now how could you have disputed that belief?

TEEN: Told myself that just because she asked to talk tomorrow does not mean that she did not want to talk to me.

THERAPIST: Good. What are some other possible reasons?

TEEN: It was late, so maybe she was tired and just wanted to go to bed.

THERAPIST: Good. What else?

TEEN: Maybe she was on an upsetting phone call and did not want to talk to anyone else.

THERAPIST: Good. What else?

TEEN: I did not tell her I was upset, so maybe she did not know that I needed to talk.

THERAPIST: Good! And would you have felt rejected if you were thinking "she is probably just tired and did not know I was upset" instead of "she does not want to talk to me."

TEEN: No. I probably would have just talked to her the next day about it.

THERAPIST: Very good. In addition to disputing, what other skill could you use to decrease the tension in your body?

TEEN: My tape?

THERAPIST: Absolutely, you could have used your relaxation tape. Very nice job! Let's go ahead and write down "disputing" and "relaxation" as the skills you could use to replace that "weak link," and also list your disputes on your worksheet.

The exercise concludes with a series of reflective questions that the adolescent is asked to answer, such as what the need was that he or she was trying to meet by engaging in dangerous behavior and how he or she can get that need met in an adaptive manner in the future. By the end of the exercise, the adolescent has a better understanding of the suicidal episode, a plan that can be used to address harm the behavior has caused, and a plan to prevent future suicidal episodes.

WORKING WITH FAMILIES

Family sessions are also necessary in addressing suicidal behavior. At a minimum, it is important to conduct a family session examining the circumstances surrounding the suicide attempt. If necessary, the therapist emphasizes that suicide attempts are serious even if the reason for the attempt was not to die. Parent and adolescent explanations for the attempt are explored, and discrepancies in their explanations are examined. If differences in perspectives are evident, then the therapist helps the parents and adolescent understand and accept each other's explanations of the suicide attempt and work together to prevent future attempts.

Family sessions can be used to help shift the focus away from the adolescent and allow the therapist to address conflictual issues that may have contributed to the development of the suicidal behavior, including poor communication (Brinkman-Sull, Overholser, & Silverman, 2000; Hurd, Wooding, & Noller, 1999). The main goals of working with the family typically are to modify communication patterns and negative interactions among family members, support adaptive attempts by the adolescent in separating from the family, and improve the family's problem-solving abilities (Berman & Jobes, 1991). Family-focused programs emphasizing communication and problem-solving skills used to address adolescent behavior problems (e.g., Robin & Foster, 1989) have also been used successfully with families of adolescent suicide attempters (e.g., Rotheram-Borus et al., 1994). Marital problems and parental psychopathology disrupt and/or prevent treatment progress and thus necessitate outside referrals.

Communication sessions typically begin with a review of both negative and positive communication habits (Robin & Foster, 1989), followed by a discussion about the communication style used by the adolescent and his or her parents. The negative or hurtful effects of negative communication behavior (e.g., anger, resentment, low self-esteem, etc.) are also reviewed. To decrease defensiveness, the therapist notes that most people use negative communication behavior when upset or frustrated. However, it is important to recognize these patterns and alter them.

One specific set of procedures for improving family communication has been developed by Clarke, Lewinsohn, and Hops (1990). In this approach, "active listening" skills are introduced as the first step in improving communication. Clarke and colleagues present three rules of active listening: (1) Restate the sender's message in your own words; (2) begin restatements with phrases such as "I hear you saying that . . . ," or "You said you feel . . . ,"; and (3) be neutral about the other person's views (think of them as neither good nor bad).

The therapist first demonstrates the use of active listening skills by having the adolescent state a problem and then restates the adolescent's message using the techniques described above. Active listening skills are then role-played by family members. The adolescent is asked to describe a minor problem, and the parent, with the therapist's guidance, is asked to demonstrate the use of active listening skills. Then the adolescent is asked to practice active listening skills in response to a minor problem described by his or her parent. Reactions from the adolescent and the parents are elicited, and the importance of using active listening skills is discussed.

The therapist shares that it is very difficult to use active listening skills, which are essential to effective communication, when upset. Therefore, it is important that all parties involved be calm before engaging in discussions. Further, the therapist discusses the importance of not forcing anyone to engage in a discussion when he or she is not ready and/or is upset. If a discussion that initially starts off in a calm tone becomes heated, family members are instructed to separate and allow adequate time to calm down. Family members only reengage in the discussion when everyone involved is ready.

In family problem-solving sessions, the therapist first facilitates discussion regarding how solving problems together can be difficult because everyone in the family may have different feelings and ideas about the problem. The problem-solving format we use with adolescents individually (SOLVE, as discussed previously) is used to address family problems. The therapist assists the family in establishing a problem-solving system and teaches the problem-solving steps.

Clarke and colleagues (1990) suggest that the therapist first provide the family with rules for selecting a problem. These rules include being specific, describing what the other person is doing or saying that is problematic, avoiding name calling when describing the problem, expressing feelings in reaction to the problem (not the person), admitting responsibility for the problem when appropriate, avoiding blaming others, and being brief in providing input.

After everyone agrees on the problem, all possible Solutions to the problem are generated. Family members are requested to withhold judgments regarding the efficacy of the different Options at this point. Next, each person rates the Likely outcome of each option with a plus or minus. Family members then choose the solution that seems most acceptable to everyone (Very best one). After employing the chosen solution, family members are encouraged to Evaluate the outcome of that particular solution. If the problem still exists, the problem-solving process is repeated. In some approaches, the problem-solving session concludes with the development of a written contract. The contract specifies the plan for addressing problems at home that have been agreed upon by family members.

Conclusions

CBT with adolescent suicide attempters can be used to address the thought processes and behavior that result in negative affect. Many of these adolescents must learn to reduce the tendency for dichotomous thinking and catastrophizing. CBT can also help the suicidal adolescent develop a wider range of adaptive coping behavior. Useful coping skills may include directly confronting a problem instead of avoiding a difficult situation, learning to generate potential solutions to problems, and encouraging persistence, hopefulness, and a sense of personal control (Overholser, 1996). Because interpersonal problems can play a major role in depression and suicide risk, it is important for therapy to focus on helping adolescents improve their social functioning. As social functioning improves, adolescents often report less depression and reduced risk of suicidal behavior. Family meetings can help improve communication within the family (Harrington et al., 1998) and increase support provided by family members.

Even if therapy has been successful, adolescent suicide attempters remain vulnerable to a sudden resurgence of suicidal feelings (Beck, 1996). It is important for the therapist to forewarn the adolescent and parents of the potential for resurgence of suicidality. Identifying subclinical levels of sadness or pessimism that can be managed before they reach crisis proportions, via individual efforts or booster sessions, is a priority.

FUTURE DIRECTIONS

Therapy with adolescent suicide attempters is challenging for clinicians and difficult for clinical researchers to test in clinical trials. The treatment outcome literature on adolescent suicide attempters is small, both because of the difficulties inherent in treating this population and investigator concerns about liability in clinical trials with such high-risk patients (Pearson, Stanley, King, & Fisher, 2001). Other factors that make it difficult to test treatments with these adolescents include their poor adherence to treatment protocols and the high likelihood of continued suicidality during a research protocol. This latter factor typically results in patients being removed from clinical trials. If removal from a trial due to continued suicidality is the standard in research with suicide attempters, a substantial percentage may never complete treatment trials, making it difficult to accumulate knowledge. In addition, the need to treat both the suicidal behavior and underlying psychiatric disorder has proven to be a substantial challenge for researchers, complicated even further by the comorbidity commonly found in these adolescents. Finally, when enrolled in trials immediately following a suicide attempt, many of these adolescents will be on one or more medications. Thus, combined psychosocial/ psychopharmacologic treatments, with a standard algorithm guiding medication use, may be the research designs best suited to address the clinical and ethical realities of studying such a high-risk population.

ACKNOWLEDGMENTS

This work was conducted at the Brown University Center for Alcohol and Addiction Studies, Providence, Rhode Island, and supported in part by grants to Anthony Spirito (No. MH01738) and Christianne Esposito-Smythers (No. AA014191 and the American Foundation for Suicide Prevention).

REFERENCES

Adams, J., & Adams, M. (1996). The association among negative life events, perceived problem solving alternatives, depression, and suicidal ideation in adolescent psychiatric patients. *Journal of Child Psychology and Psychiatry, 37*, 715–720.

Beautrais, A. L., Joyce, P. R., & Mulder, R. T. (1996). Risk factors for serious suicide attempts among youths aged 13 through 24 years. *Journal of the American Academy of Child and Adolescent Psychiatry, 35*, 1174–1182.

Beautrais, A. L., Joyce, P. R., & Mulder, R. T. (1997). Precipitating factors and life events in serious suicide attempts among youths aged 13 through 24 years. *Journal of the American Academy of Child and Adolescent Psychiatry, 36*, 1543–1551.

Beck, A. T. (1996). Beyond belief: A theory of modes, personality, and psychopathology. In P. Salkovskis (Ed.), *Frontiers of cognitive therapy* (pp. 1–25). New York: Guilford Press.

Beck, A. T., Rush, A. J., Shaw, B. F., & Emery, G. (1979). *Cognitive therapy of depression.* New York: Guilford Press.

Beck, A. T., Schuyler, D., & Herman, I. (1974). Development of Suicidal Intent Scales. In A. T. Beck, H. Resnick, & D. Lettieri (Eds.), *The prediction of suicide* (pp. 45–56). Bowie, MD: Charles Press.

Beck, A. T. & Steer, R. A. (1991). *Beck Scale for Suicide Ideation.* San Antonio, TX: Psychological Corporation.

Berman, A. L., & Jobes, D. A. (1991). *Adolescent suicide: Assessment and intervention.* Washington, DC: American Psychological Association.

Bernard, M. E., & Joyce, M. R. (1984). *Rational emotive therapy with children and adolescents: Theory, treatment strategies, preventative methods.* New York: Wiley.

Boergers, J., & Spirito, A. (2003). The outcome of suicide attempts among adolescents. In A. Spirito & J. Overholser (Eds.), *Evaluating and treating adolescent suicide attempters: From research to practice* (261–276). San Diego, CA: Academic Press.

Boergers, J., Spirito, A., & Donaldson, D. (1998). Reasons for adolescent suicide attempts: Associations with psychological functioning. *Journal of the American Academy of Child and Adolescent Psychiatry, 37*, 1287–1293.

Borst, S., Noam, G., & Bartok, J. (1991). Adolescent suicidality: A clinical developmental approach. *Journal of the American Academy of Child and Adolescent Psychiatry, 30*, 796–803.

Brent, D. A., Kolko, D. J., Allan, M. J., & Brown, R. V. (1990). Suicidality in affectively disordered adolescent inpatients. *Journal of the American Academy of Child and Adolescent Psychiatry, 29*, 586–593.

Brent, D. A., Perper, J., Moritz, G., Allman, C., Friend, A., Roth, C., et al. (1993). Psychiatric risk factors for adolescent suicide: A case-control study. *Journal of the American Academy of Child and Adolescent Psychiatry, 32*, 521–529.

Brent, D. A., Perper, J. A., Moritz, G., Liotus, L., Schweers, J., Balach, I., & Roth, C. (1994). Familial risk factors for adolescent suicide: a case-control study. *Acta Psychiatria Scandinavica, 89*, 52–58.

Brinkman-Sull, D., Overholser, J., & Silverman, E. (2000). Risk of future suicide attempts in adolescent psychiatric inpatients at 18-month follow-up. *Suicide and Life-Threatening Behavior, 30*, 327–340.

Brown, L. K., Overholser, J., Spirito, A., & Fritz, G. K. (1991). The correlates of planning in adolescent suicide attempts. *Journal of the American Academy of Child and Adolescent Psychiatry, 30*, 95–99.

Chatoor, I., & Krupnick, J. (2001). The role of non-specific factors in treatment outcome of psychotherapy studies. *European Child and Adolescent Psychiatry, 10*, 19–25.

Clarke, G., Lewinsohn, P., & Hops, H. (1990). *Adolescent coping with depression course.* Eugene, OR: Castalia.

Department of Health and Human Services (2002). *Youth Risk Behavior Surveillance—United States, 1999, Morbidity and Mortality Weekly Report.* Atlanta, GA. Centers for Disease Control and Prevention.

Donaldson, D., Spirito, A., & Esposito-Smythers, C. (2005). Treatment for adolescents following a suicide attempt: Results of a pilot trial. *Journal of the American Academy of Child and Adolescent Psychiatry, 44,* 113–120.

Donaldson, D., Spirito, A., & Overholser, J. (2003). Treatment of adolescent suicide attempters. In A. Spirito & J. Overholser (Eds.), *Evaluating and treating adolescent suicide attempters: From research to practice* (pp. 295–321). San Diego, CA: Academic Press.

Fritsch, S., Donaldson, D., Spirito, A., & Plummer, B. (2000). Personality characteristics of adolescent suicide attempters. *Child Psychiatry and Human Development, 30,* 219–235.

Goldston, D. B. (2003). *Measuring suicidal behavior and risk in adolescents.* Washington, DC: American Psychological Association.

Guertin, T., Lloyd-Richardson, E., Spirito, A., Donaldson, D., & Boergers, J. (2001). Self-mutilative behavior in adolescents who attempt suicide by overdose. *Journal of the American Academy of Child and Adolescent Psychiatry, 40,* 1062–1069.

Harrington, R., Kerfoot, M., Dyer, E., McNiven, F., Gill, J., Harrington, V., et al. (1998). Randomized trial of a home-based family intervention for children who have deliberately poisoned themselves. *Journal of the American Academy of Child and Adolescent Psychiatry, 37,* 512–518.

Huey, S., Henggeler, S. W., Rowland, M. D., Halliday-Boykins, C. A., Cunningham, P. B., Pickrel, S. G., & Edwards, J. (2004). Multisystemic therapy effects on attempted suicide by youths presenting psychiatric emergencies. *Journal of the American Academy of Child and Adolescent Psychiatry, 43,* 183–190.

Hurd, K., Wooding, S., & Noller, P. (1999). Parent–adolescent relationships in families with depressed and self-harming adolescents. *Australian Journal of Marriage and Family, 5,* 47–68.

Joiner, T., Voelz, Z., & Rudd, M. D. (2001). For suicidal young adults with comorbid depression and anxiety disorders, problem-solving treatment may be better than treatment as usual. *Professional Psychology: Research and Practice, 32,* 278–282.

Kazdin, A. E. (1996). Dropping out of child psychotherapy: Issues for research and practice. *Clinical Child Psychology and Psychiatry, 1,* 133–156.

Kessler, R., Borges, G., & Walters, E. (1999). Prevalence of and risk factors for lifetime suicide attempts in the National Comorbidity Survey. *Archives of General Psychiatry, 56,* 617–626.

LeComte, D., & Fornes, P. (1998). Suicide among youth and young adults, 15 through 24 years of age: A report of 392 cases from Paris, 1989–1996. *Journal of Forensic Sciences, 43,* 964–968.

Linehan, M. M. (1993). *Cognitive-behavioral treatment of borderline personality disorder.* New York: Guilford Press.

Marciano, P. L., & Kazdin, A. E. (1994). Self-esteem, depression, hopelessness, and suicidal intent among psychiatrically disturbed inpatient children. *Journal of Clinical Child Psychology, 23,* 151–160.

McClung, T. (2000). *Rational emotive therapy adapted for adolescent psychiatric inpatients.* Unpublished manual, West Virginia University School of Medicine.

Overholser, J. C. (1996). Cognitive-behavioral treatment of depression: VII. Coping with precipitating events. *Journal of Contemporary Psychotherapy, 26,* 337–360.

Pearson, J., Stanley, B., King, C., & Fisher, C. (2001). Intervention research with persons at high risk for suicidality: Safety and ethical considerations. *Journal of Clinical Psychiatry, 62,* 17–26.

Prinstein, M. J., Boergers, J., Spirito, A., & Little, T. D. (2000). Peer functioning, family dysfunction, and psychological symptoms in a risk factor model of adolescent inpatients' suicidal ideation severity. *Journal of Clinical Child and Adolescent Psychology, 29,* 392–405.

Rathus, J. H., & Miller, A. L. (2002). Dialectical behavior therapy adapted for suicidal adolescents. *Suicide and Life Threatening Behavior, 32,* 146–157.

Reynolds, W. M. (1988). *Suicidal Ideation Questionnaire.* Lutz, FL: Psychological Assessment Resources.

Robin, A. L., & Foster, S. L. (1989). *Negotiating parent–adolescent conflict: A behavioral–family systems approach.* New York: Guilford Press.

Rotheram-Borus, M. J., Piacentini, J., Miller, S., Graae, F., & Castro-Blanco, D. (1994). Brief cognitive-behavioral treatment for adolescent suicide attempters and their families. *Journal Of the American Academy of Child and Adolescent Psychiatry, 33,* 508–517.

Rudd, M. D., Joiner, T., & Rajab, M. H. (2001). *Treating suicidal behavior: An effective time-limited approach.* New York: Guilford Press.

Rudd, M. D., Rajab, M. H., Orman, D. T., Stulman, D. A., Joiner, T., & Dixon, W. (1996). Effectiveness of an outpatient intervention targeting suicidal young adults: Preliminary results. *Journal of Consulting and Clinical Psychology, 64,* 179–190.

Sadowski, C., & Kelley, M. L. (1993). Social problem-solving in suicidal adolescents. *Journal of Consulting and Clinical Psychology, 61,* 121–127.

Shaffer, D., Gould, M. S., Fisher, P., Trautman, P., Moreau, D., Kleinman, M., & Flory, M. (1996). Psychiatric diagnoses in child and adolescent suicide. *Archives of General Psychiatry, 53,* 339–348.

Shaffer, D., & Pfeffer, C. (2001). Practice parameter for the assessment and treatment of children and adolescents with suicidal behavior. *Journal of the American Academy of Child and Adolescent Psychiatry, 40*(Suppl. 7), 24S–51S.

Spirito, A., Boergers, J., Donaldson, D., Bishop, D., & Lewander, W. (2001). An intervention trial to improve adherence to community treatment by adolescents after a suicide attempt. *Journal of the American Academy of Child and Adolescent Psychiatry, 41,* 435–442.

Spirito, A., Sterling, C., Donaldson, D., & Arrigan, M. (1996). Factor analysis of the Suicide Intent Scale with adolescent suicide attempters. *Journal of Personality Assessment, 67,* 90–101.

Spirito, A., Williams, C. A., Stark, L. J., & Hart, K. J. (1988). The Hopelessness Scale for Children: Psychometric properties with normal and emotionally disturbed adolescents. *Journal of Abnormal Child Psychology, 16,* 445–458.

Trautman, P. D., Stewart, N., & Morishima, A. (1993). Are adolescent suicide attempters noncompliant with outpatient care? *Journal of the American Academy of Child and Adolescent Psychiatry, 32,* 89–94.

Wagner, B. M. (1997). Family risk factors for child and adolescent suicidal behavior. *Psychological Bulletin, 121,* 246–298.

Wood, A., Trainor, G., Rothwell, J., Moore, A., & Harrington, R. (2001). Randomized trial of group therapy for repeated deliberate self harm in adolescents. *Journal of the American Academy of Child and Adolescent Psychiatry, 40,* 1246–1253.

CHAPTER 7

Treating Anxiety Disorders in Youth

PHILIP C. KENDALL and CYNTHIA SUVEG

The past decade has seen an increased commitment to researching the etiology, nature, and treatment of anxiety in youth. Such research is justified when one considers that prevalence rates for anxiety disorders using community samples have ranged from 2.4 to 17% (Costello, Mustillo, Erkanli, Keeler, & Angold, 2003; Kashani & Orvaschel, 1988). Given the long-term implications of experiencing anxiety in youth (Kendall, 1992a), research has also continued to explore potential negative sequelae. Anxiety in youth places children at increased risk for comorbid diagnoses (Brady & Kendall, 1992; Last, Strauss, & Francis, 1987; Verduin & Kendall, 2003), psychopathology in adulthood (anxiety, depression, substance use; Aschenbrand, Kendall, Webb, Safford, & Flannery-Schroeder, 2003; Woodward & Fergusson, 2001), and lower adaptive functioning in the domains of academic performance, peer relations, and family relations (Last, Hansen, & Franco, 1997; Woodward & Fergusson, 2001).

From a developmental perspective, however, it is important to consider that mild fear and anxiety are part of normal development. Thus, this chapter begins by placing anxiety within a normative context. Following this, the somatic, behavioral, cognitive, and emotion-related features of anxiety disorders in youth are described. Assessment issues are discussed, with special attention to normal developmental trajectories of anxiety. Recognizing the potential impact of family stress, pathology, and individual members' interpersonal/parenting styles, we explore the role of the family in the development and maintenance of a child's anxious experience. Finally, a descriptive review of the common principles and strategies of cognitive–behavioral therapy (CBT) is presented, and recent outcome research evaluating these procedures is provided. One treatment model for anxious youth is outlined in detail and illustrated by real-life session vignettes of cases seen at the Child and Adolescent Anxiety Disorders Clinic (CAADC) at Temple University.

NORMATIVE DEVELOPMENT

Normative data provide a useful starting point for understanding the content and nature of childhood anxieties and fears, as well as for evaluating the severity of the targeted anxieties and fears (see Kendall, Marrs-Garcia, Nath, & Sheldrick, 1999). As children develop, the content of their anxieties and fears tends to reflect changes in their perceptions of reality (Campbell, 1986). Children's fears begin with a content that is more global, imaginary, uncontrollable, and powerful, and over time becomes more specific, differentiated, and realistic (Bauer, 1976). Thus, for example, fears of the diffuse "boogie man" that lurks in the dark evolve into more distinct and realistic fears that include peer acceptance and school performance concerns (Bauer, 1976; for a review of the development of fear, see Gullone, 2000).

The content of childhood fears has often been designated and described in terms of a five-factor structure based on the Fear Survey Schedule for Children—Revised (FSSC-R; Ollendick, 1983; Ollendick, Matson, & Helsel, 1985), including (1) fear of failure and criticism, (2) fear of the unknown, (3) fear of injury and small animals, (4) fear of danger and death, and (5) medical fears. Although age and gender differences exist, the factors themselves appear to be robust across age, gender, and even nationality (Ollendick, King, & Frary, 1989). However, a recent cross-cultural examination (Fonseca, Yule, & Erol, 1994) was unable to replicate the five-factor model in non-English-speaking countries, reminding us to be cautious about generalizations across cultures.

Importantly, research examining the fears of children of different ethnicities reveals that there are more similarities than differences across these ethnicities (see Ginsburg & Silverman, 1996; Neal & Turner, 1991; Treadwell, Flannery-Schroeder, & Kendall, 1994). In their broader cross-cultural review, Fonseca and colleagues (1994) concluded that the most common fears endorsed by children are remarkably similar across countries and cultures; however, when examining supplemental lists to the FSSC-R, a variety of fears were also endorsed by children in different countries. Thus, although similarities may prevail, broad generalizations should not be made. As children grow older, the number of fears they experience generally decreases (Bauer, 1976; Draper & James, 1985), and this trend has been supported cross-culturally (see Fonseca et al., 1994). Also supported are sex differences in the number of childhood fears, with maternal and self-report accounts indicating that girls often report exhibiting more fears than boys (Bauer, 1976; Gullone, 2000; Ollendick et al., 1985). Sex differences vary by culture (Fonseca et al., 1994), and, as some have cautioned, social desirability and sex-role stereotypes and expectations may affect not only reportability but also referability. This concern is reflected in the research, which suggests that girls are more likely to be referred for clinical attention than boys (e.g., Weisz & Weiss, 1991).

Although anxiety is an expected part of typical development, it becomes a disorder when the experience is exaggerated beyond that which would be expected in a given situation and interferes with the youth's functioning. There are several disorders listed within the fourth edition of the *Diagnostic and Statistical Manual of Mental Disorders* (DSM-IV; American Psychiatric Association, 1994) that may be largely or primarily associated with anxiety. Our focus is on three subtypes of childhood anxiety disorder that are identified in the DSM-IV: generalized anxiety disorder (GAD), separation anxiety disorder (SAD), and social phobia (SP).[1] Separation anxiety disorder involves extreme anxiety in anticipation of or upon separation from an attachment figure. Youth with SAD may fear that danger or harm will come to themselves or a loved one, which would prevent the youth from seeing the loved one again. Such fear often results in a refusal to be away from the caregiver for developmentally appropriate periods of time. In SP, the source of fear is social evaluation that may include a fear of embarrassing or humiliating oneself in front of others. For younger children, social fear around peers is required for the diagnosis. GAD is typified by pervasive, uncontrollable worries that can occur in an array of domains, including concern about performance, family or social relations, physical health, or ruminations about future or past behavior. Importantly, youth with GAD find the worry hard to control.

FEATURES OF ANXIETY

Anxiety is a multidimensional construct that consists of behavioral, somatic, cognitive, and emotional elements. The most prominent behavioral response to anxiety is avoidance, but other responses may include shaky voice, rigid posture, crying, nail biting, and thumb sucking (Barrios & Hartmann, 1988). In the case of a child with SAD, he or she may avoid sleepovers in an effort to stay close to a caregiver, whereas a child with SP may avoid sleepovers due to fear of evaluation by peers. Physiologically, youth with anxiety may report an increase in autonomic nervous system activity, perspiration, diffuse abdominal pain ("butterflies in the stomach"), flushed face, gastrointestinal distress, and trembling (see also Barrios & Hartmann, 1988). The cognitive distress experienced by anxious children may include rumination or excessive worry, or anxious thinking (expecting the worse will happen in a situation). Although many youth with anxiety experience cognitive distress, the particular nature of the cognitive distress varies by disorder. Fears that the youth or his or her parent may be hurt, or that caregivers may leave and never return, are common among children with separation fears. Children with SP worry about social or performance situations in which they might be humiliated or embarrassed. The anxious distress may include circumscribed social situations (e.g., speaking, eating in public) or more generalized social situations, but it must include anxiety that is present in peer settings. GAD, as its name implies, is characterized by a more generalized or diffuse sense of worry about a number of issues that may include fear of evaluation, self-consciousness, and rumination about past or future behavior. In each of these disorders, such worry, despite its target, is persistent, excessive, and often difficult for the child to control. Diagnostically, symptom duration is an important consideration. Whereas children experiencing the symptoms of separation (SAD) may receive a formal diagnosis after at least 4 weeks of such distress, both SP and GAD diagnoses require at least 6 months of symptom expression and impairment (American Psychiatric Association, 1994).

An important distinction to be made when treating youth is between *cognitive distortions* and *cognitive deficiencies* (Kendall, 1985, 1991, 2000a; Kendall, Choudhury, Chung, & Robin, 2002). Whereas deficiencies refer to an absence of a cognitive skill, distortions include thinking that is dysfunctional or biased. With deficiencies, there is a lack of forethought in situations that require some advanced consideration; with distortions, the cognitive dysfunction occurs not in the lack of information processing but in the presence of maladaptive thinking. Making such a distinction is helpful therapeutically in that it allows clinicians to target the specific nature of the dysfunction; that is, addressing cognitive deficiencies would require eliminating impulsive acting without thinking and working toward more thoughtful and meaningful problem solving. Alternately, cognitive distortions must first be identified, recognized as problematic, and subsequently corrected. The negative self-talk, preoccupation with the evaluations of others, and misperceptions of threat or danger that often plague children with anxiety, for example, seem to result from a thinking process that is primarily distorted and ultimately dysfunctional. Ehrenreich and Gross (2002) recently reviewed the literature documenting the tendency of anxious youth to focus their attention on threatening or fearful stimuli in their environments. The consequence of this disposition may be a hypervigilance to environmental cues that signal some sort of threat. It is precisely this style of maladaptive and self-defeating thinking that becomes a treatment target for anxious children.

As evidenced by terms such as "affect revolution" (Fischer & Tangney, 1995), considerable research in the past decade has been devoted to the study of emotional development. This research, although scant relative to that conducted with normative populations, has included clinical samples of anxious youth (see Southam-Gerow & Kendall, 2002). In one study that compared anxious and normal children on facets of emotional understanding, anxious children demonstrated less understanding of how to hide and change their emotions (Southam-

Gerow & Kendall, 2000). Insofar as the acts of hiding and changing emotions are methods used to manage one's emotional experiences, anxious children may be limited in their capacity to understand the regulation or modification of their emotions. Another study (Suveg & Zeman, 2004) compared emotion regulation processes in children with anxiety disorders versus nonanxious counterparts. Results indicated that anxious children (1) experienced their emotions more intensely and (2) perceived themselves as less able to successfully manage emotionally provocative situations than the nonanxious children. When particular patterns of emotion management were examined, the anxious children exhibited (1) more dysregulated management (i.e., culturally inappropriate emotional expression) and (2) less adaptive coping across anger, sadness, and worry situations than did the non-AD youth. Mothers of children with anxiety disorders also perceived their children as significantly more inflexible, labile, and emotionally negative than did mothers of nonanxious children. Therapeutically, it follows that anxious children may benefit from interventions that include efforts to improve their knowledge of and ability to regulate their emotions.

FAMILY MATTERS

The cognitive-behavioral model acknowledges and is concerned with the influence of the family and other social contexts on childhood anxiety (Ginsburg, Siqueland, Masia-Warner, & Hedtke, 2004; Kendall, 1985, 1991), and recent years have witnessed a dramatic increase in research on family factors associated with anxiety in youth (see Wood, McLeod, Sigman, Hwang, & Chu, 2003, for a review). The results of the "top-down" and "bottom-up" studies provide evidence that children with anxiety disorders are more likely to have parents with anxious symptomatology or mood disorders, and that parents with anxiety disorders are more likely to have children with anxiety disorders (e.g., Last, Hersen, Kazdin, Francis, & Grubb, 1987; Last, Phillips, & Statfeld, 1987). Further, using various methodologies, parents of anxious children have been shown to encourage potentially maladaptive patterns of responding through direct discussions with their children (Barrett, Rapee, Dadds, & Ryan, 1996; Dadds, Barrett, Rapee, & Ryan, 1996; Suvey, Zeman, Flannery-Schroeder, & Cassano, 2005), by modeling anxious behavior themselves (Whaley, Pinto, & Sigman, 1999), and by exhibiting overcontrolling and overprotective behavior (Dumas, LaFreniere, & Serketich, 1995; Hudson & Rapee, 2001; Lieb et al., 2000; Siqueland, Kendall, & Steinberg, 1996; Whaley et al., 1999). For example, Barrett and colleagues (1996) reported that anxious children interpreted ambiguous situations in a more threatening manner than did nonanxious children. Differing from both nonanxious and aggressive children in their selected responses to these situations, anxious children were more likely to respond in an avoidant manner. The parents of anxious children also had significantly higher rates of threat interpretation and higher rates of predicting their children would select an avoidant response. Further reinforcing the role of the family in possibly contributing to anxious behavior, it was found that after anxious children had the opportunity to engage in a family discussion about how to act in a given situation, their avoidant responses significantly increased, whereas oppositional children's aggressive responses increased and the nonanxious children's responses became less avoidant. This phenomenon, called the "family enhancement of avoidant and aggressive response," has implications for the types of interventions to be implemented with families of anxious youth. However, these influences are not unidirectional—the interaction between child (e.g., biological predisposition to anxiety) and parent (e.g., their own psychopathology) variables most likely contributes to the youth's anxiety (Kendall & Ollendick, 2004).

At the heart of much of the research investigating family variables in childhood anxiety is the notion of "control" or "perceived control" (see Chorpita & Barlow, 1998; Chorpita, Brown, & Barlow, 1998; Ginsburg, Silverman, & Kurtines, 1995). In essence, control refers to the extent to which children believe that their behavior can influence events and outcomes. Adults with anxiety and depressive disorders have described having family environments that were more likely to have limited experience with control over various events, with parental overprotection and discouragement of autonomy being related to subsequent anxiety and depression (Parker, 1983). Research indicates that the parents of youth with anxiety disorders are less inclined to grant them psychological autonomy than are parents of nonreferred children (Siqueland et al., 1996). Furthermore, children diagnosed with anxiety and depression are more likely to describe their families as less supportive, cohesive, and democratic in decision making and more conflictual than do other children (Stark, Humphrey, Crook, & Lewis, 1990).

In examining maternal expectations and attributions of a child's ability to cope in a stressful situation, Kortlander, Kendall, and Panichelli-Mindel (1997) reported that mothers of anxious children expected their children to be more distressed and less able to perform in a given situation than mothers of nonanxious children. Similarly, mothers of highly anxious girls, as opposed to mothers of less anxious girls, were more likely to intervene in their daughter's problem solving of a task and less likely to wait for the child to solve the task (Krohne & Hock, 1991). In a cross-cultural examination of childhood fears and anxiety by Dong, Yang, and Ollendick (1994), it was predicted that Chinese child-rearing practices and educational beliefs, which tended to be more restrictive and overprotective, should predict higher levels of anxious and depressive symptomatology in more Western contexts. The authors found support for these predictions, particularly for 11- to 13-year-old children. Considering all of these findings, each of these family factors may contribute to a child's anxious behavior. Eventually, parents must cede control, and the notion of autonomy granting is an important consideration, given that families of anxious children may be overprotective. Thus, fostering independence requires treatment consideration.

Several therapy models have attempted to target issues of parental control and the child's need for autonomy in treatment. One model, "transfer of control" (Ginsburg et al., 1995), sets up a system wherein the therapist transfers coping skills to the child, with the parents serving as a mediator. The therapist teaches skills to the parents and child and then serves as a coach for the parents as they help guide their child through distressing situations. Barriers to the transfer of control, according to these authors, include parental anxious symptomatology and deficient family relations. Including the cognitive-behavioral framework, treatment strategies include contingency management, self-control management, and exposure (as seen in Kendall, 1994), as well a dyadic intervention approach that focuses on barriers in the transfer of control and targets parental anxious symptomatology as well as the problematic family relationships (see also Ginsburg et al., 1995; Silverman & Kurtines, 1996).

Anxiety disorders in youth are multifaceted and multidetermined. How do we come to understand the experience of a child who, for example, worries excessively about the potential rejection of his or her peers, is physically sickened by it, wants to avoid school because of it, or feels all of these things at once? How do we translate a child's worries, words of fear, and feelings of dread into a clinically meaningful account? Continuing from our developmental perspective, we now turn to the topic of assessment as a critical starting point in the treatment of childhood anxiety.

ASSESSMENT

We have, thus far, described anxiety disorders in youth in a manner that is consistent with the DSM formulation: a categorical system in which a child either does or does not qualify for a diagnosis. However, the assessment of anxiety need not adopt a categorical system. Indeed, there is considerable controversy about the DSM system of classification of childhood disorders, with some mental health professionals arguing instead that the childhood disorders are best described along multiple continua (Achenbach & Edelbrock, 1978; Quay, 1977). Although a thorough review of this debate is beyond the scope of this chapter, it is noteworthy that some researchers argue that the significant overlap of symptoms among the childhood disorders raises questions regarding the discriminative validity and clinical utility of the disorders classified in the categorical system of DSM. Also, the categorical system requires that the patient display a minimum number of required symptoms in order to meet criteria for a diagnosis; a system requiring such a "threshold" for diagnosis may compromise the treatment of subclinical patients (Albano, Chorpita, & Barlow, 1996).

An alternative to a categorical system is an empirically derived dimensional system of classification, such as that developed by Achenbach and colleagues (Achenbach, 1991, 1993; Achenbach & Edelbrock, 1983, 1986). From a multivariate standpoint, Achenbach and colleagues (Achenbach, 1991; Achenbach & McConaughy, 1992) developed the Child Behavior Checklist (CBCL) and identified four specific narrowband syndromes in clinic-referred children and adolescents of various ages who present with internalizing problems: anxious–depressed, schizoid, somatic complaints, and withdrawn (this does not include the externalizing problems that can also be assessed by the CBCL). Research in this area has contributed to the delineations represented in the fourth edition of DSM. DSM-IV is based on a classification that combines features of both the categorical and dimensional approaches by identifying essential symptoms of a disorder while allowing for nonessential variations of symptoms to occur (Barlow, 1992). Nevertheless, although considerable improvement has been made over previous DSM versions, problems remain, and the classification of psychopathology in children and adolescents and some aspects of the DSM remain controversial (Albano et al., 1996).

These classification issues in combination with other factors combine to make the assessment of anxiety in youth a challenging endeavor and include: frequent comorbidity and overlapping criteria among the anxiety disorders (Costello et al., 2003), the need to distinguish between developmentally appropriate and developmentally atypical anxiety, and frequent disagreement among informants (Grills & Ollendick, 2002). The issue of disagreement among informants with respect to childhood anxiety disorders has been recognized (Grills & Ollendick, 2002, 2003), and recent empirical research has begun to investigate the nature of the reporting (Choudhury, Pimentel, & Kendall, 2003; Comer & Kendall, 2004; Silverman & Rabian, 1995).

The practice parameters for the assessment and treatment of anxiety disorders (American Academy of Child and Adolescent Psychiatry, 1997) noted important areas to emphasize in the assessment of anxiety disorders in children and adolescents. Specifically, the onset, development, and context of anxiety symptoms, as well as information regarding the child's developmental, medical, school, and social history and family psychiatric history, should be obtained (Bernstein, Borchart, & Perwein, 1996). Given these factors, instruments used to assess anxiety in children and adolescents should (1) provide reliable and valid measurement of symptoms across multiple domains (i.e., cognitive, behavioral, and psychological channels); (2) discriminate between disorders (selection/classification); (3) evaluate severity; (4) reconcile multiple observations (e.g., parent and child ratings); and (5) enable the evaluation of therapeutic change (Kendall & Flannery-Schroeder, 1998; Stallings & March, 1995). Though no instrument is perfect, several acceptable assessment tools are available. In this section, we provide an overview of some of the more commonly used instruments for assessing anxiety in children and adolescents (for a more thorough review, see Langley, Bergman, & Piacentini, 2002).

Clinical Interviews

The interview remains one of the most common methods for assessing childhood disorders in general and anxiety specifically. Numerous interview schedules designed to be administered to both children and parents have been developed and empirically tested. Interviews range from a highly structured format to an unstructured one and have the advantage of gleaning information about the child's developmental history from both child and parent perspectives. Although an unstructured clinical interview may be acceptable in some clinical settings, the absence of standardization makes this problematic for subsequent research. The semistructured interview format has been developed to provide structure while also providing opportunities for elaboration as judged appropriate by an examiner, and it serves to increase the reliability of diagnostic assignment.

The Anxiety Disorders Interview Schedule for Children (ADIS-C/P; Silverman & Albano, 1996) is a semistructured interview developed specifically to determine DSM-IV anxiety diagnoses (assessing symptomatology, course, etiology, and severity) in youth (Silverman, 1991). The ADIS-C/P relies on DSM criteria for anxiety and related disorders and utilizes an interviewer–observer format, allowing the clinician to draw information both from the interview and from clinical observation. The parent interview extracts information on the child's history, while the child interview addresses symptomatology in greater detail. Final, or composite, diagnoses are based on the level of severity endorsed in each interview and the agreement in identification of pathology between parent and child interviews. Among its strengths are favorable psychometric properties (March & Albano, 1998; Silverman, Saavedra, & Pina, 2001; Wood, Piacentini, Bergman, McCracken, & Barrios, 2002) and clear and clinically sensitive sections for diagnosing the separate anxiety disorders in youth. Additional portions of this interview have been developed to permit diagnosis of other disorders (e.g., to assess comorbid conditions).

Another commonly used semistructured interview is the Schedule for Affective Disorders and Schizophrenia in School-Age Children (K-SADS; Puig-Antich & Chambers, 1978), which requires experienced clinicians to determine diagnoses using information generated by the interview and all other available sources and material. The Diagnostic Interview for Children and Adolescents (DICA; Herjanic & Reich, 1982) and the National Institute of Mental Health (NIMH) Diagnostic Interview Schedule for Children— fourth version (DISC-IV; Shaffer, Fisher, Lucas, Dulcan, & Schwab-Stone, 2000) are other interviews designed to establish diagnoses according to a classification system.

Although these interviews are designed to elicit general diagnoses in children, not all have been developed to specifically address the diagnosing of anxiety. For general diagnoses, concordance between parent and child report during the clinical interview ranges from moderate to good, but concordance for the diagnosis of anxiety disorders is often lower (Chambers et al., 1985; Choudhury et al., 2003; Comer & Kendall, 2004; Edelbrock, Costello, Duncan, Conover, & Kalas, 1986; Edelbrock, Costello, Duncan, Kalas, & Conover, 1985; Grills & Ollendick, 2003; Hodges, McKnew, Birbach, & Roebuck, 1987). For example, a recent study by Comer and Kendall (2004) examined parent–child concordance on symptoms and diagnoses of the ADIS-IV. Results indicated greater agreement at the symptom- rather than diagnostic-level. Furthermore, the agreement was higher for observable and non-school-based symptoms than for nonobservable and school-based symptoms, respectively. Questions concerning factual, unambiguous, and concrete information produce the highest agreement between parent and child report (Herjanic, Herjanic, Brown, & Wheatt, 1975; Herjanic & Reich, 1982), whereas questions concerning subjective information and internalizing symptoms related to depression and anxiety produce the lowest (Herjanic et al., 1975; Herjanic & Reich, 1982; Verhulst, Althaus, & Berden, 1987). The reliability of parent and child reports on clinical interview also vary by developmental level—the reliability of child reports increases with age, whereas that of the parents tends to decrease with the child's age (Edelbrock et al., 1985).

Self-Reports

The most widely used method for assessing childhood anxiety is the self-report inventory. Self-report measures assess the youth's perspective on his or her symptoms, an important aspect to consider given the subjective nature of anxiety (Bernstein et al., 1996). Self-report questionnaires are also often quick to administer and inexpensive. However, one important limitation to consider for most self-report measures of general anxiety is that they are not diagnostic tools when used in isolation. The ability of the self-report measures to distinguish between anxiety and other disorders has been questioned (e.g., Perrin & Last, 1992). In part this may be due to limitations in the questionnaires themselves or the lack of conceptual distinction between the anxiety disorders in children (see Schniering, Hudson, & Rapee, 2000). Regardless, assessment should include a multimethod approach to maximize accurate diagnosis.

Although numerous self-report inventories exist, the Revised Children's Manifest Anxiety Scale (RCMAS; Reynolds & Richmond, 1978), the Fear Survey Schedule for Children—Revised (FSSC-R; Ollendick, 1983), the State–Trait Anxiety Inventory for Children (STAIC; Spielberger, 1973), and the Multidimensional Anxiety Scale for Children (MASC; March, Parker, Sullivan, Stallings, & Conners, 1997) are perhaps among the most commonly used. In addition to these instruments, we also review some less well researched, though promising, assessment measures.

The RCMAS (Reynolds & Richmond, 1978, 1997) is a 37-item scale that assesses anxiety in children and adolescents ages 6–19. The RCMAS yields a total score as well as three subscales: physiological anxiety, worry/oversensitivity, and concentration. The RCMAS also contains a scale to measure the degree to which the child may have responded socially in a desirable way. The psychometric properties of the RCMAS have been extensively studied and reflect adequate reliability and validity (e.g., Lonigan, Carey, & Finch, 1994; Muris, Merckelbach, Ollendick, King, & Bogie, 2002; Reynolds & Paget, 1983; Reynolds & Richmond, 1979).

The STAIC (Speilberger, Edwards, & Lushene, 1973) comprises two 20-item inventories: the state scale, which examines present state and situationally linked anxiety, and the trait scale, which assesses stable anxiety across situations. Normative data based on a national sample of children between ages 8 and 12 are available for the STAIC (Spielberger, 1973). Reliability for the overall scale is acceptable (Muris et al., 2000), although, as with other self-report questionnaires, the discriminant validity of the measure is questionable. For these reasons, the STAIC may be best used primarily as a general screening instrument (see Barrios & Hartmann, 1988; Perrin & Last, 1992).

The FSSC-R is the revised version of the Fear Survey Schedule for Children, developed by Scherer and Nakamura (1968). As mentioned earlier, five factors have been found to be measured with this instrument, including fear of failure, fear of death, fear of injury and small animals, medical fears, and fear of the unknown. This five-factor structure makes the scale useful in identifying specific sources of fear, severity of fearfulness, and treatment effects. Ollendick and colleagues (1985) provided normative data for the FSSC-R for children ages 7–18 that indicate high internal consistency and moderate retest reliability over a 3-month interval (Ollendick, 1983).

The Social Phobia and Anxiety Inventory for Children (SPAI-C; Beidel, Turner, & Morris, 1995) is also a reliable and commonly used self-report measure to assess anxiety in children and adolescents. The SPAI-C, a 26-item self-report that taps anxiety-arousing situations, physical and cognitive symptoms, and avoidance behavior, has demonstrated high internal consistency and high retest reliability (Beidel, Turner, Hamlin, & Morris, 2000; Beidel et al., 1995). It has also discriminated between children with social phobia and either normal children or children with externalizing problems (Beidel et al., 2000).

The Multidimensional Anxiety Scale for Children (MASC; March et al., 1997) was developed to address the issue of a multidimensional conceptualization of anxiety. The scale covers the major domains of self-reported anxiety in children and adolescents. It is a 39-item self-report inventory containing four major factors: physical symptoms (e.g., tension), social anxiety (e.g., rejection), harm avoidance (e.g., perfectionism), and separation anxiety. This factor structure has been shown to hold for boys and girls, and for younger and older youth, and retest reliability has been shown to be excellent over 3 weeks and 3 months (March & Albano, 1998).

A relatively unexplored, though promising, area of self-report in childhood anxiety is that of cognitive assessment. Cognitive contents, schemas, processes, and products have been implicated in the maintenance and etiology of anxiety (e.g., Ingram & Kendall, 1986, 1987; Kendall & Ingram, 1987, 1989) but have received little empirical attention with children (Kendall & Ronan, 1990). Although the cognitive assessment of children with anxiety disorders is a promising area, relatively few scales exist. Ronan, Kendall, and Rowe (1994) developed the Negative Affectivity Self-Statement Questionnaire (NASSQ) to assess the cognitive content of anxious/dysphoric children. A subscale for assessing anxious self-talk was evaluated, with results indicating favorable reliability and the ability to differentiate among both psychometrically defined and clinic cases of anxious and nonanxious children between 8 and 15 years old. The NASSQ consists of self-statements that participants endorse on a 1–5 scale representing the frequency that the thought occurred to them during the past week. Scale development, reliability, and validity support have been reported in Ronan and colleagues (1994) and Treadwell and Kendall (1996; see also Ronan & Kendall, 1997).

The Coping Questionnaire—Child Version (CQ-C; Kendall, 1994; Kendall et al., 1997) is another important instrument for cognitive assessment. This measure assesses the child's ability to cope with anxious distress in challenging situations. Analyses indicate adequate internal consistency and strong retest reliability and document its usefulness as a measure of improvement (Kendall & Marrs-Garcia, 1999).

Self-report measures have the advantage of being economical in both time and expense, but are limited in several ways. They do not adequately address the situational specificity of childhood anxiety disorders, and some may not capture the fears and anxieties specific to the child (Kendall & Ronan, 1990). This limitation is potentially serious, as without such information treatment can neither be individualized, nor can it address a child's unique behavioral dysfunction. The present inability of self-report inventories to account for developmental difficulties is another disadvantage. Few inventories have adequate normative data for different developmental stages, and many inventories are not modified for variations in children's comprehension abilities. For example, it is unclear whether the differences among "Never worried," "Rarely worried," and "Often worried" represent the same meaning for children at different stages of cognitive development or whether children at lower stages of development are capable of making such distinctions. Self-reports may also fail to reflect the child's internal state. The inaccuracy may result from the child's desire to respond in a nondistressed or socially desirable manner. Youth with anxiety disorders approach problems with a hypersensitive concern about self-presentation and evaluation by others (Kendall & Ingram, 1989). Their preference for a favorable self-presentation may influence their performance on tasks such as self-report assessments (Kendall & Flannery-Schroeder, 1998). Some questionnaires recognize this tendency and include scales to assess self-presentation (e.g., RCMAS; Reynolds & Richmond, 1997).

Behavioral Observations

The behavioral assessment of childhood anxiety includes many structured and unstructured observational techniques. Throughout the assessment process, especially during the clinical interview, diagnosticians observe the child and note any behavior that may be suggestive of anxiety, such as fidgeting, fingernail biting, avoiding eye contact, and speaking softly. Parent and teacher rating scales, discussed below, are based on unstructured observations of the child's behavior in naturalistic settings. Unstructured observations are important but can be limited by observer bias and, especially in the case of parent and teacher ratings, typically lack appropriate observer training.

More structured observation strategies are employed in behavioral avoidance tasks (BATs), with direct observation by trained raters in naturalistic settings such as the schoolroom or playground. As an example, consider a BAT for assessing distressing anxiety associated with eating food in public. The situation could be arranged so that there would be food available, trays for selecting foods, and several options for places to eat the food—places that are solitary, with one person, or with many others. In a BAT, the participant would enter the situation and trained observers would record the degree of approach to the distressing situation. In this case, how far along the continuum of "not eating" to "eating among people" did the participant move? Although the structured behavioral assessment methods are advantageous because trained raters assess a child's behavior against an operationalized definition, they are limited by the absence of standardized procedures. This problem hinders the comparability across studies of data obtained with these techniques. Furthermore, neither unstructured nor structured behavioral observations are sufficient assessment techniques by themselves. Although the total of several behavioral observation codes is correlated with the presence of anxiety, no single coded behavioral frequency appears to be pathognomonic to childhood anxiety. As noted earlier, there appears to be symptom overlap among the internalizing disorders (see also Kendall & Watson, 1989), and there is between-subjects variability in the behavioral expression of anxious symptomatology.

Parent, Teacher, and Clinician Rating Scales

Parent and teacher reports offer additional important perspectives; however, there are some potential limitations to using these instruments for assessing internalizing disorders in children. Parents and teachers may not know the nature or extent of the child's inner pressures and anguish. There is also often low concordance between child and parent reports of anxiety (Klein, 1991). Additionally, although not all data are consistent (see Krain & Kendall, 2000), Frick, Silverthorn, and Evans (1994) reported that mothers tend to overreport anxiety symptoms in their children, and that this is related to the increased level of maternal anxiety. This finding would suggest that clinicians should be aware of any distressing levels of parental anxiety (Bernstein et al., 1996). Among other potential limitations are the retrospective nature of the observations and the possibility of rater bias.

Among the most widely used rating scales is the Child Behavior Checklist (Achenbach, 1991), which has acceptable reliability, validity, and normative data. The 118-item CBCL assesses behavioral problems and social competencies. Items are scored 0, 1, or 2, depending on the degree to which the particular statement characterizes the child. The CBCL provides data on a child's level of disturbance on specific factors and offers discrimination between broadband externalizing disorders and internalizing disorders: The CBCL does not identify or differentiate among the subtypes of anxiety described in DSM-IV. The CBCL also provides data on the child's participation in social activities and interactions with peers for evaluation of change. Using the items from the CBCL, a set of 16 items was found to have retest reliability and internal consistency, and to reliably differentiate anxiety-disordered and nondisordered youth (Kendall, Henin, MacDonald, & Treadwell, 1999). Following additional research, the CBCL-A may be a useful subscale to the CBCL for the identification of youth with anxiety disorders.

There is also a version of the CBCL designed for teachers—the Teacher Report Form (TRF; Achenbach, 1991; Achenbach & Edelbrock, 1986). The primary teacher, using the TRF, rates the child's classroom functioning. Gathering and reviewing the TRF allows a comparison of the child's anxious behavior at home and in the school setting, and may be especially relevant for children whose fears involve social and evaluative situations. Keep in mind, however, that the classroom behavior of anxious children may not be seen as troubling to a teacher; thus, the TRF scores of some children with anxiety disorders are not necessarily extreme. The instrument provides useful information but is not linked to DSM diagnostic categories.

Recent efforts have translated child-report measures into parallel parent-report measures of child symptomatology. One such measure is the State–Trait Inventory for Children–Parent Report—Trait Version (Strauss, 1987; see also Southam-Gerow, Flannery-Schroeder, & Kendall, 2003), in which items on the STAIC were modified in order to gain the parent's perspective. Examination of the psychometric properties of the parent-report measure indicates high internal consistency, moderate retest reliability, and mixed validity.

The Pediatric Anxiety Rating Scale for Children (PARS; RUPP Anxiety Group, 2002) is a clinician-rated anxiety severity scale for use with children and adolescents. The PARS has a 50-item symptom checklist and 7 severity ratings. Unlike other anxiety checklists, the PARS specifically reflects the combined severity of symptoms of SAD, SP, and GAD. The PARS requires approximately 30 minutes to complete and has excellent interrater reliability.

The Coping Questionnaire described earlier also has a parallel parent version, called the Coping Questionnaire—Parent (CQ-P; Kendall, 1994). The parent rates the child's ability to cope with the three most anxiety-provoking situations typically identified from the diagnostic interview. The scale shows moderate interrater agreement and has been shown to be sensitive to treatment effects (Kendall & Marrs-Garcia, 1999).

Physiological Recordings

The physiological assessment of anxiety has received wide attention in the adult literature (see Himadi, Boice, & Barlow, 1985), yet little empirical data on these indicators exist in the child and adolescent population (Barrios & Hartmann, 1988; Beidel, 1988). Opponents of this method of assessing anxiety in children have cited the large imbalance between the extensive cost, in time and money, of gathering such information, and its relative yield (Barlow & Wolfe, 1981). Furthermore, the most commonly used physiological techniques, such as cardiovascular and electrodermal measures, lack adequate normative data for children. Children also appear to show idiosyncratic patterns of response during physiological assessment. Moreover, measures can be influenced by expectancy effects, emotions other than anxiety, and incidental motoric and perceptual activity (Wells & Virtulano, 1984; Werry, 1986).

Despite these somewhat daunting limitations, the physiological assessment of childhood anxiety should not be totally abandoned. Empirical investigations of autonomic responsivity in anxious children should be conducted, as the results of such work would increase our understanding of the psychophysiological expression of anxiety and help to develop normative data in this area. For a review of psychophysiological assessment of anxiety in children, see Beidel (1989).

Family Variables

Given the literature reviewed previously on family factors associated with anxiety in youth, assessing family factors can be useful clinically. Although such assessment has often run into psychometric limitations, there now exists a growing number of measures designed to try to assess family-related constructs theorized to play a role in youth anxiety (e.g., control, overprotection, etc.). For example, the Egna Minnen Betraffande Uppfostram (EMDU-C; Castro, Toro, van der Ende, & Arrindell, 1993) assesses children's perceptions of parental emotional warmth, control, and rejection, among other factors. Similarly, the Family Assessment Measure (FAM; Skinner, Steinhauer, & Santa Barbara, 1983, 1995) examines several aspects of family functioning such as involvement and control. For a thorough review of self-report and behavioral observation family assessment devices, the reader is referred to Ginsburg, Siqueland, Masia-Warner, and Hedtke (2004).

The assessment of anxiety in children requires a multimethod approach, drawing information from clinical interviews, child self-report, parent and teacher ratings, and behavioral observations, as well as family history and patterns of interaction. Each method has advantages and potential disadvantages that limit the merits of relying on a single assessment technique for diagnostic purposes. The multiple assessments should measure the child's anxiety and be sensitive to the evaluation of therapeutic change.

TREATMENT: PROCEDURES AND OUTCOMES

Interventions that target childhood anxiety disorders have received much-needed attention. The development of such treatments is consistent with the field's increasing understanding of the prevalence and impact of anxiety disorders in youth. Various forms of behavior therapy and cognitive-behavioral treatments have shown promise in treating childhood phobias and anxiety disorders. A developmentally sensitive synthesis of behavioral and cognitive treatment approaches can result in therapeutic gains for the anxious child (see Kazdin & Weisz, 1998; Ollendick, King, & Chorpita, Chapter 14, this volume). The following discussion highlights features of cognitive-behavioral treatment, such as relaxation, building a cognitive coping template, problem solving, modeling, contingency maintenance, and imaginal and *in vivo* exposure. We also discuss an integrated treatment package for youth with anxiety disorders (see Kendall, 2000a; Kendall & Hedtke, 2006a) that uses the *Coping Cat Workbook* (Kendall, 1992b; Kendall & Hedtke, 2006b). Last, a review of the research evaluations of these procedures is provided.

Overview of CBT for Anxious Children

CBT for anxiety disorders in youth integrates the demonstrated efficiencies of the behavioral approach (e.g., exposure, relaxation training, role plays) with an added emphasis on the cognitive information processing factors associated with each individual's anxieties (see treatment manuals; e.g., Kendall, 2000b; Kendall & Hedtke, 2006a; Howard & Kendall, 1996b; Flannery-Schroeder & Kendall, 1996).[2] The overall goal of the treatment program is to teach children to recognize signs of anxious arousal and to let these signs serve as cues for the use of anxiety management strategies. Typically, the structured treatment program consists of a total of 16 sessions, which are broken up into two equal treatment segments: skills training (first eight sessions) and skills practice (last eight sessions). The skills training sessions focus on the building of four basic skill areas: awareness of bodily reactions to feelings and those physical symptoms specific to anxiety; recognition and evaluation of "self-talk," or what the child thinks and says to him- or herself when anxious; problem-solving skills, including modifying anxious self-talk and developing plans for coping; and self-evaluation and reward. During the skills practice segment of treatment, youth practice the learned skills in actual anxiety-provoking situations (i.e., exposure tasks). Exposure tasks provide the child with opportunities to demonstrate his or her abilities in real-life situations and develop a sense of self-competence. Through rehearsal and multiple attempts, the child succeeds in situations that previously felt impossible and learns to rely on his or her own coping skills rather than depend on others for reassurance. The focus on cognitive processes and creating a coping template stems from an interest in helping the child internalize lessons and generalize skills across settings. The child is taught to attribute successes to his or her own burgeoning competence and to use these skills in a variety of situations, not just those practiced in session. To facilitate the learning process, the therapist assumes the posture of a collaborative coach who generates treatment goals with the child and tailors therapy interventions to the child's interests and abilities. Indeed, the importance of establishing rapport and a collaborative atmosphere to treatment outcome has recently been supported by research (Chu et al., 2004; Chu & Kendall, 2004; Creed & Kendall, 2005; see Shirk & Karver, 2003, for a review).

Throughout treatment, the therapist functions as a coping model, demonstrating the skill in each new situation. As a coping model, the therapist models an anxious experience and strategies that attempt to cope with the anxiety. The child is then invited to participate with the therapist in role playing. To make role plays less threatening, the therapist may role-play a situation first as the child follows along with him or her. Describing what he or she is feeling or thinking, the therapist asks the child if he or she is experiencing similar or different feelings. Ultimately, the child is encouraged to role-play scenes alone, practicing the newly acquired skills by him- or herself. Variations in role playing are used, depending on the child's skill level and understanding of concepts being introduced. With adolescents, the tag-along procedure is often unnecessary. Role plays should represent situations relevant to the child, and thus they may be derived from the child's organized fear hierarchy or from external events that the child has reported to have occurred.

Therapist self-disclosure may also be appropriate to demonstrate the therapist's role as a coping model. Therapist self-disclosure often takes the form of revealing past experiences that are relevant to the child's own experiences or describing out loud his or her thoughts and feelings about situations as they arise in therapy. For example, it may be appropriate for the therapist to disclose his or her own anxiety upon meeting the child for the first session. This sort of disclosure normalizes anxiety and sets the tone for sessions to be a setting in which feelings can be discussed freely. The therapist works as an opportunist, seizing upon situations in which he or she can demonstrate to the child how to cope with a distressing situation. If the therapist trips, the best he can do is express his own anxiety ("Wow, I'm glad you didn't laugh at me. That would have been embarrassing") and then describe how he made himself feel better ("But I thought that even if you had laughed at me, that wouldn't mean that you didn't like me anymore"). By modeling a general process of coping with distress, the child begins to see how a competent adult copes with daily stresses. In the next section, we (1) describe components common to most CBT programs available for youth and (2) provide an example of a CBT program utilized at the CAADC.

Components of CBT

Psychoeducation

Throughout the treatment process, youth learn about various aspects of anxiety (e.g., the nature and components of anxiety). Part of the psychoeducation component of treatment helps youth to identify and discriminate their own (and others') feelings states. Many youth with anxiety experience physical symptoms that they may attribute to an illness, as opposed to their anxiety. Youth are taught to help discriminate when their somatic symptom (e.g., stomachache) may be due to anxiety or an illness by examining the context in which the symptom occurs (e.g., only before school). The rationale is that youth will be better able to cope with their anxiety if they can identify it and differentiate it from other states.

Relaxation

Relaxation training aims to teach children to develop awareness and control over their own physiological and muscular reactions to anxiety. In this procedure, major muscle groups of the body are progressively relaxed through systematic tension-releasing exercises (e.g., King, Hamilton, & Ollendick, 1988). By tensing and relaxing various muscle groups, the individual learns to perceive sensations of bodily tension and to use these sensations as cues to begin relaxation procedures. During the initial instruction, the child is taught to identify the particular muscle groups and somatic sensations that uniquely characterize his or her own anxious states. This increased awareness of his or her own somatic reactions to anxiety enables the child to use an aroused physical state as an "early warning signal" to initiate relaxation procedures. Furthermore, greater awareness of individual responses to distress allows the child to target specific muscle groups that tense when anxious.

A therapist can also teach cue-controlled relaxation, in which the child learns to associate a relaxed state with a self-produced cue word such as "calm." While the child is totally relaxed, the cue word is subvocalized with each exhalation. The cue serves as a reminder of the relaxed state and can initiate muscle relaxation when used during a distressed state. Cue-controlled relaxation can be helpful when the child wishes to initiate muscle relaxation in a public setting but does not feel comfortable performing progressive relaxation techniques. When teaching both progressive and cue-controlled techniques, relaxation training scripts are often incorporated (e.g., Koeppen, 1974; Ollendick & Cerny, 1981;

Pincus, 2000). For example, a child is taught to tense and relax her stomach by imagining that she is squeezing through a fence or tensing and relaxing her hand muscles by pretending to squeeze the juice out of a lemon. Scripts differ, depending on the age range of the targeted clients. Scripts for younger children are typically shorter in length and offer fewer distinctions among the muscle groups than scripts for adolescents or adults. Weisman, Ollendick, and Horne (1978) demonstrated the efficacy of muscular relaxation procedures with normal 6- and 7-year-old children. They found that the procedures of both Ollendick and Cerny (1981) and Koeppen (1974) resulted in significantly reduced muscle-tension levels, as measured by electromyographic (EMG) recordings (both groups were superior to an attention–control group but did not differ from each other). This finding suggests that muscular relaxation procedures may be an effective counterconditioning agent for young children. Adding imaginal or *in vivo* exposure tasks to a relaxation training program (as in systematic desensitization) may enhance the therapeutic outcome of progressive relaxation. A recent review of controlled studies assessing the efficacy of treatments for childhood fears and phobias (see Ollendick & King, 1998) concluded that relaxation used in conjunction with gradual imaginal exposures is superior to relaxation training alone (Barabasz, 1973; Kondas, 1967; Mann & Rosenthal, 1969; Miller, Barrett, Hampe, & Noble, 1972), and the therapeutic benefit is greater still if *in vivo*, rather than imaginal, exposures are implemented (Kuroda, 1969; Ultee, Griffioen, & Schellekens, 1982). Thus, muscle relaxation may work best as a counterconditioning agent when the child first achieves an aroused emotional state, via exposure, similar to that produced by the anxiety-provoking stimulus.

Building a Cognitive Coping Template

Because cognition is theorized to be inextricably linked to emotion and behavior (Ingram, Kendall, & Chen, 1991), it is believed that dysfunction in either the behavioral or emotional realm can be ameliorated by identifying and challenging a child's distorted or unrealistic cognition. Cognitive-based therapies highlight the role of maladaptive thinking in dysfunctional behavior and operate by adjusting distorted cognitive processing to more constructive ways of thinking. Cognitive strategies typically consist of teaching the child to test out and reduce negative self-talk, generating positive self-statements, challenging unrealistic or dysfunctional negative self-statements, and creating a plan to cope with feared situations. Cognitive modeling, rehearsal, social reinforcement, and role play are all used to help the child build a coping template that helps in interpreting future interactions with feared situations in a new light. Building a cognitive coping template entails the identification and modification of maladaptive self-talk, along with building a new way to view situations a new structure that is based on coping. The therapist works with the child to (1) remove characteristic misinterpretations of environmental events and (2) gradually and systematically build a frame of reference that includes strategies for coping. Accurate assessment and conceptualization of the dysfunctional thought structure are essential. For example, a child's fear of speaking in front of others may be based on legitimate grounds if the child has had difficulty with stuttering and has been teased in the past. However, it may be less realistic for the child to conclude that, because he stutters and is teased by some children, other children will refuse to be his friends. At this level, the therapist and child can create a coping template, including helpful self-talk, that challenges this inflexible belief structure. Guiding the child in asking such questions as "Is it true that all of the other classmates will tease the child after a speech?" and "Will the child's current friends abandon him or her after being teased by others?" can help the child begin to understand that alternative perspectives exist.

The goal of building a new template for thinking is not so that the perceptions of stress will disappear forever, but so that the formerly distressing misperceptions and arousal, when seen through a cognitive coping structure, will serve as reminders for the use of coping strategies. It is also not the case that we strive to fill the anxious child with positive self-talk. Rather, it is recognized that the power lies not in positive self-talk but in the reduction of negative self-talk—a phenomenon termed "the power of non-negative thinking" (Kendall, 1984; Treadwell & Kendall, 1996). At present, cognitive-based treatment of children with anxiety disorders has shown considerable promise (e.g., Eisen & Silverman, 1993; Kane & Kendall, 1989; Ollendick, 1995). Often cognitive strategies are used in combination with other forms of behavioral therapy (e.g., Friedman & Ollendick, 1989; Graziano & Mooney, 1980, 1982; Mansdorf & Lukens, 1987), and it has been suggested that self-talk and cognitive restructuring may require operant-based reinforcement strategies when used in treatments with children (e.g., Hagopian, Weist, & Ollendick, 1990). Further study is also required to determine if cognitive procedures actually alter those processes that are conceptualized as critical in the treatment model (i.e., whether distorted cognition changes as a result of treatment; Ollendick & King, 1998). Recent evidence suggests that changes in children's negative self-talk (but not positive self-talk) does indeed mediate change in anxiety associated with treatment (Treadwell & Kendall, 1996).

Problem Solving

Another component of the cognitive-behavioral approach to anxiety is problem solving. Early on, D'Zurilla and Goldfried (1971) outlined a five-stage problem-solving sequence (see also D'Zurilla & Nezu, 1999; Spivack & Shure, 1974). The overall goal of teaching problem solving is training children to develop confidence in their own ability to help themselves meet daily challenges. In the first stage of problem solving (general orientation), the therapist focuses on helping the child understand that problems are a part of everyday life and encourages the child to inhibit his or her initial impulses (e.g., avoidance behavior). In the second stage, the child works to operationally define and formulate the problem into a workable problem with goals. The third stage in problem solving involves the generation of alternative solutions, the core of which lies in brainstorming. Here, ideas, both practical and outlandish, should be generated without judgment. Oftentimes, alternatives that appear implausible at first glance may be viable solutions once given more deliberate consideration. The therapist can model good brainstorming skills by generating both pragmatic and improbable alternatives, and encouraging the child to follow suit. In decision making, the fourth stage, the child evaluates each alternative, choosing the most appropriate solution, and then puts the action into effect. The final stage consists of evaluating the merits of the chosen solution. Training the child to ask him- or herself the following questions may help the child orient him- or herself in a problem-solving mindset: (1) What is the problem? (2) What are all the things I could do about it? (3) What will probably happen if I do those things? (4) Which solution do I think will work best? and (5) After I have tried it, how did I do? In the end, problem solving helps the child become adept at generating alternatives in what may at first seem to be hopeless situations.

Kleiner, Marshall, and Spevack (1987) reported that problem solving helps prevent posttreatment relapses in anxiety disorders. In this study, 26 agoraphobic patients were randomly assigned to either an *in vivo* exposure treatment or *in vivo* exposure plus a problem-solving skills training program. All of the patients improved significantly after 12 treatment sessions. However, those in the *in vivo*–only procedure failed to show further gains at follow-up or relapsed, but those receiving training in problem solving continued to improve at follow-up. Thus, problem solving may enhance the therapeutic gains of treatment strategies, such as with *in vivo* exposure (e.g., Arnow, Taylor, Agras, & Telch, 1985; Jannoun, Munby, Catalan, & Gelder, 1980).

Contingent Reinforcement

In contrast to relaxation, systematic desensitization, and modeling, which all assume that fear must be reduced or eliminated before approach behavior will occur, contingency reinforcement procedures, based on operant conditioning principles, operate on a different assumption. Operant based procedures focus on facilitating approach responses through appropriate reward and reinforcement, and focus less on the reduction of anxiety per se. Shaping, positive reinforcement, and extinction are the most frequently used contingency management procedures to reduce phobic or anxious behaviors.

Some children diagnosed with anxiety disorders will demonstrate a negative self-focus characterized by self-deprecating thoughts and doubts in self-confidence. Other anxious children may place exceedingly high standards for achievement on themselves and may be less forgiving than most if they fail to meet these standards. To help counter this unjustly critical belief structure, the therapist emphasizes the importance of rewarding oneself for effort and partial successes. The therapist might use the example of a dog learning a trick for the first time. When first learning to sit at its owner's command, a dog is not expected to achieve perfect success the first time, nor is it expected to perform consistently so. Likewise, the anxious child should be reminded that when he or she is initially attempting to accomplish a challenging task, perfect execution is not expected. Graduated practice and timely reinforcement will help the child develop confidence over time and lead to a growing sense of competence.

Reinforcement procedures contingent upon performance have been successful in modifying a wide variety of anxiety-related behavior, such as school phobic behavior (e.g., Ayllon, Smith, & Rogers, 1970) and avoidance of the dark (Leitenberg & Callahan, 1973). In comparison to other behavioral techniques, a contingency management program was shown to produce greater benefits for treating fear of the dark than a self-instruction group without reinforcement procedures (Sheslow, Bondy, & Nelson, 1982). Similarly, in a comparison between live modeling and reinforced practice in the treatment of children with water phobia (Menzies & Clarke, 1993), the reinforced practice condition produced statistically and clinically significant gains over live modeling procedures. Furthermore, there was no difference in efficacy between the reinforced practice condition when implemented alone or when combined with an added live modeling intervention.

Modeling

Modeling derives its conceptual roots from the social learning paradigm (Bandura, 1969, 1986), in which nonfearful behavior is demonstrated in the fear-producing situation so as to illustrate appropriate responses for the child. As a result, fear may be reduced and appropriate skills acquired. Variations of modeling include filmed (symbolic), live, and participant modeling. In filmed modeling, the anxious child watches a videotape of the model, whereas in live modeling the model is in the presence of the anxious child. In participant modeling, the live model interacts with the anxious child and guides his or her approach to the feared stimulus. Regular corrective feedback and reinforcement for effort and partial success are required to help the child match the performance of the model (Ollendick & Francis, 1988).

Ross, Ross, and Evans (1971) demonstrated a successful use of modeling procedures in treating a 6-year-old boy who feared interaction with his peers. Generalized imitation, participant modeling, and social reinforcement were the main treatment procedures. Directly following treatment and upon follow-up, the child could interact positively with his peers and displayed few avoidance behaviors. Some studies indicate that interventions that include assisted participation (child participation with therapist modeling of approach behaviors) show greater change in avoidance behavior than treatments that make use of filmed or live modeling alone (Lewis, 1974; Ritter, 1968). Overall, modeling in its various forms has received support for its clinical utility in treating anxious and fearful children (e.g., Melamed & Siegel, 1975; Murphy & Bootzin, 1973) as well as helping children placed in stressful situations (e.g., medical procedures; Peterson, 1989).

Exposure-Based Procedures

Exposure entails placing the client in a fear-evoking experience, either imaginally or *in vivo*, to help the client acclimate to the distressing situation and to provide opportunities for the client to practice coping skills within simulated or real-life situations (Francis & Beidel, 1995; Marks, 1975). Exposures can be conducted in graduated measures or by flooding. In gradual exposure, the therapist and child generate a list of feared situations in a hierarchy from least to most anxiety-provoking. The child then approaches each situation sequentially, moving up the hierarchy as his or her anxiety level permits. It is important that, at any level, the exposure is not so aversive that the experience actually reinforces the fear. Gradual exposures help the child build experience upon experience and develop a sense of mastery over time. It is important to note that the extent to which the child can discriminate between threatening and nonthreatening stimuli is linked to the exposure's effectiveness in producing fear reduction. The therapist will be careful to collaborate with the child when designing exposures so that the child has an understanding of the intended goals.

In flooding, a child participates in repeated and prolonged exposure to the feared stimulus and remains in the presence of the anxiety-provoking stimulus (either imaginal or *in vivo*) until his or her self-reported anxiety level diminishes. Typically, flooding is used in conjunction with response prevention, in which the child is prevented from engaging in avoidance behavior during exposure. Flooding and response prevention may create more distress than other exposure procedures (Francis & Beidel, 1995), and so the child's clear understanding of the treatment rationale is important. Accordingly, application with younger children should be considered thoughtfully.

In a single-case study of the utility of exposure in treating childhood anxiety, Francis and Ollendick (1990) followed a 16-year-old adolescent with generalized social phobia through a 3-month exposure intervention. The adolescent had a history of school refusal and avoidance of most social situations, and reported intense social-evaluative fears. A fear hierarchy of situations was developed that ranged from least (going to a shopping mall with someone) to most anxiety-provoking (going to school alone and staying all day). Items from the hierarchy were used as homework assignments to be practiced between sessions. Tasks were completed in a gradual fashion, with repeated practice for each one. Although the adolescent was not able to return to her previous school, the exposure intervention did enable her to attend an alternative school program, obtain her GED, and enroll in a local community college. Although she still reported anxiety in some social situations, she no longer engaged in avoidance behavior (for a more extensive discussion on the use of exposure tasks with anxious youth, see Kendall et al., 2005).

Examples from a CBT Program

These cognitive-behavioral strategies form an integrated cognitive-behavioral program, such as the one used at the Child and Adolescent Anxiety Disorders Clinic of Temple University. To facilitate learning, the CBT program presents the main principles of anxiety management using the FEAR acronym: (1) recognizing bodily symptoms of anxiety (i.e., *Feeling Frightened?*), (2) identifying anxious cognition (i.e., *Expecting bad things to happen?*), (3) developing a repertoire of coping strategies (i.e., *Attitudes and actions that can help*), and (4) contingency management (i.e., *Results and rewards*). The behavioral strategies previously reviewed are included (e.g., modeling, exposure tasks). Finally, the treatment program uses STIC (*Show That I Can*) tasks as weekly homework assignments to provide the child an opportunity to practice the skills learned in session. As noted by Hudson and Kendall (2002), STIC tasks are an essential component of the treatment process and facilitate the development of a sense of mastery over the skills learned in session and eventually the youth's anxiety. In carrying out CBT, attention to the individual needs and development level (i.e., social, emotional, and cognitive) of the child is crucial (e.g., Barrett, 2000; Kendall & Choudhury, 2003; Piacentini & Bergman, 2001; Silverman & Ollendick, 1999). In this way, the therapist is encouraged to apply the manual flexibly within the CBT model (Kendall, Chu, Gifford, Hayes, & Nauta, 1998).

The "F" Step of the FEAR Plan: *Feeling Frightened?*

In the Coping Cat program (or C.A.T. Project, for teens), youth learn that one of the first steps in managing anxiety is to recognize anxious feelings and to differentiate them from other emotions. Through affective education, youth learn to recognize facial expressions, postures, and the physiological signals that are associated with different emotions, in both themselves and others. Concepts are first introduced in the abstract or by referring to others, rather than focusing on the child's own experience. Any one of many activities can be used to facilitate learning of the "F" step and may involve the child and therapist cutting out pictures of people from magazines or books who are experiencing various emotions. In another activity, the therapist and child can role-play experiencing different emotions (e.g., feelings charades). Finally, children can learn to identify their own particular physiological expressions of anxiety by imagining themselves in an anxious situation and then drawing a very large picture of themselves experiencing the anxiety (e.g., draw a heart pounding, flushed face, etc.).

In the following example, a 10-year-old girl acts out an emotion from a feelings list. As the therapist attempts to name the feeling, she verbally describes the behavior she is using to make her guess. The therapist also uses multiple labels, which requires the child to consider each and decide whether to accept or reject the guess. In this way, she may develop a sense of the unique characteristics of each feeling and apply her own labels. At the end of the exchange, the girl associates her acted feeling to an experience she has had in the past. Children will often internalize experiences better when they have applied their own labels and to the extent that feeling is paired with a real-life experience.

THERAPIST: (*Child jumps around, looks jittery, and hits the table.*) You're drumming, you're jamming, you're breathing!

CHILD: That's not a feeling!

THERAPIST: You're right, that's not a feeling. You're breathing hard, you're intense.

CHILD: I don't know what that means.

THERAPIST: It may be that you're concentrating. You're holding your breath. You're working hard. Umm, you're stressed?

CHILD: What's that?

THERAPIST: It means like you're under a lot of pressure.

CHILD: Maybe. But it's on the list. It's a couple of things, all together.

THERAPIST: You look a little scared. Your eyes are really wide. You may be nervous.

CHILD: Nervous, scared, and worried. I'm like on stage and nervous.

THERAPIST: Oh, so you're taking deep breaths.

CHILD: Yeah, could you see my lips trembling?

THERAPIST: Yeah.

CHILD: It's like trying out for a play.

Once children begin to identify their own physical symptoms of anxiety, they can use these physical reactions as cues to begin relaxation. In general, youth are taught to take a few deep breaths as soon as they recognize they are becoming anxious. Children are then taught a modified, progressive muscle relaxation procedure, which first focuses on the three or four muscle groups most affected by their anxiety. The therapist can then model and discuss with the child the times when using the relaxation steps may be useful. For the younger child, a script that puts the exercise in a story-like scenario (e.g., Koeppen, 1974) encourages participation; a script by Ollendick and Cerny (1981) can be used for the older youth. An audiotape of the therapist going through the relaxation procedure can be given to the child, enabling him or her to practice at home. In addition, the child can demonstrate the procedure to his or her own parents, who might like to practice with the child, or help the child find a time and a place to practice at home. The therapist reminds the child that relaxation is learned; therefore, practice is very important.

The "E" Step of the FEAR Plan: *Expecting Bad Things to Happen?*

Following recognition of physiological symptoms of anxiety, youth are taught to identify thoughts that are contributing to the anxious experience. The notion of self-talk, the things children say to themselves when they are anxious, is an important concept introduced in this training program. Self-talk includes the child's expectations and attributions about him- or herself, others, and situations. For the anxious child, these expectations may include negative self-evaluation, perfectionist standards for performance, heightened self-focused attention, concern about what others are thinking, and concerns about failure or not coping. For example, when discussing an upcoming quiz in Bible study, a 12-year-old boy diagnosed with social phobia reported the following five fears: "I won't pass," "I'm going to do so badly that I'm going to be kicked out of school," "Everyone in my family is going to think I'm dumb," "I'll be really embarrassed," and "I won't have a confirmation party." Contained within this child's fears were doubts about self-competence, presupposed consequences for failure, and fears of public humiliation.

Although it may be a bit challenging to help youth, particularly younger or cognitively delayed youth, articulate their self-talk, a variety of strategies may be used to facilitate this goal. For example, the therapist might utilize cartoons with empty thought bubbles over their heads that portray simple, nonthreatening scenes in which the character's thoughts are likely to be fairly obvious. As the child becomes comfortable with the task, more ambiguous or anxiety-provoking situations can be used. Once youth are able to identify anxious thoughts, therapists assist them in generating anxiety-reducing (coping) thoughts for the characters. For example, the therapist might prompt the child with such questions as "How likely is it that that will actually happen?" "How many times has it ever happened before?" "Could there be other ways to look at it?" or "How do you know it will be as bad as you are expecting?" The therapist guides the child through an empirical hypothesis-testing process in which both work to challenge the assumptions and beliefs that lead to anxiety and distress. The goal over the course of treatment is for youth to develop an alternative information processing template that is based on coping.

In the following example, a child recounts the anxious thoughts he experienced prior to a science fair and the advice he received from a principal who noticed him worrying:

THERAPIST: Can you think of a situation where you were really nervous? Let's take the example you gave before—that science project. What kinds of things were you thinking?

CHILD: Oh, no, will I get an "F"? What about the big kids? Will they make fun of me? I'm not going to do this. Well, I have to or I'll get an "F." . . . My principal was telling me not to worry about the big kids. And I was looking at their projects, and they weren't that great, so I don't know . . .

THERAPIST: What did you think of your principal's advice?

CHILD: I don't know. I guess it was OK, I guess . . .

The child appears comfortable disclosing his anxious self-talk and demonstrates some ability in producing coping thoughts. Early in treatment, such coping thoughts may not yield immediate anxiety reduction. Throughout the treatment process, anxious youth may become skilled at producing coping self-statements even when the child may not have fully internalized a coping belief structure. In the preceding passage, the child admits that the other children should not worry him and acknowledges that an authority figure supports him for doing the best he can. However, as evidenced by his last reply, the child has difficulty believing the principal's advice—a phenomenon not uncommon with anxious youth. Although the therapist can help the child build a coping template, homework assignments (STIC tasks), role plays, and exposure tasks are needed to buttress the message that the child has the ability to handle his own distressing situations. In the case described here, the therapist might ask the child to interview others at home to see what they would think of his science project, or how they would evaluate him if he did not win the contest. If his primary fear is being singled out by bullies, he could poll friends and ask how many of them had ever been teased, or how they had coped with their fear. Gaining confidence through practice and investigation helps the anxious child develop greater faith that his or her coping template will be useful in future challenges.

The "A" Step of the FEAR Plan: Attitudes and Actions That Can Help

As children learn to identify their physiological and cognitive manifestation of anxiety, they learn easy-to-implement strategies that might help them to reduce their anxiety acutely (e.g., when learning the "F" step, youth learn to take a few deep breaths). However, at the "A" step, youth develop a more comprehensive plan to manage the anxious situation. Problem solving is emphasized in this step, where the therapist helps the child begin to generate various alternative solutions to cope with a difficult situation and to select the most appropriate solution. In order to not overwhelm youth, discussion of nonthreatening situations can be used to introduce the problem-solving concept. For example: "You have lost your shoes in the house. What are some ways you could go about trying to find them?" The therapist provides other examples of situations and helps the child to generate alternatives, to evaluate these possibilities, and to choose the preferred solution. Once the child appears comfortable in problem-solving nonthreatening situations, anxious situations can be introduced. As with the other steps, the therapist first role-plays an anxious situation that he or she experienced. Then, situations specific to the child can be generated. Solutions may involve enlisting friends or family members for support or advice, thinking about or watching how others cope with situations, or rehearsing and practicing various skills in academic, performance, or social situations. For example, a child who was afraid of going into the snake house at the zoo (on a school trip) came up with the following possibilities to deal with the situation: "Take deep breaths," "Say everything is OK," "Listen to my tape player and think about the music," or "Be with a friend who is not scared and will not tease me." The child both generates and evaluates the different possibilities as much as he or she can and decides which solution feels best.

When practicing problem solving, younger children may want to choose a cartoon (television, movie) character or hero whom he or she admires or believes can cope with difficult situations. The therapist can encourage the child to think about how that character might handle anxiety-provoking situations. As a problem-solving strategy, the child can pretend to be that character or take that character along into scary situations for support. A 10-year-old boy who was afraid to walk home from school following a confrontation with an older child, who pushed him off his bike, used this method as one of his coping strategies. The next time that he was nervous, he planned to take deep breaths and think "Nothing will happen to me" or "I can handle this," or go into a store or to someone's doorstep. He also felt more confident if he brought "X-man" (a superhero figure) along with him on the walk and imagined that he would be right behind him if he needed him.

The "R" Step of the FEAR Plan: *Results and Rewards*

Anxious children often have difficulty evaluating themselves accurately, and they often set extremely high standards for success. Thus, the final skill that youth learn to manage their anxiety is to evaluate their efforts in coping and to reward themselves accordingly. Importantly, youth are taught to rate themselves based on their effort, not the outcome of the situation. Youth learn to identify what things they liked about how they handled the situation and what things they would like to do differently. Youth are encouraged to generate a list of possible self-rewards, ranging from spending more time in an enjoyed activity (e.g., riding bikes or reading), giving themselves a pat on the back, telling themselves "I've done a good job," to spending extra time with family and friends. Therapists are also encouraged to amply reward youth for their efforts verbally.

In the following example, the therapist helps the 12-year-old boy described earlier preparing for a Bible study quiz to develop a plan to cope with the upcoming exam. Initially, the child demonstrates acumen in listing anxious thoughts and generating coping thoughts to challenge his fears. In addition to identifying anxiety-producing and anxiety-reducing thoughts, the child and therapist collaboratively draft a list of actions that the child can take in preparation for the quiz. However, typical of anxious children, the boy has difficulty separating effort from outcome and places too much emphasis on his test grade when evaluating his coping performance. The therapist attempts to help the child by distinguishing between one's effort and performance in coping and one's letter grade on a test:

THERAPIST: Let's say you do all these actions: You study by reading it, writing it, and saying it out loud.

CHILD: . . . writing it, saying it out loud, yep.

THERAPIST: And let's say you ask your parents to quiz you on it.

CHILD: They will.

THERAPIST: You make a pretend quiz up and you've checked off everything you needed to know. How are you going to rate yourself from 1 to 10?

CHILD: If I pass?

THERAPIST: No, for now, that doesn't matter. It's how well you do these things, regardless of whether you pass or fail, that you're rating yourself on.

CHILD: Oh . . . if I do really, really good, I'll give myself about a . . . a 7.

THERAPIST: (surprised) A 7? If you try at these things really hard, you're going to give yourself a 7 out of 10?

CHILD: Yeah, if I do really, really good, and I pass the test, then I'd give myself a 10, but see I'm only going to—

THERAPIST: —but see, you give this rating for how hard you tried to prepare and to cope, not on—

CHILD: —Yeah, 7—

THERAPIST: (beginning to sound exasperated)—but if you try really, really hard, then don't you deserve a 10, regardless of how you do.

CHILD: Oh, I guess, I'd give myself—

THERAPIST: So we're going to give you a 10. If you do all those things—

CHILD: If I don't, I get a zero.

THERAPIST: If you do none, then . . . then I'd give you a zero.

In the last statement, it would have been equally appropriate if the therapist had disagreed with the child and suggested that he deserved a 3, even if he had put none of his plans into action. Undoubtedly, the boy would have been surprised at this suggestion. However, the therapist could have reminded him that proceeding through the first three steps of coping (i.e., listing anxious self-talk, generating coping self-talk, generating actions that can help) is part of the battle. Although implementing his plan of action is the ultimate goal, the child should be rewarded for initiating the coping process and reminded that these are skills that take time to master.

Review of FEAR Plan and Implementation of Exposure Tasks

To help youth recall the steps to manage their anxiety when out-of-session, they are encouraged to make a sign, wallet-sized card, or decorated wall poster—each representing a personalized version of the FEAR plan. The final review of the integrated FEAR plan will also help prepare youth for the start of the exposure tasks. Through imaginal and *in vivo* exposure, the second half of the program provides opportunities for children to practice their newly acquired skills in anxiety-provoking situations. Imaginal exposure to stressful situations is used to help children begin thinking through the various coping strategies that they might use in these situations. However, imaginal exposure does not always produce much visible anxiety except in the most anxious children; thus, it is often used as an intermediate step, prior to *in vivo* exposure. When planning *in vivo* exposures, low-anxiety situations are arranged first, followed by a gradual progression to higher-anxiety-producing situations.

The therapist presents the situation to be encountered, remarks about aspects of the situation that are likely to be troubling, and models coping behavior. The therapist then helps the child think through the steps to use when approaching the situation. The therapist and child then rehearse what might occur during the *in vivo* exposure using these coping steps, until the child feels calmer and ready to try the situation. Following the exposure, the child is helped to evaluate his or her performance and to think of a reward. When possible, the therapist should elicit the child's help in designing exposure tasks. *In vivo* exposures that result from a collaborative effort between the therapist and child are often among the most memorable and meaningful to the child.

Various *in vivo* situations can be set up in the office, such as taking a math test, giving a speech, reading a poem in front of a small audience or video camera, or introducing oneself to office personnel. Other *in vivo* exposures involve taking the child outside the office, for example, to a graveyard, zoo, or shopping center. Many naturally occurring academic and social situations can be arranged in schools with the help of teachers and guidance personnel. Following the first successful *in vivo* situation, the child often experiences a new sense of competency and more willingly engages in other anxiety-provoking situations. Given the new set of skills that the child can call on if feeling anxious, much of the treatment encourages risk taking. In the process, the therapist is mindful of normalizing anxiety, stressing that fear is a normal and manageable experience.

The following example demonstrates a representative exchange between a child and therapist as they prepare for an *in vivo* exposure (first described in Kendall, 1991). The child is afraid to visit new places for fear of getting lost. When taken to a shopping mall, he came up with the following plan:

THERAPIST: So, are you feeling nervous now?

CHILD: I don't know. Not really.

THERAPIST: How would you know you were starting to get nervous?

CHILD: My heart would start beating faster.

THERAPIST: (*recalling a common somatic complaint for this child*) What about your breathing?

CHILD: I might start breathing faster.

THERAPIST: And what would you be thinking to yourself?

CHILD: I might get lost, or I don't know where I am.

THERAPIST: And what are some things you could do if you start getting nervous?

CHILD: I could take deep breaths and say everything is going to be OK.

THERAPIST: That's good, but what if you were unsure where you were or got lost?

CHILD: I could ask somebody.

THERAPIST: Yes, you could ask somebody. Would it be a good idea to ask one of the guards or policemen? How are you feeling? Do you think you are ready to give it a try?

The therapist and child agree on a number of trips to make within the mall, varying in distance and degree of familiarity. During the trip, the child was to ask the guard for directions so that he could feel comfortable doing this in the future.

Although conducted within a supportive environment, exposure tasks are intended to be challenging and anxiety-provoking. The therapist can improve chances for child participation by incorporating elements that are fun for the child when designing tasks and assignments. Situations that are typically threatening for a child can appear more manageable when livened up with creative twists. For example, a child afraid of giving a speech can pretend to give a speech after winning an Academy Award, or the therapist might arrange for a child with social phobia to visit an arcade to get change for a video game. The child overcomes a challenge of interacting with others, but the situation provides natural reinforcement. A particularly valuable exposure task is one that permits the child to engage in an activity that is ordinarily somewhat prohibited. For a child concerned about public opinion, strutting through the library singing his favorite tune is a frightening proposition. But what child would turn down the rare opportunity to create a ruckus in the library with a consenting adult nearby? The therapist adheres to the principle that the engaging and creative exposure task is the memorable and effective one (Kendall et al., 1998).

Throughout the exposure tasks portion of treatment, the therapist remains flexible in the timing and planning of *in vivo* exposures. Traditionally, the therapist plans exposures in a hierarchical fashion, progressing from easiest to hardest for the child. At times, events that occur outside the therapy call for the therapist to adjust his or her plans to take full advantage of opportunities as they present themselves. This kind of opportunity often presents itself when the child experiences a stressful situation that would have been addressed or simulated later in the exposure stage. As described in more detail in Kendall and colleagues (1998), the following case illustrates how a therapist can appropriately adapt his or her plans to a child's concern as it arises. In the following example, the clinician had planned to address separation issues with his 11-year-old female client, who feared her father might leave her after they argued. The clinician was aware of this issue and, because of the severity of the fear, had planned to simulate an argument between the child and father for an exposure task later in treatment. The clinician's plan was challenged when the child arrived for the 12th session panicked and visibly distraught because she had just had an argument with her father. The therapist was confronted with a choice: Should he initiate relaxation exercises and tell her to hold her concerns off until a later date, when they could systematically build up to a related exposure, or should he rearrange his plans and devise a task that would address the presenting crisis while matching the child's current level of coping skills? Appropriately, the therapist chose the latter approach.

THERAPIST: So, Belinda, you've told me a lot of ways that you think your dad is mean to you. Are there any other thoughts except "madness" that are running through your thought bubbles? Do you ever worry about what your dad might be thinking of you?

CHILD: Yeah, I guess. Yeah, sometimes I worry that he'll be more mad at me, that he won't like me. Like, I'll come home and tell him some bad things that happened to me today, and he'll say I complain too much. He says all I ever do is complain. He doesn't care what happens to me.

THERAPIST: Do you really think he doesn't care about you?

CHILD: Well, he says he doesn't want to spend time with me because I complain too much. Then he says, "Well, Belinda, if I stopped spending any time with you, then you'd learn to appreciate the time I do spend with you."

In this scenario, the child is worried that being open with her feelings will drive her father away. Previous meetings with the father confirmed that he often felt overwhelmed by his daughter's emphasis on negative events and wished they could spend more time engaging in mutually enjoyable activities. When the father felt frustrated by his daughter's complaining, he would distance himself from her. This behavior elicited fear from his daughter and led to further clinging behavior. Through a series of role plays, the therapist helps Belinda articulate her feelings while at the same time helping her to understand her father's perspective. The therapist and child alternate roles. First, Belinda acts the role of the distant father while the therapist models appropriate ways for Belinda to express her hurt feelings. Then, the therapist and child switch roles so that Belinda is portraying herself, and the therapist provides a realistic portrayal of a father who might become irritable but is unlikely to be condemning. After a number of these rehearsals, Belinda and the therapist devise a realistic plan that allows Belinda to communicate openly with her father, including discussions of both negative and positive events that occur during the day. By the end of the session, Belinda invites her father into the therapy room, proposes her plan to him, and sets up a required schedule that would reward successful interactions with him.

Going "Hollywood"

The program described here closes with the child contributing to the creation and production of a "commercial" about his or her experiences in the program; that is, the client is asked to help put together a video, booklet, cassette tape, or other creative expression to help tell other children about the ways to manage anxiety. Youth are encouraged to take full creative control with the development and subsequent production of the commercial and are encouraged to act as the "directors" of the commercial. In the past, commercials have included "rap" tapes and videocassettes that are both humorous and impressively informative. The goal is to set the stage for clients to endorse the program, and making a tape, for example, gives clear evidence of our interest in their support, provides a demonstration of their success, offers a tangible reward at the end of the program, and we suspect, helps to buttress the maintenance of the treatment-produced gains.

Working with Families

We recognize the importance of parental involvement in helping the child to overcome disproportionate anxiety. Although the cognitive-behavioral nature of the program focuses on helping the individual learn to think and behave differently, we also encourage parents to participate in a supportive role (see Suveg et al., in press, for a discussion of parent involvement in CBT). Though the child-focused treatment program described herein does not focus on "family" therapy, parents are actively involved from the outset of the child-focused protocol. Once treatment has begun, the therapist meets with the parents after the third session to collaborate with them on treatment plans and to solicit their cooperation. At this meeting, we provide additional information about the treatment via an outline of the program and details where the child is in the program. We give the parents an opportunity to discuss their concerns about the child and provide further information that might be helpful to the therapist. We share impressions about what specific situations provoke the child's anxiety and how the child typically reacts. Last, we offer specific ways that the parents can become involved in the program. For example, the parents are invited to sit in on part of the child's next session so that they can help the child practice relaxation skills. Also, they are invited to call the therapist if they can think of any further information that might be helpful, or if they have any questions. Depending on the age of the child and the quality of parental support, the therapist may ask the parents to help in other specific tasks assigned to the child in upcoming weeks. Given the important role that parents can play in their child's treatment, therapists should be aware of the particular problems that families of anxious children may be experiencing. These problems may range from increased rates of anxiety disorders, as well as other types of pathology, to particular problems in parenting, such as overprotectiveness and guilt about the problems that their child is experiencing (see also Chorpita & Barlow, 1998).

Although the research reviewed in the early part of the chapter suggests that families with anxious children may have increased rates of pathology, the studies provide little insight into what to expect when working with parents in a clinical setting. Given the dearth of research in this area, many of the following suggestions stem from our clinical work and observations. It is our experience that parental involvement with overanxious youth ranges from underinvolved, in which parents appear to be unaware of their children's problems, to extreme overprotectiveness. Underinvolvement can lead to problems with keeping appointments or helping the child to keep his or her therapy-related material organized. Parents benefit from being informed of the negative impact that this can have on therapy. Overprotectiveness can interfere with the child's performing important tasks that are designed to build his or her sense of confidence. For example, one mother of a 12-year-old girl who had suffered from cancer as a young child expressed concern when the therapist said that she and the girl were going to leave the building and go to a nearby bookstore. The parent wanted to go along! Rather than getting into a power struggle with the concerned parent, the therapist simply announced that she and the girl were going together, and kept walking out the door. When dealing with such an overprotective parent, the therapist needs to strike a delicate balance between helping the child to become more independent while at the same time not increasing the parent's own anxiety and hence risking alienation from the treatment. One tactic may be to get the parent initially involved in suggesting or participating in some of the *in vivo* experiences that the child will complete. This allows the parent to maintain initial involvement with the child while also encouraging the child's independent behavior, since the parent does not continue with the *in vivo* experiences. The therapist may also want to point out how parents communicate their own anxicty and overprotectiveness to their child. Parents may not be aware of how their well-intentioned communications might be interpreted by their child as cues to respond with anxiety and fear. For example, in a therapy session conducted with a mother and her 12-year-old son diagnosed with social phobia, the therapist had to demonstrate how the mother's messages about embarrassment in social situations were contributing to the child's fear of social situations. The child's self-reported goals for treatment were to make new friends and become more comfortable speaking to unfamiliar people. The child's coexisting diagnosis of expressive–receptive learning disability meant that he had real concerns about understanding and being understood by other children, which compounded his fears of talking to others.

Observing that the child was not ready for a social exposure task, the therapist chose an intermediate approach. As a STIC task, she suggested that the child begin acclimating to social environments by riding his bicycle around the neighborhood to get used to the idea of seeing unfamiliar children. The therapist recommended that the child not engage in any interactions, but simply ride down the block. Before he could respond, the mother interjected, "But if you ride down the street without saying anything, won't the other kids see you and think you're rude?" Although the parent's question was intended to help the child consider the consequences of his actions, the therapist pointed out that there are better ways to communicate this. The therapist recommended that, instead of interjecting her own fears about possible negative outcomes, she might ask the child what he thought might happen and discuss the situation within a problem-solving framework.

Parents of anxious children may also express guilt about the child's anxiety. Helping them to cope with these feelings may involve a pragmatic discussion, suggesting that how the problem developed is not the issue; rather, it is important to focus on how they can contribute to helping their child cope at the present time. If the parent's own anxiety or other problems appear to be genuinely contributing to the child's anxiety, it is discussed with the parent. Such a discussion may involve observations and suggestions about how to change the "parent–child" interaction and even recommendations for the parent's own treatment. More specifically, it may be helpful to find out what kinds of expectations the parents hold for their children both academically and behaviorally. For instance, are they overconcerned with academic performance and therefore placing a lot of pressure on their child to achieve? Parents may also have inaccurate expectations about what is appropriate behavior, given their child's developmental level. Helping parents to clarify what is and is not within the normal range of behavior may prevent inappropriate and anxiety-provoking responses to their child's normal behavior. Finally, it is important to help parents learn new ways of responding to their child's anxious behavior. The stress of dealing with an anxious child may lead parents to become sensitized to any signs of anxiety in their children. They may be hypervigilant and strongly react to any indication of anxiety, for example, by becoming anxious themselves or depressed when they feel helpless about what to do.

One therapist videotaped her session with an 8-year-old boy and his mother to make a dramatic point about the parent's hypervigilance around her son's somatic complaints and school-refusal behavior. Minutes before the child was to depart for school or other extracurricular activities, he would begin reporting a variety of physical symptoms, including stomach cramps, headaches, and diarrhea, and would claim he had to use the bathroom. In response to the child's complaints, the mother would ask a series of questions to assess the extent of his physical distress: "What's the matter?", "Does your throat hurt?", "Do your ears hurt?", "Are you going to be sick?" Once the mother began showing concern, the child's report of somatic symptoms would escalate until he became nearly incapacitated with pain, sickness, or fear. The therapist used the videotaping to demonstrate how the mother's questions contributed to the escalation of her child's physical symptoms. Presented with this evidence, the mother was able to see how her demonstrations of concern could actually contribute to her son's reported symptoms of distress. The mother admitted that she had believed she was "making it worse" in some way but was unaware of how or where the cycle began. Such demonstrations, if provided in a nonaccusatory, nonjudgmental manner, can provide parents with concrete information that helps explain current interactional patterns and gives direction for behavioral change. Given the important role that parents play in the success of child-focused treatment for childhood anxiety disorders, and given the hypothesized roles family members may play in the genesis and maintenance of anxiety disorders, it should not be surprising that, in addition to the child-focused intervention, we have also developed a family intervention. The same strategies are employed, but the sessions include parental participation. A manual describing this program is available (Howard, Chu, Krain, Marrs-Garcia, & Kendall, 2000). Initial research has been conducted with a family-focused cognitive-behavioral format (Howard & Kendall, 1996a). As discussed in greater detail later, Barrett, Dadds, and Rapee (1996) have implemented a family management component (i.e., affective education, contingent reinforcement schedules, and management of parental anxiety) for the families of anxious children and have reported positive results.

We encourage the continued development of family-focused intervention and support models that target the interactive influence of family members. For example, treatment for a separation-anxious child might address the child's need for greater independence by working on age-appropriate problem-solving or assertiveness skills in situations in which he or she may have previously unnecessarily relied on a parent, and concurrently examine and correct (testing out *in vivo*) parents' misperceptions of their child's competencies or equating good parenting with being overinvolved. One can imagine that, without coordinating efforts between parents and children, a child's gains toward greater independence and management of fears may be mislabeled as disobedience or contribute to sadness in parents because they misattribute this change to their no longer being needed. Such responses could threaten the maintenance of the child's gains. By coordinating efforts, the new behavior in the child is made consonant with new beliefs or expectancies on the part of the parents. Conversely, a parent's acquisition of new coping skills and overt behaviors, such as going to work rather than sleeping all day, will be coupled with the child's new attributions of strength to the parent and less fear for his or her own safety. Although cognitive-behavioral treatment strategies for families are incorporated into our clinical research and practice, there remains a great need for empirical evaluation of when it is best to include, or not include, parents in the treatment of anxiety disorders in children and adolescents.

Research Outcomes

The American Psychological Association (APA) Task Force on Promotion and Dissemination of Psychological Procedures (1995) has provided guidelines for what should be considered "well-established," "probably efficacious," and "experimental" treatments (see also Chambless & Hollon, 1998). For a treatment to be considered efficacious, it must be shown to be more effective than a control (i.e., no treatment) in randomized clinical trials conducted by independent researchers. A review of empirically supported treatments for children with anxiety disorders concluded that behavioral and cognitive-behavioral procedures represent the modalities that have received the most empirical support (Kazdin & Weisz, 1998; Ollendick & King, 1998; see also Albano & Kendall, 2002). For treating phobias, behavioral techniques—including imaginal and *in vivo* desensitization; live, filmed, and participant modeling; as well as contingency management strategies—were granted "probably efficacious" or "well-established" status. For treating other anxiety disorders, cognitive-behavioral procedures with and without family anxiety management were deemed "probably efficacious."

Building upon a base of promising results from single-case design studies (e.g., Eisen & Silverman, 1993; Kane & Kendall, 1989; Ollendick, 1995), three randomized clinical trials conducted by two different research groups using cognitive-behavioral techniques constitute the weight of the evidence upon which these labels were applied (Barrett, Dadds, et al., 1996; Kendall, 1994; Kendall et al., 1997). Kendall (1994) conducted the first randomized clinical trial aimed at investigating the efficacy of CBT for 9- to 13-year-old youth with anxiety disorder. In the trial comparing a manual-based CBT to a wait-list control, 64% of children treated did not receive their principal anxiety disorder diagnosis at posttreatment and maintained their treatment gains at 1-year follow-up (Kendall, 1994). Longer-term follow-up assessments documented that the gains were maintained over a 2- to 5-year period (mean of 3.35 years) (Kendall & Southam-Gerow, 1996). The efficacy of this procedure was replicated in a second randomized trial with ninety-four 9- to 13-year-olds diagnosed with a primary anxiety disorder and randomly assigned to CBT and wait-list control (Kendall et al., 1997). At posttreatment, there were positive outcomes on a variety of measures for children in the treatment group over those in the wait-list control. These treatment gains were maintained and evident at 1-year follow-up (Kendall et al., 1997).

Kendall, Safford, Flannery-Schroeder, and Webb (2004) recently reported on a long-term follow-up of the sample included in the second RCT (i.e., the sample included in the 1997 report). The maintenance of treatment effects was examined, as were the effects of treatment on potential sequelae of childhood anxiety. The follow-up sample included 86 of the 94 children in the original sample (over 90% of the original sample) with a primary diagnosis of GAD ($n =$ 55), SAD ($n = 22$), or SP ($n = 17$). Results indicated that treatment gains were maintained an average of 7.4 years after treatment, based on diagnostic interviews and both child- and parent-report for the majority of participants. With respect to effects on potential sequelae of child anxiety, results revealed that those who responded positively to treatment used alcohol and other substances less and had fewer difficulties related to substance use than less positive treatment responders. No relationship between treatment response and the later development of a mood disorder was found. Other research has also found support for group cognitive-behavioral treatment of anxiety (e.g., Flannery-Schroeder & Kendall, 2000; Manassis et al., 2002; Silverman et al., 1999).

Importantly, the positive treatment effects of CBT appear robust even in the presence of comorbid externalizing disorders. Specifically, studies have found that children with anxiety disorders who have comorbid externalizing psychopathology tend to respond similarly to treatment as do AD youth without comorbid psychopathology, at (1) posttreatment (e.g., Berman, Weems, Silverman, & Kurtines, 2000; Rapee, 2000; Southam-Gerow, Kendall, & Weersing, 2001), (2) 1-year follow-up (Kendall, Brady, & Verduin, 2001) and (3) several years (mean 7.4 years) posttreatment (Flannery-Schroeder, Suveg, Safford, Kendall, & Webb, 2004). Less is known about the effects of comorbid depressive disorders on treatment, perhaps because these youth with anxiety disorders typically qualify for depression as the principal diagnosis and thus serious depression is not included in studies of youth with principal anxiety disorders. Nevertheless, some research suggests a negative link between depressive disorders and treatment outcome (Berman et al., 2000).

Several researchers have suggested the need for additional involvement of parents or family in the treatment of childhood anxiety disorders (e.g., Barrett et al., 1996; Barrett, Duffy, Dadds, & Rapee, 2001; Medlowitz et al., 1999; Siqueland & Diamond, 1998). Barrett, Dadds, and colleagues (1996) compared a CBT intervention based on Kendall's (1992b) program to an intervention that included the CBT intervention plus a family intervention (FAM). Seventy-nine 7- to 14-year-old children who met a primary diagnosis of overanxious disorder, separation anxiety disorder, or social phobia were included and randomly assigned to a CBT group, a CBT + FAM, or wait-list control. All conditions lasted 12 weeks. The CBT condition paralleled that of Kendall (1994), whereas the CBT + FAM included a Family Anxiety Management component wherein parents were trained in contingency management strategies and communication and problem-solving skills, and taught to recognize and address their own emotional and anxious responses to stimuli. Sixty percent of both treatment conditions achieved a nondiagnosis status, compared to less than 30% of the wait-list control children. At the 12-month follow-up, no-diagnosis rates were 70% for the CBT and 95% for the CBT + FAM intervention groups. Other studies that have included parents in treatment have not yielded as positive results (e.g., Nauta, Scholing, Emmelkamp, & Minderaa, 2003; Spence, Donovan, & Brechman-Toussaint, 2000). For example, Spence and colleagues (2000) conducted a treatment outcome study of 50 youth (ages 7 through 14) diagnosed with social anxiety disorder. Youth and their parents were randomly assigned to either a parent–child group treatment, child-only treatment, or a wait-list condition. Although both active treatments yielded significant improvement in the reduction of anxiety diagnoses as compared to the wait-list condition, there was no difference between the two active conditions. Thus, although it is somewhat intuitive that adding a family component to treatment may be more effective, a review of the published reports (Barmish & Kendall, 2005) determined that the benefits of including parents in treatment are inconclusive. As the researchers have noted, the ways that parents have been included (e.g., training in parental anxiety management and contingency management) in the treatment studies have varied widely, precluding clear general conclusions regarding parental involvement. Future research is needed to guide clinicians on which treatment may be best for whom and under what conditions.

In addition to individual and family treatments for anxiety in youth, other researchers have begun to examine the effectiveness of group school-based treatment approaches (e.g., Masia, Klein, Storch, & Corda, 2001). Although researchers in this area discuss potential challenges to implementing treatment in the school setting (e.g., space, school personnel hesitancy), pilot work provides support for this area of research (Masia et al., 2001).

In recent years, research has also examined the efficacy of cognitive-behavioral prevention programs for anxiety targeted at both "at-risk" samples and universal school-age populations. Several studies (Barrett & Turner, 2001; Dadds et al., 1999; Dadds, Spence, Holland, Barrett, & Laurens, 1997) provide evidence for the effectiveness of cognitive-behavioral and family-based group treatment for the prevention of anxiety in children and adolescents at risk for anxiety disorders. For example, the Queensland Early Intervention and Prevention of Anxiety Project used a school-based screening procedure to identify children at risk for later anxiety disorders and then offered cognitive-behavioral skills training to children and parents. Educational sessions focusing on family involvement and parents managing their own anxious symptomatology were included. Both intervention and monitored groups showed improvements immediately at postintervention; however, at 6-month follow-up, only the intervention group maintained improvements, showing a reduced rate of existing anxiety disorder and preventing the onset of new anxiety disorders. At 12 months, the groups converged, but the superiority of the intervention group was evident again at 2-year follow-up (Dadds et al., 1999). Other research teams have found support for a universal prevention program using a cognitive-behavioral model for school-age youth (e.g., Barrett & Turner, 2001; Shortt, Barrett, & Fox, 2001).

ACKNOWLEDGMENTS

Portions of the work reported here were supported by a research grants from the National Institute of Mental Health (Nos. MH59087, MH64484, and MH63747). We acknowledge and thank the authors of the chapter on this topic who appeared in the first and second editions of this book. As before, the effort was collaborative and reflects the input of each author, as well as the groundwork provided by the authors of the chapter in the first two editions.

NOTES

1. Other childhood disorders, such as posttraumatic stress disorder (PTSD) and obsessive–compulsive disorder (OCD), also have anxiety as part of the central presenting problem. However, there are important differences, suggesting that PTSD and OCD require their own focused interventions. Readers interested in OCD, for example, should see Piacentini, March, and Franklin, Chapter 8, this volume; Piacentini, Gitow, Jaffer, Graae, and Whitaker (1994); March and Mulle (1998); and Henin and Kendall (1997). Regarding abuse, readers are referred to Deblinger, Behl, and Glickman, Chapter 11, this volume.
2. Readers interested in foreign language translations of the treatment manuals or the *Coping Cat Workbook* should contact the publisher, Workbook Publishing, Ardmore, Pennsylvania (www.WorkbookPublishing.com). Readers interested in adaptations and applications in other countries or languages should consult the following resources: Kendall and DePietro (1995; in Italian, Italy); Masayi Ichii, University of the Ryukyus, Okinawa, Japan; Barrett, Dadds, and Rapee (e.g., 1996; in English, Australia); John Weisz and Michael Southam-Gerow, University of California at Los Angeles, for a Spanish version used in Los Angeles; Claire Hayes, University of Dublin, Ireland; Maaki Nauta, University of Groningen, the Netherlands; Susan Bogels, University of Maastricht, the Netherlands; Dominiek Bracke and Caroline Braet, University of Ghent, Belgium; Sandra Mendlowitz and colleagues (1999), Hospital for Sick Children, Toronto, Canada. Readers interested in prevention should see the report of Dadds and colleagues (1997) and consider the ongoing work of Dena Hirshfeld, Massachusetts General Hospital, Harvard Medical School, Boston.

REFERENCES

Achenbach, T. M. (1991). *Integrative guide for the 1991 CBCL/4-18, YSR, and TRF.* Burlington: University of Vermont.

Achenbach, T. M. (1993). Implications of multiaxial empirically based assessment for behavior therapy with children. *Behavior Therapy, 24,* 91–116.

Achenbach, T. M., & Edelbrock, C. (1986). *Manual for the TRF and the Child Behavior Profile.* Burlington: University of Vermont.

Achenbach, T. M., & Edelbrock, C. S. (1978). The classification of child psychopathology: A review and analysis of empirical efforts. *Psychological Bulletin, 85,* 1275–1301.

Achenbach, T. M., & Edelbrock, C. S. (1983). *Manual for the Child Behavior Checklist and Revised Child Behavior Profile.* Burlington: University of Vermont, Associates in Psychiatry.

Achenbach, T. M., & McConaughy, S. H. (1992). Taxonomy of internalizing disorders of childhood and adolescence. In W. M. Reynolds (Ed.), *Internalizing disorders in children and adolescents* (pp. 19–60). New York: Wiley.

Albano, A. M., Chorpita, B. F., & Barlow, D. H. (1996). Childhood anxiety disorders. In E. J. Mash & R. A. Barkley (Eds.), *Child psychopathology* (pp. 196–241). New York: Guilford Press.

Albano, A. M., & Kendall, P. C. (2002). Cognitive behavioural therapy for children and adolescents with anxiety disorders: Clinical research advances. *International Review of Psychiatry, 14,* 129–134.

American Academy of Child and Adolescent Psychiatry. (1997). AACAP official action: Practice parameters for the assessment and treatment of anxiety disorders. *Journal of the American Academy of Child and Adolescent Psychiatry, 36,* 1639–1641.

American Psychiatric Association. (1994). *Diagnostic and statistical manual of mental disorders* (4th ed.). Washington, DC: Author.

American Psychological Association Task Force on Promotion and Dissemination of Psychological Procedures. (1995). Training in and dissemination of empirically-validated psychological treatments: Report and recommendations. *Clinical Psychologist, 48,* 3–24.

Arnow, B. A., Taylor, C. B., Agras, W. S., & Telch, M. H. (1985). Enhancing agoraphobia treatment outcome by changing couple communication patterns. *Behavior Therapy, 16,* 452–467.

Aschenbrand, S. G., Kendall, P. C., Webb, A., Safford, S., & Flannery-Schroeder, E. (2003). Is childhood separation anxiety disorder a predictor of adult panic disorder and agoraphobia? A seven-year longitudinal study. *Journal of the American Academy of Child and Adolescent Psychiatry, 42,* 1478–1485.

Ayllon, T., Smith, D., & Rogers, M. (1970). Behavioral management of school phobia. *Journal of Behavior Therapy and Experimental Psychiatry, 1,* 125–138.

Bandura, A. (1969). *Principles of behavior modification.* New York: Holt, Rinehart & Winston.

Bandura, A. (1986). *Social learning theory.* Englewood Cliffs, NJ: Prentice-Hall.

Barabasz, A. F. (1973). Group desensitization of test anxiety in elementary school. *Journal of Psychology, 83,* 295–301.

Barlow, D. (1992). Diagnosis, DSM-IV, and dimensional approaches. In A. Ehlers, W. Fiegenbaum, I. Florin, & J. Margraf (Eds.), *Perspectives and promises of clinical psychology* (pp. 13–21). New York: Plenum Press.

Barlow, D., & Wolfe, B. E. (1981). Behavioral approaches to anxiety disorders: A report on the NIMH–SUNY, Albany, Research Conference. *Journal of Consulting and Clinical Psychology, 49,* 448–454.

Barmish, A., & Kendall, P. C. (2005). Should parents be co-clients in cognitive-behavioral therapy for anxious youth? *Journal of Clinical Child and Adolescent Psychology, 34,* 569–581.

Barrett, P. M. (2000). Treatment of childhood anxiety: Developmental aspects. *Clinical Psychology Review, 20,* 479–494.

Barrett, P. M., Dadds, M. R., & Rapee, R. M. (1996). Family treatment of childhood anxiety: A controlled trial. *Journal of Consulting and Clinical Psychology, 64,* 333–342.

Barrett, P. M., Duffy, A. L., Dadds, M. R., & Rapee, R. M. (2001). Cognitive-behavioral treatment of anxiety disorders in children: Long-term (6-year) follow-up. *Journal of Consulting and Clinical Psychology, 69,* 135–141.

Barrett, P. M., Rapee, R. M., Dadds, M. M., & Ryan, S. M. (1996). Family enhancement of cognitive style in anxious and aggressive children. *Journal of Abnormal Child Psychology, 24,* 187–203.

Barrett, P., & Turner, C. (2001). Prevention of anxiety symptoms in primary school children: Preliminary results from a universal school-based trial. *British Journal of Clinical Psychology, 40,* 399–410.

Barrios, B. A., & Hartmann, D. P. (1988). Fears and anxieties. In E. J. Mash & L. G. Terdal (Eds.), *Behavioral assessment of childhood disorders* (2nd ed., pp. 196–264). New York: Guilford Press.

Bauer, D. (1976). An exploratory study of developmental changes in children's fears. *Journal of Child Psychology and Psychiatry, 17,* 69–74.

Beidel, D. C. (1988). Psychophysiological assessment of anxious emotional states in children. *Journal of Abnormal Psychology, 97,* 80–82.

Beidel, D. C. (1989). Assessing anxious emotion: A review of psychophysiological assessment in children. *Clinical Psychology Review, 9,* 717–736.

Beidel, D. C., Turner, S. M., Hamlin, K., & Morris, T. L. (2000). The Social Phobia and Anxiety Inventory for Children (SPAI-C): External and discriminative validity. *Behavior Therapy, 31,* 75–87.

Beidel, D. C., Turner, S. M., & Morris, T. (1995). A new inventory to assess childhood social anxiety and phobia: The Social Phobia and Anxiety Inventory for Children. *Psychological Assessment, 7,* 73–79.

Berman, S. L., Weems, C. F., Silverman, W. K., & Kurtines, W. M. (2000). Predictors of outcome in exposure-based cognitive and behavioural treatment for phobic and anxiety disorders in children. *Behaviour Therapy, 31,* 713–731.

Bernstein, G. A., Borchardt, C. M., & Perwein, A. R. (1996). Anxiety disorders in children and adolescents: A review of the past 10 years. *Journal of the American Academy of Child and Adolescent Psychiatry, 35,* 1110–1119.

Brady, E., & Kendall, P. C. (1992). Comorbidity of anxiety and depression in children and adolescents. *Psychological Bulletin, 111,* 244–255.

Campbell, S. B. (1986). Developmental issues. In R. Gittelman (Ed.), *Anxiety disorders of childhood* (pp. 24–57). New York: Guilford Press.

Castro, J., Toro, J., van der Ende, J., & Arrindell, W. A. (1993). Exploring the feasibility of assessing perceived parental rearing styles in Spanish children with the EMBU. *International Journal of Social Psychiatry, 39,* 47–57.

Chambers, W. J., Puig-Antich, J., Hirsch, M., Paez, P., Ambrosini, P. J., Tabrizi, M. A., & Davies, M. (1985). The assessment of affective disorders in children and adolescents by semistructured interview: Test–retest reliability of the Schedule for Affective Disorders and Schizophrenia for school-age children, present episode version. *Archives of General Psychiatry, 42,* 696–702.

Chambless, D., & Hollon, S. (1998). Defining empirically supported treatments. *Journal of Consulting and Clinical Psychology, 66,* 5–17.

Chorpita, B., & Barlow, D. (1998). The development of anxiety: The role of control in the early environment. *Psychology Bulletin, 124,* 3–21.

Chorpita, B. F., Brown, T. A., & Barlow, D. H. (1998). Perceived control as a mediator of family environment in etiological models of childhood anxiety. *Behavior Therapy, 29*, 457–476.

Choudhury, M. S., Pimentel, S. S., & Kendall, P. C. (2003). Childhood anxiety disorders: Parent–child (dis)agreement using a structured interview for the DSM-IV. *Journal of the American Academy of Child and Adolescent Psychiatry, 42*, 957–964.

Chu, B. C., Choudhury, M. S., Shortt, A. L., Pincus, D. B., Creed, T. A., & Kendall, P. C. (2004). Alliance, technology, and outcome in the treatment of anxious youth. *Cognitive and Behavioral Practice, 11*, 44–55.

Chu, B. C., & Kendall, P. C. (2004). Positive association of child involvement and treatment outcome within a manual-based cognitive-behavioral treatment for children with anxiety. *Journal of Consulting and Clinical Psychology, 72*, 821–829.

Comer, J. S., & Kendall, P. C. (2004). A symptom-level examination of parent-child agreement in the diagnosis of anxious youths. *Journal of the American Academy of Child and Adolescent Psychiatry, 43*, 878–886.

Costello, E. J., Mustillo, S., Erkanli, A., Keeler, G., & Angold, A. (2003). Prevalence and development of psychiatric disorders in childhood and adolescence. *Archives of General Psychiatry, 60*, 837–844.

Creed, T. A., & Kendall, P. C. (2005). Therapist alliance-building behavior within a cognitive-behavioral treatment for anxiety in youth. *Journal of Consulting and Clinical Psychology, 73*, 498–505.

Dadds, M. R., Barrett, P. M., Rapee, R. M., & Ryan, S. (1996). Family process and child anxiety and aggression: An observational analysis. *Journal of Abnormal Child Psychology, 24*, 715–734.

Dadds, M. R., Holland, D. E., Laurens, K. R., Mullins, K. R., Barrett, P. M., & Spence, S. H. (1999). Early intervention and prevention of anxiety disorders in children: Results at 2-year follow-up. *Journal of Consulting and Clinical Psychology, 67*, 145–150.

Dadds, M. R., Spence, S. H., Holland, D., Barrett, P. M., & Laurens, K. (1997). Early intervention and prevention of anxiety disorders: A controlled trial. *Journal of Consulting and Clinical Psychology, 65*, 627–635.

Dong, Q., Yang, B., & Ollendick, T. H. (1994). Fears in Chinese children and adolescents and their relations to anxiety and depression. *Journal of Child Psychology and Psychiatry, 35*, 351–363.

Draper, T. W., & James, R. S. (1985). Preschool fears: Longitudinal sequence and cohort changes. *Child Study Journal, 15*, 147–155.

Dumas, J., LaFreniere, P., & Serketich, W. (1995). "Balance of power": Transactional analysis of control in mother–child dyads involving socially competent, aggressive, and anxious children. *Journal of Abnormal Psychology, 104*, 104–113.

D'Zurilla, T. J., & Goldfried, M. R. (1971). Problem-solving and behavior modification. *Journal of Abnormal Psychology, 78*, 107–126.

D'Zurilla, T., & Nezu, A. M. (1999). *Problem-solving therapy: A social competence approach to clinical intervention* (2nd ed.). New York: Springer.

Edelbrock, C., Costello, A. J., Duncan, M. K., Conover, N. C., & Kalas, R. (1986). Parent–child agreement on child psychiatric symptoms assessed via structured interview. *Journal of Child Psychology and Psychiatry, 27*, 181–190.

Edelbrock, C., Costello, A. J., Duncan, M. K., Kalas, R., & Conover, N. C. (1985). Age differences in the reliability of the psychiatric interview of the child. *Child Development, 56*, 265–275.

Ehrenreich, J. T., & Gross, A. M. (2002). Biased attentional behavior in childhood anxiety: A review of theory and current empirical investigation. *Clinical Psychology Review, 22*, 991–1008.

Eisen, A. R., & Silverman, W. K. (1993). Should I relax or change my thoughts? A preliminary examination of cognitive therapy, relaxation training, and their combination with overanxious children. *Journal of Cognitive Psychotherapy: An International Quarterly, 7*, 265–279.

Fischer, K. W., & Tangney, J. P. (1995). Self-conscious emotions and the affect revolution: Framework and overview. In J. P. Tangney & K. W. Fischer (Eds.), *Self-conscious emotions: The psychology of shame, guilt, embarrassment, and pride* (pp. 3–22). New York: Guilford Press.

Flannery-Schroeder, E., & Kendall, P. C. (1996). *Cognitive-behavioral therapy for anxious children: Therapist manual for group treatment.* Ardmore, PA: Workbook Publishing.

Flannery-Schroeder, E., & Kendall, P. C. (2000). Group and individual cognitive-behavioral treatments for youth with anxiety disorders: A randomized clinical trial. *Cognitive Therapy and Research, 24*, 251–278.

Flannery-Schroeder, E., Suveg, C., Safford, S., Kendall, P. C., & Webb, A. (2004). Comorbid externalizing disorders and child anxiety treatment outcomes. *Behaviour Change, 21*, 14–25.

Fonseca, A. C., Yule, W., & Erol, N. (1994). Cross-cultural issues. In T. H. Ollendick, N. J. King, & W. Yule (Eds.), *International handbook of phobic and anxiety disorders in children and adolescents* (pp. 67–84). New York: Plenum Press.

Francis, G., & Beidel, D. (1995). Cognitive-behavioral psychotherapy. In J. S. March (Ed.), *Anxiety disorders in children and adolescents* (pp. 321–340). New York: Guilford Press.

Francis, G., & Ollendick, T. (1990). Behavioral treatment of social anxiety. In E. L. Feindler & G. R. Kalfus (Eds.), *Casebook in adolescent behavior therapy* (pp. 127–146). New York: Springer.

Frick, P. J., Silverthorn, P., & Evans, C. (1994). Assessment of childhood anxiety using structured interviews: Patterns of agreement among informants and association with maternal anxiety. *Psychological Assessment, 6*, 372–379.

Friedman, A. G., & Ollendick, T. H. (1989). Treatment programs for severe nighttime fears: A methodological note. *Journal of Behavior Therapy and Experimental Psychiatry, 20*, 171–178.

Ginsburg, G., & Silverman, W. (1996). Phobic and anxiety disorders in Hispanic and Caucasian youth. *Journal of Anxiety Disorders, 10*, 517–528.

Ginsburg, G. S., Siqueland, L., Masia-Warner, C., & Hedtke, K. A. (2004). Anxiety disorders in children: Family matters. *Cognitive and Behavioral Practice, 11*, 28–43.

Ginsburg, G. S., Silverman, W. K., & Kurtines, W. K. (1995). Family involvement in treating children with phobic and anxiety disorders: A look ahead. *Clinical Psychology Review, 15*, 457–473.

Graziano, A. M., & Mooney, K. C. (1980). Family self-control instruction for children's nighttime fear reduction. *Journal of Consulting and Clinical Psychology, 48*, 206–213.

Graziano, A. M., & Mooney, K. C. (1982). Behavioral treatment of "Nightfears" in children: Maintenance of improvement at 2½- to 3-year follow-up. *Journal of Consulting and Clinical Psychology, 50*, 598–599.

Grills, A. E., & Ollendick, T. H. (2002). Issues in parent–child agreement: The case of structured diagnostic interviews. *Clinical Child and Family Psychology Review, 5*, 57–83.

Grills, A. E., & Ollendick, T. H. (2003). Multiple informant agreement and the Anxiety Disorders Interview Schedule for Parents and Children. *Journal of the American Academy of Child and Adolescent Psychiatry, 42*, 30–40.

Gullone, E. (2000). The development of normal fear: A century of research. *Clinical Psychology Review, 20*, 429–451.

Hagopian, L. P., Weist, M. D., & Ollendick, T. H. (1990). Cognitive-behavior therapy with an 11-year-old girl fearful of AIDS infection, other diseases, and poisoning: A case study. *Journal of Anxiety Disorders, 4*, 257–265.

Henin, A., & Kendall, P. C. (1997). Obsessive–compulsive disorder in childhood and adolescence. In T. Ollendick & R. Prinz (Eds.), *Advances in clinical child psychology* (Vol. 19, pp. 75–131). New York: Plenum Press.

Herjanic, B., Herjanic, M., Brown, F., & Wheatt, T. (1975). Are children reliable reporters? *Journal of Abnormal Child Psychology, 1,* 41–48.

Herjanic, B., & Reich, W. (1982). Development of a structured psychiatric interview for children: Agreement between child and parent on individual symptoms. *Journal of Abnormal Child Psychology, 10,* 307–324.

Himadi, W. G., Boice, R., & Barlow, D. H. (1985). Assessment of agoraphobia: Triple response measurement. *Behaviour Research and Therapy, 23,* 311–323.

Hodges, K., McKnew, C., Burbach, D. J., & Roebuck, L. (1987). Diagnostic concordance between the Child Assessment Schedule and the Schedule for Affective Disorders and Schizophrenia for School-age Children in an outpatient sample using lay interviewers. *Journal of the American Academy of Child and Adolescent Psychiatry, 26,* 654–661.

Howard, B. L., Chu, B., Krain, A., Marrs-Garcia, A., & Kendall, P. C. (2000). *Cognitive-behavioral family therapy for anxious children: Therapist manual* (2nd ed.). Ardmore, PA: Workbook Publishing.

Howard, B. L., & Kendall, P. C. (1996a). Cognitive-behavioral family therapy for anxiety disordered children: A multiple baseline evaluation. *Cognitive Therapy and Research, 20,* 423–443.

Howard, B. L., & Kendall, P. C. (1996b). *Cognitive-behavioral therapy for anxious children: Therapist manual.* Ardmore, PA: Workbook Publishing.

Hudson, J. L., & Kendall, P. C. (2002). Showing you can do it: Homework in therapy for children and adolescents with anxiety disorders. *Journal of Clinical Psychology, 58,* 525–534.

Hudson, J. L., & Rapee, R. M. (2001). Parent–child interactions and anxiety disorders: An observational study. *Behaviour Research and Therapy, 39,* 1411–1427.

Ingram, R. E., & Kendall, P. C. (1986). Cognitive clinical psychology: Implications of an information processing perspective. In R. E. Ingram (Ed.), *Information processing approaches to clinical psychology* (pp. 3–21). New York: Academic Press.

Ingram, R. E., & Kendall, P. C. (1987). The cognitive side of anxiety. *Cognitive Therapy and Research, 11,* 523–537.

Ingram, R. E., Kendall, P. C., & Chen, A. H. (1991). Cognitive-behavioral interventions. In C. R. Snyder & D. R. Forsyth (Eds.), *Handbook of social and clinical psychology: The health perspective* (pp. 509–522). New York: Pergamon Press.

Jannoun, L., Munby, M., Catalan, J., & Gelder, M. (1980). A home-based treatment program for agoraphobia: Replication and controlled evaluation. *Behavior Therapy, 11,* 294–305.

Kane, M., & Kendall, P. C. (1989). Anxiety disorders in children: A multiple baseline evaluation of a cognitive-behavioral treatment. *Behavior Therapy, 20,* 499–508.

Kashani, J. H., & Orvaschel, H. (1988). Anxiety disorders in mid-adolescence: A community sample. *American Journal of Psychiatry, 145,* 960–964.

Kazdin, A., & Weisz, J. (1998). Identifying and developing empirically supported child and adolescent treatments. *Journal of Consulting and Clinical Psychology, 66,* 100–110.

Kendall, P. C. (1984). Behavioral assessment and methodology. In G. T. Wilson, C. M. Franks, K. D. Brownell, & P. C. Kendall, *Annual review of behavior therapy: Theory and practice* (Vol. 9, pp. 39–94). New York: Brunner/Mazel.

Kendall, P. C. (1985). Toward a cognitive-behavioral model of child psychopathology and a critique of related interventions. *Journal of Abnormal Child Psychology, 13,* 357–372.

Kendall, P. C. (1991). Guiding theory for treating children and adolescents. In P. C. Kendall (Ed.), *Child and adolescent therapy: Cognitive-behavioral procedures* (pp. 3–24). New York: Guilford Press.

Kendall, P. C. (1992a). Childhood coping: Avoiding a lifetime of anxiety. *Behaviour Change, 9*, 1–8.

Kendall, P. C. (1992b). *Coping cat workbook.* Ardmore, PA: Workbook Publishing.

Kendall, P. C. (1994). Treating anxiety disorders in children: Results of a randomized clinical trial. *Journal of Consulting and Clinical Psychology, 62*, 100–110.

Kendall, P. C. (2000a). *Childhood disorders.* London: Psychology Press.

Kendall, P. C. (2000b). *Cognitive-behavioral therapy for anxious children: Therapist manual* (2nd ed.). Ardmore, PA: Workbook Publishing.

Kendall, P. C., Brady, E. U., & Verduin, T. L. (2001). Comorbidity in childhood anxiety disorders and treatment outcome. *Journal of the American Academy of Child and Adolescent Psychiatry, 40*, 787–794.

Kendall, P. C., & Choudhury, M. S. (2003). Children and adolescents in cognitive-behavioral therapy: Some past efforts and current advances, and the challenges in our future. *Cognitive Therapy and Research, 27*, 89–104.

Kendall, P. C., Choudhury, M., Chung, H. L, & Robin, J. A. (2002). Cognitive-behavioral approaches. In M. Lewis (Ed.), *Child and adolescent psychiatry* (pp. 154–164). Philadelphia: Lippincott Williams & Wilkins.

Kendall, P. C., Chu, B., Gifford, A., Hayes, C., & Nauta, M. (1998). Breathing life into a manual: Flexibility and creativity with manual-based treatments. *Cognitive and Behavioral Practice, 5*, 177–198.

Kendall, P. C., & DiPietro, M. (1995). *Terapia scolastica dell'ansia: Guida per psicologi e insegnanti.* Trento, Italy: Edizioni Erickson.

Kendall, P. C., & Flannery-Schroeder, E. C. (1998). Methodological issues in treatment research for anxiety disorders in youth. *Journal of Abnormal Child Psychology, 26*(1), 27–38.

Kendall, P. C., Flannery-Schroeder, E., Panichelli-Mindel, S., Southam-Gerow, M., Henin, A., & Warman, M. (1997). Therapy for youths with anxiety disorders: A second randomized clinical trial. *Journal of Consulting and Clinical Psychology, 65*, 366–380.

Kendall, P. C., & Hedtke, K. (2006a). *Cognitive-behavioral therapy for anxious children: Therapist manual* (3rd ed.). Ardmore, PA: Workbook Publishing.

Kendall, P. C., & Hedtke, K. (2006b). *Coping Cat workbook* (2nd ed.). Ardmore, PA: Workbook Publishing.

Kendall, P. C., & Ingram, R. (1987). The future for cognitive assessment of anxiety: Let's get specific. In L. Michelson & L. M. Ascher (Eds.), *Anxiety and stress disorders: Cognitive-behavioral assessment and treatment* (pp. 89–104). New York: Guilford Press.

Kendall, P. C., & Ingram, R. (1989). Cognitive-behavioral perspectives: Theory and research on depression and anxiety. In P. C. Kendall & D. Watson (Eds.), *Anxiety and depression: Distinction and overlapping features* (pp. 27–54). New York: Academic Press.

Kendall, P. C., & Marrs-Garcia, A. (1999). *Psychometric analyses of a therapy-sensitive measure: The Coping Questionnaire (CQ).* Manuscript submitted for publication.

Kendall, P. C., Marrs-Garcia, A., Nath, S., & Sheldrick, R. C. (1999). Normative comparisons for the evaluation of clinical significance. *Journal of Consulting and Clinical Psychology, 67*, 285–299.

Kendall, P. C., & Ollendick, T. H. (2004). Setting the research and practice agenda for anxiety in children and adolescence: A topic comes of age. *Cognitive and Behavioral Practice, 11*, 65–74.

Kendall, P. C., Puliafico, T. C., Barmish, A. J., Choudhury, M., & Henin, A. (2005). *Assessing anxiety with the Child Behavior Checklist and the Teacher Report Form.* Manuscript in preparation.

Kendall, P. C., Robin, J. A., Hedtke, K. A., Suveg, C., Flannery-Schroeder, E., & Gosch, E. (2005). Considering CBT with anxious youth? Think exposures. *Cognitive and Behavioral Practice, 12*, 136–150.

Kendall, P. C., & Ronan, K. R. (1990). Assessment of childhood anxieties, fears, and phobias: Cognitive-behavioral models and methods. In C. R. Reynolds & R. W. Kamphaus (Eds.), *Handbook of psychological and educational assessment of children: Personality, behavior, and context* (pp. 223–244). New York: Guilford Press.

Kendall, P. C., Safford, S., Flannery-Schroeder, E., & Webb, A. (2004). Child anxiety treatment: Outcomes in adolescence and impact on substance use and depression at 7.4-year follow-up. *Journal of Consulting and Clinical Psychology, 72*, 276–287.

Kendall, P. C., & Southam-Gerow, M. (1996). Long-term follow-up of treatment for anxiety disordered youth. *Journal of Consulting and Clinical Psychology, 65*, 883–888.

Kendall, P. C., & Watson, D. (Eds.). (1989). *Anxiety and depression: Distinctive and overlapping features.* San Diego, CA: Academic Press.

King, N. J., Hamilton, D. I., & Ollendick, T. H. (1988). *Children's phobias: A behavioral perspective.* London: Wiley.

Klein, R. G. (1991). Parent–child agreement in clinical assessment of anxiety and other psychopathology: A review. *Journal of Anxiety Disorders, 5*, 187–198.

Kleiner, L., Marshall, W. L., & Spevack, M. (1987). Training in problem-solving and exposure treatment for agoraphobics with panic attacks. *Journal of Anxiety Disorders, 1*, 219–238.

Koeppen, A. S. (1974). Relaxation training for children. *Elementary School Guidance and Counseling, 9*, 12–21.

Kondas, O. (1967). Reduction of examination anxiety and "stage fright" by group desensitization and relaxation. *Behaviour Research and Therapy, 5*, 275–281.

Kortlander, E., Kendall, P. C., & Panichelli-Mindel, S. M. (1997). Maternal expectations and attributions about coping in anxious children. *Journal of Anxiety Disorders, 11*, 297–315.

Krain, A. L., & Kendall, P. C. (2000). The role of parental emotional distress in parent report of child anxiety. *Journal of Clinical Child Psychology, 29*, 328–335.

Krohne, H. W., & Hock, M. (1991). Relationships between restrictive mother–child interactions and anxiety of the child. *Anxiety Research, 4*, 109–124.

Kuroda, J. (1969). Elimination of children's fears of animals by the method of experimental desensitization: An application of learning theory to child psychology. *Psychologia, 12*, 161–165.

Langley, A. K., Bergman, L., & Piacentini, J. C. (2002). Assessment of childhood anxiety. *International Review of Psychiatry, 14*, 102–113.

Last, C. G., Hansen, C., & Franco, N. (1998). Cognitive-behavioral treatment of school phobia. *Journal of the American Academy of Child and Adolescent Psychiatry, 37*, 404–411.

Last, C. G., Hersen, M., Kazdin, A. E., Francis, G., & Grubb, H. J. (1987). Psychiatric illness in the mothers of anxious children. *American Journal of Psychiatry, 144*, 1580–1583.

Last, C. G., Phillips, J. E., & Statfield, A. (1987). Childhood anxiety disorders in mothers and their children. *Child Psychiatry and Human Development, 18*, 103–112.

Last, C. G., Strauss, C. C., & Francis, G. (1987). Comorbidity among childhood anxiety disorders. *Journal of Nervous and Mental Disease, 175*, 726–730.

Lieb, R., Wittchen, H., Höfler, M., Fuetsch, M., Stein, M. B., & Merikangas, K. R. (2000). Parental psychopathology, parenting styles, and the risk of social phobia in offspring: A prospective-longitudinal community study. *Archives of General Psychiatry, 57*, 859–866.

Leitenberg, H., & Callahan, E. J. (1973). Reinforced practice and reduction of different kinds of fears in adults and children. *Behaviour Research and Therapy, 11*, 19–30.

Lewis, S. (1974). A comparison of behavior therapy techniques in the reduction of fearful avoidant behavior. *Behavior Therapy, 5*, 648–655.

Lonigan, C. J., Carey, M. P., & Finch, A. J. (1994). Anxiety and depression in children and adolescents: Negative affectivity and the utility of self-reports. *Journal of Consulting and Clinical Psychology, 62*, 1000–1008.

Mann, J., & Rosenthal, T. L. (1969). Vicarious and direct counter-conditioning of test anxiety through individual and group desensitization. *Behaviour Research and Therapy, 7,* 359–367.

Manassis, K., Mendlowitz, S. L., Scapillato, D., Avery, D., Fiksenbaum. L., Freire, M., et al. (2002). Group and individual cognitive-behavioral therapy for childhood anxiety disorders. A randomized trial. *Journal of the American Academy of Child and Adolescent Psychiatry. 41,* 1423–1430.

Mansdorf, I. J., & Lukens, E. (1987). Cognitive-behavioral psychotherapy for separation anxious children exhibiting school phobia. *Journal of the American Academy of Child and Adolescent Psychiatry, 26,* 222–225.

March, J. S., & Albano, A. M. (1998). New developments in assessing pediatric anxiety disorders. In T. Ollendick & R. Prinz (Eds.), *Advances in clinical child psychology* (Vol. 20, pp. 213–242). New York: Plenum Press.

March, J. S., & Mulle, K. (1998). *OCD in children and adolescents: A cognitive-behavioral treatment manual.* New York: Guilford Press.

March, J. S., Parker, J., Sullivan, K., Stallings, P., & Conners, C. (1997). The Multidimensional Anxiety Scale for Children (MASC): Factor structure, reliability, and validity. *Journal of the American Academy of Child and Adolescent Psychiatry, 36,* 554–565.

Marks, I. M. (1975). Behavioral treatments of phobic and obsessive–compulsive disorders: A critical appraisal. In M. Hersen, R. M. Eisler, & P. M. Miller (Eds.), *Progress in behavior modification* (Vol. 1, pp. 65–158). New York: Academic Press.

Masia, C. L., Klein, R. G., Storch, E. A., & Corda, B. (2001). School-based behavioral treatment for social anxiety disorder in adolescents: Results of a pilot study. *Journal of the American Academy of Child and Adolescent Psychiatry, 40,* 780–786.

Melamed, B. G., & Siegel, L. J. (1975). Reduction of anxiety in children facing hospitalization and surgery by use of filmed modeling. *Journal of Consulting and Clinical Psychology, 43,* 511–521.

Mendlowitz, S. L., Manassis, K., Bradley, S., Scapillato, D., Miezitis, S., & Shaw, B. F. (1999). Cognitive-behavioral group treatments in childhood anxiety disorders: The role of parental involvement. *Journal of the American Academy of Child and Adolescent Psychiatry, 38,* 1223–1229.

Menzies, R. G., & Clarke, J. C. (1993). A comparison of *in vivo* and vicarious exposure in the treatment of childhood water phobia. *Behaviour Research and Therapy, 31,* 9–15.

Miller, L. C., Barrett, C. L., Hampe, E., & Noble, H. (1972). Comparison of reciprocal inhibition, psychotherapy, and waiting list control for phobic children. *Journal of Abnormal Psychology, 79,* 269–279.

Muris, P., Merckelbach, H., Ollendick, T., King, N., & Bogie, N. (2002). Three traditional and three new childhood anxiety questionnaires: Their reliability and validity in a normal adolescent sample. *Behaviour Research and Therapy, 40,* 753–772.

Murphy, C. M., & Bootzin, R. R. (1973). Active and passive participation in the contact desensitization of snake fear in children. *Behavior Therapy, 4,* 203–211.

Nauta, M., Scholing, A., Emmelkamp, P., & Minderaa, R. (2003). Cognitive-behavioral therapy for children with anxiety disorders in a clinical setting: No additional effect of a cognitive parent training. *Journal of the American Academy of Child and Adolescent Psychiatry, 42,* 1270–1278.

Neal, A. M., & Turner, S. M. (1991). Anxiety disorders research with African Americans: Current status. *Psychological Bulletin, 109,* 400–410.

Ollendick, T. H. (1983). Reliability and validity of the Revised Fear Survey Schedule for Children (FSSC-R). *Behaviour Research and Therapy, 21,* 685–692.

Ollendick, T. H. (1995). Cognitive behavioral treatment of panic disorder with agoraphobia in adolescents: A multiple baseline design analysis. *Behavior Therapy, 26,* 517–531.

Ollendick, T. H., & Cerny, J. A. (1981). *Clinical behavior therapy with children.* New York: Plenum Press.

Ollendick, T. H., & Francis, G. (1988). Behavioral assessment and treatment of childhood phobias. *Behavior Modification, 12,* 165–204.

Ollendick, T. H., & King, N. J. (1998). Empirically supported treatments for children with phobic and anxiety disorders: Current status. *Journal of Clinical Child Psychology, 27,* 156–167.

Ollendick, T. H., King, N. J., & Frary, R. B. (1989). Fears in children and adolescents: Reliability and generalizability across gender, age, and nationality. *Behaviour Research and Therapy, 27,* 19–26.

Ollendick, T. H., Matson, J. L., & Helsel, W. J. (1985). Fears in children and adolescents: Normative data. *Behaviour Research and Therapy, 23,* 465–467.

Parker, G. (1983). *Parental overprotection: A risk factor in psychosocial development.* New York: Grune & Stratton.

Perrin, S., & Last, C. G. (1992). Do childhood anxiety measures measure anxiety? *Journal of Abnormal Child Psychology, 20,* 567–578.

Peterson, L. (1989). Coping by children undergoing stressful medical procedures: Some conceptual, methodological, and therapeutic issues. *Journal of Consulting and Clinical Psychology, 57,* 380–387.

Piacentini, J., & Bergman, R. L. (2001). Developmental issues in cognitive therapy for childhood anxiety disorders. *Journal of Cognitive Psychotherapy, 15,* 165–182.

Piacentini, J., Gitow, A., Jaffer, M., & Graae, F., & Whitaker, A. (1994). Outpatient behavioral treatment of child and adolescent obsessive compulsive disorder. *Journal of Anxiety Disorders, 8,* 277–289.

Pincus, D. (2000). *I Can Relax! CD for children.* Boston: Child Anxiety Network.

Puig-Antich, J., & Chambers, W. (1978). *The Schedule for Affective Disorders and Schizophrenia for School-Age Children (Kiddie-SADS).* New York: New York State Psychiatric Institute.

Quay, H. C. (1977). Measuring dimensions of deviant behavior: The Behavior Problem Checklist. *Journal of Abnormal Child Psychology, 5,* 277–289.

Rapee, R. (2000). Group treatment of children with anxiety disorders: Outcome and predictors of treatment response. *Australian Journal of Psychology, 52,* 125–129.

Reynolds, C. R., & Paget, K. D. (1983). National normative and reliability data for the Revised Children's Manifest Anxiety Scale. *School Psychology Review, 12,* 324–336.

Reynolds, C. R., & Richmond, B. O. (1978). What I Think and Feel: A revised measure of children's manifest anxiety. *Journal of Abnormal Psychology, 6,* 271–280.

Reynolds, C. R., & Richmond, B. O. (1979). Factor structure and construct validity of "What I Think and Feel": The Revised Children's Manifest Anxiety Scale. *Journal of Personality Assessment, 43,* 281–283.

Reynolds, C. R., & Richmond, B. (1997). *Revised Children's Manifest Anxiety Scale.* Los Angeles: Western Psychological Services.

Ritter, B. (1968). The group desensitization of children's snake phobias using vicarious and contact desensitization procedures. *Behaviour Research and Therapy, 6,* 1–6.

Ronan, K. R., & Kendall, P. C. (1997). Self-talk in distressed youth: States-of-mind and content specificity. *Journal of Clinical Child Psychology, 26,* 330–337.

Ronan, K., Kendall, P., & Rowe, M. (1994). Negative affectivity in children: Development and validation of a self-statement questionnaire. *Cognitive Therapy and Research, 18,* 509–528.

Ross, C., Ross, S., & Evans, T. (1971). The modification of extreme social withdrawal with guided practice. *Journal of Behavior Therapy and Experimental Psychiatry, 2,* 273–279.

The RUPP Anxiety Group. (2002). The Pediatric Anxiety Rating Scale: Development and psychometric properties. *Journal of the American Academy of Child and Adolescent Psychiatry, 41,* 1061–1069.

Scherer, M. W., & Nakamura, C. Y. (1968). A Fear Survey Schedule for Children (FSS-FC): A factor analytic comparison with manifest anxiety (CMAS). *Behaviour Research and Therapy, 6,* 173–182.

Schniering, C. A., Hudson, J. L, & Rapee, R. M. (2000). Issues in the diagnosis and assessment of anxiety disorders in children and adolescents. *Clinical Psychology Review, 20,* 453–478.

Shaffer, D., Fisher, P., Lucas, C. P., Dulcan, M. K., & Schwab-Stone, M. E. (2000). NIMH Diagnostic Interview Schedule for Children—Version IV (NIMH DISC-IV): Description, differences from previous versions, and reliability of some common diagnoses. *Journal of the American Academy of Child and Adolescent Psychiatry, 39,* 28–38.

Sheslow, D. V., Bondy, A. S., & Nelson, R. O. (1982). A comparison of graduated exposure, verbal coping skills, and their combination in the treatment of children's fear of the dark. *Child and Family Behavior Therapy, 4,* 33–45.

Shirk, S. R., & Karver, M. (2003). Prediction of treatment outcome from relationship variables in child and adolescent therapy: A meta-analytic review. *Journal of Consulting and Clinical Psychology, 71,* 452–464.

Shortt, A. L., Barrett, P. M., & Fox, T. L. (2001). Evaluating the FRIENDS program: A cognitive-behavioral group treatment for anxious children and their parents. *Journal of Clinical Child Psychology, 30,* 525–535.

Silverman, W., Kurtines, W., Ginsburg, G., Weems, C., Lumpkin, P., & Carmichael, D. (1999). Treating anxiety disorders in children with group cognitive-behavioral therapy: A randomized clinical trial. *Journal of Consulting and Clinical Psychology, 67,* 995–1003.

Silverman, W. K. (1991). *Guide to the use of the Anxiety Disorders Interview Schedule for Children—Revised* (child and parent versions). Albany, NY: Graywind.

Silverman, W. K., & Albano, A. M. (1996). *The Anxiety Disorders Interview Schedule for Children (DSM-IV).* San Antonio, TX: Psychological Corporation.

Silverman, W. K., & Kurtines, W. M. (1996). *Anxiety and phobic disorders: A pragmatic approach.* New York: Plenum Press.

Silverman, W. K., & Ollendick, T. H. (1999). *Developmental issues in the clinical treatment of children.* Boston: Allyn & Bacon.

Silverman, W. K., & Rabian, B. (1995). Test–retest reliability of the DSM-III-R childhood anxiety disorders symptoms using the Anxiety Disorders Interview Schedule for Children. *Journal of Anxiety Disorders, 9,* 139–150.

Silverman, W. K., Saavedra, M. S., & Pina, A. A. (2001). Test–retest reliability of anxiety symptoms and diagnoses with the Anxiety Disorders Interview Schedule for DSM-IV: Child and parent versions. *Journal of the American Academy of Child and Adolescent Psychiatry, 40*(8), 937–944.

Siqueland, L., & Diamond, G. (1998). Engaging parents in cognitive behavioral treatment for children with anxiety disorders. *Cognitive Behavioral Practice, 5,* 81–102.

Siqueland, L., Kendall, P. C., & Steinberg, L. (1996). Anxiety in children: Perceived family environments and observed family interaction. *Journal of Child Clinical Psychology, 25,* 225–237.

Skinner, H. A., Steinhauer, P. D., & Santa-Barbara, J. (1983). The Family Assessment Measure. *Canadian Journal of Community Mental Health, 2,* 91–105.

Skinner, H. A., Steinhauer, P. D., & Santa-Barbara, J. (1995). *The Family Assessment Measure Version III—Technical manual.* Toronto, ON, Canada: Multi-Health Systems.

Southam-Gerow, M. A., Flannery-Schroeder, E. C., & Kendall, P. C. (2003). A psychometric evaluation of the parent report form of the State-Trait Anxiety Inventory for Children—Trait Version. *Journal of Anxiety Disorders, 17,* 427–446.

Southam-Gerow, M., & Kendall, P. C. (2000). A preliminary study of the emotion understanding of youths referred for treatment of anxiety disorders. *Journal of Child Clinical Psychology, 29,* 319–327.

Southam-Gerow, M. A., & Kendall, P. C. (2002). Emotion regulation and understanding: Implications for child psychopathology and therapy. *Clinical Psychology Review, 22,* 189–222.

Southam-Gerow, M. A., Kendall, P. C., & Weersing, V. R. (2001). Examining outcome variability: Correlates of treatment response in a child and adolescent anxiety clinic. *Journal of Clinical Child Psychology, 30,* 422–436.

Spence, S. H., Donovan, C., & Brechman-Toussaint, M. (2000). The treatment of childhood social phobia: The effectiveness of a social skills training-based, cognitive-behavioral intervention, with and without parental involvement. *Journal of Child Psychology and Psychiatry, 41,* 713–726.

Spielberger, C. (1973). *Preliminary manual for the State–Trait Anxiety Inventory for Children ("How I Feel Questionnaire").* Palo Alto, CA: Consulting Psychologists Press.

Spielberger, C. D., Edwards, C. D., & Lushene, R. E. (1973). *State–Trait Anxiety Inventory for Children.* Palo Alto, CA: Consulting Psychologists Press.

Spivack, G., & Shure, M. (1974). *A problem-solving approach to children's adjustment.* San Francisco: Jossey-Bass.

Stallings, P., & March, J. S. (1995). Assessment. In J. S. March (Ed.), *Anxiety disorders in children and adolescents* (pp. 125–147). New York: Guilford Press.

Stark, K. D., Humphrey, L. L., Crook, K., & Lewis, K. (1990). Perceived family environments of depressed and anxious children: Child's and maternal figure's perspectives. *Journal of Abnormal Child Psychology, 18,* 527–547.

Strauss, C. (1987). *Modification of trait portion of State–Trait Anxiety Inventory for Children—Parent Form.* Gainesville: University of Florida.

Suveg, C., Roblek, T., Robin, J., Krain, A., Ginsburg, G., & Aschebrand, A. (in press). Parental involvement when conducting cognitive-behavioral therapy for children with anxiety disorder. *Journal of Cognitive Psychotherapy: An International Journal.*

Suveg, C., & Zeman, J. (2004). Emotion regulation in children with anxiety disorders. *Journal of Clinical Child and Adolescent Psychology, 33,* 750–759.

Suveg, C., Zeman, J., Flannery-Schroeder, E., & Cassano, M. (2005). Emotion socialization in families of children with an anxiety disorder. *Journal of Abnormal Child Psychology, 33,* 145–155.

Treadwell, K. H., Flannery-Schroeder, E. C., & Kendall, P. C. (1994). Ethnicity and gender in a sample of clinic-referred anxious children: Adaptive functioning, diagnostic status, and treatment outcome. *Journal of Anxiety Disorders, 9,* 373–384.

Treadwell, K. H., & Kendall, P. C. (1996). Self-talk in anxiety-disordered youth: States-of-mind, content specificity, and treatment outcome. *Journal of Consulting and Clinical Psychology, 64,* 941–950.

Ultee, C. A., Griffioen, D., & Schellekens, J. (1982). The reduction of anxiety in children: A comparison of the effects of "systematic desensitization *in vitro*" and "systematic desensitization *in vivo.*" *Behaviour Research and Therapy, 20,* 61–67.

Verduin, T. L., & Kendall, P. C. (2003). Differential occurrence of comorbidity within childhood anxiety disorders. *Journal of Clinical Child and Adolescent Psychology, 32,* 290–295.

Verhulst, F. C., Althaus, M., & Berden, G. F. (1987). Psychopathology in the offspring of anxiety disordered patients. *Journal of Consulting and Clinical Psychology, 55,* 229–235.

Weisman, D., Ollendick, T. H., & Horne, A. M. (1978). *A comparison of muscle relaxation techniques with children.* Unpublished manuscript, Indiana State University, Terre Haute.

Weisz, J. R., & Weiss, B. (1991). Studying the "referability" of child clinical problems. *Journal of Consulting and Clinical Psychology, 59,* 266–273.

Wells, K. C., & Virtulano, L. A., (1984). Anxiety disorders in childhood. In S. E. Turner (Ed.), *Behavioral theories and treatment of anxiety* (pp. 413–439). New York: Plenum Press.

Werry, J. S. (1986). Diagnosis and assessment. In R. Gittelman (Ed.), *Anxiety disorders of childhood* (pp. 73–100). New York: Guilford Press.

Whaley, S. E., Pinto, A., & Sigman, M. (1999). Characterizing interactions between anxious mothers and their children. *Journal of Consulting and Clinical Psychology, 67,* 826–836.

Wood, J. J., McLeod, B. D., Sigman, M., Hwang, W., & Chu, B. C. (2003). Parenting and childhood anxiety: Theory, empirical findings, and future directions. *Journal of Child Psychology and Psychiatry, 44,* 134–151.

Wood, J. J., Piacentini, J. C., Bergman, R. L., McCracken, J., & Barrios, V. (2002). Concurrent validity of the anxiety disorders section of the Anxiety Disorders Interview Schedule for DSM-IV: Child and parent versions. *Journal of Clinical Child and Adolescent Psychology, 31*(3), 335–342.

Woodward, L. J., & Fergusson, D. M. (2001). Life course outcomes of young people with anxiety disorders in adolescence. *Journal of the American Academy of Child and Adolescent Psychiatry, 40,* 1086–1093.

PART IV

SPECIAL POPULATIONS

CHAPTER 8

Cognitive-Behavioral Therapy for Youth with Obsessive–Compulsive Disorder

JOHN C. PIACENTINI, JOHN S. MARCH,
and MARTIN E. FRANKLIN

Obsessive–compulsive disorder (OCD) is a chronic and often impairing condition in children and adolescents. Once thought to be rare, recent epidemiological data suggest the prevalence of childhood OCD to range from 0.5 to 2% (Apter et al., 1993; Rapoport et al., 2000; Valleni-Basile et al., 1994), and up to one-half of adults with OCD develop the disorder during childhood or adolescence (Rasmussen & Eisen, 1990). Although ample evidence supports the efficacy of both cognitive-behavioral therapy (CBT) and psychopharmacological approaches for the treatment of OCD in adults, the treatment of childhood OCD has garnered much less attention. This situation is unfortunate, given that early intervention has the potential to not only ameliorate suffering in youngsters with the disorder but also prevent the development of long-term morbidity associated with progression of the illness into adulthood. Fortunately, over the past decade, an emerging literature has demonstrated the efficacy of both CBT and psychopharmacological interventions for OCD in children and adolescents. However, findings from the head-to-head comparison of these two monotherapies in both children (de Haan, Hoogduin, Buitelaar, & Keijsers, 1998;

Pediatric OCD Treatment Study Team, 2004) and adults (Abramowitz, 1997) with regard to efficacy, safety, and durability of response have led to the consensus recommendation that CBT be considered as the initial treatment of choice for OCD across the age span (Albano, March, & Piacentini, 1999; March, Frances, Carpenter, & Kahn, 1997). Also of note, and in spite of widespread clinical use, psychodynamic, supportive, and non-CBT family treatments have not proven effective for children, adolescents, or adults with OCD (March, Leonard, & Swedo, 1995; Salzman & Thaler, 1981).

   The initial section of this chapter provides an overview of the phenomenology and assessment of childhood OCD, highlighting those aspects most relevant to cognitive-behavioral treatment. Following this, we present the cognitive-behavioral conceptualization of OCD, describe the implementation of CBT for childhood OCD, and review the evidence supporting the use of this treatment approach with these youngsters.

PHENOMENOLOGICAL ASPECTS OF CHILDHOOD OCD

The *Diagnostic and Statistical Manual of Mental Disorders*, fourth edition, text revision (DSM-IV-TR; American Psychiatric Association, 2000) describes the essential features of OCD as obsessions and/or compulsions that are distressing, time-consuming (take more than 1 hour per day), or cause significant interference in normal functioning. Obsessions are recurrent, persistent, intrusive, and distressing thoughts, images, or impulses, whereas compulsions are defined as repetitive behaviors or mental acts performed in response to an obsession and designed to reduce distress or avoid some perceived harm. Although OCD presents as a relatively heterogeneous disorder in childhood, some symptoms are more commonly seen than others. The most common obsessions in children and adolescents with OCD relate to fears of harm or other negative outcomes to self and others and concerns with germs, contamination, and illness. Sexual, religious, superstitious (e.g., lucky/unlucky numbers, colors, or words) and somatic obsessions as well as obsessions related to scrupulosity, symmetry, and fear of humiliation are less frequent but not uncommon (Geller et al., 2001; Swedo, Rapoport, Leonard, Lenane, & Cheslow, 1989). Ritualized and/ or excessive washing, cleaning, and checking are the most commonly seen compulsions, although excessive or ritualized repeating, arranging and ordering, confessing, and seeking reassurance are also relatively common. Common mental rituals include praying and mental counting or arranging. The specific content of a given child's symptoms may vary over time (e.g., repeating symptoms may give way to contamination fears), although the absolute number of symptoms may remain relatively constant (Rettew, Swedo, Leonard, Lenane, & Rapport, 1992). The vast majority of children and adolescents with OCD experience both obsessions and compulsions, with compulsions in the absence of obsessions somewhat more common than obsessions only. It is important to note that, although DSM-IV classifies OCD as an anxiety disorder, not all youngsters describe their symptoms as anxiety-related. Many children report engaging in rituals to alleviate feelings of disgust, discomfort, incompleteness, or the sense that something just doesn't feel right.

The typical age of onset reported for samples of youth meeting the criteria for OCD ranges from 8 to 11 years (Hanna, 1995; Piacentini, Bergman, Keller, & McCracken, 2003; Rapport, Swedo, & Leonard, 1992; Riddle et al., 1990), although children with an onset of as young as 2–3 years old have been reported. Boys are typically overrepresented in clinical samples by about a 3:2 ratio, although the gender distribution tends to even out beginning in adolescence (Swedo et al., 1989).

Comorbid mental health disorders are present in up to 75% of children and adolescents with OCD (Geller et al., 2000; Geller, Biederman, et al., 2001; Hanna, 1995; Rapoport et al., 2000). At a specialty clinic for youth with OCD, a consecutive series of 151 youngsters with primary OCD were found to have a psychiatric comorbidity rate of 68% (Piacentini, Bergman et al., 2003). Consistent with past reports, other anxiety disorders, most notably, generalized anxiety disorder, were the most common comorbid condition (38%), although disruptive behavioral disorders (ADHD, CD, ODD, 19%), tic disorders (13%), and major depression/dysthymia (13%) were also frequently seen. As will be discussed further in this chapter, a thorough diagnostic assessment is recommended for all youngsters presenting with OCD, because comorbidity, especially when undetected, may complicate treatment by negatively impacting the child's level of focus during treatment as well as his or her treatment motivation and/or compliance.

Childhood OCD can have a significant negative impact on psychosocial functioning (Geller et al., 2000; Piacentini, Bergman, et al., 2003). The most common impairments are seen at home and with family members (for example, doing chores, getting ready for bed, bathing and grooming, getting along with other family members) and school (for example, concentrating on schoolwork, completing homework and in-class assignments), although illness-related social problems are often seen as well (Piacentini, Bergman, et al., 2003). OCD in childhood follows a variable yet chronic course. Follow-up studies of clinical samples provide relatively consistent evidence for the chronicity of childhood-onset OCD, with approximately 40% of OCD youngsters meeting diagnostic criteria for the disorder up to 15 years after initial identification and with another 20% evidencing subclinical disturbance (Leonard et al., 1993; Stewart et al., 2004). However, because many of the youngsters in these follow-up studies did not have the benefit of adequate treatment, existing follow-up data may paint an overly pessimistic picture regarding the chronicity of OCD in children.

ASSESSMENT OF CHILDHOOD OCD

The initial evaluation of a child or adolescent with OCD should include careful evaluation of current and past OCD symptoms, current OCD symptom severity, OCD-related functional impairment, and ascertainment of any comorbid psychopathology (March & Franklin, 2006). A careful diagnostic evaluation is necessary to accurately establish the presence of OCD, rule out phenomenologically similar conditions, and identify any coexisting problems that may influence treatment planning (Langley, Bergman, & Piacentini, 2002). In addition to collecting information about symptoms and associated interference, it is also important to evaluate the strengths of the child and his or her family. Several standardized self-report and clinician-administered measures are available for these purposes and are briefly described below.

It is often helpful to mail a packet of self-report questionnaires ascertaining history of medical and mental health problems, including history of OCD symptoms and treatment, psychosocial functioning, and possible comorbid problems, for the family to complete prior to the initial appointment. Review of these materials prior to meeting with the child can facilitate the identification of potential problem areas, such as comorbid depression or hyperactivity, which can be more carefully evaluated during the intake process. The primary assessment tools for assessing OCD in children are the Anxiety Disorders Interview Schedule for DSM-IV—Parent and Child Version (ADIS-IV: PC; Silverman & Albano, 1996) to establish the OCD diagnosis as well as identify other diagnostic comorbidities and the Children's Yale–Brown Obsessive Compulsive Scale (CY-BOCS; Goodman, Price, Rasmussen, Riddle, & Rapoport, 1991; Scahill et al., 1997) to ascertain the profile of OCD symptoms and severity of the disorders. These measures, along with a handful of other instruments, are briefly described below.

Anxiety Disorders Interview for Children

The child and adolescent ADIS is a semistructured interview for assessing DSM-IV anxiety disorders and related diagnoses in youngsters, ages 8–17 years (Silverman & Albano, 1996). The child ADIS possesses excellent psychometric properties for the internalizing disorders relative to other available diagnostic instruments (Silverman, Saavedra, & Pina, 2001; Wood, Piacentini, Bergman, McCracken, & Barrios, 2002). The ADIS uses a semistructured format that allows the clinician to draw information from both independent parent- and child-reports and clinical observations. Scores are derived regarding (1) the specific diagnoses and (2) the level of diagnosis-related interference. In addition to generating diagnoses, interviewers complete an eight-point clinical severity rating (CSR) that provides a dimensional measure of severity/impairment for each positive diagnosis (Silverman & Albano, 1996). The child ADIS is the preferred instrument for treatment studies and other clinical research with anxious children and adolescents (see also Kendall & Suveg, Chapter 7, this volume).

Children's Yale–Brown Obsessive Compulsive Scale

The CY-BOCS is a clinician-rated instrument that is scored on the basis of combined information from observation and parent- and child-report (Goodman et al., 1991). The initial section of the CY-BOCS uses a checklist format to ascertain the presence or absence of a comprehensive list of obsessions and compulsions. Findings from the checklist can be used as the basis for creating a symptom hierarchy for use in sequencing exposures later in treatment. Following completion of the checklist, the clinician separately rates the child's collective obsessions and compulsions on the following five dimensions: time spent, interference, distress, resistance, and control. Separate scores, ranging from 0 to 20, are obtained for obsessions and compulsions and then combined to yield a total score ranging from 0 to 40. The CY-BOCS is considered the primary clinical measure of OCD severity and, similar to the adult version of the instrument (Goodman et al., 1989), has been shown to possess adequate overall psychometric properties (Scahill et al., 1997). However, questions remain about the factor structure of the instrument in children and adolescents as well as the reliability of the resistance and control components (McKay et al., 2003). A total score of 16 or greater is typically used to indicate clinically significant OCD.

Child OCD Impact Scale

The Child OCD Impact Scale (COIS) is a self-report questionnaire assessing OCD-related functional impairment (Piacentini, Bergman, et al., 2003). From a treatment perspective, the COIS provides complementary information to the CY-BOCS by examining the extent to which changes in symptom severity translate into enhanced psychosocial functioning. Parallel parent and child versions consist of three factors assessing OCD-related impairment in the family, academic, and social environments. A total score is generated by summing the individual factor scores. The COIS has favorable psychometric properties (Piacentini, Jaffer, Bergman, McCracken, & Keller, 2001), including sensitivity to treatment response (Geller, Hoog, et al., 2001; Liebowitz et al., 2002). A shorter version of the measure is currently undergoing additional psychometric evaluation.

Multidimensional Anxiety Scale for Children

The Multidimensional Anxiety Scale for Children (MASC; March, Parker, Sullivan, Stallings, & Conners, 1997) is a child self-report rating scale consisting of four factors and six subfactors—physical anxiety (tense/restless, somatic/auto-nomic), harm avoidance (perfectionism, anxious coping), social anxiety (humilia-tion/rejection, performance anxiety), and separation anxiety. It provides an excellent dimensional measure of comorbid anxiety severity. The MASC pos-sesses excellent psychometric properties in both clinical and school samples, as well as a nationally derived normative sample (March, Frances, Carpenter, & Kahn, 1997).

Children's Depression Inventory

The Children's Depression Inventory (CDI) is a 27-item self-report scale avail-able in both parent and child versions that measures cognitive, affective, behav-ioral, and interpersonal symptoms of depression (Kovacs, 1996). The CDI shows adequate reliability and validity and is used to assess the severity of potential comorbid depressive symptoms, which assists in tailoring the treatment plan.

TREATMENT OF CHILDHOOD OCD

Our presentation of the treatment approaches for OCD in youth will first cover the behavioral and the cognitive conceptualizations of the disorder and their related intervention strategies. The family and developmental factors associated with OCD in youth are next described and considered, followed by illustrations of the application of treatment strategies and a review of the treatment outcome literature.

Behavioral Conceptualization of OCD

The behavioral conceptualization of OCD views obsessions as intrusive, un-wanted thoughts, images, or urges that trigger a significant and rapid increase in anxiety, and views compulsions as overt behavior or cognition (covert behavior) designed to reduce these negative feelings (Albano et al., 1999). Based on learn-ing theory, compulsions are negatively reinforced over time by their ability to reduce the obsession-triggered distress. Moreover, the more successful the com-pulsive behaviors are at reducing distress, the more powerful they become (the obsessive–compulsive cycle). As an example, a child with an obsessive fear of harm befalling him or his family may become distressed when he thinks that the front door of the house is unlocked. This distress triggers a strong desire to check the door to make sure it is locked (compulsion). Each time the child carries out the compulsion (i.e., checks the lock), the resulting reduction in distress serves to strengthen the checking ritual in the same way that a positive reward can be used to strengthen the action that precedes it. The obsessive–compulsive cycle is graphically displayed in Figure 8.1.

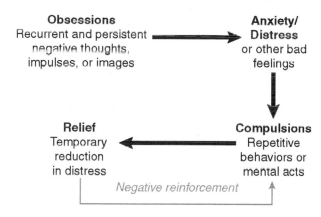

FIGURE 8.1. The obsessive–compulsive cycle. From Piacentini & Langley (2004). Copyright 2004 by Wiley Periodicals, Inc. Reprinted by permission.

Exposure plus Response Prevention

The most effective form of behavior therapy, exposure plus response prevention (ERP), was developed many years ago by Meyer (1966). ERP entails systematically triggering an individual's obsessive fear through either *in vivo* or imaginal exposure to feared objects or situations (exposure) while simultaneously encouraging him or her to not engage in the specific rituals or compulsions designed to reduce the obsession-triggered distress (response prevention) (Kozak & Foa, 1997; Meyer, 1966). Research with adult OCD patients suggests that both exposure and response prevention are necessary, with exposure reducing phobic anxiety and response prevention reducing rituals (Foa, Steketee, Grayson, Turner, & Latimer, 1984). ERP typically progresses in gradual fashion (e.g., graded exposure), based on a hierarchy of obsessive and compulsive symptoms arranged from least to most distressing (symptom hierarchy). Milder symptoms are usually exposed first, followed by more difficult exposures as treatment progresses. In most cases, exposures are developed and initially practiced in session, with the child then assigned to practice ERP in his or her natural environment. As would be expected, most treatment gains accrue from repeated practice in the natural environment.

Imaginal exposure tasks, whereby youngsters imagine themselves confronting feared situations, are used to address exposures unable to be re-created in the therapy setting. For example, a youngster with obsessive fears of harming another person might be asked to imagine him- or herself doing just that. Imaginal exposure can also be used for in-session practice of obsessions specific to a given situation or place, or as the first step in addressing symptoms the child perceives as too difficult for *in vivo* exposure. Imaginal exposure tasks are also an effective tool for addressing obsessions occurring in the absence of corresponding compulsions.

The most commonly proposed mechanism for ERP effectiveness is that, over repeated exposures, associated anxiety dissipates through the process of autonomic habituation while response prevention leads to extinction of the negative reinforcement properties of the associated compulsion. In addition, successful completion of exposures facilitates the development and storage of corrective cognitive information pertaining to the feared situation (Foa & Kozak, 1986). In other words, as their obsession-triggered fear dissipates in the absence of the associated compulsion, youngsters come to learn that the feared consequence of not ritualizing is not going to happen.

Cognitive Conceptualization of Childhood OCD

Salkovkis (1985, 1989) and other cognitive theorists (e.g., Freeston & Ladouceur, 1993; Shafran, 1997) emphasize cognitive factors as important etiological and maintaining factors for OCD in adults. The most important of these factors include distorted cognitive appraisals of risk, an inflated sense of responsibility for harm, and pathological levels of self-doubt. OCD in adults has also been related to the concept of thought–action fusion (TAF), which is defined as the tendency for individuals to view negative thoughts and actions as equivalent and see both as equally bad (Rachman, 1993). As a result of these processes, individuals with OCD are thought less able to ignore intrusive negative thoughts and more likely to react with increased anxiety and the strong desire to engage in neutralizing behavior. Numerous studies using adult samples have demonstrated reasonable support for the relationship between the cognitive biases of increased responsibility, probability, and severity of harm and clinical levels of OCD or subclinical OCD characteristics (Foa & Kozak, 1986; Lopatka & Rachman, 1995; Rheaume, Ladouceur, Freeston, & Letarte, 1994, 1995; Steketee & Frost, 1994).

The extent to which existing cognitive theories apply to childhood OCD is less clear but in need of further investigation (Comer, Kendall, Franklin, Hudson, & Pimentel, 2004). Barrett and Healy (2003) found that youngsters with OCD demonstrate the same pattern of cognitive distortions as adults; however, the OCD group was relatively indistinguishable from a comparison group of children with non-OCD anxiety. Moreover, these authors did not find an association between higher levels of experimentally induced perceived responsibility and increases in perceived distress or threat probability and harm (Barrett & Healy-Farrell, 2003). Although likely complicated by differences in the level of cognitive development between children and adults, the cognitive processes potentially underlying childhood OCD remain complicated. Given the potential treatment ramifications of a greater understanding of these processes, additional research in this area is sorely needed.

Cognitive Intervention for Childhood OCD

Despite of the level of support for existing cognitive models of OCD, at least in adults, the incremental validity of adding a cognitive intervention to ERP remains unclear. Although some studies of adult OCD have found cognitive intervention to be efficacious (e.g., Abramowitz, 1997; van Balkom et al., 1998), more recent work (Vogel, Stiles, & Gotestam, 2004) comparing ERP plus cognitive therapy to ERP plus relaxation training found that ERP/cognitive therapy reduced treatment dropout but did not enhance outcomes, using an intent-to-treat analytic strategy. The incremental efficacy of cognitive therapy for childhood OCD has yet to be examined. Barrett and Healy-Farrell (2003) found a family CBT intervention to significantly reduce child ratings of perceived responsibility for harm; however, all youngsters received both behavioral and cognitive aspects of the intervention, making it impossible to determine the specific impact of individual treatment components.

In spite of limited empirical support, however, the inclusion of cognitive techniques, primarily as a means of enhancing compliance with ERP (Soechting & March, 2002), has become somewhat standard in the treatment of childhood OCD. The most commonly used strategies include (1) constructive self-talk, (2) cognitive restructuring, and (3) cultivating nonattachment (i.e., minimizing the obsessional aspects of thought suppression) (March & Franklin, 2006). The overall goals of cognitive intervention are to teach youngsters how to more accurately evaluate the likelihood that the feared consequences of not ritualizing will occur and how to recognize and relabel obsessions in a nonreactive fashion. It is important that the cognitive intervention be individualized to match the specific symptoms of the child in question as well as his or her cognitive abilities and developmental stage. Moreover, cognitive techniques are used to support and complement ERP for a given child rather than to serve as a replacement for it (Franklin & Foa, 2002).

Family Factors in the Treatment of Childhood OCD

Although the empirical literature examining familial aspects of childhood OCD is limited, findings from recent studies are consistent with observations derived from substantial clinical experience attesting to the impact of family context on OCD expression and the impact of the child's symptoms on family functioning (Piacentini & Langley, 2004; Waters & Barrett, 2000). OCD, especially the child-onset variant, is considered to have a strong genetic component (Nestadt et al., 2000, 2001), with claims of up to 50% of childhood cases being familial in nature (Pauls & Alsobrook, 1999). These children also have a shared environment. Thus, there is a significant likelihood that youngsters presenting for treatment of OCD will have a parent or other immediate family member who is similarly affected. Parental OCD, or other anxiety disorders, can seriously complicate treatment for the child, especially if the parent either inadvertently or intentionally reinforces the child's fears and ritualistic or avoidant behavior. Families of children with OCD have been shown to be less likely to use positive problem solving and reward independence in their children than the families of comparison youngsters (Barrett, Shortt, & Healy, 2002) and to exhibit higher rates of expressed emotion and parent–child conflict (Hibbs, Hamburger, & Lenane, 1991; Riddle et al., 1990). In addition, both children with OCD and their parents report that the illness has a significant negative impact on parent–child and child–sibling relationships (Barrett, Rasmussen, & Healy, 2001; Piacentini, Bergman, et al., 2003). Children with OCD quite commonly involve other family members, typically parents, in their rituals, with excessive reassurance seeking most commonly seen. In severe cases, such involvement can result in distorted family roles and relationships, negative feelings toward the affected child by family members, and heightened levels of family conflict.

Although not well studied in youngsters with OCD, family functioning may be an important predictor of both initial response to treatment and long-term outcome. Leonard and colleagues (1993) found the presence of parental psychopathology to predict a poorer long-term outcome in children with OCD, whereas high emotional reactivity and negative family perceptions about OCD have both been associated with worse treatment response for adults with the disorder (Livingston-Van Noppen, Rasmussen, Eisen, & McCartney, 1990; Steketee, 1990). Although Knox, Albano, and Barlow (1996) concluded from a multiple baseline design study with four subjects that parental involvement enhanced child response to treatment, the incremental benefit of involving parents or other family members in the child's treatment for OCD remains to be fully evaluated in a randomized controlled evaluation. Nevertheless, in situations where the child's OCD is complicated by parental or sibling OCD or other psychopathology, a negative pattern of parent–child interaction, or other maladaptive aspects of the family environment, some level of family participation in the child's treatment is likely necessary (Albano, Knox, & Barlow, 1995; Barrett, Healy, Piacentini, & March, 2004; Piacentini & Langley, 2004). The exact nature of the family intervention will vary from case to case, but the most important targets include correcting negative attributions about the affected child, reducing parent and/or sibling involvement in the child's OCD symptoms, minimizing reinforcement of the child's avoidant behavior, and enhancing family communication and problem-solving strategies (Barrett, Healy, et al., 2004; Piacentini & Langley, 2004).

Developmental Factors in the Treatment of Childhood OCD

As with other disorders in youth, treatment success for youngsters with OCD is highly dependent on the developmental appropriateness of the intervention in question (Clarke, 1995). Although some of the current CBT protocols for child

OCD were largely derived from adult treatment models, the most successful have been adapted to address the developmental considerations inherent in working with children and adolescents (March & Franklin, 2006; Piacentini, 1999). Cognitive behavior therapy can be complicated by the difficulty many young children have in describing specific obsessions or recognizing the role obsessions play in triggering rituals. Since young children are typically more present-oriented than adults, they may also be initially less willing to engage in exposure exercises regardless of the potential for future symptom reduction. Younger children, especially those with a very early onset of the disorder, may also be less likely to recognize or describe their symptoms as excessive and/or unrealistic, which can also reduce motivation for treatment. In addition to the presence of comorbid disorders noted earlier, poor frustration tolerance and coping abilities can also serve to complicate treatment. However, the correlation between age and readiness for treatment is not exact. We have seen a number of children as young as 6 or 7 years of age who have demonstrated good insight into their symptoms and excellent motivation for treatment and an equal number of older adolescents with high levels of denial, limited insight, poor frustration tolerance, and minimal motivation for treatment. Therefore, optimal treatment planning requires careful evaluation of these factors.

The most successful CBT treatment packages for childhood OCD have included elements to address the complicating factors noted above, including (1) behavioral reward systems for treatment compliance, (2) an increased emphasis on psychoeducation, (3) the use of age-appropriate metaphors to facilitate cognitive restructuring and, as described earlier, (4) greater family involvement in treatment (Barrett, Healy-Farrell, & March, 2004; March & Mulle, 1998; Piacentini et al., 2002). Using a developmentally sensitive approach, we have been able to successfully treat children with OCD as young as 4 or 5 years of age. Although we maximize the developmental appropriateness of our interventions by allowing for considerable flexibility in treatment, this flexibility is achieved within the constraints of a careful cognitive behavioral conceptualization of OCD and fixed goals for each treatment session. Perhaps the most important consideration is the need to adjust the level of therapist discourse to the cognitive functioning, social maturity, and capacity for sustained attention of each patient (March & Franklin, 2006; Piacentini & Bergman, 2001). Younger patients—and many of those with comorbid disorder—require more redirection and activities in order to sustain attention and motivation, whereas adolescents are generally more sensitive to the impact of OCD on social and academic functioning and may require additional intervention in these areas. Cognitive interventions are likely to be particularly sensitive to developmental level (e.g., Piacentini & Bergman, 2001). For example, younger children are more likely to benefit from giving OCD a "nasty nickname" than are older adolescents. The use of metaphors relevant to a child's area of interest or knowledge can also be quite helpful (March & Mulle, 1998). We have found sports metaphors to be quite useful for youngsters so inclined; for example, one young basketball player was taught to consider OCD as a defender blocking his way to the basket (Piacentini & Langley, 2004), while a teenager who played football was better able to conceptualize his treatment by considering it in the context of offensive and defensive schemes (March & Franklin, 2006).

TREATMENT STRATEGIES: A SELECTIVE ILLUSTRATION

Several treatment strategies will be illustrated. Specifically, we provide examples of psychoeducation, creating a symptom hierarchy, exposure and response prevention, addressing obsessions, and contingency management.

Psychoeducation

During the initial phase of treatment, typically the first session, the therapist focuses on educating the patient and family about OCD, presenting a cognitive-behavioral conceptualization of OCD and describing what treatment will entail. Most of these activities are conducted jointly with the child and parents, although this can vary with the developmental level of the child. The goal of psychoeducation is to address feelings of stigma and embarrassment on the part of the child, address any feelings of anger, blame, or hopelessness on the part of the family, and give the family a sense of confidence in the therapist. Describing the prevalence of OCD in the context of the size of the child's school (e.g., a prevalence rate of 1–2% suggests that 10–20 children in a school of 1,000 students will be affected) can help to reduce stigma about being different from others or "the only one in the world with this problem" (Piacentini & Langley, 2004).

Presenting the concept of OCD as a neurobehavioral disorder can also help to reduce feelings of blame and conflict among family members who may perceive the child's symptoms as totally willful or intentional. It is also worth sharing that, although OCD is a neurobehavioral disorder, environmental determinants play an important role in the development and/or expression of specific symptoms (March & Mulle, 1998; Piacentini, Langley, Roblek, Chang, & Bergman, 2003).

> "OCD is really no different than some medical or physical conditions, like asthma, diabetes, or even poor eyesight. Asthma is a problem affecting breathing and diabetes is a problem with how your body handles sugar, whereas OCD is a problem with how you control your thoughts, feelings, and behavior. We have different chemicals in our bodies that control how we think, feel, and act. People with OCD may have slightly too much or

too little of these chemicals, which can make it difficult to tell the difference between things that are really dangerous and things that aren't. However, even though we think of OCD as a medical problem, psychological approaches (i.e., CBT) can be a very effective way for helping you to learn how to control your fears and compulsions, hopefully for a long time. However, just as asthma sometimes gets worse when you are sick or stressed out or some other big changes are happening, some OCD symptoms may come back. The good news is that, if this happens, you can use what you will learn in CBT to help get them under control again.

"Sometimes OCD symptoms may be related to things that have actually happened to you or to other people you know. For example, getting stuck in an elevator has led some people to get really scared of elevators. In some cases, whenever they need to go on an elevator or even see an elevator, they feel the need to do rituals like praying or counting or other things to make the bad feeling go away."

As noted earlier, metaphors are often useful ways to present information to both children and their parents (March et al., 1994). The metaphor of obsessions as a "false fire alarm" can be helpful in further destigmatizing OCD and presenting youngsters and their families with a framework for conceptualizing OCD and the way he or she experiences anxiety (Piacentini, Langley, et al., 2003).

"We all feel anxious or frightened at times. Anxiety is a normal feeling that everyone—even animals—experience. It helps to protect us from dangerous things or situations. If nothing ever frightened us, then what would keep us from doing dangerous things like walking into traffic or driving our cars (or riding our bikes) way too fast? However, although a little anxiety is a good thing, too much anxiety, as with OCD, can be a problem.

"We can use the example of a fire alarm to understand how OCD works. The fire alarm is designed to alert you to a possibly dangerous situation—a fire. When most people hear a fire alarm go off, they get concerned or anxious—they may start to sweat, their heart may beat faster, and their thoughts may race—does this sound familiar? Just like when you start to worry that you may be contaminated. And when everyone has left the building where the fire alarm was, they calm down because they are no longer in danger—just like you feel better after you wash your hands. However, have you ever heard the fire alarm go off unexpectedly when there was no fire—perhaps it was a drill or an accident or even a prank by someone. A false alarm. What happens? That's right, even though there is no fire, the loud noise makes everyone nervous as if there was a fire, and they want to leave the building. People think they are in a dangerous situation even when they aren't.

"OCD is just like a false fire alarm. When you start to worry about germs, it's like a fire alarm going off—you feel nervous and think something bad is going to happen. However, just like the false alarm, nothing bad is going to happen. In treatment, you will learn that your OCD fears are false alarms and that if you ignore them they will go away and nothing bad will happen."

The final major component of psychoeducation is to present the child and family with the rationale for CBT. The extent to which the family understands and accepts the rationale for treatment can be an important determinant of treatment compliance and, ultimately, the success of the intervention.

"Did you know that the more you do your rituals, the stronger they become? Each time you give in to your OCD, you may actually be suggesting to yourself—not on purpose, of course—that you need to do your rituals to make the obsessions go away (*refer to Figure 8.1*). In CBT, you will learn how to make your anxiety go away without needing to do your rituals. In fact, the more you resist giving in to your OCD, the weaker it will get.

"Although it may be difficult at first, it should get easier as we go along. It's just like when you jump into a cold swimming pool. At first it feels really cold, but after a few minutes your body gets used to it, or habituates, and then it doesn't feel so bad anymore. The same thing will happen in treatment. You may feel pretty anxious or uncomfortable at first, but your body will habituate, just like in the pool, and you will feel better—without having to do your ritual."

Creation of Symptom Hierarchy

The symptom hierarchy provides a template for designing individual exposure tasks (see next section) and determining the sequence in which they will be attempted. The symptom checklist from the CY-BOCS is often a good starting point for creating the hierarchy. Each symptom is individually rated and ranked in terms of associated distress, using a fear thermometer (see Figure 8.2) or other developmentally appropriate ranking system. The level of parental involvement in the development of the symptom hierarchy is negotiated by the therapist, child, and parents, with younger children typically needing more parental input than older children and adolescents. Once the hierarchy has been completed, the therapist and patient select an initial symptom for ERP. Most often, the starting symptom should be a concrete behavior that is associated with relatively low distress and is easily re-created in the therapeutic session.

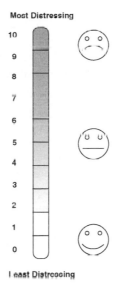

FIGURE 8.2. OCD fear thermometer. From Piacentini & Langley (2004). Copyright 2004 by Wiley Periodicals, Inc. Reprinted by permission.

Exposure plus Response Prevention

It is important that in-session exposure tasks be as realistic as possible in order to efficiently trigger distress and lead to generalization at home and/or other relevant environmental settings (see also Kendall et al., 2005). Once a given exposure task begins, the youngster is encouraged to remain in contact with the feared stimulus and resist all related rituals or other anxiety-reduction actions over the entire exposure period. Distress ratings using the fear thermometer are typically assessed every 30–60 seconds at first and then less frequently over the exposure period to monitor the pace and pattern of the child's habituation. It is often helpful to graph the child's distress ratings over the course of the exposure task. Graphing provides a visual demonstration of habituation and can be highly reinforcing to the child as well as identifying difficult spots that may require more intensive exposure or the addition of other treatment techniques (e.g., additional cognitive intervention).

Therapist modeling of both the exposure task and adaptive coping strategies is helpful in reducing anticipatory anxiety and enhancing child self-talk before and during ERP. Shaping procedures are also used to address difficult exposures. For example, a child who anticipates difficulty in completing a contamination exposure may first be asked to touch a contaminated object with one finger and then not wash. Once his or her anxiety level has dropped at least 50%, the next step might be to touch the object with two fingers, then the entire hand, then touch the hand to the arm, then to the face, etc. Once an exposure task has been practiced in session, the child is instructed to practice the exposure at least several times per week in his or her natural environment. The child is also instructed to resist ritualizing to the targeted fear, should it occur naturalistically.

Addressing Obsessions

Exposure tasks are used to address obsessions occurring in the absence of compulsions (e.g., thoughts of harming someone or being harmed, or sexual obsessions). A shaping procedure, similar to that described earlier, is used to facilitate exposure to these symptoms. Typical shaping steps include imagining the feared scenario, writing out the feared scenario, describing it out loud, having the therapist describe the scenario to the child, and recording the scenario and then listening to it repeatedly. Although youngsters may deny the presence of any ritualistic behaviors associated with obsessions such as those described above, associated avoidance behaviors are quite common (e.g., avoiding contact with a given individual for fear of triggering an aggressive or sexual thought). In such instances, the avoidance behaviors are added to the symptom hierarchy and exposed at the appropriate time.

Other strategies may be used to change the emotional valence of an obsessional thought or image. These include singing, rapping, or rhyming the obsession or changing feared images into innocuous or humorous ones (e.g., substituting a carrot for a knife). As an example, one patient was able to change an image of his father and him in a sexual situation to an image of the two of them playing a sport. In another case, a boy with unwanted images of himself stabbing his parents with a knife was able to facilitate successful habituation by stabbing a picture of his parents with a plastic knife while imagining the feared situation.

Contingency Management

Contingency management, both behavioral reward programs and liberal social reinforcement, are used to encourage treatment compliance (March & Franklin, 2006; Owens & Piacentini, 1998). Note that structured reward programs target treatment compliance (attempting or completing exposure tasks and other treatment requirements) and not habituation per se. The nature of specific rewards depends on the age and preference of the child, with some adolescents reporting minimal interest in or need for concrete reinforcers. Over time, as treatment draws to a close, the goal is to fade out tangible rewards in favor of increased emphasis on praise and positive encouragement from the therapist, parents, and other important individuals in the child's life.

EMPIRICAL SUPPORT: THE STATE OF THE RESEARCH EVIDENCE

The present consideration of the literature on the outcomes from treatment for OCD will consider, separately, open clinical trials and controlled outcome trials.

Open Clinical Trials

As with many other child anxiety and mood disorders, initial treatment approaches for childhood OCD were drawn from those shown to be efficacious with adult patients. Many of these early approaches involved single-case studies or a small series of cases that, although flawed methodologically, when taken as a whole provided initial support for the use of ERP in treating childhood OCD (March, 1995). These early studies were followed by a series of open clinical trials involving more sophisticated, developmentally sensitive, and structured CBT protocols (e.g., Franklin et al., 1998; March et al., 1994; Piacentini et al., 2002). Although there have been methodological differences, collectively, these trials yielded remarkably similar findings supporting CBT, both individual and group, as an efficacious and durable treatment for OCD in children and adolescents (see Table 8.1).

The open trials provided some preliminary evidence regarding additional treatment-related questions. March and colleagues (1994) found that improvement persisted in six of nine responders withdrawn from medication following completion of CBT—a finding that is consistent with the notion that CBT may prevent relapse to medication discontinuation. Both Franklin and colleagues (1998) and Piacentini and colleagues (2002) reported that baseline medication status was not related to treatment outcome. In addition, Piacentini and colleagues found that a poorer response to CBT was associated with a higher baseline CY-BOCS obsessions score and poorer pretreatment social functioning.

Controlled Outcome Trials

Four controlled trials have evaluated the outcomes associated with CBT for childhood OCD (Barrett, Healy-Farrell, et al., 2004; de Haan et al., 1998; Pediatric OCD Treatment Study Team, 2004; Piacentini, 2005). Barrett and colleagues (2004) compared individual cognitive-behavioral family-based therapy (CBFT, $n = 24$), group CBFT (GCBFT, $n = 29$), and wait-list control (WL, $n = 24$) in 77 youngsters (ages 7–17 years) with OCD. Both active treatments consisted of a 14-week manualized protocol that included both parent and sibling components. Participants in the WL group were assessed at baseline and 4–6 weeks later. Both active treatments were associated with significant improvement as compared to the WL group. At posttreatment, 88% of CBFT, 76% of GCBFT, and 0% of WL youngsters no longer met criteria for OCD, according

TABLE 8.1. Open Clinical Trials of CBT for Childhood OCD

Study	Sample size	Mean age (yr)	On stable medication	Type of treatment[a]	No. of sessions	Response rate	Follow-up
March et al. (1994)	15	14.3	93%	ICBT	16	80%	3–21 mo
Piacentini et al. (1994)	5[b]	13.0	20%	ICBT	10	80%	0–12 mo
Scahill et al. (1996)	7	13.1	71%	ICBT	15	100%	3 mo
Franklin et al. (1998)	14	14.1	57%	ICBT[c]	16–18	86%	9 mo
Benazon et al. (2002)	16	13.5	0%	ICBT	12	79%	None
Piacentini et al. (2002)	42	11.8	52%	ICBT	12	79%	None
Knox et al. (1996)	4	10.8	25%	ICBT+Fam	12	[d]	3 mo
Waters et al. (2001)	7	12.0	nr	FCBT	14	86%	3 mo
Thienemann et al. (2001)	18	15.2	83%	GCBT	14	50%	None
Himle et al. (2003)	19	14.6	68%	GCBT	7	56%[e]	6 mo

Note. Wever and Rey (1997) openly treated 57 youngsters with OCD and reported a 68% remission rate after 2 weeks of medication followed by 4 weeks of daily CBT. Given the design, it is not possible to determine the contribution of CBT by itself to outcome.
[a]ICBT, individual CBT with varying degrees of family involvement; ICBT+Fam, individual CBT plus systematic family involvement; GCBT, group CBT; FCBT, family-based CBT; nr, not reported.
[b]Includes two additional cases completed as part of this case series but not included in the original publication.
[c]Seven subjects received 16 weekly sessions over 4 months, and seven received 18 sessions over 1 month. Assignment was not random. There were no significant differences in outcome between the two treatment conditions.
[d]Multiple-baseline design indicated parental involvement in treatment associated with better outcome.
[e]Response rate not reported but calculated as follows: number of participants estimated to have had > 30% decrease in CY-BOCS at posttreatment (n = 9)/number of participants with CY-BOCS > 15 at baseline (n = 16).

to parental report on the ADIS. CBFT was associated with a 65% reduction on the CY-BOCS, according to child-only reports, as compared to 61% for GCBFT and no change for WL. Observed gains were largely maintained at a 6-month follow-up. Of interest, though a tad surprising, there were no treatment-related gains on any of the family measures.

A recently completed randomized controlled trial (Piacentini, 2005) compared individual CBT (ERP plus cognitive therapy) supplemented with a weekly manualized family intervention (F/ERP, $n = 49$) to a psychosocial comparison condition (relaxation training/psychoeducation, P/RT) in 22 youth. Participants ranged in age from 8 to 17 years. The family intervention was designed to (1) reduce the level of conflict and feelings of anger, blame, and guilt; (2) facilitate disengagement from the child's OCD symptoms; (3) rebuild normal (OCD-free) family interaction patterns; and (4) foster an environment conducive to maintaining treatment gains. Both treatments consisted of 14 manualized sessions delivered over 12 weeks. Participants responding to either treatment were reassessed at 1-month and 6-month follow-ups. Initial results from this study indicate that F/ERP was superior to P/RT in terms of clinician-rated response rate (a clinical global improvement score of much improved or very much improved), but not all differences on primary continuous outcome measures (e.g., CY-BOCS), although favoring F/ERP, reached statistical significance. The lack of significant differences on the continuous outcomes is somewhat surprising, given that relaxation training has not been shown effective for adult OCD (Fals-Stewart, Marks, & Schaeffer, 1993). However, these findings are consistent with results from Silverman and colleagues (1999) and Last, Hansen, and Franco (1998), both of whom found CBT and a psychosocial comparison condition (psychoeducation/support) to be effective for non–OCD child anxiety disorders.

The remaining two controlled trials involved comparison of CBT to medication. de Haan and colleagues (1998) randomly assigned 22 children (mean age of 13.7 years, 50% female) to 12 weeks of clomipramine (mean dose = 2.5 mg/kg) or CBT (ERP plus cognitive restructuring). The study did not include a control group. Both treatments led to significant improvement; however, ERP was significantly more efficacious than clomipramine in terms of response rate (66.7% vs. 50%) and reduction in symptom severity (59.9% vs. 33.4% decrease in the CY-BOCS).

The Pediatric OCD Treatment Study (POTS) is the largest controlled child OCD trial to date (Pediatric OCD Treatment Study Team, 2004). This multicenter trial of 112 youngsters (ages 7–17, 28 in each treatment group) with OCD compared CBT, an SSRI (sertraline [SER]) and their combination (COMB) to a pill placebo (PBO). Treatment was provided according to manuals over a 12-week period (Stage I). Stage I responders advanced to an additional 4 weeks of open treatment followed by discontinuation of all active treatment and follow-up evaluations at weeks 16, 20, 24, and 28 (Stage II) (Franklin, Foa, & March, 2003).

Using an intent-to-treat analytic strategy, all three active treatments were found to have significantly outperformed pill placebo. In addition, the combined treatment (CBT plus medication) was found to be superior to both CBT and medication (SER), which did not differ from each other. However, an examination of "excellent responders," those with a posttreatment score on the CY-BOCS, revealed a significant advantage for the CBT conditions. The combined treatment was associated with a 54% excellent response rate, compared to 39% for CBT but only 21% for medication (SER) and 3% for pill placebo. A significant site by treatment interaction was identified such that CBT alone at one site (i.e., University of Pennsylvania) was superior to CBT at another site (i.e., Duke University), with the reverse being true for the medication-alone (SER) condition. These latter results suggest to us that in some cases CBT alone may be as effective as the combined treatment. Collectively the results of these controlled trials provide support for the efficacy of CBT, both alone and in combination with medication, for the treatment of childhood OCD.

REFERENCES

Abramowitz, J. (1997). Effectiveness of psychological and pharmacological treatments for obsessive–compulsive: A quantitative review. *Journal of Consulting and Clinical Psychology, 65*, 44–52.

Albano, A., Knox, L., & Barlow, D. (1995). Obsessive-compulsive disorder. In A. R. Eisen, C. A. Kearney, & C. E. Schaefer (Eds.), *Clinical handbook of anxiety disorders in children and adolescents* (pp. 282–316). Northvale, NJ: Jason Aronson.

Albano, A., March, J., & Piacentini, J. (1999). Cognitive behavioral treatment of Obsessive–Compulsive Disorder. In R. E. Ammerman (Ed.), *Handbook of prescriptive treatments for children and adolescents* (pp. 193–213). Boston: Allyn & Bacon.

American Psychiatric Association. (2000). *Diagnostic and statistical manual of mental disorders* (4th ed., text rev.). Washington, DC: Author.

Apter, A., Pauls, D. L., Bleich, A., Zohar, A. H., Kron, S., Ratzoni, G., et al. (1993). An epidemiologic study of Gilles de la Tourette's syndrome in Israel. *Archives of General Psychiatry, 50*, 734–738.

Barrett, P., & Healy, L. (2003). An examination of the cognitive processes involved in childhood obsessive–compulsive disorder. *Behaviour Research and Therapy, 41*, 285–299.

Barrett, P., & Healy-Farrell, L. (2003). Perceived responsibility in juvenile obsessive–compulsive disorder: An experimental manipulation. *Journal of Clinical Child and Adolescent Psychology, 32*, 430–441.

Barrett, P., Healy-Farrell, L., & March, J. (2004). Cognitive-behavioral family treatment of childhood obsessive-compulsive disorder: A controlled trial. *Journal of the American Academy of Child and Adolescent Psychiatry, 43*, 46–62.

Barrett, P., Healy, L., Piacentini, J., & March, J. (2004). Treatment of OCD in children and adolescents. In P. Barrett & T. Ollendick (Eds.), *Handbook of interventions that work with children and adolescents* (pp. 187–216). West Sussex, UK: Wiley.

Barrett, P., Rasmussen, P. J., & Healy, L. (2001). The effect of obsessive–compulsive disorder on sibling relationships in late childhood and early adolescence: Preliminary findings. *The Australian Educational and Developmental Psychologist, 17*, 82–102.

Barrett, P., Shortt, A. L., & Healy, L. (2002). Do parent and child behaviours differentiate families whose children have obsessive–compulsive disorder from other clinic and non-clinic families? *Journal of Child Psychology and Psychiatry and Allied Disciplines, 43*, 597–607.

Benazon, N. R., Ager, J., & Rosenberg, D. R. (2002). Cognitive behavior therapy in treatment-naive children and adolescents with obsessive-compulsive disorder: An open trial. *Behavior Research and Therapy, 40*, 529–539.

Clarke, G. N. (1995). Improving the transition from basic efficacy research to effectiveness studies: Methodological issues and procedures. *Journal of Consulting and Clinical Psychology, 63*, 718–725.

Comer, J., Kendall, P. C., Franklin, M., Hudson, J., & Pimentel, S. (2004). Obsessing/worrying about the overlap between obsessive–compulsive disorder and generalized anxiety disorder in youth. *Clinical Psychology Review, 24*, 663–683.

de Haan, E., Hoogduin, K. A., Buitelaar, J., & Keijsers, G. (1998). Behavior therapy versus clomipramine for the treatment of obsessive–compulsive disorder. *Journal of the American Academy of Child and Adolescent Psychiatry, 37*, 1022–1029.

Fals-Stewart, W., Marks, A., & Schafer, J. (1993). A comparison of behavioral group therapy and individual behavior therapy in treating obsessive–compulsive disorder. *Journal of Nervous and Mental Disorders, 181*, 189–193.

Foa, E., & Kozac, M. (1986). Emotional processing of fear: Exposure to corrective information. *Psychological Bulletin, 99*, 450–472.

Foa, E., Steketee, G., Grayson, J., Turner, R., & Latimer, P. (1984). Deliberate exposure and blocking of obsessive compulsive rituals: Immediate and long term effects. *Behavior Therapy, 15*, 450–472.

Franklin, M. E., Kozak, M. J., Cashman, L. A., Coles, M. E., Rheingold, A. A., & Foa, E. B. (1998). Cognitive-behavioral treatment of pediatric obsessive–compulsive disorder: An open clinical trial. *Journal of the American Academy of Child and Adolescent Psychiatry, 37*, 412–419.

Franklin, M. E., & Foa, E. B. (2002). Cognitive behavioral treatment of obsessive compulsive disorder. In P. Nathan & J. Gorman (Eds.), *A guide to treatments that work* (2nd ed., pp. 367–386). Oxford, UK: Oxford University Press.

Franklin, M. E., Foa, E. B., & March, J. S. (2003). The Pediatric OCD Treatment Study (POTS): Rationale, design and methods. *Journal of Child and Adolescent Psychopharmacology, 13*(Suppl. 1), 39–52.

Freeston, M. H., & Ladouceur, R. (1993). Appraisals of cognitive intrusions and response style: Replication and extension. *Behaviour Research and Therapy, 31*, 185–191.

Geller, D. A., Biederman, J., Faraone, S., Agranat, A., Cradock, K., Hagermoser, L., et al. (2001). Developmental aspects of obsessive compulsive disorder: Findings in children, adolescents, and adults. *Journal of Nervous and Mental Disease, 189*, 471–477.

Geller, D. A., Biederman, J., Faraone, S., Frazier, J., Coffey, B., Kim, G., & Bellordre, C. (2000). Clinical correlates of obsessive compulsive disorder in children and adolescents referred to specialized and non-specialized clinical settings. *Depression and Anxiety, 11*, 163–168.

Geller, D. A., Hoog, S. L., Heiligenstein, J. H., Ricardi, R. K., Tamura, R., Kluszynski, S., & Jacobson, J. G. (2001). The fluoxetine pediatric OCD study team, U.S. fluoxetine treatment for obsessive–compulsive disorder in children and adolescents: A placebo-controlled clinical trial. *Journal of the American Academy of Child and Adolescent Psychiatry, 40*, 773–779.

Goodman, W., Price, L., Rasmussen, S., Riddle, M., & Rapoport, J. (1991). *Children's Yale–Brown Obsessive Compulsive Scale (CY-BOCS)*. New Haven, CT: Yale University.

Goodman, W., Price, L. H., Rasmussen, S. A., Mazure, C., Fleischmann, R. L., Hill, C. L., et al. (1989). The Yale–Brown Obsessive Compulsive Scale: Development, use and reliability. *Archives of General Psychiatry, 46,* 1006–1011.

Hanna, G. (1995). Demographic and clinical features of obsessive–compulsive disorder in children and adolescents. *Journal of the American Academy of Child and Adolescent Psychiatry, 34,* 19–27.

Hibbs, E., Hamburger, S., & Lenane, M. (1991). Determinants of expressed emotion in families of disturbed and normal children. *Journal of Child Psychology and Psychiatry, 32,* 757–770.

Himle, J. A., Fischer, D. J., Van Etten, M., Janeck, A., & Hanna, G. L. (2003). Group behavioral therapy for adolescents with tic-related and non tic-related obsessive–compulsive disorder. *Depression and Anxiety, 17,* 73–77.

Kendall, P. C., Robin, J., Hedtke, K., Suveg, C., Flannery-Schroeder, E., & Gosch, E. (2005). Considering CBT with anxious youth? Think exposures. *Cognitive and Behavioral Practice, 12,* 136–148.

Knox, L., Albano, A., & Barlow, D. (1996). Parental involvement in the treatment of childhood OCD: A multiple-baseline examination involving parents. *Behavior Therapy, 27,* 93–114.

Kovacs, M. (1996). *The Children's Depression Inventory.* Toronto, ON, Canada: Multi-Health Systems.

Kozak, M. J., & Foa, E. B. (1997). *Mastery of obsessive–compulsive disorder: A cognitive-behavioral approach* (therapist guide). San Antonio, TX: Psychological Corporation.

Langley, A., Bergman, R. L., & Piacentini, J. (2002). Assessment of childhood anxiety. *International Review of Psychiatry, 14,* 102–113.

Last, C., Hansen, C., & Franco, N. (1998). Cognitive-behavioral treatment of school phobia. *Journal of the American Academy of Child and Adolescent Psychiatry, 37,* 404–411.

Leonard, H., Swedo, S., Lenane, M., Rettew, D., Hamburger, S., Bartko, J., & Rapoport, J. (1993). A two- to seven-year follow-up study of 54 obsessive–compulsive children and adolescents. *Archives of General Psychiatry, 50,* 429–439.

Liebowitz, M., Turner, S., Piacentini, J., Beidel, D., Clarvit, S., Davies, S., et al. (2002). Fluoxetine in children and adolescents with OCD: A placebo-controlled trial. *Journal of the American Academy of Child and Adolescent Psychiatry, 41,* 1431–1438.

Livingston-Van Noppen, B., Rasmussen, S. I., Eisen, J., & McCartney, L. (1990). Family function and treatment in obsessive–compulsive disorder. In M. A. Jenike, L. Baer, & W. E. Minichiello (Eds.), *Obsessive–compulsive disorders: Theory and management* (pp. 118–131). Littleton, MA: Year Book Medical Publishers.

Lopatka, C., & Rachman, S. (1995). Perceived responsibility and compulsive checking: An experimental analysis. *Behaviour Research and Therapy, 33,* 673–684.

March, J. (1995). Cognitive-behavioral psychotherapy for children and adolescents with OCD: A review and recommendations for treatment. *Journal of the American Academy of Child and Adolescent Psychiatry, 34,* 7–18.

March, J., Frances, A., Carpenter, D., & Kahn, D. (1997). Expert consensus guidelines: Treatment of obsessive–compulsive disorder. *Journal of Clinical Psychiatry, 58,* 1–72.

March, J., & Franklin, M. E. (2006). Cognitive-behavioral therapy for pediatric OCD. In B. O. Rothbaum (Ed.), *Pathological anxiety: Emotional processing in etiology and treatment* (pp. 147–165). New York: Guilford Press.

March, J., Leonard, H., & Swedo, S. (1995). Obsessive compulsive disorder. In J. S. March (Ed.), *Anxiety disorders in children and adolescents* (pp. 251–275). New York, Guilford Press.

March, J. S., & Mulle, K. (1998). *OCD in children and adolescents: A cognitive-behavioral treatment manual.* New York: Guilford Press.

March, J., Mulle, K., & Herbel, B. (1994). Behavioral psychotherapy for children and adolescents with OCD. *Journal of the American Academy of Child and Adolescent Psychiatry, 33,* 333–341.

March, J., Parker, J. D. A., Sullivan, K., Stallings, P., & Conners, C. K. (1997). The Multidimensional Anxiety Scale for Children (MASC): Factor structure, reliability, and validity. *Journal of the American Academy of Child and Adolescent Psychiatry, 36,* 554–565.

McKay, D., Piacentini, J., Greisberg, S., Graae, F., Jaffer, M., Miller, J., et al. (2003). The Children's Yale–Brown Obsessive Compulsive Scale: Item structure in an outpatient setting. *Psychological Assessment, 15,* 578–581

Meyer, V. (1966). Modification of expectations in cases with obsessive rituals. *Behavioral Research and Therapy, 4,* 270–280.

Nesdadt, G., Samuels, J., Riddle, M., Bienvenu, J. O., Llang, K. Y., LaBuda, M., et al. (2000). A family study of obsessive compulsive disorder. *Archives of General Psychiatry, 57,* 358–363.

Nestadt, G., Samuels, J., Riddle, M. A., Liang, K. Y., Bienvenu, O. J., Hoehn-Saric, R., et al. (2001). The relationship between obsessive–compulsive disorder and anxiety and affective disorders: Results from the Johns Hopkins OCD Family Study. *Psychological Medicine, 31,* 481–487.

Owens, E., & Piacentini, J. (1998). Behavioral treatment of obsessive–compulsive disorder in a boy with comorbid disruptive behavior problems. *Journal of the American Academy of Child and Adolescent Psychiatry, 37,* 443–446.

Pauls, D., & Alsobrook, J. (1999). The inheritance of obsessive–compulsive disorder. *Child and Adolescent Psychiatric Clinics of North America, 8,* 481.

Pediatric OCD Treatment Study Team. (2004). Cognitive-behavioral therapy, sertraline, and their combination for children and adolescents with obsessive–compulsive disorder: The Pediatric OCD Treatment Study (POTS) randomized controlled trial. *Journal of the American Medical Association, 292,* 1969–1976.

Piacentini, J. (1999). Cognitive behavioral therapy of childhood OCD. *Child and Adolescent Psychiatric Clinics of North America, 8,* 599–616.

Piacentini, J. (2005). *Controlled comparison of exposure plus response prevention and relaxation training for children and adolescents with obsessive–compulsive disorder.* Manuscript in preparation.

Piacentini, J., & Bergman, R. L. (2001). Developmental issues in cognitive therapy for childhood anxiety disorders. *Journal of Cognitive Psychotherapy, 15,* 165–182.

Piacentini, J., Bergman, R. L., Jacobs, C., McCracken, J., & Kretchman, J. (2002). Cognitive-behaviour therapy for childhood obsessive–compulsive disorder: Efficacy and predictors of treatment response. *Journal of Anxiety Disorders, 16,* 207–219.

Piacentini, J., Bergman, R. L., Keller, M., & McCracken, J. (2003). Functional impairment in children and adolescents with obsessive compulsive disorder. *Journal of Child and Adolescent Psychopharmacology, 13,* 61–70.

Piacentini, J., Gitow, A., Jaffer, M., Graae, F., & Whitaker, A. (1994). Outpatient behavioral treatment of child and adolescent obsessive compulsive disorder. *Journal of Anxiety Disorders, 8,* 277–289.

Piacentini, J., Jaffer, M., Bergman, R. L., McCracken, J., & Keller, M. (2001). Measuring impairment in childhood OCD: Psychometric properties of the COIS. *Proceedings of the American Academy of Child and Adolescent Psychiatry Meeting, 48,* 146.

Piacentini, J., & Langley, A. (2004). Cognitive-behavioral therapy for children who have obsessive–compulsive disorder. *Journal of Clinical Psychology, 60,* 1181–1194

Piacentini, J., Langley, A., Roblek, T., Chang, S., & Bergman, R. (2003). *Multimodal CBT treatment for childhood OCD: A combined individual child and family treatment manual* (3rd rev.). Los Angeles: UCLA Department of Psychiatry.

Rachman, S. (1993). Obsessions, responsibility, and guilt. *Behaviour Research and Therapy, 31,* 149–154.

Rapoport, J., Inoff-Germain, G., Weissman, M. M., Greenwald, S., Narrow, W. E., Jensen, P. S., et al. (2000). Childhood obsessive–compulsive disorder in the NIMH MECA

Study: Parent versus child identification of cases. *Journal of Anxiety Disorders, 14*, 535–548.

Rapoport, J., Swedo, S. E., & Leonard, H. L. (1992). Childhood obsessive–compulsive disorder. *Journal of Clinical Psychiatry, 53*, 11–16.

Rasmussen, S., & Eisen, J. (1990). Epidemiology of obsessive compulsive disorder *Journal of Clinical Psychiatry, 51*(2, Suppl.), 10–13.

Rettew, D., Swedo, S. E., Leonard, H. L., Lenane, M. C., & Rapport, J. L. (1992). Obsessions and compulsions across time in79 children and adolescents with obsessive–compulsive disorder. *Journal American Academy of Child and Adolescent Psychiatry, 31*, 1050–1056.

Rheaume, J., Ladouceur, R., Freeston, M., & Letarte, H. (1994). Inflated responsibility in obsessive–compulsive disorder: Psychometric studies of a semi-idiographic measure. *Journal of Psychopathology and Behavioural Assessment, 16*, 265–276.

Rheaume, J., Ladouceur, R., Freeston, M., & Letarte, H. (1995). Inflated responsibility in obsessive–compulsive disorder: validation of an operational definition. *Behavioural Research and Therapy, 88*, 159–169.

Riddle, M. A., Scahill, L., King, R., Hardin, M. T., Toublin, K. E., Ort, S. I., et al. (1990). Obsessive compulsive disorder in children and adolescents: phenomenology and family history. *Journal of the American Academy of Child and Adolescent Psychiatry, 29*, 766–772.

Salkovskis, P. M. (1985). Obsessional compulsive problems: A cognitive-behavioural analysis. *Behaviour Research and Therapy, 23*, 571–583.

Salkovskis, P. M. (1989). Cognitive behavioural factors and the persistence of intrusive thoughts in obsessional problems. *Behaviour Research and Therapy, 27*, 677–682.

Salzman, L., & Thaler, F. (1981). Obsessive–compulsive disorders: A review of the literature. *American Journal of Psychiatry, 138*, 286–296.

Scahill, L., Riddle, M. A., McSwiggan-Hardin, M. T., Ort, S. I., King, R. A., Goodman, W. K., et al. (1997). Children's Yale–Brown Obsessive Compulsive Scale: Reliability and validity. *Journal of the American Academy of Child and Adolescent Psychiatry, 36*, 844–852.

Scahill, L., Vitulano, L. A., Brenner, E. M., Lynch, K. A., & King, R. A. (1996). Behavioral therapy in children and adolescents with obsessive–compulsive disorder: A pilot study. *Journal of Child and Adolescent Psychopharmacology, 6*, 191–202.

Shafran, R. (1997). The manipulation of responsibility in obsessive–compulsive disorder. *British Journal of Clinical Psychology, 36*, 397–407.

Silverman, W., & Albano, A. M. (1996). *Anxiety Disorders Interview Schedule for DSM-IV: Parent Version.* San Antonio, TX: Graywing.

Silverman, W., Kurtines, W., Ginsburg, G., Weems, C., Rabian, B., & Serafini, L. (1999). Contingency management, self-control, and education support in the treatment of childhood phobic disorders: A randomized clinical trial. *Journal of Consulting and Clinical Psychology, 67*, 675–687

Silverman, W., Saavedra, L., & Pina, A. (2001). Test–retest reliability of anxiety symptoms and diagnoses with anxiety disorders interview schedule for DSM-IV: Child and parent versions. *Journal of the American Academy of Child and Adolescent Psychiatry, 40*, 937–944.

Soechting, I., & March, J. (2002). Cognitive aspects of obsessive compulsive disorder in children. In R. Frost & G. Steketee (Eds.), *Cognitive approaches to obsessions and compulsions: Theory, assessment, and treatment* (pp. 299–314). Amsterdam, Netherlands: Pergamon/Elsevier Science.

Steketee, G. (1990). Personality traits and disorders in obsessive–compulsives. *Journal of Anxiety Disorders, 4*, 351–364.

Steketee, G., & Frost, R. O. (1994). Measurement of risk-taking in obsessive–compulsive disorder. *Behavioural and Cognitive Psychotherapy, 22*, 287–298.

Stewart, S., Geller, D., Jenike, M., Pauls, D., Shaw, D., Mullin, B., & Faraone, S. (2004).

Long-term outcome of pediatric obsessive–compulsive disorder: A meta-analysis and qualitative review of the literature. *Acta Psychiatrica Scandinavica, 110,* 4–13.

Swedo, S., Rapoport, J., Leonard, H., Lenane, M., & Cheslow, D. (1989) Obsessive–compulsive disorder in children and adolescents: Clinical phenomenology of 70 consecutive cases. *Archives of General Psychiatry, 46,* 335–341.

Thienemann, M., Martin, J., Cregger, B., Thompson, H. B., & Dyer-Freidman, J. (2001). Manual driven group cognitive-behavioral therapy for adolescents with obsessive–compulsive disorder: A pilot study *Journal of American Academy of Child and Adolescent Psychiatry, 40,* 1254–1260.

Valleni-Basile, L., Garrison, C., Jackson, K., Waller, J., McKeown, R., Addy, C., & Cuffe, S. (1994). Frequency of obsessive–compulsive disorder in a community sample of young adolescents. *Journal of the American Academy of Child and Adolescent Psychiatry, 33,* 782–791.

van Balkom, A., de Haan, E., van Oppen, P., Spinhoven, P., Hoogduin, K. A., & van Dyck, R. (1998). Cognitive and behavioral therapies alone versus in combination with fluvoxamine in the treatment of obsessive compulsive disorder. *Journal of Nervous and Mental Disorder, 186,* 492–499.

Vogel, P. A., Stiles, T. C., & Gotestam, K. G. (2004). Adding cognitive therapy elements to exposure therapy for obsessive compulsive disorder: A controlled study. *Behavioural and Cognitive Psychotherapy, 32,* 275–290.

Waters, T., & Barrett, P. (2000). The role of the family in childhood obsessive–compulsive disorder. *Clinical Child and Family Psychology Review, 3,* 173–184.

Waters, T., Barrett, P., & March, J. (2001). Cognitive-behavioural family treatment of childhood obsessive–compulsive disorder: An open clinical trial. *American Journal of Psychotherapy, 55,* 372–387.

Wever, C., & Rey, J. M. (1997). Juvenile obsessive–compulsive disorder. *Australian and New Zealand Journal of Psychiatry, 31,* 105–113.

Wood, J., Piacentini, J., Bergman, R. L., McCracken, J., & Barrios, V. (2002). Concurrent validity of the anxiety disorders section of the Anxiety Disorders Interview Schedule for DSM IV: Child and parent version. *Journal of Clinical Child Psychology, 31,* 335–342.

CHAPTER 9

Cognitive-Behavioral Therapy for Youth with Eating Disorders and Obesity

DENISE E. WILFLEY, VANDANA A. PASSI,
JORDANA COOPERBERG, and RICHARD I. STEIN

Although eating disorders (EDs) and obesity are often classified as disparate conditions, we have chosen to address them together, given their common factors. In particular, high rates of occurrence during adolescence, issues relating to hunger and satiety, body dissatisfaction, the use of unhealthy weight-loss methods, binge eating, and dieting are all common issues (Fairburn & Brownell, 2002) that must be addressed in treatment. In addition, there appears to be a strong interplay between ED psychopathology and obesity, such that the development of either condition makes the other more likely. Specifically, childhood adiposity is a risk factor for the development of eating-disordered pathology (Fairburn, Welch, Doll, Davies, & O'Conner, 1997), and binge eating in adolescence is a risk factor for developing obesity (Stice, Presnell, & Sprangler, 2002).

We begin with current data on the prevalence, associated medical complications, and psychosocial features of each condition. This overview is followed by a review of controlled treatment trials involving cognitive-behavioral therapy (CBT), a discussion of these findings, and their application to youth. Finally, a summary is provided and future directions are discussed.

EATING DISORDERS

EDs are well-recognized psychological conditions affecting adolescents. These disorders include anorexia nervosa (AN), characterized by extremely low body weight; bulimia nervosa (BN), characterized by recurrent eating binges followed by compensatory behaviors; and binge-eating disorder (BED; classified under eating disorders not otherwise specified [EDNOS]), characterized by recurrent eating binges without any compensatory behaviors (see Table 9.1). Current epidemiological data indicate that young females are the group most at risk for developing an ED (Hoek, 2002). In fact, EDs are the third most common chronic illness among females 15–19 years old (Lucas, Beard, O'Fallon, & Kurland, 1991). Typical age of onset is during adolescence, and it is estimated that approximately 3% of young women meet full diagnostic criteria for an ED (Becker, Grinspoon, Klibanski, & Herzog, 1999). In addition, youth diagnosed with EDs face numerous medical and psychological comorbidities.

To date no randomized controlled clinical trials have been conducted with children or adolescents with BN or BED; whereas four randomized controlled treatment studies on adolescents with AN have been conducted, none has investigated the effects of CBT. Thus far, the majority of research on CBT for EDs has been with adults, although these samples sometimes include older adolescents. It is unclear why there is such a dearth of literature on CBT for youth with EDs. Perhaps because EDs typically develop during adolescence, parents view the symptoms as more of a transitory phase rather than an established pattern requiring treatment. Another possibility is that adolescents are not as motivated as adults to seek help (Fisher, Schneider, Burns, Symons, & Mandel, 2001) and thus intentionally hide their ED from those that would seek treatment (e.g., family). Although adults also often hide their ED from others, it does not preclude them from seeking treatment. Adolescents, on the other hand, often cannot transport themselves and thus are dependent on adults to bring them to therapy. This could particularly be the case in BN, where the symptoms are not overtly obvious. In AN, however, the physical weight loss associated with this condition is difficult to overlook, which may explain why numerous treatments other then CBT have been developed (e.g., inpatient hospitalization, family therapy, pharmacotherapy) for this population. In terms of BED, the lack of studies with adolescents may be due to the novelty of our awareness of this condition and the absence of any abnormal physical symptoms (other than weight gain). With its inclusion into the DSM only within the last decade, adolescents, their families, and health care providers may not have recognized the behavioral symptoms of BED as an actual ED.

For AN, efficacy studies on CBT even for adults are sparse. This lack of data is likely due to the low base rate of AN and the inherent difficulty involved in treating this population (Agras et al., 2004; Wilson, 1999). Adults with AN are especially difficult to treat, as longer duration of illness in AN is associated with

TABLE 9.1. DSM-IV-TR Diagnostic Criteria for Eating Disorders

Anorexia nervosa	Bulimia nervosa	Binge-eating disorder
A. Refusal to maintain body weight at or above a minimally normal weight for age and height (e.g., weight loss leading to maintenance of body weight less than 85% of that expected; or failure to make expected weight gain during period of growth, leading to body weight less than 85% of that expected).	A. Recurrent episodes of binge eating. An episode of binge eating is characterized by both of the following: (1) eating, in a discrete period of time (e.g., within any 2-hour period), an amount of food that is definitely larger than most people would eat during a similar period of time and under similar circumstances (2) a sense of lack of control over eating during the episode (e.g., a feeling that one cannot stop eating or control what or how much one is eating)	A. Recurrent episodes of binge eating. An episode of binge eating is characterized by both of the following: (1) eating in a discrete period of time (e.g., within any 2-hour period), an amount of food that is definitely larger than most people would eat during a similar period of time and under similar circumstances (2) a sense of lack of control over eating during the episode (e.g., a feeling that one cannot stop eating or control what or how much one is eating)
B. Intense fear of gaining weight or becoming fat, even though underweight.	B. Recurrent inappropriate compensatory behavior in order to prevent weight gain, such as self-induced vomiting; misuse of laxatives, diuretics, enemas, or other medications; fasting; or excessive exercise.	B. The binge-eating episodes are associated with three (or more) of the following: (1) eating much more rapidly than usual (2) eating until uncomfortably full (3) eating large amounts of food when not feeling physically hungry (4) eating alone because of being embarrassed by how much one is eating (5) feeling disgusted with oneself, depressed, or very guilty after overeating
C. Disturbance in the way in which one's body weight or shape is experienced, undue influence of body weight or shape on self-evaluation, or denial of the seriousness of the current low body weight.	C. The binge eating and inappropriate compensatory behaviors both occur, on average, at least twice a week for 3 months.	C. Marked distress regarding binge eating is present.
D. In postmenarcheal females, amenorrhea, i.e., the absence of at least three consecutive menstrual cycles.	D. Self-evaluation is unduly influenced by body shape and weight.	D. The binge eating occurs, on average, at least 2 days a week for 6 months.
	E. The disturbance does not occur exclusively during episodes of anorexia nervosa.	E. The binge eating is not associated with the regular use of inappropriate compensatory behaviors (e.g., purging, fasting, excessive exercise) and does not occur exclusively during the course of anorexia nervosa or bulimia nervosa.

Note. From American Psychiatric Association (2000). Copyright 2000 by the American Psychiatric Association. Reprinted by permission.

poorer outcome (Fairburn & Harrison, 2003; Lask & Bryant-Waugh, 1993), higher dropout rates (Agras et al., 2003; Halmi et al., 2005), and more resistance to treatment as compared to those with a shorter duration of illness (i.e., adolescents). In 2002, numerous researchers specializing in EDs convened at the National Institutes of Health (NIH) to discuss overcoming these barriers to treatment in the AN population. A primary recommendation from this meeting was early detection and treatment for patients with AN (Agras et al., 2004). Note that this scarcity of studies is not the case for BN and BED, where extensive randomized controlled trials (RCTs) of CBT have been conducted for adults diagnosed with these disorders.

As CBT has been developed and evaluated only for adults with EDs, we begin with a description of CBT and an overview of the treatment literature for adults with AN, BN, and BED. This section is followed by a review of current adolescent ED treatments that contain cognitive and/or behavioral components. Based on these treatment models, we then discuss the various ways in which CBT strategies can be employed for youth with EDs.

BULIMIA NERVOSA

Prevalence, Medical Complications, and Psychosocial Features in BN

Age of onset for BN is typically in late adolescence, and the lifetime prevalence rate is 1–3% (American Psychiatric Association, 1994). Medical complications can arise from vomiting and the abuse of laxatives, diuretics, and/or enemas. Adolescents employing these compensatory behaviors repeatedly for prolonged time periods can develop electrolyte disturbances, gastric ruptures, gastric and esophageal irritation and bleeding, Mallory–Weiss tears (a syndrome characterized by esophageal bleeding caused by a mucosal tear in the esophagus as a result of forceful vomiting or retching), Barret esophagus (abnormal growth of intestinal-type cells between the esophagus and stomach), large bowel abnormalities including permanent impairment of colonic function, erosion of dental enamel, parotid enlargement, hyperamylasemia, and acute pancreatitis (Fisher et al., 1995; Pomeroy & Mitchell, 2002).

Comorbid psychological conditions include anxiety disorders (most commonly, social phobia and generalized anxiety disorder), major depression (Bulik, 2002), borderline personality disorder, and substance abuse disorders (O'Brien & Vincent, 2003).

CBT for BN

The first CBT manual for BN was developed in the 1980s (Wilson, Fairburn, & Agras, 1997). An expanded version of this manual appeared in 1993 (Fairburn, Marcus, & Wilson, 1993) and is currently considered the treatment of choice for

BN (Fairburn, 2002; Garner, Vitousek, & Pike, 1997; Wilson, 1999). The underlying theory of CBT for BN is that societal pressures to be thin lead to an overvalued focus on body weight and shape. As a result of these pressures, some individuals begin to severely restrict their dietary intake, resulting in increased hunger and feelings of deprivation, which, in turn, create an increased psychological and physiological susceptibility to binge eat. In an effort to compensate for binge eating, these individuals employ extreme forms of weight control, most often self-induced vomiting. This binge–purge cycle is thought to cause extreme distress and decreased self-esteem, which perpetuates further dietary restraint (Wilson et al., 1997). The primary goal of CBT is to eliminate the binge–purge cycle by restoring normal dietary intake and modifying the dysfunctional thoughts associated with weight and shape (Wilson et al., 1997). Protocol-based CBT advances through three additive and sequential stages and is broken down into 19 sessions over a 20-week period. In the initial phase, the goals are to establish a solid therapeutic relationship and provide education on BN and an orientation to the structure and the rationale underlying CBT for BN. Behavioral techniques such as weekly weighing and self-monitoring of food intake are introduced to interrupt the cycle of dietary restraint, binge eating, and resultant compensatory behaviors. In the second stage, behavioral techniques are continued while cognitive techniques including problem solving and cognitive restructuring are initiated to challenge the dysfunctional thoughts maintaining the disorder. The final stage is focused on relapse prevention, where the objective is to prepare the patient for any future setbacks, including high-risk situations and triggers (Wilson et al., 1997).

Empirical Support

CBT for BN has been studied extensively in the United States and abroad. Currently, over 20 randomized controlled trials have been conducted, with substantial evidence to support its efficacy in reducing the core features of BN (Fairburn & Harrison, 2003; Stein et al., 2001; Wilson, 1999). Specifically, CBT for BN has been found superior to both pharmacological therapy and most other psychotherapy it has been compared with; it has been shown to significantly improve binge eating, purging, dietary restraint, and abnormal attitudes about weight and shape, as well as improving mood and social functioning; the effects are evident within the first few weeks and usually maintained at 6-month and 1-year follow-up (Wilson, 1999). CBT combined with antidepressant medication has also been shown to be more effective than CBT or medication alone (Wilson, 1999). In terms of treatment outcome, currently the most robust predictor in CBT for BN is early response to treatment, where a reduction in behavioral symptoms by week 4 is associated with better outcome. In addition, rapid reduction in dietary restraint has clearly been shown to mediate treatment outcome (Wilson, Fairburn, Agras, Walsh, & Kraemer, 2002). As mentioned already, all of these studies have been with adults, and to date there are no published controlled trials regarding the efficacy of CBT in youth with BN.

ANOREXIA NERVOSA

Prevalence, Medical Complications, and Psychosocial Features in AN

Age of onset for AN is typically between the ages of 14 and 18, and the prevalence rate in the general population is approximately 0.5% (American Psychiatric Association, 1994). Medical conditions associated with AN are usually a result of starvation and in the most severe cases of AN can lead to death. One meta-analysis on this topic reported that the mortality rate for females with AN between 15 and 24 years old was more than 12 times higher than the annual death rate for all causes in the general population (Sullivan, 1995). Medical conditions unique to adolescents with AN include increased chance for significant growth retardation, interruption or delay of pubertal development, and peak bone-mass reduction (Fisher et al., 1995; Lock, le Grange, Agras, & Dare, 2001; Pomeroy & Mitchell, 2002). Conditions affecting both adults and adolescents with AN include dehydration, bradycardia, cardiac arrhythmias, hypotension, hypothermia, lanugo hair (a fine hair that develops on the face, back, or arms and legs), failure to develop or loss of secondary sexual characteristics, poor peripheral circulation, acrocyanosis, occasional ulceration, and gangrenous changes in the toes (Lask, Waugh, & Gordon, 1997). Although most of these conditions can be reversed with weight gain, effects on growth in particular can be permanent if the disorder continues for a prolonged period of time (Fisher et al., 1995). Finally, further medical complications can arise from vomiting and the abuse of laxatives, diuretics, and/or enemas, which are symptoms of the binge–purge subtype of AN (see the BN section, above).

Comorbid psychological disorders and symptoms often found in this population include major depression, social withdrawal, obsessive–compulsive tendencies, poor peer relations, and loss of sexual libido (Beumont, 2002).

CBT for AN

The underlying theory of CBT for AN is that self-worth is primarily defined through body weight and shape. It is thought that these beliefs develop from an interaction between specific personality variables (e.g., perfectionism, mood instability) and an internalization of the sociocultural model of female beauty (Vitousek, 1998). Individuals with AN resort to extreme forms of weight control to achieve and maintain their low weight, often resulting in starvation (Vitousek, 2002). Some of the variables thought to maintain the disorder include an intense fear of weight gain, fears of sexuality, and family issues, as well as feelings of success and sense of self-control from achieving weight loss and positive social reinforcement (Garner, Vitousek, & Pike, 1997).

In their CBT treatment manual for AN, Garner and colleagues (1997) noted that treatment issues specific to this population require "variations in the style, pace, and content of CBT" as compared to CBT for BN (p. 95). Specifically, whereas in CBT for BN clients are told that their body weight will likely remain stable, in AN weight gain is a priority and the primary goal of treatment. Because fear of weight gain is a core symptom of AN, motivation to begin and/or continue treatment is often poor and must be addressed within the first stage of treatment (Garner et al., 1997). Other unique factors contributing to the difficulty in treating this population include denial of illness and egosyntonic symptomatology, leading to a strong resistance to change (Vitousek, Watson, & Wilson, 1998).

Although there are several overlaps between CBT for AN and that for BN, there are also important differences. Specifically, cognitive interventions are focused on a broader range of interpersonal and personal areas than in BN. In addition, weight must be regularly checked, and any recorded changes (increases or decreases) can influence the direction and structure of therapy sessions. Based on these variables, duration of treatment is substantially longer (1–2 years) than CBT for BN, as more time is needed to achieve substantial weight gain, address and resolve motivational obstacles, and incorporate any needed inpatient or partial hospitalizations to address medical complications that often occur in this population and in order for cognitive intervention to be possible (Garner et al., 1997). As in CBT for BN, treatment for AN is divided into three phases. The first phase partly focuses on psychoeducation as clients are taught the repercussions of starvation and provided information on nutrition. Other important strategies employed during this stage include self-monitoring, structured techniques on how to alter food intake, and motivational enhancement skills. During the second stage, distorted beliefs are operationalized, examined, and empirically tested, using standard cognitive techniques. The third stage is focused on relapse prevention techniques and termination preparation (Garner et al., 1997).

An alternative theory has been proposed to explain the maintenance of AN (Fairburn, Shafran, & Cooper, 1998). Specifically, this model hypothesizes that the core feature of AN is an extreme need to control one's eating that perpetuates dietary restriction through three primary feedback mechanisms: dietary restriction enhances the sense of being in control; aspects of starvation further encourage dietary restriction; and extreme concerns about shape and weight encourage dietary restriction. Fairburn and colleagues (1998) describe their work as a synthesis and extension of Slade's (1982) theory of self-control as central to the development and maintenance of AN, and the central premise of CBT for AN of overvaluation of weight and shape (Fairburn et al., 1998). In particular, they view "the extreme need to control eating" (p. 8) as primary to the maintenance of AN, and argue that this should be the organizing factor through which other issues (i.e., concerns about weight and shape) are addressed. Based on this model, Fairburn and colleagues note two treatment implications: treatment should (1) primarily focus on the excessive need for self-control and the mechanisms operating to maintain the disorder, and

(2) address the relation between general self-control needs and the control being exerted over weight, shape, and food.

Empirical Support

To our knowledge, only four (three published and one unpublished) controlled outcome studies have been conducted investigating CBT in the AN adult population. In the first study (Channon, de Silva, Helmsley, & Perkins, 1989), CBT was compared with behavioral therapy (BT) and an eclectic-based therapy, with eight subjects in each treatment condition; increases in weight and psychosocial functioning were reported in all groups. In a second study, Ball (1998) compared CBT ($n - 13$) with a behavioral family therapy ($n - 12$), which will be described in the following section. At the 6-month follow-up, 78% of subjects who had completed either treatment were rated as having good to intermediate outcomes. However, both of these studies used small sample sizes, making interpretations very difficult. A third study compared CBT with nutritional counseling (Serfaty, Turkington, Heap, Ledsham, & Jolley, 1999). Interestingly, the study could not be completed due to the large drop-out rate in the nutrition condition. This trend was not the case in the CBT condition, where over 90% of participants completed treatment. Similar findings were reported in a study evaluating CBT in AN posthospitalization (Pike, Walsh, Vitousek, Wilson, & Bauer, 2003). More specifically, AN participants were randomly assigned to 1 year of either outpatient CBT or nutritional counseling. Results indicated that more participants in the CBT condition had favorable outcomes (e.g., weight regain, resumed menstruation), and CBT participants dropped out significantly less, than did those in the nutritional condition. Finally, one treatment outcome study (Halmi, 1999) comparing CBT, fluoxetine, and their combination released 6-month data indicating that CBT with fluoxetine is more effective than fluoxetine alone. In addition, these data suggest that this combination may offer improvements in self-esteem over and above those provided by CBT alone. Due to the high drop-out rate in this study, long-term data were not available (Halmi et al., 2005). It is important to note that these findings are preliminary and based on a small number of treatment completers. There are currently no published randomized controlled studies investigating CBT exclusively in adolescents with AN.

BINGE-EATING DISORDER

Prevalence, Medical Complications, and Psychosocial Features in BED

Age of onset for BED is usually during late adolescence through the early twenties, with prevalence in the general population ranging between 0.4 and 0.7% (American Psychiatric Association, 1994). Among obese individuals in weight-control programs, the prevalence reports have varied considerably, ranging from

5 to 40%, depending on the assessment methods used; studies using more stringent assessment methods have reported rates between 5 and 10% (Grilo, 2002). A medical complication associated with BED is obesity (Yanovski, 2002). Psychological comorbidities of BED include major depressive disorder (MDD), alcohol use disorders, anxiety disorders, borderline personality disorder, avoidant personality disorder, and obsessive–compulsive personality disorder (Grilo, 2002; Wilfley et al., 2000; Wilfley, Wilson, & Agras, 2003).

CBT for BED

CBT for BED is a modified version of the CBT model for BN (Marcus, 1997). As with AN, the treatment has been adapted to address the specific behaviors and cognitions associated with BED. For example, whereas in BN and AN high dietary restraint is a central behavior thought to maintain the binge–purge cycle, in BED chaotic eating patterns (involving overrestriction and underrestriction) are more typical, and thus therapy is focused on healthy restraint (overall moderation of food intake rather than decreasing dietary restraint) (Wilfley et al., 2002). In addition, distorted cognition about shape/weight, low self-esteem, and negative affectivity, which are addressed in CBT for BN and AN as well, are thought to perpetuate binge-eating episodes. Thus, the general treatment model of CBT for BED is focused on normalizing the pattern of eating, encouraging moderate caloric intake, and changing dysfunctional thoughts related to the diet–binge cycle (Stein et al., 2001). The same general format of three phases is used and can be conducted individually over 24 weeks (Marcus, 1997) or in a group format over 20 weeks (Wilfley et al., 2002). During phase 1 of treatment, behavioral strategies are introduced, which include adopting a regular pattern of eating and self-monitoring to identify patterns of over- and underrestriction (Marcus, 1997; Wilfley et al., 2002). Phase 2 is focused on identifying and challenging beliefs perpetuating the binge cycle. In addition, cognitive skills are taught to counteract the negative thoughts associated with and predisposing individuals to binge eating (Marcus, 1997; Wilfley et al., 2002). In the final phase, treatment progress is identified and relapse prevention skills (e.g., coping with high-risk situations, problem solving) are taught (Marcus, 1997; Wilfley et al., 2002).

Empirical Support

CBT for BED has been tested in both individual (Marcus, Wing, & Fairburn, 1995) and group formats (Telch, Agras, Rossiter, Wilfley & Kenardy, 1990; Wilfley et al., 1993, 2002). When compared to a wait-list condition, CBT has consistently resulted in significantly greater reductions in binge eating (Telch et al., 1990; Wilfley et al., 1993). CBT has also been compared with interpersonal psychotherapy (IPT) in two randomized controlled trials (Wilfley et al., 1993, 2002). In both cases, CBT and IPT demonstrated equivalent and substantial improvement in binge eating and psychosocial functioning at posttreatment and

1-year follow-up. In the Wilfley and colleagues (2002) study, some relapse was noted from posttreatment to 1-year follow-up; however, the majority of participants were abstinent at the 1-year follow-up (CBT = 59%; IPT = 62%). Although studies comparing CBT with behavioral weight loss treatment (BWL) (Agras et al., 1994; Marcus et al., 1995; Nauta, Hospers, Kok, & Jansen, 2000) have demonstrated comparable reductions in binge eating at posttreatment, data from 6- and 12-month follow ups indicate that CBT is more effective than BWL in rates of abstinence from binge eating and reduction of concerns related to eating, weight, and shape (Nauta et al., 2000). Finally, CBT for BED has also been compared and found superior to pharmacological therapy (Grilo, Masheb, & Wilson, 2005; Ricca et al., 2001). Across studies, CBT for BED has resulted in rates of abstinence from binge eating around 50% (Stein et al., 2001). To date no published randomized controlled studies have investigated CBT in adolescents diagnosed with BED.

CBT AND RELATED TREATMENTS FOR ADOLESCENTS WITH EDs

CBT Modified for Adolescents with BN

Recently, Lock and colleagues modified Fairburn and colleagues' (1993) adult model of CBT for BN, for use with adolescents (Lock, 2002). The authors first treated youth with BN in a series of case studies using an unmodified version of CBT to determine which segments would be appropriate for this population. They found motivation for treatment low, family involvement necessary, and that adolescents responded well to parental involvement (Lock, 2002). Their modified version of CBT includes these factors and is divided into three stages designed to be completed over a 6-month period. During the first stage, CBT behavioral techniques are introduced. Parents are given the role of encouraging their child to participate in treatment, making sure their child attends therapy sessions, providing regular meal structure, limiting access to "trigger foods" to prevent binges, and staying with their child after meals to prevent purge episodes (Lock, 2002). Stage 2 involves cognitive techniques and continuing the behavioral strategies introduced in stage 1. Here, parents' involvement is to provide their observations of the adolescent's behavior to the therapist, offer insight on the problem-solving techniques from the family perspective, and provide their adolescent with assistance at home, if needed (Lock, 2002). Maintenance is the focus for the final phase. Parents are involved at this stage and beyond, in order to prevent or assist their child in any high-risk situations (Lock, 2002).

Empirical Support

Lock and colleagues have pilot tested (uncontrolled) their model of CBT for youth with BN on 16 adolescents. At posttreatment, binge eating or purging was reduced on average by 77%. Ten participants were abstinent, and two dropped out (Lock, 2002); these findings are consistent with the literature on CBT for adults with BN. Additional data are required before we can reach conclusions. Current results are only preliminary.

Family-Based Therapies

The first family models of AN were developed by Minuchin, Rosman, and Baker (1978), followed in 1989 by Mara Selvini Palazzoli and colleagues (Stein et al., 2001; see le Grange, 1999, for details). Two primary models of family therapy have been developed: the Maudsley approach and Behavioral Family Systems Therapy (BFST). The Maudsley approach, which is divided into three clear stages and is routinely delivered in 20 sessions over a 1-year time period, is based on the assumption that individual, family, and sociocultural influences interact to maintain the disorder (Dare & Eisler, 1997). The first phase lasts approximately 4–6 months and involves educating the family on the dangers of severe malnutrition, as well as enlisting the parents to help the child begin eating again. In case the parents have difficulty in going against their child's wishes, the therapist will attempt to help the family perceive the AN symptoms as separate from the child. More specifically, the goal is to have the child and parents perceive the illness (AN) as disparate from the child rather than a part of him or her. For example, the therapist may have the parents remember what their child was like prior to developing AN. In doing so, the family can begin to gather the necessary strength to fight the symptoms of AN without feeling like they are attacking their child. As another step within this stage of treatment, an actual family meal is brought to a therapy session. The family is told to eat as they do at home, thus offering the therapist a more objective view of the family dynamics (Lock, 2002). Phase 2, which lasts approximately 3–4 months, begins once the adolescent is eating properly and some weight gain is maintained. During this phase, the focus is on the symptoms of disordered eating, continued weight gain, and any other family issues that are pertinent to these topics. Although weight gain is of primary importance, the therapist is careful not to apply such excessive pressure on the child as to elicit conflict. Once the adolescent reaches 95% of his or her ideal body weight and the parents feel the child is able to prepare meals and eat independently, phase 3 is initiated. This final phase lasts 2–3 months and addresses issues related to adolescence in areas ranging from puberty to socialization. Other issues addressed include appropriate family boundaries and increased personal autonomy for the adolescent (Lock, 2002). Due to the numerous CBT components, some have described the Maudsley approach as a CBT treatment (Bowers, Evans, le Grange, & Anderson, 2003); however, because of the family-based format, we have described this treatment under family therapies.

Behavioral family systems therapy (BFST), developed by Robin, Siegel, Koepke, Moye, and Tice (1994), is similar to the Maudsley approach in design and content and is divided into four phases: (1) assessment, (2) control rationale,

(3) weight gain, and (4) weight maintenance (Robin, 2003). Because of the procedural overlap between these family-based approaches, we have chosen not to elaborate further on BFST (for details, see Robin, 2003).

Empirical Support

Both BFST and the Maudsley approach to family therapy for individuals diagnosed with AN have been subjected to randomized controlled clinical trials. The first randomized controlled study compared the Maudsley approach with individual supportive therapy (Russell, Szmukler, Dare, & Eisler, 1987). Russell and colleagues grouped 80 adolescents and adults diagnosed with AN based on early (<18 years) or late (>19 years) onset and short (<3 years) and long (>3 years) duration of illness. Family therapy was found to be superior to individual therapy for adolescents with short duration of illness, whereas adults responded equally well to both treatments on general outcome measures (e.g., weight gain and resuming menstruation). At the 5-year follow-up, approximately half of the participants were found to have good or intermediate outcomes (Eisler et al., 1997). In another follow-up study, le Grange, Eisler, Dare, and Russell (1992) investigated whether family therapy where the parents and child are seen together would be differentially more effective than family therapy where the parents and child are seen separately. Participants included 18 adolescents with early-onset AN randomly assigned to treatment condition. The results indicated improvement in both groups and no significant differences on weight gain or general outcome measures between the treatment formats.

The only randomized treatment outcome study involving BFST was conducted by Robin and colleagues (1999). They compared BFST to ego-oriented therapy within a sample of 37 adolescent females with AN. At posttreatment, weight gain was significantly greater in the BFST condition; however, at the 1-year follow-up this difference was no longer significant. In terms of general outcome, both treatments were found to be effective in treating adolescents with AN.

HOW CBT CAN BE APPLIED TO YOUTH WITH AN, BN, OR BED

In numerous psychological conditions affecting youth, CBT has been applied, evaluated, and found to be effective (see Kendall, 2000; Kendall & Choudhury, 2003). Based on our review of the literature on CBT for adults with EDs, it is clear that CBT is effective for BN and BED, and promising for AN. The question arises as to which components from these models (CBT for AN, BN, and BED) are appropriate for youth with EDs and what modifications are necessary. Several authors have suggested techniques that would be helpful in treating youth and abilities that make a particular youth more likely to respond to CBT.

For example, in their 2004 clinical guidelines for EDs, the National Institute for Clinical Excellence (NICE), the British organization responsible for providing national guidance on treatments and care, stated that once CBT is adjusted based on age, level of development, and appropriate family involvement, it is suitable for adolescents with BN.

As already described, CBT for ED diagnoses is broken into three stages emphasizing behavioral techniques (stage 1), cognitive techniques (stage 2), and relapse prevention (stage 3). This structure has been successful with adults and may be used with appropriate modifications for adolescents. Our recommendations include approaching CBT from a developmental perspective, placing a heightened emphasis on the context in which the ED has developed and is maintained, and recognizing the issues unique to the adolescent population. In addition, modifying specific cognitive and behavioral techniques to match the cognitive capabilities and interests of adolescents is also recommended. Finally, parental involvement is strongly encouraged. Our recommendations for applying CBT for youth with EDs are based on (1) empirical evidence from family therapy for adolescents with EDs; (2) empirical evidence from CBT for youth across conditions; and (3) clinical recommendations from experts working with this population. In the following section, we elaborate on these recommendations.

Approach

Adolescents face a range of developmental issues. In particular, dramatic physical, social, cognitive, behavioral, and affective changes are known to occur during this stage and are likely to impact the nature and frequency of problems experienced (Reinecke, Dattilio, & Freeman, 2003). EDs typically develop during adolescence and may be perpetuated by developmental factors such as postpubertal changes and associated weight gain, beginning awareness of sexuality, self-esteem, heightened self-awareness, and the struggle to create one's own separate identity. Because of the potential salience of these factors in the development of an ED, it is our recommendation that CBT address these developmental issues. For example, one suggestion is to educate the adolescent about the natural progression of weight gain and physical changes associated with puberty, and the discrepancy between these changes and the societal standard of beauty (Pike & Wilfley, 1996); this topic may be particularly relevant for those adolescents maturing earlier than their peers. In general, approaching CBT from this developmental perspective is unlikely to change specific CBT techniques. Instead, it will require familiarity with the developmental psychopathology of EDs (see Smolak, Levine, & Striegel-Moore, 1996) and sensitivity to the key issues noted above.

In determining whether CBT is appropriate for a given child, the level of cognitive development must also be considered. Given that both the theory and treatment of CBT is centralized around cognitions, Piaget's stages of cognitive development (Piaget, 1926) provide some insight into this question. Research has supported a great many of Piaget's central propositions (Siegler, 1986), although there are of course individual differences from child to child. Based on this model, between the ages of 7 and 11 children demonstrate organized and logical thought. In addition, thinking is less egocentric than at younger ages, and the youth is capable of concrete problem solving. From the ages of 11 to 15, thoughts become more abstract, integration of formal logic principles become possible, the ability to create theoretical intentions emerges, and numerous hypotheses and their potential outcome become apparent. Based on clinical experience, Robin, Gilroy, and Dennis (1998) suggest that CBT can be applied successfully in youth with EDs as long as the cognitive abilities of the child allow him or her to think abstractly about the meaning of ED concepts (e.g., appearance), consider alternative explanations, and are willing to test them out. They note that adolescents age 14 and older typically have acquired these abilities and that in some cases younger children may have, as well. Indeed, with normal development, adolescents as young as 11 are at a cognitive stage where they could benefit from typical CBT interventions.

For children who do not meet these criteria, we suggest using cognitive and behavioral techniques that have been adapted to meet their cognitive level. Perhaps one of the best examples of how CBT has been modified for children (ages 9–12 years) is the Coping Cat program (Kendall, 1990), for treating children with anxiety disorders. In this evidence-based program (Kendall, 1994; Kendall et al., 1997; see Albano & Kendall, 2002), behavioral techniques including modeling, exposure tasks, and role play are used and reinforced through homework assignments. Cognitive techniques include cognitive restructuring (e.g., identify and challenge anxious thoughts; develop coping thoughts to counter anxious thoughts) and problem solving (e.g., in an anxiety-provoking situation children are taught to use self-statements to reduce anxiety). New Beginnings (Lustig, Wolchik, & Weiss, 1999) is another evidence-based program using modified CBT for children (Weiss & Wolchik, 1998; Wolchik et al., 1993). This preventative intervention program is specifically for children (ages 9–12 years) of divorced parents and is designed for a group format. Coping skills are introduced through teaching (i.e., presenting the skill), modeling via role play and/or videotape, and practicing using structured activities. Specific modifications include explaining and labeling cognitive techniques with more understandable terms (e.g., negative self-talk labeled "doom and gloom"; challenging negative self-talk labeled "thoughtbusting") and using creative ways to explicate important concepts (e.g., puppet show, feelings thermometer). In both programs, positive reinforcement (e.g., stickers as a reward for homework completion; therapist/group leader giving positive feedback when appropriate) is used to increase compliance and to improve feelings of self-efficacy. We recommend that similar techniques be adapted for children with EDs.

A second modification of CBT for youth with EDs is to incorporate the social context in which development takes place (Bowers et al., 2003; Lock, 2002; Reinecke et al., 2003). Cognitive development of adolescents occurs in the social context through modeling and reinforcement; this adolescent social framework predominantly includes family (parents and siblings), peers, school environment, community, and role models (Bandura, 1977; Lock, 2002; Reinecke et al., 2003). In the context of EDs, perceived pressure to be thin (a known risk factor for developing an ED) is reinforced through mass media and social peer groups. For example, research shows that glorification of ultra-thin fashion models (role models) and comparing one's weight and shape with peers promotes negative body image and eating disturbances in adolescent females (Stice, Maxfield, & Wells, 2003). Among peers, direct (e.g., weight-related teasing) and indirect (e.g., "fat talk") forms of social pressures to be thin have also been found to contribute to eating disturbances in female adolescents (Wertheim, Paxton, Schutz, & Muir, 1997). In addition, family eating patterns, family dieting practices, and parental attitude toward the adolescent's weight and shape are variables that can also affect an adolescent's cognitions and beliefs toward food and his or her body (Thelen & Cormier, 1995; Wertheim, Mee, & Paxton, 1999). Pressures emanating from peers are particularly relevant for therapy, as adolescent girls have reported comparing their bodies with their friends and girls at school more than with family members and women in the media (Wertheim et al., 1997).

Therapists treating youth with EDs might adapt CBT to incorporate this psychosocial context. As the degree of influence from these variables will vary for each adolescent, it is up to the therapist to determine which social relationships are significantly contributing to the ED in each individual case. For example, if the parents' eating patterns and attitude are involved in maintaining the ED, the therapist might either include them during sessions with the adolescent or separately during the same time frame (see "Parental Involvement," below). To address the influence of media on the ED it is useful to be well informed of the current popular teen role models (i.e., models, actresses, and musicians). This knowledge will not only prepare the therapist for the adolescent's standard of comparison but also strengthen the therapeutic alliance by providing the adolescent with a feeling of being understood. Given that a great proportion of media influence is through fashion magazines, it may also be constructive to include teen magazine photographs and articles in therapy. In particular, these pictures and articles can be used to stimulate discussion and to eventually help the adolescent identify and counter the persuasion tactics attached to them (e.g., thinness is equated with success). Finally, in most cases, CBT for youth with EDs must also address the influence of peers. Useful techniques may include role playing and assertiveness training to combat teasing from schoolmates. Additionally, same-gender adolescent support groups focused on body acceptance and healthy eating may be needed to supplement CBT.

Parental Involvement

Parental involvement in treatment is highly recommended. CBT for youth across disorders (e.g., Albano, 2003; Heflin & Deblinger, 2003; Kendall & Choudhury, 2003; Pardini & Lochman, 2003) and family therapy for youth with EDs most often utilize parents in therapy, ranging from consultants to co-clients (see also Barmish & Kendall, 2005). Family members (including siblings) of adolescents with any ED should be included in the treatment process to share information, assist in communication, and offer advice on behavioral management; this is particularly the case for adolescents with AN, due to the impact the disorder often has on the entire family (National Institute for Clinical Excellence, 2004). Parental attendance during sessions can aid adolescents who have deficits in cognitive abilities (either age-based or as a result of the ED itself) and ensure treatment compliance if motivational issues are present (Lock, 2002). Parental involvement outside sessions can be vital as well, as parents can facilitate and encourage a family environment where behavioral modifications can occur (e.g., providing the adolescent with a regular meal pattern and shopping for food that fits into that pattern). Although familial involvement may be important for treatment adherence, treatment also needs to work toward adolescent independence (Young, 1990). Thus, some have suggested that for older adolescents treatment should begin in a family context but shift toward individual sessions as adolescent self-initiation is sustained over a period of time (Young, 1990). In general, for treatment of EDs parental involvement is recommended; however, the nature of involvement (e.g., included in sessions or seen separately) should be determined based on the adolescent's age, severity of the ED, parental level of support, and presence of any parental psychopathology.

Issues and Adaptations Specific to the Adolescent ED Population

Motivation is a critical component for treatment compliance. As noted earlier, lack of motivation for change is a common problem in the AN population in general, and the CBT protocol has been developed accordingly. Adolescents with AN and BN often lack motivation to participate in treatment and to recover, as they do not see their behavior as problematic (Bowers et al., 2003). In addition, adolescents with EDs are more likely to deny having an illness and less likely to desire help as compared to young adults with EDs (Fisher et al., 2001). To overcome these treatment barriers, several strategies are recommended. First, rather than force their child into therapy, parents are encouraged to bring him or her in willingly. One way to accomplish this task is to enlist the help of an individual the adolescent respects and with whom the adolescent has a positive relationship (e.g., older sibling, teacher, religious leader) (Pike & Wilfley, 1996). Second, if the adolescent does not feel an alliance with the therapist, it is unlikely that any significant changes can be made. Thus, it is critical that the therapist establish a positive working relationship during the first few meetings (see Creed & Kendall, 2005). One example of how one might build rapport is to devote the majority of the initial session to discussing feelings toward treatment and the ED from the adolescent's perspective. Other goals for this session might be to normalize the adolescent's concerns by highlighting commonalities between him or her with other youth who have been treated successfully. Third, to communicate acceptance, understanding, and empathy, the therapist is encouraged to maintain a nonjudgmental stance and use the same phrasing and examples as the adolescent.

CBT behavioral techniques to modify eating patterns will often need to be adjusted to accommodate the adolescents' capabilities in addition to their school and home environments. In terms of meal patterns, parental support is recommended to help the adolescent follow a prescribed regular pattern of eating (i.e., three meals and two to three snacks per day). In particular, to ensure compliance, the therapist might instruct the parents to provide the recommended meals and snacks for the adolescent. In addition, during stage 1 of CBT, families are discouraged from buying "dangerous" foods (i.e., foods that might increase the likelihood of binges) and instructed to keep an adequate quantity of "safe" foods in the house. Prescribed morning and afternoon snacks may also be difficult to integrate into the school setting (e.g., no eating in the classroom). In this instance, the therapist will need to problem-solve with the adolescent on how to incorporate the snacks into his or her schedule (e.g., eating a larger breakfast to compensate for the lack of a morning snack; having a somewhat late afternoon snack after returning home from school).

Additional modifications are recommended for implementing cognitive treatment strategies. As adolescents are more likely to identify with someone their age dealing with similar issues as compared to an authoritative figure (i.e., parent or therapist) (Berndt, 1996; Laursen, 1996), we recommend using videos or vignettes involving other adolescents with EDs to enhance the effectiveness of traditional cognitive techniques. For example, to further clarify the concept of reality testing automatic thoughts, the therapist might refer to a vignette of a young girl with an ED identifying an automatic thought (e.g., "If I gain weight, no one will like me") and then providing an alternative response (e.g., "Last summer, when I weighed more, I had the same number of friends"). By supplementing cognitive techniques with vignettes and/or written stories, adolescents may be more likely to attempt the technique themselves.

Specific cognitive techniques used in family therapy for youth with EDs include emphasizing alternative ways of thinking rather than challenging the adolescent's thinking, and having the adolescent keep a journal to identify automatic thoughts and maladaptive assumptions (Bowers et al., 2003). These modifications are applicable for CBT. Due to their lack of motivation and/or cognitive-developmental stage, some adolescents may be completely resistant to or incapable of engaging in cognitive techniques. In the CBT manual for adults with BN, Fairburn and colleagues (1993) recommend that in this situation the therapist abandon cognitive therapy and instead focus primarily on implementing behavioral techniques that are cognitively oriented (e.g., thought monitoring); this suggestion is applicable for youth as well.

PEDIATRIC OVERWEIGHT

Pediatric overweight is rising in prevalence at a rapid rate, with approximately 31% of children and adolescents ages 6–12 currently classified as overweight or at risk for overweight (Hedley et al., 2004). For youth, the CDC defines *at risk for overweight* as a Body Mass Index (BMI—kilograms divided by height in meters squared) between the 85th and 95th percentiles and *overweight* as a BMI at or above the 95th percentile for sex and age. Considered one of the leading health problems worldwide, the World Health Organization declared obesity a global epidemic in 1998, with the rate for children increasing at a faster level than that of adult obesity (Henderson & Brownell, 2003). Sadly, obesity in childhood tracks into adulthood, as do the associated psychosocial and medical sequelae (Serdula et al., 1993).

Numerous randomized controlled studies have been conducted testing treatments for pediatric overweight. Studies examining the effectiveness of family-based behavioral therapy provide empirical support for its effectiveness. In one of the earliest studies, Epstein and colleagues (1985) found that children in a family-based behavioral program showed better reductions in weight than a control group receiving equal education and attention. These differences were found in the short term (i.e., at 6- and 12-month follow-ups) and maintained in the long term (i.e., at 5- and 10-year follow-ups) (Epstein, McCurley, Wing, & Valoski, 1990; Epstein, Valoski, Wing, & McCurley, 1994; Epstein, Wing, Koeske, Andrasik, & Ossip, 1981). A review of the literature included 42 randomized studies targeting childhood and adolescent overweight (Jelalian & Saelens, 1999). However, if one selects only randomized controlled studies with a minimum of a 6-month follow-up, only 18 studies meet criteria (Summerbell et al., 2003). Although several studies have shown long-term improvement after behavioral treatment, Summerbell and colleagues (2003) concluded that because most studies had relatively small sample sizes, their results are not generalizable. While results are clearly promising, further study and replication are required. In addition, studies are needed to identify which components of treatment are the most helpful.

We begin this section with current data on the prevalence, associated medical complications, and psychosocial features of pediatric overweight. We then provide an overview of CBT for pediatric overweight, followed by a detailed discussion of the main behavioral components for treating childhood overweight. We then discuss the role of parents in treating childhood overweight. Finally, we describe what cognitive components have been included thus far in CBT for overweight youth and discuss potential future directions.

Prevalence, Medical Complications, and Psychosocial Features of Childhood Overweight

Data from the third National Health and Nutrition Examination Survey (NHANES III) found that 16% of children (ages 6–11 years) and 16% of adolescents (ages 12–17 years) in the United States were overweight (Hedley et al., 2004). Several health problems are associated with child and adolescent overweight. Overweight children have more cardiovascular risk factors, such as higher total cholesterol and serum lipoprotein ratios, than their normal-weight counterparts (Freedman, Dietz, Srinivasan, & Berenson, 1999; Berenson, Srinivasan, Wattigney, & Harasha, 1993). Also, the recent increase in the number of cases of type-2 diabetes found in adolescents has been linked to the increase in those who are overweight (Pinhas-Hamiel et al., 1996; Rosenbloom, Joe, Young, & Winter, 1999). Pediatric overweight is also associated with various health complications that emerge in the long term (Must, Jacques, Dallal, Bajema, & Dietz, 1992). An overweight child is six to seven times more likely to become an overweight adult, as compared to a non–overweight child (Serdula et al., 1993). Adult overweight has been linked to several severe health problems, such as hypertension, cardiovascular disease, type-2 diabetes, and an increased risk for developing cancer (Faith & Allison, 1996).

Perhaps just as damaging as the physical effects of childhood overweight are the psychosocial effects, which have been well documented. Discrimination, prejudice, and teasing are commonly directed at overweight children (Dietz, 2002; Goldfield & Chrisler, 1995; Gortmaker, Must, Perrin, Sobol, & Dietz, 1993; Hayden-Wade et al., 2005). Discrimination against overweight children has been persistent over time, and this stigmatization has increased in the past 40 years (Latner & Stunkard, 2003). Overweight children are perceived as being less competent than normal-weight children in social and athletic situations (Banis et al., 1988). Severely overweight children and adolescents have a lower quality of life as compared to normal-weight counterparts, in the areas of physical, emotional, social, and school functioning. These quality-of-life ratings were similar to those found in children and adolescents diagnosed with cancer and were consistent across sex, ethnicity, and socioeconomic status (Schwimmer, Burwinkle, & Varni, 2003). Overweight children are also considered less attractive and have worse body image than their non–overweight counterparts (Striegel-Moore et al., 2000), with childhood overweight documented as one of the most robust risk factors for later development of eating disorder psychopathology (Fairburn et al., 1997, 1998). Thus, along with reducing physical and psychosocial problems, treating childhood overweight can be one of the most important prevention tools for eating disorders as well as adult overweight and all of the associated negative sequelae (Golan, Fainaru, & Weizman, 1998).

CBT for Childhood Overweight

The behavioral methods used to treat childhood overweight parallel those used for the treatment of adult overweight (Wilson, 1994); yet, treatment of pediatric overweight has shown significantly better outcomes than that of adult overweight in both the short and long term (e.g., Epstein, Valoski, et al., 1995). Several reasons have been suggested for the increased treatment effect in children. First, weight loss in children may require less self-motivation, as parents can assist children in making changes, such as modifying the types of foods available in the home to healthier options. Second, diet and exercise patterns may not be as entrenched in children as in adults, so that these habits will respond better to modification programs. Third, natural increases in height make it easier for children to show a reduction in percent overweight even if they do not lose weight (Wilson, 1994).

Behavior change components are central in almost all forms of overweight treatment for children and adolescents. Typical behavioral weight-loss methods include stimulus control strategies and self-monitoring of eating and physical activity behaviors (Epstein, Myers, Raynor, & Saelens, 1998; Graves, Meyers, & Clark, 1988). Stimulus control refers to a restructuring of the home to promote desired behavior and limit undesirable behavior for both food and activity. For example, healthier foods are placed in more accessible areas, while accessibility to high-fat and high-sugar foods is limited. Similarly, equipment used for physical activity is made more accessible while that used for sedentary activities is placed in less reachable areas. Programs differ in the specific dietary modification plan used and the type of physical activity instruction. However, some form of both is typically included as the main focus of behavior modification. Programs that include both a dietary and physical activity component have shown long-term success as compared to exercise modification alone (Jelalian & Saelens, 1999).

As noted above, family-based behavioral treatment programs have been the most studied intervention for childhood overweight and have produced the best short- and long-term results (Jelalian & Saelens, 1999). Parental involvement is considered crucial, but the degree and nature of that involvement vary by program. Effective treatments not only lead to reduced weight but are also associated with significant health benefits, better physical fitness, and improved lipid profiles (Faith, Saelens, Wilfley, & Allison, 2001).

Currently, full inclusion of cognitive components in the treatment of pediatric overweight is rare, though some programs have now expanded to include problem solving and cognitive restructuring about self-esteem and feelings of self-efficacy (Graves et al., 1988). In an attempt to improve long-term effectiveness of treatment, Wilfley and colleagues (2005) developed behavioral skills-based maintenance (BSM), a treatment plan that teaches cognitive strategies to help improve weight maintenance. The underlying theory is that, while behavioral components are effective in reducing weight, cognitive components may be necessary to help prevent weight regain (see "Cognitive Components," below, for details). A large-scale randomized controlled trial evaluating behavioral skills-based maintenance has recently been completed, and data analysis is underway (Wilfley et al., 2005).

Dietary Modification

No consistent evidence has shown that overweight children consume more calories than do normal-weight counterparts. However, reducing caloric intake is primary for successful weight loss. Several behavioral components are central to dietary modification. Self-monitoring is a recommended first step to help increase the child's awareness of current eating habits and of ongoing changes (Wilfley & Saelens, 2002). Participants are instructed in self-monitoring of various aspects of their eating, such as daily diet and caloric intake. In addition, weekly weight monitoring helps children to learn the association between their eating behaviors and changes in their weight. Self-monitoring continues throughout treatment as a means of keeping track of food intake. Additional strategies include contracting, where rewards are given for having met behavioral goals, with the rewards often contingent on weight loss. Participants are also taught to praise one another for positive eating practices. In particular, parents are encouraged to praise their children.

While several diets have been studied, Epstein's traffic light diet (Epstein & Squires, 1988; Epstein et al., 1998) is the main dietary behavioral change program evaluated across studies. The traffic light diet was developed by Epstein and colleagues and is used mainly with preadolescent children, although a recent study included a modified version of the traffic light diet with adolescents (Saelens et al., 2002). Using the USDA's Food Guide Pyramid as its foundation, the diet uses a color-coded food exchange system, mainly based on fat content and nutritional value, with some coding based on sugar content. Foods are grouped into one of three color categories, indicating the recommended frequency of each food. "Red" foods (e.g., French fries and donuts) are foods to mostly avoid, "yellow" foods (e.g., pasta and lower-fat varieties of cheese) can be eaten in moderation, and "green" foods (e.g., most fruits and vegetables) may be eaten freely (Epstein et al., 1998). Families are provided with detailed lists of healthy (i.e., green and yellow) alternatives within each food guide pyramid category, although the top level of the pyramid contains only red foods. Children are educated as to how to meet their nutritional needs by decreasing their total fat and calorie intake and by selecting nutrient-dense foods based on the color codes (Epstein et al., 1994). Children are given an individualized calorie range goal, approximately 1,000–1,200 calories per day, and a limited number of servings of red foods, aimed at producing a half-pound weight loss per week. The range is adjusted if necessary, depending on the child's rate of weight loss. Consistent with the aims of the intervention, outcomes of this approach show reduced caloric intake and a decreased number of red foods (Epstein et al., 1981).

More recent work by Epstein and colleagues focuses on lifestyle changes rather than caloric restriction. Results showed that, by using the traffic light diet but only reinforcing an increase in fruit and vegetable consumption, children not only increased their intake of fruits and vegetables but also decreased consumption of high-fat, high-sugar foods. Of note, this study included normal-weight children who were considered at risk because they had an overweight parent (Epstein et al., 2001).

Physical Activity

Targeting changes in physical activity augments the long-term effects of dietary interventions (Epstein et al., 1994). Targeting either increases in physical activity or reductions in sedentary activity leads to successful weight loss (Epstein, Paluch, Gordy, & Dorn, 2000). Reduction in sedentary activity is promoted by positively reinforcing decreases in leisure-time activities such as television watching, computer time, and playing video games. Previous studies indicated that targeting reductions in sedentary behavior produced more effective weight-loss results (Epstein, Wing, Koeske, & Valoski, 1985). However, the most recent study by Epstein and colleagues (2000), comparing reductions in sedentary activity to increases in physical activity in children ages 8–12, found that both groups showed similar decreases in percent overweight and increases in fitness at 2-year follow-up. These findings increase treatment options, as either approach to modifying physical activity can be successful. Similar to dietary modification, self-monitoring of children's physical and sedentary activity is a reasonable first step and should continue throughout treatment (Faith et al., 2001).

Parent Participation

Parental involvement has been a main feature of treatment, stemming from the idea that childhood overweight is a result of maladaptive behaviors that are learned and reinforced by the child's surroundings. Having an overweight parent, which is likely due to a combination of genetics and environment (e.g., the parents maintain higher-fat foods around the house) increases the risk of being an overweight child (Whitaker, Wright, Pepe, Weidel, & Dietz, 1997). Whether or not they are overweight, parents can play a crucial role in treatment because of their ability to directly change the home environment through stimulus control (Golan et al., 1998). Parents can help their children lose weight by supporting healthy eating behavior (e.g., serving healthy meals and limiting child access to fast-food restaurants), supporting healthy physical activity changes (e.g., planning fun family activities), and supporting healthy lifestyle changes (e.g., modeling and praising healthy behaviors). The nature of parental involvement varies across studies, with treatments including parent and child together, parent and child simultaneously but separately, and most recently only the parents.

Epstein's family-based treatment targets behavioral modification of the parent and child together, teaching them the necessary skills to establish and maintain healthier eating and physical activity. Participating family members typically sign a behavioral contract, which stipulates the child's behavioral goals and the reinforcements provided by the parent that will be used to help achieve those goals. Parents are taught that reinforcements should never be rewards in the form of food or money but ideally should be interpersonal in nature—for example, family outings, adding special privileges, or sometimes buying something like a favorite CD. Along with these, praise is used on an ongoing basis to encourage positive change, and attention to negative behavior is minimized. These interventions teach more positive parenting skills, such as reinforcement and environmental restructuring, using stimulus control techniques described above. Additionally, parents are instructed in behavioral changes similar to their children, including self-monitoring and changing diet and physical activity behavior, so the parents can serve as models for their children. Typically, parents and children are seen together as an individual dyad, followed by separate group sessions for the parents and children. Reductions in parental BMI are significant predictors of a child's BMI change both in treatment and at follow-up, although this relation decreases over time (Wrotniak, Epstein, Paluch, & Roemmich, 2004).

Targeting only the parents as the agents of change for childhood overweight has also been found to be effective. Golan and colleagues (1998) adapted a family-based approach to treating childhood overweight such that only parents participated in the treatment. In the parent-only intervention, parents attended group sessions and five short individual sessions, with no direct involvement by the children. Parents were instructed in behavior modification for the entire family, such as decreasing family sedentary behaviors, improving diet, and decreasing availability of more fattening foods in the home. In addition, parents were taught parenting skills, such as better coping techniques and setting appropriate child responsibilities. Golan's program places responsibility in the hands of the parents, teaching that it is the parent's responsibility to offer proper foods, and children must be empowered to make their own decisions. This treatment was compared to one in which children were seen alone (Golan et al., 1998). Results showed that children in the parent-only group evidenced significantly greater weight loss than children targeted exclusively. At 1-year, 2-year, and 7-year follow-ups, the decrease in percent overweight for the children in the parent-only group was significantly greater than that in the child-only group (Golan & Crow, 2004a, 2004b). Similarly, a recent study by Epstein and colleagues (2001) found that changes in the eating habits of normal-weight children could be obtained by targeting just the parents.

Targeting the parent only may be more effective with younger children, as parents have more control over their child's food intake and activity level. However, different approaches may be more successful depending on the age of the child. For older children, it may be more effective to target the parent and child separately. A study by Brownell, Kelman, and Stunkard (1983) indicated that for overweight adolescents the most effective results are seen when parents and children are treated separately. It is recommended that programs tailor the degree of parental involvement based on the age of the youth.

Cognitive Components

A limited number of studies have evaluated the addition of cognitive components, and thus far the results are inconclusive as to whether they enhance weight loss. To date, the added component has mainly focused on incorporating problem-solving skills into treatment. In addition, cognitive restructuring has been included in some studies, but this has not been studied in detail as a specific component of treatment. Graves and colleagues (1988) found that the addition of problem solving to family-based behavioral therapy did improve weight loss. Forty overweight children and their parents were assigned to one of three treatment groups, either family-based behavioral therapy with or without problem-solving or a family-based education-only weight-loss group. Children in both family-based behavioral programs decreased their BMI and percent overweight, but decreases were significantly greater for the problem-solving group. In a similar study, Epstein, Paluch, Gordy, and Dorn (2000) looked at three family-based behavioral treatment programs that differed in whether problem-solving techniques were included as a program component. Sixty-seven families were assigned to one of three groups: problem solving taught to parent and child, problem solving taught only to the child, and standard family-based behavioral treatment. All three groups reduced their mean weights at 6 months.

In contrast to the earlier findings of Graves and colleagues (1988), Epstein and colleagues (2000) reported that the addition of problem solving did not appear to add any benefit to weight reduction. The apparent contradiction in results between these two studies might be understood by the difference in length of treatment: Participants in the earlier study received 8 weeks of training, while the more recent study provided 6 months of treatment. Besides the different effects of extended treatment, it is possible that a longer treatment includes some discussion on how to handle barriers even without direct instruction in problem solving. Further research should continue to assess whether there is any added benefit to including cognitive components in treatment for pediatric overweight.

Toward this end, Wilfley and colleagues (2005) developed a comprehensive CBT intervention that expands family-based weight-loss treatment by incorporating a focus on weight maintenance. In daily life, children are exposed to numerous situations that are not conducive to persisting with weight maintenance behaviors, such as birthday parties, bad weather for physical activities, or peer pressure to play video games instead of engaging in physical activity. BSM teaches children and parents to identify high-risk situations, preplan to avoid these situations, or problem-solve to cope more effectively with them. Instruction in cognitive restructuring (e.g., avoiding all-or-nothing thinking such as

"I've blown it for today, so I might as well eat whatever I want," or "I'm off the program this week") is essential to decrease the likelihood that inevitable behavioral slips will result in full relapse. Without adequate long-term coping skills, negative cognitions make the change in goal from weight loss to weight maintenance difficult; also, feelings of a lack of self-efficacy and continued exposure to high-risk situations will likely lead to an increase in weight (Perri, 2002). The BSM intervention attempts to improve long-term outcomes through CBT strategies, including (1) motivation enhancement skills, such as helping children and parents to view maintenance as a viable goal, since it may seem to be less inherently rewarding than losing weight; (2) cognitive restructuring; and (3) relapse prevention, teaching parents and children coping skills for avoiding or recovering from lapses in the face of high-risk situations. Using these strategies has the potential to limit behavioral lapses and improve children's self-efficacy for coping with difficult situations, likely resulting in improved long-term success (Wilfley et al., 2005).

SUMMARY AND FUTURE DIRECTIONS

The empirical testing of CBT for youth with obesity and EDs is at different stages of development. In terms of EDs, CBT has been well established for adults with BN and BED, where a considerable number of randomized controlled studies have confirmed its efficacy in comparison to wait-list, other empirically based psychotherapies, and medication. Fewer studies have been conducted with AN, likely due to the recalcitrant nature of the disorder. EDs are commonly found in the female adolescent population, and there are numerous comorbid physical and psychological conditions linked with these disorders. In spite of the development of most EDs during adolescence, as well as the finding that shorter duration of illness is predictive of better outcome, there is a dearth of research evidence on CBT specifically for youth with EDs. With the demonstrated effectiveness of CBT with BN and BED in adults, it is ripe to be adapted and evaluated for youth with these disorders. For example, a model of CBT for adolescents with BN was recently developed with promising initial findings. It is imperative that future studies focus on developing empirically supported CBT treatments for youth with EDs. We have offered some preliminary recommendations that we hope will be useful in the formulation stages.

Although CBT is considered the treatment of choice for BN and BED (NICE, 2004), it is not a panacea. For example, abstinence rates across treatment trials for adults with BN receiving a full course of CBT range between 40 and 50% (Wilson et al., 2002). This recurrent finding raises a natural question, namely, Which subgroups does CBT not impact and why? Perhaps, for some, the chronicity of ED symptoms limits the chance of a full recovery. Targeting younger populations and hence shortening the time period between onset of the disorder and initiation of treatment is likely to lead to a greater probability of success. Another possibility is that CBT in its current form is too narrowly focused on the symptoms of the ED. Broadening CBT to incorporate other pertinent issues (e.g., interpersonal difficulties) has recently been proposed for adults (Fairburn, Cooper, & Shafran, 2003) and may be germane for adolescents with EDs as well. Finally, it is unclear whether the current classification system for diagnosing EDs in adults is applicable to youth. Further research is needed to determine the clinically significant threshold and nature of EDs in children and adolescents.

In contrast to the limited testing of ED treatment specifically for youth, promising long-term effects have been found with overweight children who receive behavioral family-based weight-loss treatment. However, although studies indicate that the treatment of childhood overweight can be highly successful, pediatric weight control programs have mostly been studied with carefully selected homogeneous samples of Caucasian middle- and upper-income families in research clinical laboratories (Crawford, Story, Wang, Ritchie, & Sabry, 2001; Summerbell et al., 2003; Zeller, Saelens, Roehrig, Kirk, & Daniels, 2004). They have rarely been studied in community-based settings or settings that serve diverse populations (Summerbell et al., 2003), and only to a limited degree among adolescents (Jelalian & Saelens, 1999).

Treatments must continue to be tested and enhanced to improve the long-term maintenance of weight loss in children. The primary areas that might lead to more effective treatments would include (1) adding and specifically evaluating cognitive components, (2) understanding which family members should be included in treatment for optimal results, and (3) potentially improving long-term outcomes by capitalizing on the peer environment. Additionally, intervention should begin as early as possible, since the older a child is when overweight, the greater the risk of becoming an overweight adult (Epstein, Valoski, Koeske, & Wing, 1986). Further research could be done targeting children younger than the typically studied age group of 8–12; in such programs, targeting the parent as the agent of change would be necessary, as children this young are likely not developmentally capable of making the changes themselves. Across age groups, parent-only interventions are a promising research direction, particularly as they are more cost-effective and can avoid the potential stigma a child might feel from participating in a weight-loss program (Epstein et al., 2001).

REFERENCES

Agras, W. S., Brandt, H. A., Bulik, C. M., Dolan-Sewell, R., Fairburn, C. G., Halmi, K. A., et al. (2004): Report of the National Institutes of Health workshop on overcoming barriers to treatment research in anorexia nervosa. *International Journal of Eating Disorders, 35*(4), 509–521.

Agras, W. S., Telch, C. F., Arnow, B., Eldredge, K., Wilfley, D. E., Raeburn, S. D., et al.

(1994). Weight loss, cognitive-behavioral, and desipramine treatments in binge eating disorder: An additive design. *Behavior Therapy, 25,* 225–238.

Albano, A. M. (2003). Treatment of social anxiety disorder. In M. A. Reinecke, F. M. Dattilio, & A. Freeman (Eds.), *Cognitive therapy with children and adolescents: A casebook for clinical practice* (2nd ed., pp. 128–161). New York: Guilford Press.

Albano, A. M., & Kendall, P. C. (2002). Cognitive behavioural therapy for children and adolescents with anxiety disorders: Clinical research advances. *International Review of Psychiatry, 14,* 129–134.

American Psychiatric Association. (1994). *Diagnostic and statistical manual of mental disorders* (4th ed.). Washington, DC: Author.

American Psychiatric Association. (2000). *Diagnostic and statistical manual of mental disorders* (4th ed., text rev.). Washington, DC: Author.

Ball, J. R. (1998). *A controlled evaluation of psychological treatments for anorexia nervosa (cognitive behavior therapy, behavioral family therapy).* Unpublished doctoral dissertation, University of New South Wales, Sydney, Australia.

Ball, J., & Mitchell, P. (2004). A randomized controlled study of cognitive behavior therapy and behavioral family therapy for anorexia nervosa patients. *Eating Disorders, 12,* 303–314.

Bandura, A. (1977). *Social learning theory.* New York: General Learning Press.

Banis, H. T., Varni, J. W., Wallander, J. L., Korsch, B. M., Jay, S. M., Adler, R., et al. (1988). Psychological and social adjustment of obese children and their families. *Child: Care, Health, and Development, 14,* 157–173.

Barmish, A. & Kendall, P. C. (2005). Should parents be co-clients in treating anxious youth? *Journal of Clinical Child and Adolescent Psychology, 34,* 569–581.

Becker, A. E., Grinspoon, S. K., Klibanski, A., & Herzog, D. B. (1999). Current concepts: Eating disorders. *New England Journal of Medicine, 340*(14), 1092–1098.

Berenson, G. S., Srinivasan, S. S. Wattigney, W. A., & Harasha, D. W. (1993). Obesity and cardiovascular risk in children. *Annals of the New York Academy of Sciences, 699,* 93–103.

Berndt, T. J. (1996). Transitions in friendship and friends' influence. In J. A. Graber & A. C. Petersen (Eds.), *Transitions through adolescence: Interpersonal domains and context* (pp. 57–84). Hillsdale, NJ: Erlbaum.

Beumont, P. J. V. (2002). Clinical presentation of anorexia nervosa and bulimia nervosa. In C. G. Fairburn & K. Brownell (Eds.), *Eating disorders and obesity: A comprehensive handbook* (2nd ed., pp. 162–170). New York: Guilford Press.

Bowers, W. A., Evans, K., le Grange, D., & Anderson, A. E. (2003). Treatment of adolescent eating disorders. In M. A. Reinecke, F. M. Dattilio, & A. Freeman (Eds.), *Cognitive therapy with children and adolescents: A casebook for clinical practice* (2nd ed., pp. 247–280). New York: Guilford Press.

Brownell, K. D., Kelman, J. H., & Stunkard, A. J. (1983). Treatment of obese children with and without their mothers: Changes in weight and blood pressure. *Pediatrics, 71,* 515–523.

Bulik, C. M. (2002). Anxiety, depression, and eating disorders. In C. G. Fairburn & K. Brownell (Eds.), *Eating disorders and obesity: A comprehensive handbook* (2nd ed., pp. 193–198). New York: Guilford Press.

Channon, S., de Silva, P., Helmsley, D., & Perkins, R. (1989). A controlled study of cognitive-behavioral and behavioral treatment of anorexia. *Behaviour Research and Therapy, 27,* 529–535.

Creed, T. A., & Kendall, P. C. (2005). Therapist alliance-building behaviour within a cognitive-behavioral treatment for anxiety in youth. *Journal of Consulting and Clinical Psychology, 73,* 498–505.

Dare, C., & Eisler, I. (1997). Family therapy for anorexia nervosa. In D. M. Garner & P. E.

Garfinkel (Eds.), *Handbook of treatment for eating disorders* (2nd ed., pp. 307–324). New York: Guilford Press.

Dietz, W. H. (2002). Medical consequences of obesity in children and adolescents. In C. G. Fairburn & K. D. Brownell (Eds.), *Eating disorders and obesity: A comprehensive handbook* (2nd ed., pp. 473–476). New York: Guilford Press.

Eisler, I., Dare, C., Russell, G., Szmuckler, G., le Grange, D., & Dodge, E. (1997). Family and individual therapy in anorexia nervosa: A five-year follow-up. *Archives of General Psychiatry, 54*, 1025–1030.

Epstein, L. H., Gordy, C. C., Raynor, H. A., Beddome, M., Kilanowski, C. K., & Paluch, R. (2001). Increasing fruit and vegetable intake and decreasing fat and sugar intake in families at risk for childhood obesity. *Obesity Research, 9*(3), 171–178.

Epstein, L. H., McCurley, J., Wing, R. R., & Valoski, A. M. (1990). Five-year follow-up of family-based behavioral treatments for childhood obesity. *Journal of Consulting and Clinical Psychology, 58*(5), 661–664.

Epstein, L. H., Myers, M. D., Raynor, H. A., & Saelens, B. E. (1998). Treatment of pediatric obesity. *Pediatrics, 101*, 554–570.

Epstein, L. H., Paluch, R., Gordy, C. C., & Dorn, J. (2000). Decreasing sedentary behaviors in treating pediatric obesity. *Archives of Pediatric Adolescent Medicine, 154*, 220–226.

Epstein, L. H., & Squires, S. (1988). *The stoplight diet for children.* Boston: Little, Brown.

Epstein, L. H., Valoski, A. M., Koeske, R., & Wing, R. R. (1986). Family-based behavioral weight control in obese young children. *Journal of the American Dietetic Association, 86*, 481–484.

Epstein, L. H., Valoski, A. M., Wing, R. R., & McCurley, J. (1994). Ten-year outcomes of behavioral family based treatment for childhood obesity. *Health Psychology, 13*, 373–383.

Epstein, L. H., Valoski, A. M., Vara, L. S., McCurley, J., Wisniewski, L., Kalarchian, M. A., et al. (1995). Effects of decreasing sedentary behavior and increasing activity on weight change in obese children. *Health Psychology, 14*, 109–115.

Epstein, L. H., Wing, R. K., Koeske, R., & Valoski, A. M. (1985). A comparison of lifestyle exercise, aerobic exercise, and calisthenics on weight loss in obese children. *Behavior Therapy, 16*, 345–356.

Epstein, L. H., Wing, R. R., Koeske, R., Andrasik, F., & Ossip, D. J. (1981). Child and parent weight loss in family-based behavior modification programs. *Journal of Consulting and Clinical Psychology, 49*(5), 674–685.

Epstein, L. H., Wing, R. R., Woodall, K., Penner, B. D., Kress, M. J., & Koeske, R. (1985). Effects of family-based behavioral treatment on obese 5- to 8-year-old children. *Behavior Therapy, 16*, 205–212.

Fairburn, C. G. (2002). Cognitive-behavioral therapy for bulimia nervosa. In C. G. Fairburn & K. D. Brownell (Eds.), *Eating disorders and obesity: A comprehensive handbook* (2nd ed., pp. 302–307). New York: Guilford Press.

Fairburn, C. G., & Brownell, K. D. (Eds.) (2002). *Eating disorders and obesity: A comprehensive handbook* (2nd ed.). New York: Guilford Press.

Fairburn, C., Cooper, Z., & Shafran, R. (2003). Cognitive behavior therapy for eating disorders: A "transdiagnostic" theory and treatment. *Behaviour Research and Therapy, 41*, 509–528.

Fairburn, C. G., & Harrison, P. J. (2003). Eating disorders. *The Lancet, 361*, 407–416.

Fairburn, C. G., Marcus, M. D., & Wilson, G. T. (1993). Cognitive-behavioral therapy for binge eating and bulimia nervosa: A comprehensive treatment manual. In C. G. Fairburn & T. G. Wilson (Eds.), *Binge eating: Nature, assessment, and treatment* (pp 361–404). New York: Guilford Press.

Fairburn, C. G., Shafran, R., Cooper, Z. (1998). A cognitive behavioral theory of anorexia nervosa. *Behaviour Research and Therapy, 37*, 1–13.

Fairburn, C. G., Welch, S. L., Doll, H. A., Davies, B. A., & O'Conner, M. E. (1997). Risk factors for bulimia nervosa: A community-based case-control study. *Archives of General Psychiatry, 54,* 509–517.

Faith, M. S., & Allison, D. B. (1996). Obesity and physical health: Looking for shades of grey. *Weight Control Digest, 6,* 539–540.

Faith, M. S., Saelens, B. E., Wilfley, D. E., & Allison, D. B. (2001). Behavioral treatment of childhood and adolescent obesity: Current status, challenges, and future directions. In J. K. Thompson & L. Smolak (Eds.), *Body image, eating disorders, and obesity in youth: Assessment, prevention, and treatment* (pp. 313–340). Washington, DC: American Psychological Association.

Fisher, M., Golden, N. H., Katzman, D. K., Kreipe, R. E., Rees, J., Schebendach, J., et al. (1995). Eating disorders in adolescents: A background paper. *Journal of Adolescent Health, 16,* 420–437.

Fisher, M., Schneider, M., Burns, J., Symons, H., & Mandel, F. (2001). Differences between adolescents and young adults at presentation to an eating disorders program. *Journal of Adolescent Health, 28*(3), 222–227.

Freedman, D. S., Dietz, W. H., Srinivasan, S. R., & Berenson, G. S. (1999). The relation of overweight to cardiovascular risk factors among children and adolescents: The Bogalusa Heart Study. *Pediatrics, 103,* 1175–1182.

Garner, D. M., Vitousek, K. M., & Pike, K. M. (1997). Cognitive-behavioral therapy for anorexia nervosa. In D. M. Garner & P. E. Garfinkel (Eds.), *Handbook of treatment for eating disorders* (2nd ed., pp. 94–144). New York: Guilford Press.

Golan, M., & Crow, S. (2004a). Parents are key players in the prevention and treatment of weight-related problems. *Nutrition Reviews, 62*(1), 39–50.

Golan, M., & Crow, S. (2004b). Targeting parents exclusively in the treatment of childhood obesity: Long-term results. *Obesity Research, 12*(2), 357–361.

Golan, M., Fainaru, M., & Weizman, A. (1998). Role of behavior modification in the treatment of childhood obesity with the parents as the exclusive agents of change. *International Journal of Obesity, 22,* 1217–1224.

Goldfield, A., & Chrisler, J. C. (1995). Body stereotyping and stigmatization of obese persons by first graders. *Perceptual and Motor Skills, 81,* 909–910.

Gortmaker, S. L., Must, A., Perrin, J. M., Sobol, A. M., & Dietz, W. H. (1993). Social and economic consequences of overweight in adolescence and young adulthood. *New England Journal of Medicine, 329,* 1008–1012.

Graves, T., Meyers, A. W., & Clark, L. (1988). An evaluation of parental problem solving training in the behavioral treatment of childhood obesity. *Journal of Consulting and Clinical Psychology, 56*(2), 246–250.

Grilo, C. M. (2002). Binge eating disorder. In C. G. Fairburn & K. D. Brownell (Eds.), *Eating disorders and obesity: A comprehensive handbook* (2nd ed., pp. 178–182). New York: Guilford Press.

Grilo, C. M., Masheb, R. M., & Wilson, G. T. (2005). Efficacy of cognitive behavioral therapy and fluoxetine for the treatment of binge eating disorder: A randomized double-blind placebo-controlled comparison. *Biological Psychiatry, 57,* 301–309.

Halmi, K. (1999, November). *A multi-site study of AN treatment involving CBT and fluoxetine treatment in prevention of relapse: A 6-month treatment analysis.* Paper presented at the annual meeting of the Eating Disorders Research Society, San Diego, CA.

Halmi, K. A., Agras, W. S., Crow, S., Mitchell, J., Wilson, G. T., Bryson, S. W., & Kraemer, H. C. (2005). Predictors of treatment acceptance and completion in anorexia nervosa. *Archives of General Psychiatry, 62,* 776–781.

Hayden-Wade, H. A., Stein, R. I., Ghaderi, A., Saelens, B. E., Zabinski, M. F., & Wilfley, D.

F. (2005). Prevalence, characteristics, and correlates of teasing experiences among overweight children versus non overweight peers. *Obesity Research, 13,* 1381–1392.

Hedley, A. A., Ogden, C. L., Johnson, C. L., Carroll, M. D., Curtin, L. R., & Flegal, K. M. (2002). Prevalence of overweight and obesity among U.S. children, adolescents, and adults, 1999–2002. *Journal of American Medical Association, 23,* 2847–2850.

Heflin, A. H., & Deblinger, E. (2003). Treatment of a sexually abused adolescent with posttraumatic stress disorder. In M, A. Reinecke, F. M. Dattilio, & A. Freeman (Eds.), *Cognitive therapy with children and adolescents: A casebook for clinical practice* (2nd ed., 214–246). New York: Guilford Press.

Henderson, K. E., & Brownell, K. D. (2003). The toxic environment and obesity: Contribution and care. In J. K Thompson (Ed.), *Handbook of eating disorders and obesity* (pp. 339 348). New York: Wiley.

Hoek, H. W. (2002). Distribution of eating disorders. In C. G. Fairburn & K. D. Brownell (Eds.), *Eating disorders and obesity: A comprehensive handbook* (2nd ed., pp. 233–237). New York: Guilford Press.

Jelalian, E., & Saelens, B. E. (1999). Empirically supported treatments in pediatric psychology: Pediatric obesity. *Journal of Pediatric Psychology, 24*(3), 223 248.

Kendall, P. C. (1990). *Coping Cat workbook.* Ardmore, PA: Workbook Publishing.

Kendall, P. C. (1994). Treating anxiety disorders in children: Results of a randomized clinical trial. *Journal of Consulting and Clinical Psychology, 62,* 100–110.

Kendall, P. C. (2000). *Child and adolescent therapy: Cognitive-behavioral procedures* (2nd ed.). New York: Guilford Press.

Kendall, P. C., & Choudhury, M. S. (2003). Children and adolescents in cognitive-behavioral therapy: Some past efforts and current advances, and the challenges in our future. *Cognitive Therapy and Research, 27*(1), 89–104.

Kendall, P. C., Flannery-Schroeder, E., Panicelli-Mindel, S. M., Southam-Gerow, M. A., Henin, A., & Warman, M. (1997). Therapy for youths with anxiety disorders: A second randomized clinical trial. *Journal of Consulting and Clinical Psychology, 65,* 366–380.

Lask, B., & Bryant-Waugh, R. (1993). *Childhood onset anorexia nervosa and related eating disorders,* Hillsdale, NJ: Erlbaum.

Lask, B., Waugh, R., & Gordon, J. (1997). Childhood-onset anorexia nervosa is a serious illness. In M. S. Jacobson & J. M. Rees (Eds.), *Adolescent nutritional disorders: Prevention and treatment* (pp. 120–126). New York: New York Academy of Sciences.

Latner, J. D., & Stunkard, A. J. (2003). Getting worse: The stigmatization of obese children. *Obesity Research, 11,* 452–456.

Laursen, B. (1996). Closeness and conflict in adolescent peer relationships: Interdependence with friends and romantic partners. In W. M. Bukowski, A. F. Newcomb, & W. W. Hartup (Eds.), *The company they keep: Friendship in childhood and adolescence* (pp. 186–210). New York: Cambridge University Press.

le Grange, D. (1999). Family therapy for adolescent anorexia nervosa. *Journal of Clinical Psychology, 55,* 727–739.

le Grange, D., Eisler, I., Dare, C., & Russell, G. F. (1992). Evaluation of family treatments in adolescent anorexia nervosa: A pilot study. *International Journal of Eating Disorders, 12,* 347–357.

Lock, J. (2002). Treating adolescents with eating disorders in the family context: Empirical and theoretical considerations. *Child and Adolescent Psychiatry Clinics of North America, 11,* 331 342.

Lock, J., le Grange, D., Agras, W. S., & Dare, C. (2001). *Treatment manual for anorexia nervosa: A family-based approach.* New York: Guilford Press.

Lucas, A. R., Beard, C. M., O'Fallon, W. M., Kurland, L. T. (1991). 50-year trends in the incidence of anorexia nervosa in Rochester, Minn.: A population-based study. *American Journal of Psychiatry, 148*(7), 917–922.

Lustig, J. L., Wolchik, S. A., & Weiss, L. (1999). The New Beginnings parenting program for divorced mothers: Linking theory and intervention. In C. A. Essau & F. Petermann (Eds.), *Depressive disorders in children and adolescents: Epidemiology, risk factors, and treatment* (pp. 361–381). Northvale, NJ: Jason Aronson.

Marcus, M. D. (1997). Adapting treatment for patients with binge-eating disorder. In D. M. Garner & P. E. Garfinkel (Eds.), *Handbook of treatment for eating disorders* (2nd ed., pp. 484–493). New York: Guilford Press.

Marcus, M. D., Wing, R. R., & Fairburn, C. G. (1995). Cognitive behavioral treatment of binge eating vs. behavioral weight control on the treatment of binge eating disorder. *Annals of Behavioral Medicine, 17*, S090.

Minuchin, S., Rosman, B. L., & Baker, L. (1978). *Psychosomatic families: Anorexia nervosa in context.* Cambridge, MA: Harvard University Press.

Must, A., Jacques, P. F., Dallal, G. E., Bajema, C. J., & Dietz, W. H. (1992). Long-term morbidity and mortality of overweight adolescents: A follow-up of the Harvard Growth Study of 1922 to 1935. *New England Journal of Medicine, 327*, 1350–1355.

Nauta, H., Hospers, H., Kok, G., & Jansen, A. (2000). A comparison between cognitive and a behavioral treatment for obese binge eaters and obese non-binge eaters. *Behavior Therapy, 31*, 441–461.

National Institute for Clinical Excellence. (2004). *Eating disorders: Core interventions in the treatment and management of anorexia nervosa, bulimia nervosa and related eating disorders: A national clinical practice guideline.* London: Author.

O'Brien, K. M., & Vincent, N. K. (2003). Psychiatric comorbidity in anorexia and bulimia nervosa: Nature, prevalence, and causal relationships. *Clinical Psychology Review, 23*, 57–74.

Pardini, D. A., & Lochman, J. E. (2003). Treatments for oppositional defiant disorder. In M. A. Reinecke, F. M. Dattilio, & A. Freeman (Eds.), *Cognitive therapy with children and adolescents: A casebook for clinical practice* (2nd ed., 43–69). New York: Guilford Press.

Perri, M. G. (2002). Improving maintenance in behavioral treatment. In C. G. Fairburn & K. D. Brownell (Eds.), *Eating disorders and obesity: A comprehensive handbook* (2nd ed., pp. 593–598). New York: Guilford Press.

Piaget, J. (1926). *The language and thought of the child.* Oxford, UK: Harcourt, Brace.

Pike, K. M., Walsh, T. B., Vitousek, K., Wilson, T. G., & Bauer, J. (2003). Cognitive behavior therapy in the posthospitalization treatment of anorexia nervosa. *American Journal of Psychiatry, 160*(11), 2046–2049.

Pike, K. M., & Wilfley, D. E. (1996). The changing context of treatment. In L. Smolak, M. P. Levine, & R. Striegel-Moore (Eds.), *The developmental psychopathology of eating disorders: Implications for research, prevention, and treatment* (pp. 365–397). Mahwah, NJ: Erlbaum.

Pinhas-Hamiel, O., Dolan, L. M., Daniels, S. R., Staniford, D., Khoury, P., & Zeitler, P. (1996). Increased incidence of non-insulin-dependent diabetes mellitus among adolescents. *Journal of Pediatrics, 128*, 608–615.

Pomeroy, C., & Mitchell, J. E. (2002). Medical complications of anorexia nervosa and bulimia nervosa. In C. G. Fairburn & K. D. Brownell (Eds.), *Eating disorders and obesity: A comprehensive handbook* (2nd ed, pp. 278–285). New York: Guilford Press.

Reinecke, M. A., Dattilio, F. M., & Freeman, A. (2003). What makes for an effective treatment? In M. A. Reinecke, F. M. Dattilio, & A. Freeman (Eds.), *Cognitive therapy with children and adolescents: A casebook for clinical practice* (2nd ed., pp. 1–18). New York: Guilford Press.

Ricca, V., Mannucci, E., Mezzani, B., Moretti, S., Di Bernardo, M., Rotella, C. M., &

Faravelli, C. (2001). Fluoxetine and fluvoxamine combined with individual cognitive-behaviour therapy in binge eating disorder: A one-year follow-up study. *Psychotherapy and Psychosomatics, 70,* 298–306.

Robin, A., Gilroy, M., & Dennis, A. B. (1998). Treatment of eating disorders in children and adolescents. *Clinical Psychology Review, 18*(4), 421–446.

Robin, A., Siegel, P., Koepke, T., Moye, A. W., & Tice, S. (1994). Family therapy versus individual therapy for adolescent females with anorexia nervosa. *Journal of Developmental and Behavioral Pediatrics, 15,* 111–116.

Robin, A., Siegel, P., Moye, A., Gilroy, M., Dennis, A. B., & Sikand, A. (1999). A controlled comparison of family versus individual therapy for adolescents with anorexia nervosa. *Journal of the American Academy of Child and Adolescent Psychiatry, 38*(12), 1482–1489.

Robin, A. L. (2003). Behavioral family systems therapy for adolescents with anorexia nervosa. In A. E. Kazdin & J. R. Weisz (Eds.), *Evidence-based psychotherapies for children and adolescents* (pp. 358–373). New York: Guilford Press.

Rosenbloom, A. L., Joe, J. R., Young, R. S., & Winter, W. E. (1999). Emerging epidemic of type 2 diabetes in youth. *Diabetes Care, 22,* 345–354.

Russell, G. F., Szmukler, G. I., Dare, C., & Eisler, I. (1987). An evaluation of family therapy in anorexia nervosa and bulimia nervosa. *Archives of General Psychiatry, 44,* 1047–1056.

Saelens, B. E., Sallis, J. F., Wilfley, D. E., Patrick, K., Cella, J. A., & Buchta, R. (2002). Behavioral weight control for overweight adolescents initiated in primary care. *Obesity Research, 10,* 22–32.

Schwimmer, J. B., Burwinkle, T. M., & Varni, J. W. (2003). Health-related quality of life in severely obese children and adolescents. *Journal of American Medical Association, 289*(14), 1813–1819.

Serdula, M., Ivery, D., Coates, R., Freedman, D., Williamson, D., & Byers, T. (1993). Do obese children become obese adults? A review of the literature. *Prevention Medicine, 22,* 167–177.

Serfaty, M. A., Turkington, D., Heap, M., Ledsham, L., & Jolley, E. (1999). Cognitive therapy versus dietary counseling in the outpatient treatment of anorexia nervosa: Effects of the treatment phase. *European Eating Disorders Review, 5,* 102–114.

Siegler, R. S. (1986). *Children's thinking.* Englewood Cliffs, NJ: Prentice-Hall.

Slade, P. D. (1982). Towards a functional analysis of anorexia nervosa and bulimia nervosa. *British Journal of Clinical Psychology, 21,* 167–179.

Smolak, L., Levine, M. P., & Striegel-Moore, R. (Eds.). (1996). *The developmental psychopathology of eating disorders: Implications for research, prevention, and treatment.* Hillsdale, NJ: Erlbaum.

Stein, R. I., Saelens, B. E., Dounchis, J.Z., Lewczyk, C. M., Swenson, A. K., & Wilfley, D. E. (2001). Treatment of eating disorders in women. *The Counseling Psychologist, 29*(5), 695–732.

Stice, E., Maxfield, J., & Wells, T. (2003). Adverse effects of social pressure to be thin on young women: An experimental investigation of the effects of "fat talk." *International Journal of Eating Disorders, 34,* 108–117.

Stice, E., Presnell, K., & Sprangler, D. (2002). Risk factors for binge eating onset in adolescent girls: A 2-year prospective investigation. *Health Psychology, 21,* 131–138.

Striegel-Moore, R. H., Schreiber, G. B., Lo, A., Crawford, P., Obarzanek, E., & Rodin, J. (2000). Eating disorder symptoms in a cohort of 11- to 16-year-old black and white girls: The NHLBI growth and health study. *International Journal of Eating Disorders, 27,* 49–66.

Sullivan, P. (1995). Mortality in anorexia nervosa. *American Journal of Psychiatry, 152*(7), 1073–1074.

Summerbell, C. D., Ashton, V., Campbell, K. J., Edmunds, L., Kelly, S., & Waters, E. (2004).

Interventions for treating obesity in children (Cochrane Review). In *The Cochrane Library*, Issue 2. Chichester, UK: Wiley.

Telch, C. F., Agras, W. S., Rossiter, E. M., Wilfley, D. E., & Kenardy, J. (1990). Group cognitive – behavioral treatment for the nonpurging bulimic: An initial evaluation. *Journal of Consulting and Clinical Psychology, 58,* 629–635.

Thelen, M. H., & Cormier, J. F. (1995). Desire to be thinner and weight control among children and their parents. *Behavior Therapy, 26,* 85–99.

Vitousek, K. B. (2002). Cognitive-behavioral therapy for anorexia nervosa. In C. G. Fairburn & K. Brownell (Eds.), *Eating disorders and obesity: A comprehensive handbook* (2nd ed., pp. 308–313). New York: Guilford Press.

Vitousek, K., Watson, S., & Wilson, G. T. (1998). Enhancing motivation for change in treatment-resistant eating disorders. *Clinical Psychology Review, 18*(4), 391–420.

Vitousek, K. M. (1998). The current status of cognitive-behavioral models of anorexia nervosa and bulimia nervosa. In P. M. Salkovskis (Ed.), *Frontiers of cognitive therapy: The state of the art and beyond* (pp. 383–418). New York: Guilford Press.

Weiss, L., & Wolchik, S. A. (1998). New Beginnings: An empirically-based intervention program for divorced mothers to help their children adjust to divorce. In J. M. Briesmeister, & C. E. Schaefer (Eds.), *Handbook of parent training: Parents as co-therapists for children's behavior problems* (2nd ed., pp. 445–478). New York: Wiley.

Wertheim, E. H., Mee, V., & Paxton, S. J. (1999). Relationships among adolescent girls' eating behaviors and their parents' weight-related attitudes and behaviors. *Sex Roles, 41*(3/4), 169–187.

Wertheim, E. H., Paxton, S. J., Schutz, H. K., & Muir, S. L. (1997). Why do adolescent girls watch their weight? An interview study examining sociocultural pressures to be thin. *Journal of Psychosomatic Research, 42,* 345–355.

Whitaker, R. C., Wright, J. A., Pepe, M. S., Weidel, K. D., & Dietz, W. H. (1997). Predicting obesity in young adulthood from childhood and parental obesity. *New England Journal of Medicine, 337,* 869–873.

Wilfley, D. E., Agras, W. S., Telch, C. F., Rossiter, E. M., Schneider, J. A., Cole, A. G., et al. (1993). Group cognitive-behavioral therapy and group interpersonal psychotherapy for the nonpurging bulimic individual: A controlled comparison. *Journal of Consulting and Clinical Psychology, 61*(2), 296–305.

Wilfley, D. E., Friedman, M. A., Dounchis, J. Z., Stein, R. I., Welch, R. R., & Ball, S. A. (2000). Comorbid psychopathology in binge eating disorder: Relation to eating disorder severity at baseline and following treatment. *Journal of Consulting and Clinical Psychology, 68*(4), 641–649.

Wilfley, D. E., & Saelens, B. E. (2002). Epidemiology and causes of obesity in children. In C. G. Fairburn & K. D. Brownell (Eds.), *Eating disorders and obesity: A comprehensive handbook* (2nd ed., pp. 429–432). New York: Guilford Press.

Wilfley, D. E., Stein, R. I., Saelens, B. E., Mockus, D. S., Matt, G. E., Hayden-Wade, H. A., et al. (2005). *Maintenance approach to childhood obesity treatment.* Manuscript in preparation.

Wilfley, D. E., Welch, R. R., Stein, R. I., Spurrell, E. B., Cohen, L. R., Saelens, B. E., et al. (2002). A randomized comparison of group cognitive-behavioral therapy and group interpersonal psychotherapy for the treatment of overweight individuals with binge-eating disorder. *Archives of General Psychiatry, 59,* 713–721.

Wilfley, D. E., Wilson, G. T., & Agras, W. S. (2003) The clinical significance of binge eating disorder. *International Journal of Eating Disorders, 34*(Suppl.), S96–S106.

Wilson, G. T. (1994). Behavioral treatment of childhood obesity: Theoretical and practical implications. *Health Psychology, 13*(5), 371–372.

Wilson, T. (1999). Cognitive behavior therapy for eating disorders: progress and problems. *Behaviour Research, 37,* S79–S95.

Wilson, G. T., Fairburn, C. G., & Agras, W. S. (1997). Cognitive-behavioral therapy for bulimia nervosa. In D. M. Garner & P. E. Garfinkel (Eds.), *Handbook of treatment for eating disorders* (2nd ed., pp 67–93). New York: Guilford Press.

Wilson, T., Fairburn, C., Agras, W. S., Walsh, B. T., & Kraemer, H. C. (2002). Cognitive-behavioral therapy for bulimia nervosa: Time course and mechanisms of change. *Journal of Consulting and Clinical Psychology, 70*(2), 267–274.

Wiser, S., & Telch, C. (1999). Dialectical behavior therapy for binge-eating disorder. *Journal of Clinical Psychology, 55*, 755–768.

Wolchik, S. A., West, S. G., Westover, S., Sandler, I. N., Martin, A., Lustig, J., et al. (1993). The children of divorce parenting intervention: Outcome evaluation of an empirically based program. *American Journal of Community Psychology, 21*(3), 293–331.

Wrotniak, B. H., Epstein, L. H., Paluch, R. A., & Roemmich, J. N. (2004). Parent weight change as a predictor of child weight change in family-based behavioral obesity treatment. *Archives of Pediatric Adolescent Medicine, 158*, 342–347.

Yanovski, S. Z. (2002). Binge eating in obese persons. In C. G. Fairburn & K. Brownell (Eds.), *Eating disorders and obesity: A comprehensive handbook* (2nd ed., pp. 403–407). New York: Guilford Press.

Young, F. (1990). Strategic adaptations of cognitive-behavioral therapy for anorexic and bulimic adolescents and their families. In R. McMahon & R. Peters (Eds.), *Behavior disorders of adolescence: Research, intervention, and policy in clinical and school settings* (pp. 111–123). New York: Plenum Press.

Zeller, M. H., Saelens, B. E., Roehrig, H., Kirk, S., & Daniels, S. R. (2004). Psychological adjustment of obese youth presenting for weight management treatment. *Obesity Research, 12*, 1576–1586.

CHAPTER 10

Treating Children and Adolescents Affected by Disasters and Terrorism

ANNETTE M. LA GRECA and WENDY K. SILVERMAN

Devastating natural disasters (e.g., hurricanes, earthquakes, floods, brush-fires, tsunamis), human-made disasters (e.g., plane crashes, ship sinkings, nuclear waste accidents), and acts of violence (e.g., school shootings, bombings, terrorist attacks) have focused tremendous attention and concern on how disasters affect children and adolescents. In fact, it has become apparent that children's exposure to such events can lead to reactions that may interfere substantially with their day-to-day functioning and cause significant distress and impairment (e.g., Gurwitch, Sitterle, Young, & Pfefferbaum, 2002; La Greca, Silverman, Vernberg, & Prinstein, 1996; La Greca, Silverman, & Wasserstein, 1998; Lonigan, Shannon, Finch, Daugherty, & Taylor, 1991; Pynoos et al., 1987; Vernberg, La Greca, Silverman, & Prinstein, 1996).

Understanding children's and adolescents' reactions to disasters and to terrorism, and developing appropriate interventions to treat children who are severely traumatized by these events, has become an incredibly challenging, important, and timely mental health concern. For example, it has only been within the past 15 years that empirical reports have begun to document the severe and often persistent trauma reactions that are evident among children exposed to devastating natural disasters, such as hurricanes (e.g., La Greca et al.,

1996, 1998; Lonigan et al., 1991; Vernberg et al., 1996). At the present time, the United States is in an active era of hurricane activity, which could last for the next 10–30 years, and will bring more hurricanes, and more of the stronger hurricanes (Category 3 or higher, with sustained winds above 110 miles per hour) to the United States each year (report of the National Oceanic and Atmospheric Administration, *The Miami Herald*, September 8, 2004, p. 1). In fact, the 2004 hurricane season produced five hurricanes that affected the United States—Alex, Charley, Frances, Ivan, and Jeanne—and three of these hurricanes were a Category 3 or higher. Moreover, as we finalize this chapter, the tremendous devastation, massive relocation, and extensive loss of life are still unfolding from Hurricane Katrina, which struck Florida in late August 2005 and subsequently decimated a massive area along the Gulf Coast of the United States, including New Orleans. This terrifying and catastrophic event affected millions of children and families, and it will likely take years for recovery and reconstruction.

In addition to unpredictable and devastating natural disasters, the terrorist attacks of September 11, 2001, on the World Trade Center and Pentagon have led to increasing concerns within the United States and abroad about the possibility of future attacks and how to deal with their mental health repercussions. Surveys of New York City school children taken 6 months after the attacks on the World Trade Center estimated that as many as 75,000 children and youth might have posttraumatic stress disorder, thereby representing a tremendous public mental health concern (Applied Research & Consulting LLC and the Columbia University Mailman School of Public Health, 2002). Considering these recent events, it is a critical time for understanding disasters' effects on children and adolescents, and how to help them cope with and recover from such events.

In this chapter we describe the symptoms and prevalence of posttraumatic stress disorder (PTSD) in children and adolescents as well as other reactions that may result from exposure to disasters and terrorism. We also outline factors that contribute to the development and course of children's posttraumatic stress. We then turn our attention to the current state of prevention and intervention research, including cognitive-behavioral treatments, for assisting children and adolescents who are affected by disasters. We end with a discussion of "best practices" for implementation.

HOW DISASTERS AFFECT CHILDREN AND ADOLESCENTS

Accumulating evidence from a variety of sources indicates that disasters and acts of terrorism represent traumatic events for children and adolescents that can result in posttraumatic stress (PTS) symptoms and posttraumatic stress disorder (see American Academy of Child and Adolescent Psychiatry, 1998; Gurwitch et al., 2002; La Greca & Prinstein, 2002; Silverman & La Greca, 2002; Yule, Udwin, & Bolton, 2002). Immediately following a disaster or terrorist attack, there may be a brief period of "shock" or numbing, or sometimes even elation and relief at being alive (Vogel & Vernberg, 1993). Beyond these initial shock reactions, however, children and adolescents commonly report symptoms of PTSD within the first few weeks or months postdisaster.

Findings also reveal that children's reactions to disasters can be severe and are not merely transitory events that dissipate quickly (see Gurwitch et al., 2002; La Greca & Prinstein, 2002; Yule et al., 2002). Moreover, because some children and adolescents display severe and persistent reactions, efforts to provide interventions for children and adolescents following disasters represent an important, but frequently overlooked, mental health need.

Posttraumatic Stress Disorder

Diagnosis

In DSM-IV (American Psychiatric Association, 1994), PTSD refers to a set of symptoms that develop following exposure to an unusually severe stressor or event, one that causes or is capable of causing death, injury, or threat to the physical integrity of oneself or another person. To meet criteria for a diagnosis of PTSD, a child's reaction to the traumatic event must include intense fear, helplessness, or disorganized behavior (American Psychiatric Association, 1994). In addition, specific criteria must be met for three symptom clusters: reexperiencing, avoidance/numbing, and hyperarousal. For a diagnosis of PTSD, these symptoms must be manifest for at least 1 month (acute PTSD) and be accompanied by significant impairment in functioning (e.g., problems in school, social, or family relations); when symptoms persist more than 3 months, the diagnosis is for chronic PTSD.

Symptoms of *reexperiencing* include recurrent or intrusive thoughts or dreams about the event and intense distress at cues or reminders of the event. For young children, reexperiencing also may be reflected in repetitive play with traumatic themes or by a reenactment of traumatic events in play, drawings, or verbalizations. Following acts of violence (e.g., shootings), children have described a specific vivid image or sound that disturbed them, or reported traumatic dreams with a strong feeling of life threat (Nader & Mello, 2002; Pynoos & Nader, 1988). Such findings may explain why many children are afraid to sleep alone after a traumatic event.

Symptoms of *avoidance or numbing* include efforts to avoid thoughts, feelings, or conversations about the traumatic event, avoiding reminders of the event, diminished interest in normal activities, and feeling detached or removed from other people. For example, children may report a lessened interest in play (or their usual activities—such as Play Station, video games, etc.), and may report feeling distant from parents and friends.

Symptoms of *hyperarousal* include difficulty in sleeping or concentrating, irritability, angry outbursts, hypervigilance, and an exaggerated startle response.

These behaviors must be newly occurring since the traumatic event. Startle reactions are especially persistent after exposure to violent events, like shootings (Nader & Mello, 2002) or bombings (Gurwitch et al., 2002).

Prevalence

It is difficult to estimate the prevalence of PTSD in children and adolescents following disasters and acts of terrorism because studies have been extremely diverse with respect to the type of trauma evaluated, assessment methods and sampling procedures used, and the length of time since the target event. Community studies suggest that approximately 24–39% of children and adolescents exposed to trauma (such as community violence or a natural disaster) meet the criteria for a PTSD diagnosis during the *first few weeks or months* following the trauma (e.g., Berman, Kurtines, Silverman, & Serafini, 1996; Vernberg et al., 1996; see also the American Academy of Child and Adolescent Psychiatry, 1998). However, when subclinical levels of PTS are considered, more than 50% of the children in large community samples have reported at least moderate levels of PTSD during the first 2–4 months following a traumatic event (e.g., Vernberg et al., 1996). In general, symptoms of PTSD appear to be common among children and adolescents exposed to natural disasters and community violence, although fewer children meet the criteria for a full PTSD diagnosis.

Rates of PTSD and PTS symptoms have been reported to be even higher among children and adolescents who witness death and physical injury in conjunction with acts of violence or following natural disasters associated with mass casualties. For example, in reviewing studies on the aftermath of terrorism, Gurwitch and colleagues (2002) estimated that rates of PTSD varied from 28 to 50% among children exposed to terrorist events (e.g., kidnappings, hostage situations; see also Ayalon, 1993). Following a devastating earthquake in Armenia that killed over 25,000 people, Goenjian and colleagues (1995, 1997) found that rates of "likely PTSD" in adolescents exceeded 50%, even a year or more after the disaster.

Types of PTS Symptoms Reported

Community studies indicate that child trauma victims most commonly report symptoms of reexperiencing. For example, up to 90% of children exposed to Hurricane Andrew, a devastating natural disaster, reported symptoms of reexperiencing 3 months after the disaster (Vernberg et al., 1996), and 78% reported such symptoms nearly a year after the disaster (La Greca et al., 1996). In contrast, symptoms of avoidance and numbing were the least commonly reported symptoms of PTSD (49% of children 3 months postdisaster, and 24% at 10 months postdisaster). Because of this, the presence of symptoms of avoidance and numbing may be good markers for the presence of a PTSD diagnosis in children and adolescents (e.g., Lonigan, Anthony, & Shannon, 1998).

Developmental Course

Although little is known about the course of PTSD symptoms in children over time, it does appear that such symptoms may emerge in the days or weeks following a traumatic event, and can take months or years to dissipate in some children and adolescents (e.g., Green et al., 1994; Gurwitch et al., 2002; La Greca et al., 1996, 1998; Shaw, Applegate, & Schorr, 1996; Vincent, 1997; Yule et al., 2000, 2002). In the absence of reexposure to trauma or the occurrence of other traumatic events, the typical developmental course of symptoms appears to be one of lessening frequency and intensity over time. For example, 3 months after Hurricane Andrew, 39% of the children surveyed informally met criteria for PTSD, but by 7 months postdisaster this was reduced to 24%, and further reduced to 18% by 10 months postdisaster (La Greca et al., 1996). For adolescents who survived the sinking of the cruise ship *Jupiter* in 1988, 51.5% were estimated to develop PTSD at some point in time after the disaster (compared with 3.4% of the matched controls); the duration of PTSD was less than a year for 30% of the survivors, with additional youth "remitting" each subsequent year (see Yule et al., 2000, 2002).

Despite the tendency for PTS symptoms to decline over time, children who show *persistent* symptoms of PTSD over the year following a disaster may be at risk for long-term PTSD reactions. Vincent (1997) followed children who reported moderate to severe PTS symptoms 10 months after Hurricane Andrew ("high-risk" youth), and compared them with a control sample of youth who reported very few PTS symptoms at 10 months postdisaster. When the children were reevaluated in early adolescence, 42 months postdisaster, findings revealed that 40% of the "high-risk" youth continued to report moderate to severe levels of PTS symptoms as well as impairment in their day-to-day functioning. Only one of the children who reported mild levels of symptoms at 10 months postdisaster reported significant PTS symptoms later on. Also alarming were the findings of a study of adolescent survivors of the *Jupiter* sinking at 5–8 years postdisaster. Even after this extended time period, Yule and colleagues (2000, 2002) found that PTSD was still present in 17.5% of the youth (or 34% of the initial cases of PTSD).

Together, these data suggest a steady reduction in PTS symptoms and diagnoses of PTSD over time (with no further exposure to similar disasters), although a significant minority of youth do not "recover" and report substantial difficulties years later. Across studies, the findings also suggest that it is highly unusual for children to report significant elevations in PTS symptoms or a PTSD diagnosis over a long-term period if such symptoms were not evident in the first few months or year following a traumatic event. Thus, children and adolescents who display persistent and elevated symptoms of PTS or meet criteria for a diagnosis of chronic PTSD following disasters are important to target for psychological interventions.

Other Disaster Reactions

In addition to PTSD, other trauma reactions have been identified in children and adolescents (see Vogel & Vernberg, 1993). In fact, rates of comorbidity are extremely high among youth who display PTSD (American Academy of Child and Adolescent Psychiatry, 1998). Evaluating and understanding these other reactions to trauma can aid mental health providers in delivering more effective interventions to children and adolescents.

Regardless of whether PTSD symptoms are present, children's *anxiety levels* appear to be affected by exposure to trauma. Traumatic events have long been viewed as a potential pathway to the development of phobias and other anxiety-based disorders in youth (see Silverman & Ginsburg, 1995). Evidence also suggests that exposure to disasters is associated with high levels of anxiety in youth (e.g., Goenjian et al., 1995; La Greca et al., 1998; Lonigan, Shannon, Taylor, Finch, & Sallee, 1994; Yule et al., 2002). Recent studies of the adolescent survivors of the *Jupiter* sinking at 5–8 years postdisaster (Bolton, O'Ryan, Udwin, Boyle, & Yule, 2000; Yule et al., 2002) found higher rates of anxiety disorders relative to matched controls; these disorders included specific phobia (23.6% vs. 9.2%), panic disorder (12.0% vs. 2.3%), separation anxiety (6.8% vs. 0%), and "any" anxiety disorder (40.7% vs. 18.4%). Similarly, a survey of children and adolescents in the New York City Public Schools at 6 months after the terrorist attacks of September 11, 2001, revealed significant elevations in several anxiety disorders relative to epidemiological data collected prior to the attacks (Applied Research & Consulting LLC and the Columbia University Mailman School of Public Health, 2002). Specifically, high rates were observed for agoraphobia (15%), separation anxiety (12.3%), and panic (9%).

Significant symptoms of *depression* have also been reported following natural disasters and acts of terrorism (e.g., Bolton et al., 2000; Goenjian et al., 1997; Gurwitch et al., 2002; McDermott & Palmer, 2002; Nolen-Hoeksema & Morrow, 1991). Depressive reactions especially are common following disasters that involve the loss of friends and loved ones (Goenjian et al., 1995, 1997; Gurwitch et al., 2002; Yule et al., 2002). In such cases, depression may be a secondary disorder arising from bereavement and unresolved PTSD (Vernberg & Varela, 2001). For example, in the long-term follow-up of adolescent survivors of the *Jupiter* sinking (Bolton et al., 2000; Yule et al., 2002), 61 youth developed both major depression and PTSD; in 93% of these cases, depression developed at the same time or after PTSD.

Safety and security concerns also are common reactions to disasters (Silverman & La Greca, 2002). In young children, these concerns may be manifested by fear of separation from parents or loved ones. For example, following the bombing of the Federal Building in Oklahoma City, Gurwitch and colleagues (2002) observed high levels of children's separation fears (e.g., clinging to parents); in addition, children had a heightened sense of vigilance and a decreased sense of safety and security. With sniper shootings, terrorist attacks, and other "unpredict-able" acts of violence, fears of reoccurrence, ongoing security concerns, and pre-occupation with revenge may be evident (Gurwitch et al., 2002; Nader & Mello, 2002; Pynoos & Nader, 1988).

Many children and adolescents evidence increased *fears* following a disaster (Gurwitch et al., 2002; Vogel & Vernberg, 1993; Yule et al., 2002). Usually (but not always) these fears are directly linked to the kind of trauma that is experi-enced. For example, fears of water, thunder, and rainstorms have been reported following hurricanes (Vogel & Vernberg, 1993).

Summary

In addition to PTSD, other anxiety disorders and depressive disorders constitute the most common types of clinical problems documented in children and adoles-cents following disasters, and may be comorbid with PTSD. Even at subclinical levels, it is common for children and adolescents to report anxiety, fears, security concerns, and depressive symptoms, in addition to PTS symptoms. Conse-quently, in most clinical situations it is desirable to obtain a comprehensive assess-ment of youngsters' functioning following disasters, in addition to evaluating symptoms of PTSD. Treatments for children and adolescents affected by disasters need to consider adjunct procedures for addressing significant symptoms of anxi-ety (see Kendall & Suveg, Chapter 7, this volume), depression (see Stark et al., Chapter 5, this volume), and/or fears—or possibly other behavior problems that may have been evident before the disaster—in addition to treating posttraumatic stress. In this regard, other chapters in this volume will be useful in delineating effective treatments for the variety of comorbid psychological problems youth may display following disasters.

UNDERSTANDING FACTORS THAT CONTRIBUTE TO CHILDREN'S AND ADOLESCENTS' DISASTER REACTIONS

Before describing interventions, we briefly review factors that play a role in chil-dren and adolescents' disaster reactions, as this literature provides the basis for "empirically informed" intervention efforts. Moreover, as will be discussed later, there is a dearth of well-controlled intervention studies of children and adoles-cents affected by disasters and terrorism. Thus, the material highlighted in this section may serve as a resource for the development of effective intervention and prevention programs to assist youth who are affected by disasters and terrorism.

Across a wide range of studies and types of disasters, the variables that have been linked with the development of PTSD symptoms in youth can be concep-tualized as falling within one of the following categories: (1) *aspects of traumatic exposure*, (2) *preexisting characteristics of the child*, (3) characteristics of the *postdisaster recovery environment,* and (4) the *child's psychological resources.* These variables are contained within a conceptual model developed by Korol (1990) and Green and colleagues (1991) and later modified (La Greca et al., 1996; Vernberg et al., 1996).

Some of the categories in the model (and the variables within them) are best viewed as risk factors that might be useful for identifying children and adolescents who are most likely to develop PTSD reactions following a disaster, but might not be as useful for developing disaster-related interventions because they are not modifiable (e.g., age, gender). In contrast, most aspects of the recovery environment (e.g., social support, parental reactions) and of children's resources (e.g., coping skills) *are* modifiable and could be targeted in treatment efforts.

Aspects of Traumatic Exposure

Several aspects of traumatic exposure are important for the emergence of children's disaster reactions. First and foremost is the *presence or perception of a life threat* (Green et al., 1991; see also Kendall, Chapter 1, this volume). The more children and adolescents perceive that their lives or the lives of loved ones are threatened, the higher their reports of PTSD symptoms (e.g., La Greca et al., 1996; Lonigan et al., 1991).

Disasters that lead to the *death of a loved one* (parent, friend, classmate), especially a violent death as through a shooting or terrorist act, are strongly linked to the development of PTSD symptoms (see Ayalon, 1993; Gurwitch et al., 2002; Nader & Mello, 2002). Stress reactions arising from such events are complicated by feelings of grief and guilt. Children who lose a parent in a terrorist attack, for example, not only have to deal with the complicated task of bereavement but also must reconcile why they survived and the loved one did not. This may lead to impairing and interfering thoughts regarding whether they could have done more to prevent the death from occurring in the first place.

Loss of possessions and disruption of everyday life, including displacement from home, school, and community, also contribute to PTSD symptoms following disasters (La Greca et al., 1996; Vernberg et al., 1996). Following destructive natural disasters, children and adolescents are faced with a cascading series of life stressors that are set into motion by the disaster, which may last for months or years, such as the loss of one's home and/or possessions, a change of schools, shifts in parental employment and finances, friends moving away, altered leisure activities, and so on. These stressors may seriously challenge children's adaptation and coping.

Children's *proximity* to the event is another important aspect of traumatic exposure (e.g., Gurwitch et al, 2002; Pynoos & Nader, 1988). Specifically, evidence suggests that the more proximal children are to the disaster, the more intense or severe their reactions.

The duration and intensity of life-threatening events are additional aspects of traumatic exposure associated with children's symptom severity (Nader & Mello, 2002; Vernberg & Verela, 2001). For example, the prolonged nature of certain disasters (i.e., floods), in which no immediate relief is in sight, is very distressing to children (Jacobs et al., 2002). Disaster reactions are further influenced by exposure to either *single or multiple incidents*, with greater distress often (but not always) following multiple exposures (Robin, Chester, Rasmussen, Jaranson, & Goldman, 1997).

Preexisting Characteristics of the Child

Children's predisaster functioning may put them at risk for greater postdisaster reactions. The most widely studied predisaster child characteristics are those that do not change as a result of a disaster (and are easy to assess), such as demographic variables (age, gender, ethnicity).

Sociodemographic Variables

It is difficult to make generalizations regarding children's vulnerability to disasters at different *ages*, because findings have been inconsistent and few studies have had sufficiently large samples of youth of different ages to adequately evaluate developmental differences. Systematic investigation of developmental differences is further hampered by the fact that diverse manifestations of PTSD are likely to exist at different ages (American Academy of Child and Adolescent Psychiatry, 1998).

Some studies indicate that girls report more PTSD symptoms than boys following disasters (Gurwitch et al., 2002; Yule et al., 2002), although the evidence is mixed (La Greca & Prinstein, 2002; Korol, Kramer, Grace, & Green, 2002). Even when *gender* differences have emerged, their magnitude is modest and their clinical meaningfulness is uncertain (Vernberg et al., 1996).

Ethnicity, race, and cultural background have been relatively understudied (see Rabalais, Ruggiero, & Scotti, 2002). Community studies following natural disasters generally show that minority youth report higher levels of PTSD symptoms and have more difficulty in recovering from such events than nonminority youth (e.g., La Greca et al., 1996, 1998; Lonigan et al., 1994; see Rabalais et al., 2002). It is possible that, following destructive natural disasters, families from minority backgrounds possess less financial resources and/or less adequate insurance to deal with the rebuilding and recovery process; this could prolong the period of life disruption that ensues after natural disasters. Also, minority youth may have higher levels of predisaster trauma exposure, which could sensitize them to the effects of disasters (Berton & Stabb, 1996).

Overall, the role of sociodemographic characteristics in predicting youngsters' disaster reactions is not well understood. However, such variables may be viewed as markers for other variables that play a more direct role in the development of children's reactions, and could also be used to identify children at high risk for adverse postdisaster reactions.

Psychological Functioning

Children's prior psychosocial functioning predicts their stress reactions (Earls, Smith, Reich, & Jung, 1988; La Greca et al., 1998; Lonigan et al., 1994; Nolen-Hoeksema & Morrow, 1991), although the available evidence is scant due to the difficulty of obtaining accurate information on predisaster psychological functioning. In particular, preexisting *anxiety* is a significant risk factor for postdisaster PTSD symptoms (e.g., Asarnow, 1999; La Greca et al., 1998; Lonigan et al., 1994). In fact, anxious children may be vulnerable to developing PTSD symptoms even with low levels of disaster exposure (La Greca et al., 1998).

Other findings point to predisaster *depression, stress, and ruminative coping styles* as risk factors for postdisaster reactions. Following the 1989 Loma Prieta earthquake, Nolen-Hoeksema and Morrow (1991) found that youth who had elevated levels of depression, stress, and ruminative coping before the earthquake reported more depression and stress symptoms at two follow-up periods postdisaster.

Aspects of the Recovery Environment

Various aspects of the postdisaster recovery environment may magnify or attenuate disaster reactions. These aspects include the availability of social support, the presence of parental psychopathology or of parental distress, and the occurrence of additional life events or stressors.

Given the numerous stressors that accompany a disaster, *social support* should help to minimize youngsters' postdisaster distress. In fact, social support from significant others has been found to mitigate the impact of natural disasters on children and adolescents (see La Greca & Prinstein, 2002) and to predict fewer PTSD symptoms in adolescents who are exposed to community violence (see Kupersmidt, Shahinfar, & Voegler-Lee, 2002). Such findings indicate that enhancing children's social support following disasters is an important mental health goal.

Parents' psychosocial functioning, including their levels of psychopathology and their own reactions to the disaster, are likely to affect children's postdisaster functioning. Green and colleagues (1991) found that parental psychopathology predicted higher levels of PTSD symptoms in children and adolescents following the Buffalo Creek dam collapse (see also Korol et al., 2002). In addition, mothers' distress in the aftermath of Hurricane Hugo was associated with the persistence of their children's postdisaster emotional and behavioral difficulties (Swenson et al., 1996). Other research has supported a linkage between children's symptoms of PTSD and parents' trauma-related symptoms (Foy, Madvig, Pynoos, & Camilleri, 1996).

Major life events (e.g., death or hospitalization of a family member; parental divorce or separation) occurring in the months following a disaster appear to significantly impede children's postdisaster recovery and are associated with greater persistence of PTSD symptoms in children over time (La Greca et al., 1996). Children and adolescents who encounter major life events following a disaster, in addition to disaster-related life stressors, represent a high-risk group for severe and persistent posttraumatic stress reactions. Because of this, such youth bear close monitoring and may need to learn effective ways of coping with stressors.

The *psychological resources of the child* have been linked to children's postdisaster reactions and recovery (Vernberg, 2002). In particular, children's *coping skills* have received the most attention. Community studies find that children with more negative coping strategies for dealing with stress (e.g., anger, blaming others) show higher levels of PTSD symptoms after natural disasters (La Greca et al., 1996) and community violence (Berman et al., 1996; Kupersmidt et al., 2002). Moreover, children with negative coping strategies evidence greater persistence in PTSD symptoms over time (La Greca et al., 1996). As a result, efforts to promote adaptive coping may be useful for interventions with children following disasters.

TRANSLATING RESEARCH INTO INTERVENTION STRATEGIES

Among the numerous challenges to treating children and adolescents following disasters is the dearth of outcome studies on the effectiveness of post-disaster interventions (Vernberg, 2002; Vernberg & Vogel, 1993). However, there are promising leads based on the literature on disasters' effects, as reviewed earlier. Many of these interventions focus on efforts to process the event, increase social support, and improve problem solving and coping with the event and its aftermath.

This chapter section reviews interventions for children and adolescents following disasters. We focus predominantly on interventions that are appropriate for the "recovery and reconstruction" period (3 months or more after the disaster) because, for most disasters, the recovery period ensues for months or even years following the event, and this is the most common time for persistent symptoms of PTSD to emerge (see La Greca, 2001, and Vernberg, 2002, for summaries of interventions that are appropriate earlier in the disaster recovery process).

Prior to describing psychosocial interventions, including cognitive-behavioral treatments that have been used to treat children and adolescents with moderate to severe PTS, we briefly review interventions that have been utilized during the first few weeks after a disaster (postimpact phase). We next review universal and selected interventions that have been implemented during the recovery and reconstruction phase to provide a broad context and understanding of the kinds of interventions that are used with children and adolescents following disasters and terrorism.

Postimpact Phase

The postimpact phase begins with the disaster (hurricane, earthquake, terrorist attack) and continues for several weeks (Vernberg, 2002). Community- or school-based interventions that target all youth in affected areas have been rec ommended. Vernberg and Vogel (1993) note that interventions might include classroom and small-group activities, family approaches, and individual treat-ment. The purpose of these interventions is to provide information and help to normalize individuals' reactions to the disaster (normalizing reactions can help reduce anxiety; see Kendall & Suveg, Chapter 7, this volume); to provide a sense of safety and security; and to return to a sense of routine and normalcy. Efforts to provide information to professionals and the public (e.g., via fact sheets, web sites, mass media) are also useful (Vernberg & Vogel, 1993).

The short-term interventions that have been evaluated during this post-impact phase primarily involve "debriefing," also referred to as critical incident stress debriefing (CISD). CISD is a crisis intervention designed to relieve and prevent trauma-related distress in normal individuals who are experiencing abnormally stressful events (Chemtob, Tomas, Law, & Cremniter, 1997; Mitch-ell, 1983). CISD provides opportunities for children and adolescents to express feelings, normalize their responses to the disaster, and learn about common reac-tions to the disaster in the context of a supportive group (Chemtob et al., 1997). However, at present, little support exists for the effectiveness of debriefing (Rose & Bisson, 1998). Although CISD may benefit some youth, these brief interven-tions may be insufficient to address the multiple, complex, and cascading stressors that result from disasters, which may last for months or years. It is possible that multiple applications of CISD may be required for it to be effective (Horowitz & Schreiber, 1999).

Similar to debriefing, several authors have described "psychological first-aid" that can be implemented in schools or community crisis centers, to help children and adolescents initially with the postdisaster crises (Amaya-Jackson & March, 1995; Eth, Silverstein, & Pynoos, 1985; Pynoos & Nader, 1988). These first-aid efforts provide children with an opportunity to express their feelings (through drawings or storytelling), clarify confusion, and identify areas of need (Amaya-Jackson & March, 1995). Such efforts also can help professionals identify children who are having severe reactions, so that they may receive more inten-sive interventions.

Aside from formal interventions, literature from the American Red Cross (1999a, 1999b) and other sources (Federal Emergency Management Agency, 1989; National Organization for Victim Assistance, 1991) suggests that, follow ing a disaster, parents, teachers, and mental health professionals should encourage children and adolescents to *express their feelings* in developmentally appropriate ways (e.g., through discussion, drawings, storytelling, or journal writing) *and address any fears, worries, and security concerns* that children may have. Efforts to return children and youth to their *normal roles and routines* may help youngsters to renormalize their lives following disasters (Prinstein, La Greca, Vernberg, & Silverman, 1996).

Recovery and Reconstruction Phase

There is a paucity of controlled investigations of psychosocial interventions, including cognitive-behavioral interventions, for use with children and adolescents following disasters, even though a significant proportion of youngsters report moderate to severe levels of PTS symptoms and even PTSD that persists for a year or more following a disaster (as discussed earlier). In the initial section below, we describe promising community-based efforts to intervene with children and adolescents following disasters. We then provide a summary of the psychosocial interventions that have been empirically evaluated, including cognitive-behavioral interventions. Because the number of studies is small, we describe them in some detail. In this way, we hope to convey the strengths and weaknesses of the studies conducted, which should be helpful to readers who are interested in pursuing this area of research. We conclude with a wrap-up of what would represent "best practices" to follow in assisting children and adolescent following their exposure to disasters, based on the current available knowledge base.

Promising Community-Based Interventions following Disasters

Although most community interventions have not been evaluated empirically, we view them as promising because they are "empirically informed." That is, they have been developed from research on factors associated with youth's stress levels and/or their recovery following disasters (as described).

Several investigators have developed manuals for use in schools or group settings to help children or adolescents cope with large-scale disasters, and these are available directly from the authors and/or Internet websites (see Table 10.1). Manuals that focus on natural disasters include *The Bushfire and Me: A Story of What Happened to Me and My Family* (McDermott & Palmer, 2002; Storm, McDermott, & Finlayson, 1994); *After the Storm* (LaGreca, Sevin, & Sevin, 2004); and *Helping Children Prepare for and Cope with Natural Disasters* (La Greca & Prinstein, 2002; La Greca, Vernberg, Silverman, Vogel, & Prinstein, 1994), developed after Hurricane Andrew. Manuals that focus on coping with acts of violence include *Healing after Trauma Skills* (Gurwitch & Messenbaugh, 1998; Gurwitch et al., 2002), developed following the bombing in Oklahoma City; *Helping America Cope: A Guide to Help Parents and Children Cope with the September*

TABLE 10.1. Helping Children Cope with Disasters: Selected Resources for Fact Sheets, Brochures, or Manuals

Web materials[a]	Brief description
www.fema.gov/kids/	Child-oriented website on disasters, developed by the Federal Emergency Management Agency. It contains information on different types of disasters, how to prepare for them, and how to cope
www.disastereducation.org/guide.html	Brochure developed by the American Red Cross and other agencies, *Talking about Disaster* (2004). Check the main website for the American Red Cross (www.redcross.org) and related pages (www.redcross.org/disaster/safety/guide.html) for additional information on disasters.
www.apa.org/practice/kids.html	Website developed by the American Psychological Association. Contains a fact sheet on "Helping Children Cope: A Guide to Helping Children Cope with the Stress of the Oklahoma City Explosion." Useful for a wide range of disasters. Check the main website for additional information: www.apa.org.
www.aacap.org/publications/DisasterResponse/index.htm	Website of the American Academy of Child and Adolescent Psychiatry that contains many "fact sheets" for children and families, including how to help children cope with disasters and terrorism.
www.nctsn.org	Website of the National Child Traumatic Stress Network, which contains information for parents and professionals on treating children following disasters and terrorist events.

Selected manuals[b]	Request copies in writing from:
Helping Children Prepare and Cope with Natural Disasters (La Greca et al., 1994); *Keeping Children Safe* (La Greca et al., 2002)	Annette M. La Greca, PhD, University of Miami, P.O. Box 249229, Coral Gables, FL 33124
The Bushfire and Me (Storm et al., 1994)	VBD Publications, P.O. Box 741, Newtown NSW 2042, Australia
Healing after Trauma: Skills Manual for Helping Children (Gurwitch & Messenbaugh, 1998)	Robin H. Gurwitch, PhD, Child Study Center, 1100 NE 13th Street, Oklahoma City, OK 73117
After the Storm	Available from www.7-dippity.com
Helping America Cope	Available from www.7-dippity.com

[a] Web addresses begin with http://.
[b] All contain activities for adults (parent, school personnel, or counselors) to use with children.

11th Terrorist Attacks (La Greca, Sevin, & Sevin, 2001, 2002); and *Keeping Children Safe* (La Greca, Perez, & Glickman, 2002), developed to help children cope with community violence events.

What these manuals share in common are strategies for helping children talk about or "process" the traumatic events in a supportive, structured manner; ways to develop effective coping strategies for dealing with feelings of distress and with ongoing stressors that result from the trauma; and ideas for maintaining regular roles and routines, increasing social support, and preparing for other "predictable" disasters (e.g., fires, hurricanes, etc.). These manuals contain "lessons" that teachers, parents, or mental health providers could use with children and adolescents in disaster-affected areas, and they also review "risk factors" to help parents and/or mental health professionals identify children with severe stress reactions.

Other suggestions for helping children, adolescents, and families cope with the long-term aftermath of disasters include having public ceremonies, memorials, or other disaster-related rituals that provide an opportunity for disaster survivors to both remember the event and place it in the proper context (Vernberg & Vogel, 1993). Rituals may serve several important psychological functions, including public expression of shared grief and support, reassurance that disaster victims are remembered, review and interpretation of disaster experiences, and obtaining closure on a difficult life event (Vernberg & Vogel. 1993). The anniversary of a disaster is an especially common time for community-based ceremonies. Group meetings for families of disaster victims also have been arranged by mental health professionals on the anniversary of the event (Yule & Williams, 1990). Vernberg and Vogel (1993) note that there is little research on the value of rituals, yet "the timelessness of human rites to mark deaths and tragedies bears witness to their appeal" (p. 496). Rituals and commemorative activities are especially suitable for disasters that affect large numbers of children and families or that bring together families from different geographic areas that share a disaster in common (e.g., a memorial event for family members and survivors of plane crashes or for families of individuals killed in the attacks on the World Trade Center).

Exposure-Based Cognitive-Behavioral Interventions

The psychosocial intervention that has the strongest and most consistent empirical base at present for use with individuals who are experiencing PTSD is exposure-based cognitive-behavioral treatment (CBT). Foa and colleagues (e.g., Foa & Rothbaum, 1997) expanded emotional-processing theory initially developed in working with anxiety disorders (Foa & Kozak, 1986; see Kendall & Suveg, Chapter 7, this volume) to encompass PTSD. Specifically, starting from a common observation that exposure to trauma alters cognitive beliefs about the world and self (e.g., Janoff-Bulman, 1992), Foa and Rothbaum (1997) proposed that two sets of dysfunctional beliefs underlie PTSD: (1) The world is a very dangerous place, and (2) the individual is extremely incompetent. In exposure-based CBT for anxiety disorders, pathological elements of the fear structure, as well as dysfunctional beliefs and evaluations, are targeted. This is accomplished primarily through the client's systematic carrying out of therapist-prescribed exposures—either imaginal or *in vivo*—to provide information that is incompatible with the pathological elements that underlie the fear structure. In treating PTSD, exposure to memories of the traumatic event is thought to promote habituation via targeting stimulus–response associations and by correcting distorted cognitions.

A considerable number of studies have been conducted with adults who have experienced a wide range of traumatic exposures, including war combat (Fairbank & Keane, 1982) and sexual and physical assault (e.g., Foa et al., 1999), which provide strong empirical support for the efficacy of exposure-based CBT procedures. Foa, Rothbaum, and Furr (2003) recently reported that prolonged exposure with or without CBT was consistently most effective. Prolonged exposure involves psychoeducation, breathing retraining, imaginal exposure to the trauma memory, and *in vivo* exposure to the trauma reminders. Treatment is delivered in 9–12 sessions (each 90–120 minutes in duration), administered once or twice a week. Despite the promising findings of exposure-based CBT with adults, *no* study has focused on adults exposed to disasters.

The situation is no better in the child disaster area. Of the small number of randomized clinical trials on the efficacy of exposure-based CBT for youth with PTSD, *all* have focused on treating child sexual abuse (Feeny, Foa, Treadwell, & March, in press; see also Deblinger, Behl, & Glickman, Chapter 11, this volume). Indeed, we could locate only *one* study (March, Amaya-Jackson, Murray, & Schulte, 1998) that evaluated an exposure-based CBT intervention for youth who suffered from PTSD that was not due to sexual abuse.

March and colleagues (1998) evaluated the efficacy of an intervention that they refer to as Multi-Modality Trauma Treatment (MMTT) for children and adolescents who displayed PTSD after exposure to a single-stressor traumatic incident. Some of the single incidents to which the youths were exposed were disaster related, including severe storms and fires. Additional incidents included car accidents, gunshot injury, and accidental injuries. Participants were 17 children and adolescents between the ages of 10 and 15 years (mean age = 12.1 years). The average duration of PTSD symptoms for the younger participants was 1.5 years, and 2.5 years for the older participants. Fourteen of the 17 participants completed the intervention.

Participants were assessed for PTSD using the Child and Adolescent Trauma Survey and the Clinician Administered PTSD Scale—Child and Adolescent Version. Additional outcome measures included a clinician rating of global functioning, a teacher rating scale of externalizing behavior problems, and child self-rating scales of depression, anxiety, and anger.

Adapting emotional processing theory (Foa & Rothbaum, 1997), MMTT was designed as a group-administered CBT that focused on (1) habituating conditioned anxiety through narrative exposures, (2) modifying maladaptive trauma-related cognitions through positive self-talk and cognitive restructuring, (3) teaching adaptive coping strategies for disturbing feelings and physiological reactions, and (4) reducing co-occurring symptoms such as anxiety, anger, depression, grief, and disruptive behaviors through problem-solving and self-management strategies. The treatment sessions also included youth's practicing of imaginal exposures and the introduction of *in vivo* exposures to be completed by the participants as homework. MMTT was conducted over 18 weekly sessions, with an individual "pull-out session" at week 10 (when exposure was introduced). The study used a single-case design controlling for extraneous variables using a multiple baseline by phasing in treatment across time (start date offset by 4 weeks) across location (two adjacent towns) and across school type (elementary school and junior high school).

Participants showed significant improvement on both clinician-reported PTSD outcome measures from pre- to posttreatment, and improvements were maintained at 6-month follow-up. Significant improvements also were observed on the child-rating scales of depression, anxiety, and anger from pre- to posttreatment, which were maintained at 6-month follow-up. Only the teacher ratings of child externalizing behavior problems did not show significant improvement, but were stable. Of the treatment completers, 8 (57%) no longer met criteria for PTSD at posttreatment, and 12 (86%) no longer met criteria at 6-month follow-up. These findings represent important but only initial evidence for the efficacy of exposure-based CBT for youths with PTSD, especially given that most of the participants had PTSD for 1 year or longer and because the study's analyses controlled history effects, using a single-case experimental design. Despite the importance of the findings, it remains an unanswered empirical research question whether similar positive effects would be obtained via a more rigorous, randomized controlled trial and using a larger sample of children who have been exposed to disaster-related traumatic events.

Other Psychosocial Interventions

Additional psychosocial interventions have been evaluated in the aftermath of disasters. Many of the components of these interventions are actually very similar to what would be included in an exposure-based CBT intervention. Despite this, the investigators testing these interventions do not directly refer to the interventions as "exposure-based CBT," and that is why we summarize them in this section.

Galante and Foa (1986) is an early study that we summarize for its historical significance, as it is the first report of a school-based psychosocial intervention in the aftermath of a disaster. These investigators surveyed 300 Italian elementary school children who were victims of a devastating earthquake in central Italy. Using the Children's Rutter Behavior Questionnaire for Completion by

Teachers, a score of nine or greater was viewed as indicating that a child is "at risk of developing neurotic or antisocial disturbances" (p. 353). Children found to be "at risk" were then included in a psychosocial intervention. The intervention contained seven sessions, which focused on communication, drawing, education about earthquakes, "active discharge of feelings," emphasizing future events, and that one is "not a victim of the fates" (p. 357).

Unfortunately, it is difficult to draw valid inferences from the findings, not only because the study was uncontrolled but also because the results focused primarily on providing anecdotes about how the children's reactions showed improvements from session to session. Moreover, the information presented that was quantitative in nature was limited to pre- to posttreatment changes on the Rutter Behavior Questionnaire for Completion by Teachers across six of the villages from which the participants were obtained. Significant differences were obtained in three of the six villages sampled. The authors also indicated that the "frequency of expressed fears dropped significantly," but the fears were not assessed using an objective fear inventory. Despite the study's limitations, it is one of the first reports of an intervention for children exposed to disaster. Certainly, it paved the way for the interesting studies, discussed next.

Goenjian and colleagues (1997) evaluated a "brief trauma/grief focused school-based psychotherapy" (p. 536) among adolescents (mean age = 13.2 years, 3 years postdisaster) who experienced a devastating earthquake in Armenia. The intervention was delivered 1.5 years after the earthquake. The adolescents were assessed for PTS reactions (using the Child PTSD Reaction Index) and depressive reactions (using the Depression Self-Rating Scale) prior to receiving the intervention and were reassessed again 18 months later (3 years postdisaster). All participants had been exposed to life threats, mutilating injuries, or horrific deaths during the earthquake, and all continued to live in the same urban area where the earthquake occurred.

The intervention included classroom groups (four half-hour sessions) and individual psychotherapy (an average of two 1-hour sessions) conducted over a 3-week period. The intervention addressed five main areas. *Trauma* was addressed by reconstructing and reprocessing traumatic experiences and associated feelings, clarifying distorted thinking and guilt, addressing avoidance, and legitimizing PTS reactions. *Traumatic reminders* were addressed by identifying reminders and cues to past traumatic events, helping with discrimination of these reminders, improving tolerance for reactivity, and enhancing social support-seeking behaviors. *Postdisaster stresses and adversities* were addressed by helping the youth to accept and adapt to changes and loss, and to use proactive coping strategies. *Bereavement and the interplay of trauma and grief* were addressed by helping the youth to reconstitute a nontraumatic mental representation of any deceased persons. Finally, *developmental impact* involved identifying missed developmental opportunities and promoting positive youth development. (As noted earlier in this section, this intervention has components that appear congruent with an exposure-based CBT intervention, such as the reprocessing of the traumatic experiences, handling of traumatic reminders, etc. Yet, the authors do not make any mention or cite emotional processing theory or CBT to explain or justify why their intervention contained the components that it did.)

A total of 64 adolescents from four schools were selected for inclusion in the study, based on showing high levels of PTS and depressive reactions. Because study personnel were limited, students from the two schools closest to the authors' clinics participated in the brief grief-focused treatment ($n = 35$); students from the two schools farthest from the clinic were not treated ($n = 29$). Thus, participants were not randomized to conditions.

On the main outcome measure, the Child PTSD Reaction Index, the treated group reported significantly lower PTS reactions than the no-treatment group at 18 months posttreatment; the untreated group had significantly higher PTS reactions at this time point. Moreover, the observed improvements in PTS reactions appeared to be due to overall improvement across the PTSD clusters (i.e., reexperiencing, avoidance, and hyperarousal). Further, using a score of 40 or above on the Child PTSD Reaction Index as indicating a diagnosis of PTSD, the estimated rates of PTSD at 1.5 years among treated and untreated youths were 60% and 52%, respectively. After three years (posttreatment), rates for the two groups were 28% and 69%, respectively.

Mean scores on the Depression Self-Rating Scale did not differ from pre- to posttreatment for the treated group, but scores *increased* significantly for the untreated group. Similarly, using a score of 17 or above on the Depression Self-Rating Scale as indicating a depressive diagnosis, the estimated rates of depression at 1.5 years among youth treated and untreated were 46% and 35%, respectively. After 3 years (posttreatment), rates for the two groups were 46% and 75%, respectively. Despite the limits in drawing conclusions from this nonrandomized trial, the findings are perhaps most important in showing that youths *who do not receive any intervention* for their postdisaster reactions are likely to show persistent and deleterious effects, thereby highlighting the importance of developing and evaluating randomized trials in this area.

To date, the first, largest, and most systematic attempt to evaluate the efficacy of a combined school-based screening and psychosocial intervention to identify and treat children with persistent disaster-related trauma symptoms has been reported by Chemtob, Nakashima, and Hamada (2002). Specifically, 3,864 children enrolled across all 10 public elementary schools in second through sixth grades on the Hawaiian island of Kauai, struck by Hurricane Iniki on September 11, 1992, were screened for high levels of trauma-related symptoms 2 years after the disaster. The screening instrument was the Kauai Recovery Inventory, a child-rating scale adapted from the PTSD Reaction Index that assessed the frequency of PTSD symptoms in the preceding week. The authors note that an "arbitrary cut-off score corresponding to the 94th percentile was used to identify the children reporting the most severe trauma symptoms" (p. 212). Four questions about the children's hurricane exposure also were administered.

The screening resulted in a sample size of 248 children, who were then randomly assigned to one of three consecutively treated cohorts. Children in the cohorts awaiting treatment served as wait-list controls. Within each cohort, children were randomly assigned to either individual or group treatment, to allow comparison of the efficacy of the two treatment modalities. The screening results further suggested a number of risk factors for developing the highest level of symptoms, including being female, of younger age, of lower SES, reporting reacting with panic during the hurricane event, and fearing for the physical safety of family and self during the hurricane.

Treatment was manual-based and consisted of four weekly sessions that focused on helping children to master disaster-related psychological challenges. Sessions included restoring a sense of safety (session 1), grieving losses and renewing attachments (session 2), adaptively expressing disaster-related anger (session 3), and achieving sufficient closure about the disaster to move forward (session 4). The intervention was designed to provide a context in which children would be prompted to review their experiences in a structured way while receiving support to master the psychological tasks that had not been completed. The manual outlined each session's contents and listed activities to help review the material relevant to that session. Therapists also were provided a standard box of play and art materials to use. For example, in session 2 ("Loss") children were engaged in play, art, and talk aimed at helping them identify any losses, express feelings about the losses, and identify forward-looking ways of integrating the loss into the present (which could be construed as an exposure-based procedure). Similar activities were used in the individual and group treatment approaches, with the group approach involving cooperative play and discussion.

Treatment was completed by 214 (86.3%) of the children experiencing high trauma-related symptoms. The main outcome measure was the child-completed Kauai Reaction Inventory. The Child Reaction Index, completed by clinicians blinded to children's treatment status, was completed on small random samples of treated ($n = 21$) and untreated ($n = 16$) children.

Children reported significant reductions in their trauma-related symptoms that were maintained at 1-year follow-up. The Child Reaction Index further revealed that treated children had fewer trauma symptoms as compared with untreated children. The group and individual treatment approaches did not differ, although fewer children dropped out of the group treatment approach. Overall, despite the only "partial" controlled nature of this study (i.e., there were no untreated children with the same levels of symptoms who had treatment withheld throughout the full course of the study period) and the overreliance on child-report, the study represents the first demonstration of the feasibility of conducting a screen to a large population of children at 2 years postdisaster. It also represents the first demonstration of both feasibility and initial efficacy of a brief school-based psychosocial intervention.

Chemtob, Nakashima, and Carlson (2002) reported the results of another brief treatment for school-age children with disaster-related PTS symptoms. The participants were 32 children (6–12 years; $M = 8.4$ years) who, at 1-year follow-up of a prior intervention for disaster-related symptoms (presumably the intervention described above): (1) were treatment nonresponders, (2) met criteria for disaster-related PTSD, and (3) had parental consent for treatment. The treatment used was eye movement desensitization and reprocessing (EMDR). EMDR was used because (1) a treatment manual could be readily developed, (2) possible alternative treatments, such as CBT, would require a larger number of sessions and were not manualized, and (3) efficacy data using EMDR with single-event trauma appeared promising. The study was conducted using two groups in an ABA design plus follow-up. Group 1 was assessed at pretreatment, provided treatment and reassessed at posttreatment. Group 2, consisting of wait-listed children, was assessed at baseline and then, following treatment for group 1 (about 1 month later), was reassessed at pretreatment, provided treatment, and reassessed at posttreatment. Both groups were administered 6-month follow-up assessments.

In EMDR participants identify a distressing memory and related imagery and sensations, and assess its subjective distress. Trauma-related negative self-cognitions and positive self-cognitions are then identified. Sets of eye movements are then induced by asking the participant to track the back-and-forth movements of the therapist's hand while concentrating on memory-related images, thoughts, and sensations. With young children whose eye coordination is not fully developed, "hand tapping" may be substituted, during which the therapist taps each hand in a left–right–left sequence. The client reports the content of thoughts, images, feelings, and sensations between sets of eye movements. In the "reprocessing" stages of treatment, the client is asked to focus on positive cognitions regarding the memory during further sets of eye movements. EMDR was administered in this study in three weekly treatment sessions.

On the main outcome measures (the Child Reaction Index, the Revised Children's Manifest Anxiety Scale, and the Children's Depression Inventory) both the "immediate" and "delayed" treatment groups showed significant declines from pre- to posttreatment that were maintained at 6-month follow-up. Despite encouraging findings, the authors note that inferences cannot be drawn about the efficacy of EMDR per se because the study was not designed as a comparative evaluation. The ingredients of EMDR, including imaginal exposure, rehearsal of the trauma-related experience, and support by a trained clinician, all could account for the positive results. In light of the growing evidence for exposure-based CBT for use with children who have been exposed to other types of traumatic events (e.g., child sexual abuse), it seems likely that the other active ingredients of EMDR (e.g., the exposure component) might be most critical for positive treatment response. This requires further empirical study.

SUMMARY OF PSYCHOSOCIAL INTERVENTIONS AND CONCLUSIONS

At present, the field is in need of quality data on the efficacy or effectiveness of psychosocial interventions, including CBT, for children and adolescents affected by disasters. Nevertheless, we discussed what appear to be the "best practices" to implement based on the available literature.

In the immediate aftermath of a disaster, efforts should focus on reassuring children, providing information, and "normalizing" disaster reactions. In addition, encouraging children to express their feelings, addressing any fears, worries, or security concerns they may have, and helping them resume normal roles and routines are especially important. Parents, teachers, and clinicians also should identify children with the most severe reactions, so that they can provide additional help. The materials gleaned from websites of various professional organizations (see Table 10.1) contain fact sheets, activities, and information that should facilitate this process.

Even weeks or months postdisaster, many children will exhibit subclinical levels of PTSD and difficulties coping with disaster-related experiences and their aftermath. For large-scale community-wide disasters, efforts to deal with children, adolescents, and families in community settings, such as schools, may be most productive from a preventive standpoint. Several school-based manuals (see Table 10.1), as well as the school interventions reviewed above, are suitable for community settings. In addition, it is desirable to identify those children and adolescents who display severe PTS reactions for additional mental health services.

Because disasters affect large numbers of people, intensive individualized interventions, such as CBT, may only be feasible for children and adolescents who show marked signs of disaster-related distress or who have multiple risk factors for poor mental health outcomes (e.g., high life adversity, multiple comorbid conditions) (Vernberg, 2002). In light of the consistent and strong empirical support for exposure-based CBT for use with adults with PTSD and with youth with PTSD resulting from child sexual abuse, such interventions represent the "best practices" for youth exposed to the trauma of a disaster *and* who are also suffering from PTSD reactions. Nevertheless, we recognize that this recommendation remains tentative, as the March and colleagues (1998) study represents the only evaluation of a full-fledged exposure-based CBT, and this study is limited (only 14 children treated; not all exposed to disasters; and not a randomized trial).

Although it is disheartening that so little systematic research has evaluated CBT interventions for PTSD in youth exposed to disasters, this reflects the inherent challenges in conducting controlled outcome research following disasters. The challenges in conducting postdisaster research are formidable (see La Greca, 2001; La Greca, in press). For example, schools and community systems are often in chaos after a disaster and may have more pressing priorities than conducting research. This is especially true for community-wide disasters, where rebuilding efforts are likely to take precedence. Another major difficulty is that the significant adults in children's lives—including parents and teachers—may also be affected by the disaster. In many cases, these adults are not aware of the extent of children's distress and the need for treatment, perhaps because they are also affected by the trauma event. Furthermore, it is difficult to conduct controlled outcome research without considerable resources and funding; yet, it has been our experience that current funding mechanisms are often inadequate or insufficient.

As a final point, we emphasize that children and adolescents exposed to disasters and acts of terrorism or violence are likely to need *more than* interventions that focus exclusively on PTSD reactions, because youngsters' reactions are often complex, multifaceted, and include other problems in addition to PTSD (i.e., grief, depression, anxiety). In light of this, the intervention components that were described for several of the "community interventions" and "other psychosocial interventions" in this chapter (e.g., dealing with grief, handling anger, seeking social support, promoting positive coping skills) are also likely to be important additions to any comprehensive and effective intervention. Children and adolescents with complex comorbid postdisaster reactions might also profit from associated CBT treatments that focus on comorbid psychological reactions, in addition to PTSD. We hope that the current chapter might serve as a catalyst for the development and evaluation of complex, multifaceted interventions in the future.

REFERENCES

Amaya-Jackson, L., & March, J. S. (1995). Posttraumatic stress disorder. In J. S. March (Ed.), *Anxiety disorders in children and adolescents* (pp. 276–300). New York: Guilford Press.

American Academy of Child and Adolescent Psychiatry. (1998). AACAP Official Action: Practice parameters for the assessment and treatment of children and adolescents with posttraumatic stress disorder. *Journal of the American Academy of Child and Adolescent Psychiatry, 37*(Suppl.), 4S–26S.

American Psychiatric Association. (1994). *Diagnostic and statistical manual of mental disordersx* (4th ed.). Washington, DC: Author.

American Red Cross. (1999a). *Children and disasters.* Retrieved on February 7, 2005, from www.redcross.org/services/disaster/0,1082,0_602_,00.html

American Red Cross. (1999b). *Talking about disaster: Guide for standard messages.* Washington, DC: National Disaster Education Coalition.

Applied Research & Consulting LLC and the Columbia University Mailman School of Public Health. (2002). *Effects of the World Trade Center attack on NYC public school students: Initial* report to the New York City Board of Education. Retrieved on January 25, 2005, from www.nycenet.edu/offices/spss/wtc_needs/firstrep.pdf

Asarnow, J. (1999). When the earth stops shaking: Earthquake sequelae among children diagnosed for pre-earthquake psychopathology. *Journal of the American Academy of Child and Adolescent Psychiatry, 38,* 1016–1023.

Ayalon, O. (1993). Posttraumatic stress recovery of terrorist survivors. In J. Wilson & B. Raphael (Eds.), *International handbook of traumatic stress syndromes* (pp. 855–866). New York: Plenum Press.

Berman, S. L., Kurtines, W. M., Silverman, W. K., & Serafini, L. T. (1996). The impact of exposure to crime and violence on urban youth. *American Journal of Orthopsychiatry, 66,* 329–336.

Berton, M. W., & Stabb, S. D. (1996). Exposure to violence and post-traumatic stress disorder in urban adolescents. *Adolescence, 31,* 489–498.

Bolton, D., O'Ryan, D., Udwin, O., Boyle, S., & Yule, W. (2000). The long-term psychological effects of a disaster experienced in adolescence: II. General psychopathology. *Journal of Child Psychology and Psychiatry, 41,* 513–523.

Chemtob, C. M., Nakashima, J., & Carlson, J. G. (2002). Brief treatment for elementary school children with disaster-related posttraumatic stress disorder: A field study. *Journal of Clinical Psychology, 58,* 99–112.

Chemtob, C. M., Tomas, S., Law, W., & Cremniter, D. (1997). Postdisaster psychosocial intervention: A field study of the impact of debriefing on psychological distress. *American Journal of Psychiatry, 154,* 415–417.

Earls, F., Smith, E., Reich, W., & Jung, K. G. (1988). Investigating the psychopathological consequence of disaster in children: A pilot study incorporating a structured diagnostic interview. *Journal of the American Academy of Child and Adolescent Psychiatry, 27,* 90–95.

Eth, S., Silverstein, S., & Pynoos, R. S. (1985). Mental health consultation to a preschool following the murder of a mother and child. *Hospital and Community Psychiatry, 36,* 73–76.

Fairbank, J. A., & Keane, T. M. (1982). Flooding for combat-related stress disorders: Assessment of anxiety reduction across traumatic memories. *Behavior Therapy, 13,* 499–510.

Federal Emergency Management Agency. (1989). *Coping with children's reactions to hurricanes and other disasters.* Washington, DC: U.S. Government Printing Office.

Feeny, N. C., Foa, E. B., Treadwell, K. R., & March, J. S. (2004). Posttraumatic stress disorder in youth: A critical review of the cognitive and behavioral treatment outcome literature. *Professional Psychology: Research and Practice, 35,* 466–476.

Foa, E. B., Dancu, C. V., Hembree, E. A., Jaycox, L. H., Meadows, E. A., & Street, G. P. (1999). A comparison of exposure therapy, stress inoculation training, and their combination for reducing posttraumatic stress disorder in female assault victims. *Journal of Consulting and Clinical Psychology, 67,* 194–200.

Foa, E. B., & Kozak, M. J. (1986). Emotional processing of fear: Exposure to corrective information. *Psychological Bulletin, 99,* 20–35.

Foa, E. B., & Rothbaum, B. O. (1997). *Treating the trauma of rape: Cognitive-behavioral therapy for PTSD.* New York: Guilford Press.

Foa, E. B., Rothbaum, B. O., & Furr, J. M. (2003). Augmenting exposure therapy with other CBT procedures. *Psychiatric Annals, 33,* 47–53.

Foy, D. W., Madvig, B. T., Pynoos, R. S., & Camilleri, A. J. (1996). Etiologic factors in the development of posttraumatic stress disorder in children and adolescents. *Journal of School Psychology, 34,* 133–145.

Galante, R., & Foa, D. (1986). An epidemiological study of psychic trauma and treatment effectiveness for children after a natural disaster. *Journal of the American Academy of Child Psychiatry, 25,* 357–363.

Goenjian, A. K., Karayan, I., Pynoos, R. S., Minassian, D., Najarian, L. M., Steinberg, A. M.,

& Fairbanks, L. A. (1997). Outcome of psychotherapy among early adolescents after trauma. *American Journal of Psychiatry, 154*, 536–542.

Goenjian, A. K., Pynoos, R. S., Steinberg, A. M., Najarian, L. M., Asarnow, J. R., Karayan, I., et al. (1995). Psychiatric comorbidity in children after the 1988 earthquake in Armenia. *Journal of the American Academy of Child and Adolescent Psychiatry, 34*, 1174–1184.

Green, B. L., Korol, M. S., Grace, M. C., Vary, M. G., Kramer, T. L., Gleser, G. C., & Leonard, A. C. (1994). Children of disaster in the second decade: A 17-year follow-up of Buffalo Creek survivors. *Journal of the American Academy of Child and Adolescent Psychiatry, 33*, 71–79.

Green, B. L., Korol, M. S., Grace, M. C., Vary, M. G., Leonard, A. C., Gleser, G. C., & Smitson-Cohen, S. (1991). Children and disaster: Gender and parental effects on PTSD symptoms. *Journal of the American Academy of Child and Adolescent Psychiatry, 30*, 945–951.

Gurwitch, R. H., Sitterle, K. A., Young, B. H., & Pfefferbaum, B. (2002). The aftermath of terrorism. In A. M. La Greca, W. K. Silverman, E. M. Vernberg, & M. C. Roberts (Eds.), *Helping children cope with disasters and terrorism* (pp. 327–358). Washington, DC: American Psychological Association.

Gurwitch, R. H., & Messenbaugh, A. K. (1998). *Healing after trauma: Skills manual for helping children.* Oklahoma City, OK: Author.

Horowitz, L., & Schreiber, M. (1999). *Psychological and behavioral aspects of emergency medical services for children.* Washington, DC: American Psychological Association.

Janoff-Bulman, R. (1992). *Shattered assumptions: Towards a new psychology of trauma.* New York: Free Press.

Korol, M. S. (1990). *Children's psychological responses to a nuclear waste disaster in Fernald, Ohio.* Unpublished dissertation, University of Cincinnati.

Korol, M. S., Kramer, T. L., Grace, M. C., & Green, B. L. (2002). Dam break: Long-term follow-up of children exposed to the Buffalo Creek Disaster. In A. M. La Greca, W. K. Silverman, E. M. Vernberg, & M. C. Roberts (Eds.), *Helping children cope with disasters and terrorism* (pp. 241–258). Washington, DC: American Psychological Association.

Kupersmidt, J. B., Shahinfar, A., & Voegler-Lee, M. E. (2002). Children's exposure to community violence. In A. M. La Greca, W. K. Silverman, E. M. Vernberg, & M. C. Roberts (Eds.), *Helping children cope with disasters and terrorism* (pp. 381–402). Washington, DC: American Psychological Association.

La Greca, A. M. (2001). Children experiencing disasters: Prevention and intervention. In J. N. Hughes, A. M. La Greca, & J. C. Conoley (Eds.), *Handbook of psychological services for children and adolescents* (pp. 195–222). New York: Oxford University Press.

La Greca, A. M. (in press). School-based studies of children following disasters. In F. Norris, S. Galea, M. Friedman, D. Reissman, & P. Watson (Eds.), *Research methods for studying mental health after disasters and terrorism: Community and public health approaches.* New York: Guilford Press.

La Greca, A. M., Perez, L., & Glickman, A. (2002). *Keeping children safe: A program to help children cope with community violence.* Miami, FL: Authors.

La Greca, A. M., & Prinstein, M. J. (2002). Hurricanes and tornadoes. In A. M. La Greca, W. K. Silverman, E. M. Vernberg, & M. C. Roberts (Eds.), *Helping children cope with disasters and terrorism* (pp. 107–138). Washington, DC: American Psychological Association.

La Greca, A. M., Sevin, S., & Sevin, E. (2001). *Helping America Cope: A guide for parents and children in the aftermath of the September 11th national disaster.* Miami, FL: Sevendippity. Retrieved on February 7, 2005, from www.7-dippity.com/other/op_freedownloads.html

La Greca, A. M., Sevin, S., & Sevin, E. (2002). *Helping America cope: Anniversary edition.* Miami, FL: Sevendippity. Retrieved on February 7, 2005, from www.7-dippity.com/other/op_freedownloads.html

LaGreca, A. M., Sevin, S., & Sevin, E. (2004). *After the storm: A guide to help children cope with the psychological effects of a hurricane.* Miami, FL: Sevendippity, Inc. Retrieved on September 14, 2005, from www.7-dippity.com

La Greca, A. M., Silverman, W. K., Vernberg, E. M., & Prinstein, M. (1996). Symptoms of posttraumatic stress after Hurricane Andrew: A prospective study. *Journal of Consulting and Clinical Psychology, 64,* 712–723.

La Greca, A. M., Silverman, W. K., & Wasserstein, S. B. (1998). Children's predisaster functioning as a predictor of posttraumatic stress following Hurricane Andrew. *Journal of Consulting and Clinical Psychology, 66,* 883–892.

La Greca, A. M., Vernberg, E. M., Silverman, W. K., Vogel, A., & Prinstein, M. (1994). *Helping children cope with natural disasters: A manual for school personnel.* Miami, FL: A. Vogel.

Lonigan, C. J., Anthony, J. L., & Shannon, M. P. (1998). Diagnostic efficacy of posttraumatic symptoms in children exposed to disaster. *Journal of Clinical Child Psychology, 27,* 255–267.

Lonigan, C. J., Shannon, M. P., Finch, A. J., Daugherty, T. K., & Taylor, C. M. (1991). Children's reactions to a natural disaster: Symptom severity and degree of exposure. *Advances in Behaviour Research and Therapy, 13,* 135–154.

Lonigan, C. J., Shannon, M. P., Taylor, C. M., Finch, A. J., & Sallee, F. R. (1994). Children exposed to disaster. II. Risk factors for the development of post-traumatic symptomatology. *Journal of the American Academy of Child Psychiatry, 33,* 94–105.

March, J. S., Amaya-Jackson, L., Murray, M. C., & Schulte, A. (1998). Cognitive-behavioral psychotherapy for children and adolescents with posttraumatic stress disorder after a single-incident stressor. *Journal of the American Academy of Child and Adolescent Psychiatry, 37,* 585–593.

McDermott, B. M., & Palmer, L. J. (2002). Postdisaster emotional distress, depression and event-related variables: Findings across child and adolescent developmental stages. *Australian and New Zealand Journal of Psychiatry, 36,* 754–761.

Mitchell, J. (1983). When disaster strikes: The critical incident stress debriefing process. *Journal of Emergency Medical Services, 8,* 36–39.

Nader, K., & Mello, C. (2002). Shootings, hostage takings, and children. In A. M. La Greca, W. K. Silverman, E. M. Vernberg, & M. C. Roberts (Eds.), *Helping children cope with disasters and terrorism* (pp. 301–326). Washington, DC: American Psychological Association.

National Organization for Victim Assistance. (1991). *Hurricane! Issues unique to hurricane disasters.* Washington, DC: Author.

Nolen-Hoeksema, S., & Morrow, J. (1991). A prospective study of depression and posttraumatic stress symptoms after a natural disaster: The 1989 Loma Prieta Earthquake. *Journal of Personality and Social Psychology, 61,* 115–121.

Prinstein, M. J., La Greca, A. M., Vernberg, E. M., & Silverman, W. K. (1996). Children's coping assistance after a natural disaster. *Journal of Clinical Child Psychology, 25,* 463–475.

Pynoos, R. S., Frederick, C., Nader, K., Aroyo, W., Steinberg, A., Eth, S., et al. (1987). Life threat and posttraumatic stress in school-age children. *Archives of General Psychiatry, 44,* 1057–1063.

Pynoos, R. S., & Nader, K. (1988). Psychological first aid and treatment approach to children exposed to community violence: Research implications. *Journal of Traumatic Stress, 1,* 115–173.

Rabalais, A. E., Ruggiero, K. J., & Scotti, J. R. (2002). Multicultural issues in the response of children to disasters. In A. M. La Greca, W. K. Silverman, E. M. Vernberg, & M. C. Roberts (Eds.), *Helping children cope with disasters and terrorism* (pp. 73–100). Washington, DC: American Psychological Association.

Rose, S., & Bisson, J. (1998). Brief early psychological interventions following trauma: A systematic review of the literature. *Journal of Traumatic Stress, 11,* 697–709.

Shaw, J. A., Applegate, B., & Schorr, C. (1996). Twenty-one-month follow-up study of school-age children exposed to Hurricane Andrew. *Journal of the American Academy of Child and Adolescent Psychiatry, 35,* 359–364.

Silverman, W. K., & Ginsburg, G. S. (1995). Specific phobia and generalized anxiety disorder. In J. S. March (Ed.), *Anxiety disorders in children and adolescents* (pp. 276–300). New York: Guilford Press.

Silverman, W. K., & La Greca, A. M. (2002). Children experiencing disasters: Definitions, reactions, and predictors of outcomes. In A. M. La Greca, W. K. Silverman, E. M. Vernberg, & M. C. Roberts (Eds.), *Helping children cope with disasters* (pp. 11–34). Washington, DC: American Psychological Association.

Storm, V., McDermott, B., & Finlayson, D. (1994). *The bushfire and me: A story of what happened to me and my family.* Newtown, Australia: VBD Publications.

Swenson, C. C., Saylor, C. F., Powell, M. P., Stokes, S. J., Foster, K. Y., & Belter, R. W. (1996). Impact of a natural disaster on preschool children: Adjustment 14 months after a hurricane. *American Journal of Orthopsychiatry, 66,* 122–130.

Vernberg, E. M. (2002). Intervention approaches following disasters. In A. M. La Greca, W. K. Silverman, E. M. Vernberg, & M. C. Roberts (Eds.), *Helping children cope with disasters and terrorism* (pp. 55–72). Washington, DC: American Psychological Association.

Vernberg, E. M., La Greca, A. M., Silverman, W. K., & Prinstein, M. (1996). Predictors of children's post-disaster functioning following Hurricane Andrew. *Journal of Abnormal Psychology, 105,* 237–248.

Vernberg, E. M., & Varela, R. E. (2001). Posttraumatic stress disorder: A developmental perspective. In M. W. Vasey & M. R. Dadds (Eds.), *The developmental psychopathology of disaster* (pp. 386–406). New York: Oxford University Press.

Vernberg, E. M., & Vogel, J. M. (1993). Interventions with children after disasters. *Journal of Clinical Child Psychology, 22,* 485–498.

Vincent, N. R. (1997). *A follow-up to Hurricane Andrew: Children's reactions 42 months postdisaster.* Unpublished doctoral dissertation, University of Miami.

Vogel, J., & Vernberg, E. M. (1993). Children's psychological responses to disaster. *Journal of Clinical Child Psychology, 22,* 464–484.

Yule, W., Bolton, D., Udwin, O., Boyle, S., O'Ryan, D., & Nurrish, J. (2000). The long-term psychological effects of a disaster experienced in adolescence: I. The incidence and course of PTSD. *Journal of Child Psychology and Psychiatry, 41,* 503–512.

Yule, W., Udwin, O., & Bolton, D. (2002). Mass transportation disasters. In A. M. La Greca, W. K. Silverman, E. M. Vernberg, & M. C. Roberts (Eds.), *Helping children cope with disasters and terrorism* (pp. 223–240). Washington, DC: American Psychological Association.

Yule, W., & Williams, R. (1990). Posttraumatic stress reactions in children. *Journal of Traumatic Stress, 3,* 279–295.

CHAPTER 11

Treating Children Who Have Experienced Sexual Abuse

ESTHER DEBLINGER, LEAH E. BEHL,
and ALISSA R. GLICKMAN

Child sexual abuse is frequently defined as contacts or interactions between a child and an adult or significantly older child, in which the child is used for the sexual stimulation of the perpetrator or another person. Although most researchers acknowledge the seriousness of child sexual abuse, the scope of the problem is debated. Reported estimates of the incidence and prevalence rates of child sexual abuse in the United States vary considerably, and are perhaps related to the varying definitions of child sexual abuse, response rates, sample sizes, sample characteristics, and different survey approaches across studies. Estimates of sexual abuse prevalence rates have been reported to range from 2 to 62% for females and from 3 to 62% for males in the United States and Canada (Center for the Future of Children, 1994). The best estimates of sexual abuse prevalence rates come from adult retrospective studies that utilize large representative samples. In a published review of retrospective prevalence studies in the United States and Canada, Finkelhor (1994) concluded that approximately 1 of every 4 females (20–25%) and 1 of every 7 males (5–15%) experience contact sexual abuse before 18 years of age. Finkelhor in his review only included individuals who reported direct sexual contact before the age of 18. Consequently, when noncontact sexual abuse is considered, these percentages are likely an underestimate of overall sexual abuse prevalence rates.

Perhaps one of the best estimates of incidence rates in the United States is the statistical report published annually by the National Center on Child Abuse and Neglect (NCCAN). The 2002 NCCAN report indicated that 86,656 cases of child sexual abuse, approximately 1.2% of the child population of the United States, were confirmed by child protection agencies. This number is likely an underestimate of sexual abuse incidence rates, as it does not include children who have been sexually abused by someone other than a caretaker and the large percentage of children whose abuse has not been discovered and/or reported.

IMPACT AND MODERATORS OF CHILD SEXUAL ABUSE

Children and adults who have experienced child sexual abuse often exhibit symptoms of psychopathology and impairment in many areas of functioning (see Kendall-Tackett, Williams, & Finkelhor, 1993; Putnam, 2003; Saywitz, Mannarino, Berliner, & Cohen, 2000, for reviews). Numerous studies document an association between sexual abuse and depression, suicidality, anxiety disorders, conduct disorder, and substance abuse. Many of these symptoms emerge during childhood and continue into adulthood. Among children symptoms can include poor self-esteem, heightened self-blame, reduced interpersonal trust, school and learning difficulties, and behavior problems (e.g., Kendall-Tackett et al., 1993). Victims of sexual abuse may also experience weight dissatisfaction and/or eating disorders, somatization disorder, dissociative identity disorder, and borderline personality disorder (see Putnam, 2003, for review).

Developmentally, child sexual abuse interferes with normal social, emotional, and sexual developmental trajectories. Sexual abuse may affect a child's ability to develop appropriate affect regulation and social support networks. Furthermore, reviews of the literature have found that sexual abuse is associated with an increased risk for early puberty, risky sexual behavior, and teenage pregnancy (MacMillan & Munn, 2001; Putnam, 2003). In addition, female children who have experienced sexual abuse have been found to be at an increased risk for sexual victimization as adults (e.g., Arata, 2002; Gladstone et al., 2004; Marx, Calhoun, Wilson, & Meyerson, 2001).

As child sexual abuse is often a traumatic event in a child's life, it is not surprising that over 50% of children who have suffered sexual abuse meet partial or full criteria for posttraumatic stress disorder (PTSD; see Kendall-Tackett et al., 1993; McLeer, Deblinger, Henry, & Orvaschel, 1992). There is some concern that PTSD may be underdiagnosed in children, as some of the diagnostic criteria are not easily measured in young children, and developmental manifestations of the symptoms are not taken into account (Saywitz et al., 2000). However, the association between adults with histories of childhood sexual abuse and PTSD is well documented and suggests that the impact of child sexual abuse can be severe and persist over many years. In fact, numerous retrospective surveys have found a history of childhood sexual abuse to be associated with later psychological difficulties including anxiety, depression, sexual, and substance abuse difficulties (Cunningham, Pearce, & Pearce, 1988; Fry, 1993; Laws, 1993; Thakkar & McCanne, 2000). Studies have also found survivors of child sexual abuse to be at increased risk for violent victimization in adulthood (Chewning-Korpach, 1993; Wyatt, Guthrie, & Notgrass, 1992).

Although it is clear that sexual abuse can have a variety of significant detrimental effects on children's physical, psychological, and social well-being and development, not all victims of sexual abuse experience significant negative outcomes. In a review of the literature, research has revealed that some children do not experience any significant symptoms or psychopathology following sexual abuse (e.g., Beitchman, Zucker, Hood, daCosta, & Akman, 1992; Browne & Finkelhor, 1986; Kendall-Tackett et al., 1993). However, some researchers have reported evidence for a "sleeper effect," whereby some survivors do not experience distress immediately following the abuse but may experience symptoms of distress at a much later time (Kendall-Tackett et al., 1993). Several studies have identified factors associated with increased risk of impairment in children who have experienced sexual abuse. More chronic, invasive abuse (e.g., penetration), the use of physical force or psychological coercion, and a close relationship to the perpetrator have been associated with increased levels of distress. Furthermore, and perhaps most importantly, a negative parental response to the child's disclosure of abuse has been associated with increased stress for the child, whereas family support appears to buffer the negative effects of child sexual abuse (Kendall-Tackett et al., 1993; Spaccarelli, 1994).

An individual's coping style is another important factor that may impact psychological outcomes of child sexual abuse. Specifically, positive coping skills such as constructive coping, seeking emotional support, and cognitive restructuring have been associated with fewer symptoms of distress, whereas negative coping skills such as self-destructive and avoidant coping have been associated with increased symptoms of distress (Spaccarelli, 1994). Other factors related to preabuse functioning may moderate the impact of child sexual abuse. Specifically, attributional style, feelings of shame, preexisting psychopathology, and temperament may affect postabuse functioning (Feiring, Taska, & Lewis, 2002). Family factors including parenting practices, parental psychopathology, strained parent–child relationships, and family conflict may also be associated with increased symptomatology following child sexual abuse (Deblinger, Steer, & Lippmann, 1999; Saywitz et al., 2000; Spaccarelli, 1994).

In sum, the impact of child sexual abuse varies from individual to individual. However, it is clear that there are numerous negative developmental, physiological, and psychosocial outcomes frequently associated with child sexual abuse. It is important to understand these potential moderating factors, as they often help to guide treatment.

TREATMENT OUTCOME RESEARCH

Given the frequently disruptive aftereffects of child sexual abuse, it is not surprising that much has been written about the prevention and treatment of these difficulties. The clinical literature is replete with instructive case studies, creative treatment descriptions, and therapy books from a wide array of theoretical orientations (Friederich, 1994, 2002; Friedrich, Berliner, Urquiza, & Beilke, 1988; Gil, 1991, 1996; James, 1989). However, scientific efforts to objectively evaluate the impact of treatments specifically designed to help children cope with the aftermath of child sexual abuse only began to appear in the literature in the past 15 years (Deblinger, McLeer, & Henry, 1990; Friedrich, Luecke, Beilke, & Place, 1992; Sullivan, Scanlan, Brookhouser, Schulte, & Knutson, 1992; Lanktree & Briere, 1995). Although a variety of treatment approaches have been studied (e.g., supportive counseling approaches, client-centered treatment, play therapy, community treatment, family and psychodynamic approaches), recent reviews of the child sexual abuse treatment outcome literature find that trauma-focused cognitive-behavioral treatment (CBT) has the most empirical support for its effectiveness in treating PTSD and related difficulties with this population of children (American Academy of Child and Adolescent Psychiatry, 1998; National Registry of Evidence-based Programs and Practices, Substance Abuse and Mental Health Services Administration, 2005; Putnam, 2003; Saunders, Berliner, & Hanson, 2003).

This chapter offers an outline of a trauma-focused CBT consistent with a series of outcome investigations (Cohen & Mannarino, 1996, 1998; Deblinger, Lippmann, & Steer, 1996; Deblinger, Stauffer, & Steer, 2001). The early research demonstrated the superior efficacy of trauma-focused cognitive-behavioral treatment models as compared to nondirective, supportive counseling, and community therapy approaches in both individual and group therapy formats. In addition, the findings of these investigations revealed the significant influence nonoffending parents have in terms of their children's outcomes and responsiveness to treatment. Cohen and Mannarino (1998) reported that parental levels of abuse-specific distress and support mediated children's responsiveness to treatment. More specifically, Deblinger and colleagues (1996) found that parental participation in the CBT was particularly advantageous in helping children overcome behavior problems and self-reported depression. Recently, these investigators combined their highly similar CBT models and collaborated in conducting the first multisite randomized controlled trial with children and adolescents who had experienced sexual abuse (Cohen, Deblinger, Mannarino & Steer, 2004). Children and their nonoffending parents were randomly assigned to trauma-focused CBT or client-centered treatment. The findings of this investigation demonstrated that, although children in both conditions showed significant improvements over time, families assigned to the trauma-focused CBT approach, in comparison to the client-centered approach, showed significantly greater improvements with respect to both child and parent functioning. Specifically, children assigned to CBT showed significantly greater improvements with respect to levels of PTSD, depression, behavior problems, feelings of shame, interpersonal trust, and credibility. Similarly, parents in the CBT condition showed significantly greater improvements with respect to general depression, abuse-specific distress, parenting practices, and parental support of the child. In sum, studies of trauma-focused CBT not only have demonstrated its efficacy but also have produced positive results across different sites and diverse populations (Cohen et al., 2004; King et al., 2000).

Although this empirically supported treatment was grounded and developed on the basis of cognitive-behavioral principles, some of the major components are found in approaches from diverse theoretical orientations designed to help individuals overcome trauma. The approach is not rigid; it is a rational amalgam. Over the years we have integrated aspects of humanistic, attachment, family empowerment, and developmental models to optimally address the therapeutic needs of children who have suffered abuse (Cohen et al., 2004). Perhaps unique to the CBT model, however, is the step-by-step approach that encourages structured sessions in the context of a trusting therapeutic relationship. Guided by the principles of the treatment, therapists are encouraged to utilize their skills and creativity while working collaboratively with the child and parent(s) in individual and conjoint parent–child sessions to accomplish the identified treatment goals in a relatively short time frame (see also Kendall, Chapter 1, this volume).

ASSESSMENT

Careful assessment is critical to the development of an individually tailored treatment plan. The pretreatment assessment provides a diagnostic picture of the client, begins case conceptualization, and determines whether sexual abuse treatment is currently appropriate. After the pretreatment assessment is completed, ongoing informal assessment continues throughout treatment to guide treatment goals. Finally, a posttreatment assessment is completed to assure that the child and family are ready to be terminated or discharged. It is important to include both the child and the parent in the assessment process, as parental involvement can provide important information regarding the child's and parent(s)' behavioral and emotional functioning.

Pretreatment Assessment

Even prior to the first assessment meeting, it is important to establish whether trauma-focused treatment for child sexual abuse is appropriate for the child. A first step would be to obtain a history of sexual abuse, confirming that the sexual abuse allegations have been found to be credible by an appropriate agency (i.e., child protection, law enforcement, a child advocacy unit and/or an independent child abuse professional). If the sexual abuse allegations have not been reported or investigated, following the state law, a report should be made to the appropriate agency and/or the family should be referred for an independent medical and/or psychological evaluation to help determine the veracity of allegations prior to initiating treatment. Once it is clear that the child has experienced sexual abuse, the pretreatment assessment and subsequent treatment can begin.

The purpose of the pretreatment assessment is to obtain information so that the clinician can develop a case conceptualization to guide treatment. Therefore, it is important to gather as much pertinent information as possible from as many sources as practical. Consequently, one obtains a full psychosocial history for the child and pertinent history for the parent (e.g., parental history of abuse) and administers standardized measures to assess general and abuse-specific levels of functioning for both the child and parent. After obtaining a history of the child's experiences of sexual abuse and/or other trauma(s) from the parent, it is also advisable to question the child about his or her history of trauma exposure as well. The child's ability to disclose or at a minimum acknowledge the abuse and/or other traumas provides the clinician with valuable information regarding the level of avoidance the child may be experiencing regarding the abuse (see Faller, 1996, for interviewing techniques). This information assists in the development of the case conceptualization of the child, which allows the clinician to develop hypotheses about pertinent issues as well as potential strengths and barriers to treatment.

During the pretreatment assessment, it is important to consider whether treatment needs to be initiated immediately or delayed due to a judgment that treatment may place the child at a greater risk of harm. Sexual abuse treatment may not be the best initial course of action when the child is still in contact with the perpetrator, when the child is actively suicidal, and/or when the child is actively using substances. The safety of the child is the highest priority, and when applicable the clinician works closely with the nonoffending parent, the child protection agency, and law enforcement to assure the child's safety.

Standardized Assessment

During the pretreatment assessment, the use of standardized measures provides a baseline level of functioning, compared to the general population, for both the parent and child. Furthermore, standardized measures provide a means for the objective measurement of clinical improvement at posttreatment to determine the necessity of further treatment. Consequently, the same measures should be utilized in both pre- and posttreatment assessments.

When evaluating the child's general level of functioning, it is important to assess symptoms that are often elevated among children who have suffered sexual abuse, including PTSD, depression, behavior problems, shame, anger, and anxiety. The Child Behavior Checklist (CBCL; Achenbach, 1991) and the Behavior Assessment System for Children (BASC; Reynolds & Kamphaus, 1992) are parent-report measures that address a multitude of internalizing and externalizing symptoms among children. If desired, there are also youth and teacher report versions of the CBCL and the BASC that can be used to gain additional information.

Although parents and teachers are often the best reporters of children's externalizing symptoms, research has shown that children may be the best reporters of their own internalizing symptoms (Rey, Schrader, & Morris-Yates, 1992). Any of a number of self-report normed measures can be used to assess internalizing symptoms, such as the Child Depression Inventory (Kovacs, 1985; ages 7–12), the Beck Depression Inventory–II (Beck, Steer, & Brown, 1996; ages 13 or older), or the State–Trait Anxiety Inventory for Children (Spielberger, 1973). Furthermore, it is important to assess symptoms of PTSD in children who have been sexually abused. PTSD symptoms can be assessed using a semistructured interview (e.g., K-SADS PTSD module; Kaufman, Birmaher, & Brent, 1997; parent- and child-report) and/or by utilizing standardized measures such as the UCLA PTSD Index (Rodriguez, Steinberg, & Pynoos, 1999).

It is useful to evaluate abuse-specific perceptions, attitudes, and behavior. The Children's Impact of Traumatic Events Scales (CITES; Wolfe, Gentile, & Wolfe, 1989) and the Children's Attributions and Perceptions Scale (CAPS; Mannarino, Cohen, & Berman, 1994) are self-report measures of the child's abuse-related perceptions. Assessing sexualized behavior is also paramount, and the Child Sexual Behavior Inventory (CSBI; Friedrich, Grambsch, et al., 1992) is a standardized measure that assesses parental report of children's sexual behavior problems.

An assessment of parental functioning can be important in planning treatment. Parental levels of depression can be assessed using the Beck Depression Inventory–II (Beck et al., 1996), and abuse-specific parental distress can be examined by self-report questionnaires such as the Impact of Events Scale (Joseph, Williams, Yule, & Walker, 1992) and/or the Parental Emotional Reaction Questionnaire (Mannarino & Cohen, 1996).

Ongoing Informal Assessment

The assessment process is more than the pretreatment and posttreatment assessments. Informal assessment continues throughout treatment and is used for several reasons: to test the validity of the hypotheses formulated during the pretreatment assessment, to clarify questions about case conceptualization, and to determine areas that may need additional focus. Reevaluation of treatment goals can facilitate treatment.

TREATMENT

The treatment model, described in the efficacy studies cited earlier, has been applied in both individual and group therapy formats that have consisted of approximately 12 90-minute sessions. This chapter describes how the individual therapy format may be applied in clinical settings in which the standard 60-minute session is utilized and the course of treatment is more variable (i.e., 12–40 sessions). Note, however, that many children with comorbid diagnoses and histories of multiple traumas do quite well in response to a relatively short course of treatment (i.e., 12–18 sessions) (Cohen et al., 2004). In cases where legal proceedings are expected to occur at a later time and/or family reunification is anticipated, it is helpful to plan for timely booster sessions to address these issues sometime after the initial course of treatment is completed.

Treatment is structured such that initial sessions involve the child and nonoffending parent(s) meeting separately with the therapist for 30–45 minutes each. During the early individual sessions, parents and children are working in parallel, receiving education and skills that will assist them in communicating more comfortably and effectively as sessions proceed (see Table 11.1 for general therapy session guidelines). As parents and children progress and develop effective coping skills, increasingly more time can be devoted to conjoint parent–child sessions (30–40 minutes). The initial session with parents offers an explanation of the assessment findings and an overview of the treatment plan. To inspire a sense of hopefulness in parents, it is important to highlight the child's strengths while also explaining how the treatment model will address the child's particular difficulties. Given the value of parental participation in treatment on behalf of the child, it helps to share the well-documented positive influence that parental support can have on children's postabuse adjustment.

Individual Child Sessions

Coping Skills Training

Affective Expression and Regulation Skills. Sexual abuse can often lead to intense and confusing emotions for children, which may create additional anxiety for them. Providing education about emotions and why people have emotions can be very helpful. Explaining that people experience emotions when there is something in their environment that they need to pay attention to may help the child understand that there is a reason why he or she has troubling emotions (e.g., when you are angry, you may need to stand up for yourself). Labeling emotions and understanding physiological responses that occur during intense emotions helps alleviate children's fear that something is wrong with their bodies. Normalizing children's emotional reactions to their experience of sexual abuse may also reduce anxiety. The reduction of anxiety and the increased ability

TABLE 11.1. General Therapy Session Guidelines

Child	Parent	Joint
Early stages		
Rapport building	Rapport building	None or brief joint session; exchange praise
Introduce session structure	Introduce session structure	
	Offer treatment overview and rationales	
Skills building	Skills building	
Psychoeducation: Emotions, cognitive coping	Psychoeducation	
	Behavior management	
	Introduction to praise	
Middle stages		
Begin gradual exposure/ narrative development	Encourage parents to share details of discovery of sexual abuse	Skills building
Process thoughts and feelings	Process thoughts and feelings	
Identify and dispute abuse-related distortions	Share child's narrative and/or other gradual exposure product	Psychoeducation
Prepare for joint sessions	Prepare for joint sessions	Child shares narrative and/or other gradual exposure with parent
Final stages		
	Behavior management continued—effective communication and discipline strategies	Address questions and cognitive distortions
Healthy sexuality	Healthy sexuality	Healthy sexuality
Personal safety	Personal safety	Personal safety
Prepare for graduation	Prepare for graduation	Celebrate graduation

to express emotions may help reduce behavioral problems in children who previously did not know how to deal with their emotions appropriately.

Developing a feelings vocabulary helps children accept their feelings, increases their ability to recognize emotions, and allows them to express what they are feeling more effectively. The therapist can help the child develop a list of words that describe as many feelings as possible. With younger children, the therapist may find it easier to review feelings words by reading such books as *The*

Way I Feel, by Janan Cain (2000) and *Today I Feel Silly*, by Jamie Lee Curtis (1998).

After the child has developed an expanded vocabulary for emotions, the therapist may move into helping the child identify emotions in both others and in him- or herself. Various tools such as photographs, pictures, puppets, and role playing can be used to help children learn this concept. Children are asked to talk about their own feelings. The therapist and child may take turns talking about a time when they felt different emotions. The child may be encouraged to think about how others look, act, and sound when they experience different emotions. Children can be taught to "Look, listen, and ask" when trying to understand how someone else is feeling. Teaching children to ask how someone else is feeling is important—to avoid inaccurate conclusions based solely on observations. For example, when children disclose their sexual abuse, many of them misperceive the emotions exhibited by their nonoffending parent. It is beneficial to help children realize that *asking* is the only way they will know for sure how the parent is feeling.

Once children are comfortable identifying feelings, they are encouraged to express their emotions in appropriate ways. The importance of sharing feelings with someone is emphasized, and children identify who they can talk to about their feelings. Role plays using puppets or dolls can also be utilized to practice appropriate methods of emotional expression.

Finally, children are asked to talk about abuse-related feelings. If the child has previously created a list of feelings, he or she can circle (in different colors) the feelings experienced during the sexual abuse, after the abuse, during the investigation, and today. As feelings of confusion are common, children can be directly asked if they have felt confused or mixed up about the sexual abuse, if they do not mention it themselves. Children are strongly encouraged to talk to an adult they trust about confusing feelings. The therapist emphasizes that if the first person the child goes to does not listen, he or she should continue to seek out someone who will.

Cognitive Coping Skills. After children have developed emotional expression skills, cognitive coping skills are introduced. In the early stages of treatment, the focus in terms of cognitive coping is on encouraging the identification and sharing of underlying or automatic thoughts. Many children are not aware that most people talk to themselves all the time, and these thoughts influence how we think and behave. This knowledge may help children gain a greater understanding and feeling of control over their emotions and behaviors. Initially, however, the objective is simply to help children understand the importance of identifying, monitoring, and sharing (particularly with the therapist) things they usually do not say out loud. Thus, the therapist may begin by asking a child, for example, to share what she said to herself when she first woke up in the morning before saying anything out loud. With some assistance most children can acknowledge that they might have said, "I don't want to get up," or "I'm hungry." Having the child practice sharing his or her thoughts in a variety of different positive or neutral situations will prepare the child for sharing thoughts in the context of trauma-focused exercises later in treatment.

Cognitive coping skills enable the child to understand that, by changing the way he or she thinks about something, the child can change the way he or she feels. This can also provide the child with a greater sense of control over emotions. The first step in explaining cognitive coping to an older child or parent is to illustrate the interrelationship between thoughts, feelings, and behaviors using the cognitive coping triangle (a triangle with feelings, thoughts, and behavior at the points and dual-direction arrows for the sides). Typically, children are presented with an ambiguous scenario such as the following:

"One day, you are walking down the street, and you see your very best friend across the street. You wave to your best friend, but he or she does not wave back at you. What are you saying to yourself?"

The therapist then elicits thoughts from the child as to what he or she might be thinking in the scenario presented above. Typical responses can include "My friend must be mad at me" or "Maybe he or she has something else on his or her mind." The therapist's role is to help the child understand how each of these thoughts could lead the child to experience different feelings and ultimately to behave in different ways. For example, the child who thinks "I can't believe my friend is so rude" might feel angry at the friend and might then aggressively confront the friend the next time they see each other. On the other hand, the child who thinks "Maybe he or she has something else on his or her mind" might feel somewhat concerned for the friend and might caringly approach the friend at their next meeting. This concept can be summarized by stating that when you think about a problem in a negative way you often feel bad for something that might not be true. It is better to consider all possible explanations and choose to replace the negative thought with a more accurate statement that may lead to more positive feelings.

When the child understands that the same situation can be looked at in different ways, the therapist can begin to teach the child to dispute negative thoughts. Cognitive coping is presented as a skill that can help people change negative, unproductive thoughts into more positive, productive thoughts. It is explained to the child that our thoughts are not permanent, no matter how strong they are, and that people can learn to change their thoughts if they practice doing it enough. However, it is emphasized that changing thoughts is hard, but with time and practice it can help one feel better.

After the child has a clear understanding of how to dispute negative thoughts using examples, the focus can be shifted to the child's thoughts. Initially, the therapist will help the child identify and dispute negative thoughts that are not related to the abuse. Many children are not aware of their own dysfunctional thoughts, so the therapist should help the child identify these negative thoughts and coach him or her through disputing the thought. The therapist can help the child dispute the negative thoughts in several ways, including examining contradictory evidence, testing the accuracy of thoughts, using the Socratic method, and using role plays, including the "best friend" role play.

The "best friend" role play (Deblinger & Heflin, 1996; similar to the Mr. Puppet game, Seligman, 1991) is a technique used in which children imagine that their best friend has negative thoughts (e.g., thoughts presented by the child) and they need to try to make their best friend feel better by challenging the negative thoughts. The role of the best friend can be played by the therapist, a doll, or a puppet. This procedure has the child dispute his or her own negative thoughts in order to help the "best friend." Later the therapist should explain to the child that he (or she) can be his own best friend by challenging his own thoughts and helping himself feel better.

After learning to dispute thoughts that are not related to the abuse, the therapist will help the child dispute negative abuse-related thoughts. However, it is important to note that this is typically done after the child has completed the trauma narrative or participated in other gradual exposure exercises. During these trauma-focused activities, the child will be expressing feelings and thoughts that he or she experienced at the time of the abuse. After the child has had an opportunity to fully share his or her most disturbing experiences and thoughts, the therapist can help to identify inaccurate and/or dysfunctional thoughts that can be disputed during the processing that follows the exposure. This process will be discussed further below (see "Gradual Exposure and Processing").

Finally, younger children may have difficulty understanding the concept of cognitive coping, as they may not be able to conceptualize identifying and disputing negative thoughts. The process of cognitive coping may be simplified for use with younger children. The therapist can explain what thoughts are and help the child identify "helpful" or "hurtful" thoughts. Subsequent to this, the therapist may wish to teach the child a series of positive self-statements that can replace dysfunctional thoughts. For example, a child who seems to be fearful or withdrawn might be encouraged to say simple statements like "I can do this" or "I was brave for telling." It is important to involve the child in behavioral rehearsal of these statements, as they will be better retained and more likely utilized in relevant situations.

Relaxation Skills. Although some children can begin the trauma-focused work (i.e., gradual exposure) without learning or utilizing relaxation exercises, many children benefit from learning how to relax their bodies and minds. Relaxation skills, for example, may help anxious, avoidant children to more effectively modulate their emotions, thereby giving them a sense of control and consequently reducing their tendency to avoid anxiety-provoking abuse-related memories and other stimuli (see also Kendall & Suveg, Chapter 7, this volume).

Relaxation and/or mindfulness exercises should be taught at the child's developmental level. Deep-breathing exercises can be taught to younger children by having them imagine that they are a blowfish making their belly get slowly bigger as they breathe in and then smaller as they breathe out. Younger children typically enjoy imagery exercises and can grasp the concept of tense versus relaxed using images such as a "tin soldier" and a "wet noodle." Older children may be taught progressive muscle relaxation, focusing on the major muscle groups (feet, legs, stomach, hands, arms, shoulders, face). Older children can learn focused breathing similarly to adults, by giving them instruction to breathe in through their noses and out through their mouths while counting slowly to 5.

Psychoeducation

Child sexual abuse education may provide a good starting point for a child who is uncomfortable talking about his or her own sexual abuse experience. Potentially, education will provide an introduction to the sexual abuse topic, decrease anxiety, and ease future discussion about the personal sexual abuse experiences. The education also often helps to reassure children that they are not alone in their experiences and emotions.

It can be helpful to discuss what child sexual abuse is, who sexually abuses children, how many children are sexually abused, how children feel when they are sexually abused, why children are sexually abused, and why children don't tell after they have been sexually abused. Information can be provided in a fun, informative manner. Young children are often engaged by reading. The book *Please Tell! A Child's Story about Sexual Abuse* (Jessie, 1991), a child's account of her sexual abuse experience, is an excellent resource. After reading this book, many children during gradual exposure can be encouraged to write a book about their own sexual abuse experiences. Older children may enjoy creating an educational "game show" about sexual abuse. For teenagers and older children, the board game *Survivor's Journey* by Kidsrights (Burke, 1994) addresses general sexual abuse information and the child's feelings related to his or her own sexual abuse.

Gradual Exposure and Processing

After children experience a traumatic event such as sexual abuse, they may later reexperience the same intense emotions that they had during the actual abuse whenever abuse-related memories are evoked. The process of gradual exposure helps to disconnect the intense emotional reactions that children often have from the actual memory of their abuse. This is done by exposing the child to memories of the abuse in a safe environment so that they may learn that the memory cannot harm them. In addition to diminishing the connection between the memory and the intense emotions, gradual exposure and processing establishes new connections by demonstrating that they can feel calm and even a sense of pride in recounting or writing about their experiences. During the processing phase of treatment, it is important to identify and challenge maladaptive beliefs that the child may have had at the time of the abuse, eventually allowing the child to formulate healthier views of themselves and the world (see the earlier section "Cognitive Coping Skills").

Through careful observation during the initial assessment the therapist formulates a tentative distress hierarchy for the child that can guide gradual exposure exercises. Therapists need not make an explicit hierarchy, as they might with an adult patient. In each session, the therapist provides the child with two choices (e.g., talking about the first episode of abuse or when he or she told about the abuse) so that the child can have some control over what he or she will discuss during each session. As children typically choose the experience that was less anxiety-provoking, their abuse narrative is created step by step with support and guidance to allow them to gain confidence in their ability to talk about the most difficult and disturbing experiences (i.e., the top of the hierarchy).

It is important to warn parent(s) that their children may become more resistant to attending treatment once gradual exposure exercises have been introduced. Abuse recollections may cause distress; however, reassurances can be made that talking about the abuse will help the child feel better in the long run. An analogy of a scary movie can be used (i.e., the more you watch it, the less scary it becomes). The goal of exposure is to have the child reexperience and endure the distressing feelings in a safe place until the distressing feelings diminish naturally. However, it is important to time gradual exposure tasks well so that children have time to regain their composure with a positive or relaxing activity before the treatment session ends.

Throughout the process of gradual exposure, the child is asked to confront and share his or her memories, thoughts, and feelings about the sexual abuse. Over time, the child will be able to tolerate discussions of more and more distressing abuse-related cues and memories. This process may be done using a creative medium, such as using dolls or puppets, poems, drawing pictures, creating songs, and/or writing a book about what happened. By having a product like a book or narrative that can be saved and reviewed from session to session, the process of repeated exposure is simplified, and the child has a final product that he or she can take pride in. Furthermore, this product can be shared with the (nonoffending) parent to work on his or her own reactions and responses to the child's experiences.

Preparation for Gradual Exposure: Narrative Training. Gradual exposure and processing refers to the process of gradually examining and processing increasingly disturbing traumatic memories, thoughts, and other reminders. It may be most effective when the child is able to provide a fairly spontaneous narrative that incorporates the details of what happened as well as the associated thoughts, feelings, and bodily sensations. However, even young children can share their experiences and work through their thoughts and feelings about the trauma through reenactment of the experience by using dolls, puppets, or the creation of a picture book (with some verbal descriptions) about what happened. It is helpful for children to practice providing a detailed narrative of events. Teaching the child how to give a narrative with a non-abuse-related event informs the child what type of information to provide and it allows the clinician to determine the level of detail to expect in a child's abuse narrative.

The method described by Sternberg and colleagues (1997) outlines a useful approach designed to help children provide a more detailed disclosure in the context of an investigation. In the treatment context, it is similarly used to give children practice in sharing details about a positive experience before they are asked to tell about their abusive experience(s). However, we have modified this approach to also give children practice sharing feelings, thoughts, and bodily sensations in relation to a positive or exciting experience. The child thinks of a fun event that occurred recently (such as a birthday party) and is asked to relate the event details, including their thoughts and feelings, from the time they arrived until a specified time. A positive event narrative provides a baseline for the child's ability to narrate an event that they are not avoiding. Their effectiveness in sharing a positive or neutral narrative will provide developmental information in terms of their ability to articulate details as well as their skills in sharing thoughts and feelings. A child may be prompted to share a positive narrative as follows:

"I understand you had a lot of fun going bowling this past weekend. I would like you to tell everything about going bowling, from the moment you got to the bowling alley to the end of the first game. I would like to hear everything about what happened, including how you were feeling and what you were thinking or what you were saying to yourself (remember inside your head)."

When there is a long pause during the child's sharing of the narrative, the therapist can provide open-ended prompts, such as "What happened next?," "What were you thinking?," or "What were you feeling?"

After training the child how to relate a narrative, the therapist can ask the child to talk about a part of the abuse using the same narrative process. Giving the child choices ("Do you want to talk about the first time you were abused, or the time you told your mom about the abuse?") allows the child some feeling of control. The child will likely tell a less detailed narrative of the abuse-related experience as compared to their positive experience, thus providing some information about the child's level of distress and avoidance.

Gradual Exposure and Processing: The Trauma Narrative. After the child has demonstrated the skills necessary to express their trauma-related feelings and thoughts and has shown some comfort discussing less distressing sexual abuse cues (such as general information about sexual abuse) and/or his or her own experience, the child can be encouraged to discuss the abusive experiences in greater detail. During gradual exposure and processing, there are two primary goals: for the child to become more comfortable and less avoidant of their sexual abuse memories; and to identify and correct any maladaptive thoughts.

Beginning each gradual exposure session, the child can choose between two abuse-related experiences to discuss in session. After the child chooses the experience to be shared, the child can be asked to provide the information in the narrative style described above. It is important to avoid suggesting details that the child has not provided. Furthermore, if there are details that are clearly fantasy (i.e., "and then I tied him up with my jump rope and locked him in the basement"), interject and ask the child if that really happened or if that is something he or she wanted to happen. One can allow the child to complete the narrative before asking further open-ended questions. Some children do not provide much information about thoughts and feelings during the first abuse narrative. After the child has provided the initial narrative, the therapist can revisit the information provided and ask the child to share additional thoughts and feelings (see the example below).

THERAPIST: Last week you did such a great job writing about the sexual abuse. Let's read over what you wrote about what happened with your uncle.

CHILD: (*pause*) Do I have to?

THERAPIST: I think it would be a good idea, because the more we talk about this the easier it will get. So, would you like to read it to me, or would you like me to read it to you?

CHILD: You can read it.

THERAPIST: OK. Great, but while I'm reading, I want you to listen very carefully so that you can get back there in your mind and get in touch with what you were thinking and feeling at the time. When I pause I'll ask you to share a little bit more about what you were thinking and feeling at that moment in time.

CHILD: OK.

THERAPIST: (*reading slowly*) "The first time it happened I was at my cousin's house. My uncle called me over to sit next to him on the couch. My uncle put a blanket on us and then he put his hand down my pants and started touching my penis." (*pause*) Now, what were you feeling and thinking right then?

CHILD: (*long pause*) I was feeling really scared and sort of icky. I thought, what is he doing? Get me out of here. I shouldn't have let him put the blanket on us, but I couldn't move.

THERAPIST: (*writing and repeating what the child said*) Thank you for sharing that. Let's see if I got that right. You said, "I was feeling really scared and sort of icky I thought, what is he doing? Get me out of here. I shouldn't have let him put the covers on us, but I couldn't move." Do you have anything you want to add here?

CHILD: No.

THERAPIST: OK, that was helpful. I'll keep reading.

Throughout gradual exposure, maintain focus on the child's memories of the abuse. During this process the child may need reassurance that the distressing feelings will go away after repeated discussion. Some children will become avoidant of therapy, and it is important to be prepared for this. Avoidant behaviors can be managed by several means, such as giving choices of the topic, mode, timing, and length of discussion, or making contracts ("after we talk about this for 10 minutes we can play cards"). Finally, reassurance and reminders of the rationale behind talking about the abuse may help an avoidant child get through a hard session.

By eliciting thoughts experienced at the time of the abuse, dysfunctional beliefs that are developing can be identified or hypothesized. When children who experience sexual abuse attempt to understand the abuse, they frequently lack the information or knowledge to make sense of their experience. Consequently, they may develop confusing, inaccurate, and/or dysfunctional thoughts about the abuse. These maladaptive thoughts can become the basis of their views and beliefs about themselves and the world around them, which can lead to anxiety and/or depression. Thus, it is important to elicit these often idiosyncratic thoughts in the context of exposure tasks so that they can be reviewed later during processing exercises. Challenging these maladaptive thoughts can help alleviate children's negative views about themselves or the world around them, often relieving anxious or depressive symptoms. It is important, however, to postpone the disputing of dysfunctional thoughts and beliefs until the child has shared his or her traumatic memories. The exposure exercises are intended initially to capture the actual experience, including the thoughts and feelings experienced at the time of the abuse. Thus, processing exercises (e.g., disputing thoughts or best-friend role plays) are most often engaged in after the child has completed at least several gradual exposure tasks or chapters of their book. Later, in reviewing the child's book, the child can be encouraged to correct any maladaptive thoughts while adding new, more accurate, thoughts in order to help him or her internalize more productive, optimistic thinking. For example, in the narrative above, the child seemed to be assuming the responsibility for the sexual abuse by blaming himself for allowing the perpetrator to put a blanket over them while watching television. When the narrative is complete, the therapist might help the child process this thought as follows:

THERAPIST: I think you should be very proud of the book you wrote, Jason.

CHILD: Thanks, it is pretty long.

THERAPIST: It is long and it is very well written too! I want to review the book one more time with you because there were a couple of thoughts you had at the time of the abuse that I want to go back to because I am wondering if you still think that way. Let's look at what you wrote about your uncle putting the blanket on you. You wrote: "I was feeling really scared and sort of icky. I thought, what is he doing? Get me out of here. I shouldn't have let him put the blanket on us but I couldn't move." Do you still think that you should not have let him put the blanket on you?

CHILD: Well, yeah, if I didn't do that, he wouldn't have touched me. I'll never let anyone put a blanket on me like that again.

THERAPIST: Have you ever been under the blankets with anyone else?

CHILD: You mean did someone else sexually abuse me?

THERAPIST: No, I mean did you ever sit on the couch or on a bed with someone under a blanket.

CHILD: Yeah, lots of times.

THERAPIST: Really, with whom?

CHILD: My mom, my dad, even with my friends when we had a sleepover.

THERAPIST: Did any of them touch your penis or sexually abuse you?

CHILD: No way!

THERAPIST: So, maybe the sexual abuse didn't happen because you let someone put a blanket on you. Maybe it didn't have anything to do with the blanket or what you did. Maybe it happened because your uncle has a problem.

CHILD: Yeah, but if I didn't let him put the blanket on me, he wouldn't have done that.

THERAPIST: I certainly think it wouldn't be a good idea to let your uncle put a blanket over you again, and it wouldn't even be a good idea to spend time alone with your uncle, because the sexual abuse happened because of what your uncle wanted to do, not because of the blanket. If he didn't do that right then, do you think he might have found a different time that he would have sexually abused you without a blanket?

CHILD: Yeah. He did do it other times without a blanket.

THERAPIST: So, was it being under a blanket with someone that caused the sexual abuse to happen, or was it your uncle?

CHILD: I guess, when you say it that way, it was my uncle that made it happen.

THERAPIST: Do you think it would be OK to sit under a blanket with someone else like your mom or dad or a friend whom you are comfortable with?

CHILD: Yeah, I guess it would be OK.

Finally, it is important to assist the child in organizing the narrative in the proper chronological order, incorporating different episodes of abuse as well as events that occurred in the context of the disclosure and investigation. It is also critical to help the child create a positive, hopeful ending that may summarize what he or she has learned in therapy. This process may help to more effectively encode traumatic memories so that reminders trigger more productive healthy thoughts and feelings (e.g., "That was sad, but I'm proud of how I coped with it") as opposed to shameful or frightening feelings and thoughts about the abuse.

Healthy Sexuality. Education about healthy sexuality is generally provided to children after they have completed their trauma narrative. Providing children with accurate information about sexuality in an age-appropriate manner may help to correct or prevent potential maladaptive beliefs that the child may have or may develop. First, children need to know the names for all of their body parts to ease communication and, at times, embarrassment. Therefore, the first step in discussing healthy sexuality and in developing personal safety skills is to teach children the names for their sex organs, or "private parts." With young children, it is helpful to identify private parts as those body parts that are covered by a bathing suit (i.e., penis, vagina, breasts, and buttocks).

Prior to discussing healthy sexuality with the child, it is important to determine the parents' views and values surrounding sexuality and what they wish their children to know. Furthermore, the parent can be shown sex education materials prior to use with the child, to determine if they feel comfortable with the use of those materials. The therapist and parent can also work together to determine the best approach for providing this information. In fact, therapists are encouraged to provide sexuality education with the parent when possible. Further discussion of this is presented below.

Personal Safety Skills. Education about personal safety skills is generally provided after children have completed most of their narrative or other gradual exposure exercises. The narrative reflects what they experienced, including how they actually responded and not how they think they should have responded based on personal safety education. Personal safety skills education teaches children what to do in possible future situations to keep themselves safe. This education not only safeguards against future victimization but also provides children with a greater sense of self-efficacy regarding their ability to protect themselves.

Body ownership is an important part of personal safety skills education. Children can be taught that their body belongs to them, that they have the right to decide how they do or do not want to be touched. They are also taught that all body parts are important and that nobody has any right to hurt any part of their body.

After teaching body ownership, children can be educated on the difference between OK touches and not-OK touches. It is useful to help the child generate a list of touches that are OK, such as hugs, handshakes, high fives, and so on. The therapist also may role-play how to ask for an OK touch, such as a high five or a hug. Depending on the child's developmental level and parental values, the list of OK touches may also include touching one's own private parts and adults touching each other's private parts when they both want to. Next, the child can be encouraged to generate a list of not-OK touches, such as hitting and punching, as well as sexual touches by an adult or another child.

Help children understand that sometimes it is not clear if a touch is OK or not OK, and that can be very confusing. The therapist can ask the child to tell about a time they were touched in a way that made them feel confused. If the child cannot think of anything, the therapist may provide examples of confusing touches, such as a hug from a stranger or someone the child does not know well. In addition, this can be a good time to discuss how sexual touches might feel good physically, even if they are not OK, which can be confusing. Children can be encouraged to talk to adults about both not-OK touches and confusing touches.

Children can also be encouraged to think about what they might do if someone tried to touch them again in a way that was not OK. Remember to try not to make the child feel bad if he or she did not use personal safety skills when earlier abused. Providing reassurance that most kids do not know what to do can be helpful. Also, acknowledge that what he or she *did* do kept the child safe and that "telling someone about what happened" (which he or she is doing now) is the most important safety skill. Practicing personal safety skills will help the child feel more confident if something like this should happen in the future, but he or she should be proud of how he or she handled this experience prior to knowing anything about child sexual abuse.

At this point, children can be taught that they have power and control of their body and they have the right to say "No" if they do not want to be touched, even if someone wants to give them an OK touch that they do not want that moment—and especially with not-OK touches. Children can practice saying "No" in a strong, loud voice while making direct eye contact. Many children need the therapist to model this for them.

After learning to say "No," children are encouraged to try to get away from the person doing the inappropriate touching. Some children may want to fight the perpetrator. However, it is important to inform them that this may be dangerous and that it is most important to get away to a safe place and to tell someone. However, the therapist can acknowledge that there are times when the child may be unable to get away quickly, and in this case the child should tell someone about the not-OK touch as soon as they feel safe.

Learning to tell someone about a not-OK or confusing touch is a very important part of safety skills training. The therapist can help children identify who they can talk to, both in their family and outside of their family, if they were to receive a not-OK touch. Children should be taught to keep telling until someone understands and helps. Finally, the therapist should discuss appropriate and inappropriate "secrets," so that the child can learn that it is important to tell inappropriate secrets. With younger children, this can be explained in the context of surprises versus secrets, where surprises are fun because the person will learn soon about the surprise, but a secret is something that you are told never to tell. Children can be told to tell someone, even if they promised to keep the secret. There are a number of children's books and videos that can be valuable in teaching children these concepts (Chaiet, Russell, & Gee, 1998; Freeman, 1982; Stauffer & Deblinger, 2003).

All components of personal safety skills are best internalized by rehearsal during session and at home with parents. Role plays, puppets, and dolls are useful methods of behavioral rehearsal. The therapist can generate situations relevant to each aspect of personal safety skills and rehearse with the child so the child has the opportunity to practice the skills. This also allows for coaching the child on the tone of voice, body posture, and eye contact, as well as verbal skills that reflect assertiveness and comfort in communicating their concerns to a helpful adult.

Individual Nonoffending Parent Sessions

As noted earlier, during the early stages of treatment, parents are participating in parallel individual sessions with the therapist. During these sessions, parents have an opportunity to share the myriad emotions they may be experiencing while receiving educational information and practicing the same coping skills their children are learning. These sessions are intended to help parents cope with their own distress and effectively respond to their children's behavioral and emotional difficulties.

Psychoeducation

Child Sexual Abuse. Early on in treatment, it can be very helpful to provide parents with basic information about child sexual abuse including its prevalence, characteristics, and etiology, as well as children's common emotional reactions. Much like the work with children, this education will be called upon in helping parents dispute dysfunctional and/or inaccurate thoughts identified later in treatment. Psychoeducation about sexual abuse and related issues, in fact, will continue throughout the course of treatment with issues like healthy sexuality and personal safety being addressed in the final stages of therapy.

Coping Skills Training

Affective Expression and Regulation Skills. Sexual abuse can lead to intense and often confusing emotions for the parent as well as the child. The ability to recognize, label, and express feelings is an important skill. Providing parents with an outlet to discuss their feelings about their child's abuse is important, particularly in terms of helping parents normalize their reactions and paving the way for the identification of potentially maladaptive beliefs and misattributions that they may have developed. Also, providing the parent with an understanding of what emotions their child may be experiencing and how that may impact their behavior may help parents appropriately empathize with their child while learning to model and encourage effective emotional regulation skills.

As with the child intervention, parents can be asked to enumerate the many feelings that they may have experienced upon discovering that their child was sexually abused, as well as the feelings that they currently have when they think about their child's abuse. A discussion of these feelings may follow, and it is important for the therapist to validate and show acceptance of the parents' feelings, even if they include less "socially desirable feelings" such as anger at their child or disbelief concerning the allegations. Over time these feelings may change, and it is most important that the parent feel supported by the therapist.

Parents are encouraged to monitor their feelings related to the abuse for homework during the week. It is, however, important that parents understand that they should avoid sharing intense abuse-related feelings directly with the child, including being very careful when talking on the phone or in another room of the house where the child may overhear the parent. The parent can identify people whom they feel that they can talk to about their feelings with no danger of the child's overhearing the discussions. Eventually, with the therapist's guidance, the parent may share or clarify some of his or her feelings with the child during conjoint parent–child sessions later in the course of treatment. For example, the parent may explain to a child that his or her intense reaction of anger at the time of the disclosure did not mean that the parent was angry with the child, but rather that the parent was angry with the perpetrator.

Cognitive Coping Skills. Cognitive coping skills are introduced to parents for similar reasons and in a very similar manner as they are introduced to the children. Parents are taught about the interrelationship between thoughts, feelings, and behaviors. They are educated that if they can change their dysfunctional thoughts that this will ultimately change the way they feel and respond to their children. To illustrate this concept the therapist can use the same example of walking down the street and seeing a friend who does not wave back, described in the section of the child intervention on cognitive coping.

Parents can then be encouraged to talk about their emotions related to their child's abuse and the thoughts associated with those emotions. The therapist can then help the parent learn how to dispute thoughts that are inaccurate or nonproductive, with the objective of replacing inaccurate thoughts with more accurate thoughts about child sexual abuse. For example, a parent who states that "I should have been able to tell that Mr. Jones was a sexual abuser" can be provided with education that it is not possible to tell just by looking at someone that he or she is a sexual perpetrator. That parent's thought can be changed to "There was no way I or anyone else could have been able to tell that Mr. Jones was a sexual abuser. Sexual perpetrators don't look any different than anyone else." Nonproductive thoughts (i.e., thoughts focusing on the perpetrator) may also be replaced with more productive thoughts (i.e., thoughts focusing on how well the child is doing in therapy) with some guidance from the therapist.

Finally, parents are educated that viewing a problem as permanent, pervasive, and personal is characteristic of pessimistic thinking (Seligman, 1991). It should be pointed out to parents that most problems are actually changeable rather than permanent, specific rather than pervasive, and nonpersonal rather than personal. The therapist can help parents examine their own thoughts related to the abuse to see whether they reflect any of these qualities. If so, the therapist can empathically help the parent reexamine the thought and replace it with a more helpful, accurate thought. Some common areas of emotional distress and dysfunctional thoughts among nonoffending parents are that of responsibility or guilt for the child's abuse, sadness and grief regarding their child's sexual abuse experience, anger at the child, themselves, and/or the perpetrator, and anxiety about the potential impact of the abuse on the child's future well-being.

Relaxation Skills. As with the child intervention, relaxation skills training may be helpful to introduce to parents experiencing significant distress that does not diminish following the development of cognitive coping skills. Parents may be taught deep-breathing exercises, progressive muscle relaxation, and mindfulness and/or imagery exercises that will help them relax so that they can tolerate a discussion of the child's abusive experiences. In addition, some parents may find these exercises helpful in coping with daily stress and/or warding off tension headaches and other physical manifestations of stress.

Behavior Management Skills

The therapist introduces behavior management skills during the early stages of treatment by educating the parent on how children learn (i.e., modeling, association, and consequences). Providing this rationale can help parents understand how and why their child's behavior may have changed since the sexual abuse.

Furthermore, it is explained to parents that behavioral changes need not be permanent. Rather, most behaviors are learned and can be unlearned. The behavior management skills taught may not only help parents effectively respond to abuse-related behavioral difficulties but also may be useful for non–abuse-related difficulties exhibited by the child client as well as his or her siblings. It is important to start behavior management by encouraging parents to refocus their attention on their child's strengths and prosocial behaviors instead of the symptoms or behavioral changes that they are concerned about. This will then set the stage for teaching, perhaps, the most essential parenting skill: differential attention. This skill requires parents to actively notice and effectively praise positive behaviors while reducing the attention they give to negative behaviors. In addition, parents are taught basic behavior management skills, including active listening, giving effective instructions, and setting limits and consequences for negative behaviors. Education and practice with respect to these skills are interspersed throughout the course of treatment, and the conjoint sessions provide excellent opportunities to coach parents in utilizing the skills effectively. For example, early on in treatment, therapists may end the treatment with a brief conjoint session during which the parents and children practice sharing specific and global praise. Specific praise refers to identifying and expressing appreciation for a specific behavior (e.g., "Thank you for helping me make dinner last night—it was really fun working together"), and global praise refers to expressing unconditional love (e.g., "I love you; I'm so proud to be your mom").

Many parents do not want to give consequences to the child who was sexually abused. Parents are encouraged *not* to treat their child differently by relaxing rules or limits simply because the child has been through a traumatic event. It is explained to parents that children need structure and consistency in their world, and setting rules and limits helps them to have this structure and consistency. Despite their experience of abuse, children still should be expected to follow family and school rules and should receive praise for appropriate behaviors and consequences for inappropriate behaviors. It may be necessary to use cognitive coping skills with parents who are resistant to implementing behavior management strategies at home, as there are likely dysfunctional thoughts getting in the way. Once those dysfunctional thoughts are addressed and replaced, the parent may be more willing to enforce rules and limits.

Gradual Exposure and Processing

Gradual exposure with the parent is very similar to gradual exposure with the child. Initially, the therapist should review the rationale for exposing and processing traumatic memories. Furthermore, the parent should be made aware that the child may become more resistant to attending therapy during the process of gradual exposure, and that this resistance is to be expected, so the parent should not give in to the child's requests to cancel sessions. Parents can be reassured that the child's resistance will diminish as the treatment progresses and the child begins to feel less distress and greater pride in his or her therapy efforts.

For parents, gradual exposure begins with the sharing of their own experiences upon discovering that their child had been sexually abused. In this context, parents are also encouraged to share not only what happened but also what they were feeling and thinking at that time. Eventually, however, the exposure exercises involve the sharing of the child's accounts of the abuse with the parent(s).

The process of gradual exposure with the nonoffending parent is often parallel to the process of gradual exposure with the child. As the child discloses more information about the abuse in treatment sessions, the therapist, with the child's permission, gradually begins sharing this information in individual sessions with the parent and encouraging the parent to experience any emotions and share any thoughts that the child's statements evoke. The process of cognitive and affective processing is essential here, as this is the parent's opportunity to express thoughts and feelings openly in reaction to the child's abusive experiences, without the child being present. The therapist can then help the parent process these thoughts and emotions, using the coping skills described above. If the child has created a product, such as drawings, poems, or a book, the therapist can gradually share this with the parent as a catalyst for the discussion of the child's abusive experiences. With gradual but repeated discussions of the child's abusive experiences, the parents' levels of distress typically diminish, enabling them to develop the emotional composure that will be critical to the success of the conjoint parent–child sessions.

Psychoeducation

Healthy Sexuality. When initiating a discussion of education regarding healthy sexuality with a parent, the therapist should begin by presenting the rationale for providing sex education to the child. The therapist can explain to the parent that the child has received inaccurate information regarding sexuality as a result of his or her sexually abusive experiences, and that the therapist wants to help the parent provide the child with a positive view of healthy adult sexuality. Parents should be encouraged to share their value system with the therapist so that it can be incorporated into the sex education that will be provided by both the therapist and the parent. The therapist may help the parent explore his or her own feelings about sexuality in order to become more comfortable with the idea of educating his or her child about sex. Once again, cognitive coping skills may be used to help dispute dysfunctional thoughts.

When the parent is more comfortable with the idea of educating the child about sexuality, the therapist can offer several guidelines on how best to proceed. Parents are encouraged to begin sex education early by using everyday opportunities such as bath time to teach young children the names of their sex organs or the pregnancy of a family member to teach the child about where babies come from.

The therapist can help parents to focus sex education on the child's developmental level, so that it is appropriate for that particular child. Furthermore parents should not wait for children's questions to arise before discussing sexuality with their children. They are encouraged to approach sex education in a positive manner, and even to use humor when appropriate. Interactive discussion is recommended, along with sex education materials such as books for parents and children.

Several different books may be useful for providing education regarding healthy sexuality, depending on the child's age and developmental level. For young children, *Where Did I Come From?* by Peter Mayle (1995) is a humorous book that describes how babies are conceived and delivered. Preteens may benefit from reading *Asking about Sex and Growing Up* (Cole, 1988), a factual book with common questions asked by preteens and straightforward answers. *The Quest for Excellence* (Hatcher, Wong, Wade, & Golden, 1993) is a book for older adolescents that discusses identity development as well as sexual development and desires, contraception, and sexually transmitted diseases. The book *How to Talk with Your Child about Sexuality* (Planned Parenthood, 1986) can be helpful for parents of children of all ages.

Therapists help parents prepare for difficult questions and issues that may emerge as the child develops. For instance, parents need to be aware of certain obstacles that parents of children who have been sexually abused may face: The child may be particularly avoidant of any discussions about sexuality, and the therapist can help the parent develop a more gradual manner in which to present the sex education material. For a child that is particularly anxious and avoidant, sex education may be introduced as part of the gradual exposure process.

Personal Safety Skills. The therapist involves the parent in the personal safety skills training component of therapy. Parents and children can often practice safety skills together in session and at home. In addition, parents may be encouraged to read a book about body safety with their child for homework between sessions (Stauffer & Deblinger, 2003). It is helpful to inform the parent of what is being taught to the child, as this prepares the parent for how the child might respond to inappropriate behaviors from others, especially those of a perpetrator who may have foreseeable contact with the child. Parental understanding of the skills being taught is paramount, as it is the parent who is going to be reinforcing the use of these behaviors once therapy is completed.

Conjoint Parent–Child Sessions

Preparing for Conjoint Parent–Child Sessions

During the process of gradual exposure and processing with the parent, the therapist may begin to focus on helping the parent learn how to communicate with his or her child about the abuse and other issues more effectively. Parents are encouraged to practice active listening skills that may be used in conjoint sessions as well as at home. These skills can be particularly difficult, as they require parents to suppress their desire to give advice. However, when parents are encouraged to notice how much their children seem to appreciate simply "being heard," they are often sold on the value of serving as a sounding board and support resource for children. Parents' use of active listening, in fact, may enhance children's desire to talk to their parents regarding sensitive issues so that this type of open communication may continue after treatment ends. Using behavioral rehearsal to prepare for discussions that will occur during conjoint therapy sessions and for situations that may occur at home will help the parent to feel confident and capable of handling such discussions with the child.

Conducting Conjoint Parent–Child Sessions

Both the parent and child's readiness for each conjoint session should be assessed prior to their initiation. The parent is ready when he or she manifests (1) minimal emotional reactions to discussions of the child's abuse, (2) an ability to be actively supportive of the child, (3) reduced parental anxieties and concerns, and (4) a reasonable comfort level with general discussions about child sexual abuse, sex education, and personal safety. The child's readiness is determined by his or her ability to engage in the requisite educational activities and to discuss the abuse with relatively little distress. Both parents and children are prepared for conjoint sessions by the therapist, who informs them of what will be accomplished during each session.

The first conjoint session may involve a simple skill-building exercise such as emotional expression charades, in which the parent or child acts out a feeling and the other guesses what feeling is being displayed. Depending on their skills and readiness, the parents and children may jump right into playing a question-and-answer game about child sexual abuse. To encourage a relaxing and fun atmosphere, in collaboration with their child clients, therapists may create a competitive game-show format by serving as the host and giving points for correct answers. Parents are encouraged prior to the conjoint session to let the child answer many questions but also to actively participate, in order to model their comfort in discussing sexual abuse. Children are prepared by reviewing the questions for the game show so that they are confident in answering them in front of their parents. This session can help parents and children begin to feel at ease discussing sexual abuse openly with one another.

Subsequent conjoint sessions can focus on sharing the child's narrative or other work products with the parent. During the parents' individual sessions, they have already processed their own reactions to the child's accounts of the sexual abuse. To prepare for conjoint gradual exposure sessions, the therapist helps the parent to respond to any concerns that may have emerged in the child's gradual exposure. The therapist elicits from the parent what he or she would like to say to the child and then helps the parent refine the statement so that it is supportive and affirming. It is also important to minimize the likelihood of the parent saying anything that could be viewed by the child as judgmental or blaming. Most parents respond quite well to this coaching process. In addition, parents are encouraged to respond to what the child shares with reflective listening and supportive statements, such as praising the child for telling about the abuse, for the hard work in therapy, and so on. Such responses encourage the child to be more comfortable talking to the parent about sensitive issues. In addition, children sometimes are concerned about their parent being hurt by their disclosure and will keep quiet to protect their parents. The conjoint gradual exposure session allows the child to understand that the parent knows about the abuse and he or she does not have to protect the parent by not discussing the abuse.

During the conjoint sessions, the child is encouraged to share the gradual exposure product (e.g., story, poems, song) with the parent. Some children will prefer to have the therapist read their account of the abuse, and some children will prefer to read it themselves. The parent will then have the opportunity to respond to the child with the clarifications or supportive statements rehearsed earlier with the therapist. The sharing of the details of the abusive experiences with the parent, and the parent's supportive response, can be a very powerful positive experience for the child therapeutically.

Additional conjoint sessions may focus on sex education, often utilizing educational materials that the parent(s) and the therapist have discussed and agreed upon in advance. A discussion of healthy sexuality provides children an opportunity to ask any questions they might have relating to sexuality that may be troubling them (e.g., "Could I still get pregnant from the sperm that got in me? Does someone kissing your breasts give you breast cancer?"). A discussion of sexuality often helps children to put the sexual abuse in perspective, differentiating it from loving, healthy sexual interactions between consenting adults.

Finally, children and parents review personal safety skills together. The therapist can engage both the parent and child in a series of role plays rehearsing saying "No" and telling after someone tries to touch the child in a not-OK way. It can be very meaningful for the parents to play themselves in the role play so that the child can come and tell the parent about a not-OK touch. The parent is prepared before the conjoint session on how to respond to such a disclosure. This provides an opportunity for the parent to practice a supportive response, as well as for the child to have an opportunity to be on the receiving end of a supportive parental reaction. This can be particularly powerful if the parent was unable to provide such a response when the child initially disclosed the actual abuse. Practicing personal safety through these role plays with parents is particularly important, given the research that suggests that these skills are more effectively retained and utilized when personal safety training involves the parent(s) and actively encourages behavior rehearsal (Deblinger et al., 2001; Finkelhor, Asdigian, & Dziuba-Leatherman, 1995).

Preparing for Termination

During the final stages of therapy, parents are encouraged to facilitate open lines of communication with their child surrounding the topic of the sexual abuse by encouraging questions from their child, reinforcing the child for sharing problems with the parents, encouraging the expression of feelings in an appropriate manner, and spending one-on-one time with their child. Parents are also encouraged to model open communication with their child regarding the sexual abuse. By showing the child that the parent is comfortable with talking about the abuse, the child will be more comfortable bringing it up to the parent. The therapist helps the parent to be prepared to respond to children's questions or concerns about the abuse in a positive manner that will encourage further discussion. Furthermore, when parents themselves are coping more effectively, they may be encouraged to initiate dialogues with their child about the sexual abuse naturally and gradually. For example, rather than turning off the TV if something comes on about sexual abuse, they might take the opportunity to talk about what was reported, while also encouraging their child to ask questions and share feelings.

Parents are cautioned to avoid overreacting or catastrophizing when the child discusses the sexual abuse with them. Finally, the therapist can encourage the parents to be open to having differing points of view from their child regarding the perpetrator, as the child may not view the offender in the same way as the parent. Parents are cautioned from describing the offender as all good or all bad, as this can be very confusing for a child. Instead, parents are encouraged to talk with their children about the specific behaviors that were not OK, explaining that sometimes people do things even though they know they are wrong.

The final individual and conjoint sessions provide opportunities for some continued discussion about the abuse and a review of skills and education acquired and progress achieved. This can help to prepare for termination and facilitate ongoing parent–child communication beyond the end of treatment. Parents and children are encouraged to use the skills they have learned to address temporary symptom relapses that may occur during times of stress. They can also be encouraged to call the therapist in the future to discuss concerns and determine whether additional therapy may be needed. Booster sessions, in fact, can be quite helpful prior to the initiation of family reunification if that is planned or prior to the child's participation in a criminal trial. After completing a post-treatment assessment, the final therapy session is typically planned as a graduation celebration that acknowledges the progress made and the strength and commitment demonstrated by the family's completion of the therapy process. Given the celebratory nature of the termination session, it is not unusual for children and parents to arrive for the final session with presents, cake, and occasionally even balloons!

CONCLUSION AND FUTURE DIRECTIONS

As noted earlier, new research studies continue to document the debilitating and often long-lasting difficulties suffered by many children and adolescents who have experienced sexual abuse. In fact, children who have experienced sexual abuse appear to be at high risk for a host of difficulties, including posttraumatic stress, depression, suicidal and self-injurious behavior, substance abuse, violent revictimization, and other psychosocial difficulties. It is not unusual for children who have experienced sexual abuse to have suffered numerous traumatic sexual episodes as well as other types of traumas (e.g., traumatic loss, physical abuse, exposure to domestic violence, community violence, etc.). Recent research suggests that children who have suffered sexual abuse and other traumas and who are experiencing PTSD and/or depression may be more responsiveness to a structured treatment model, as opposed to a more nondirective client-centered approach (Deblinger, Mannarino, Cohen, & Steer, 2005). The empirically supported structured approach described here is designed to short-circuit the snowballing of trauma-related difficulties by helping children and their nonoffending parent(s) gain the needed skills and strength to cope with the aftermath of child sexual abuse and other traumas. This model also applies to other traumas, including exposure to domestic and community violence, and traumatic grief (Cohen, Berliner, & Mannarino, 2003; Cohen & Mannarino, 2004; Cohen, Mannarino, & Deblinger, 2001). With assistance from the U.S. Department of Health and Human Services–SAMHSA and the National Child Traumatic Stress Network, work is underway to adapt, evaluate, and expand dissemination efforts to implement this treatment in a variety of community treatment settings for diverse populations of children and their families.

Finally, given the limited length and scope of this chapter, it was not possible to discuss the many complex mental health, medical, legal, and child protection issues that one needs to be familiar with to effectively address the therapeutic needs of this population. Thus, readers are referred to comprehensive texts on the subject (Cohen et al., 2001; Deblinger & Heflin, 1996; Dubowitz & DePanfilis, 1999; Myers et al., 2002) and are encouraged to obtain the necessary professional training and related consultation to effectively treat these children and their families.

REFERENCES

Achenbach, T. M. (1991). *Manual for the Child Behavior Checklist/4–18 and 1991 profile.* Burlington: University of Vermont, Department of Psychiatry.

American Academy of Child and Adolescent Psychiatry. (1998). Practice parameters for the assessment and treatment of children and adolescents with posttraumatic stress disorder. *Journal of the American Academy of Child and Adolescent Psychiatry, 37*(Suppl. 10), 4–26.

Arata, C. M. (2002). Child sexual abuse and sexual revictimization. *Clinical Psychology: Science and Practice, 9,* 135–164.

Beck, A. T., Steer, R. A., & Brown, G. K. (1996). *BDI–II: Beck Depression Inventory manual* (2nd ed.). San Antonio, TX: Psychological Corporation.

Beitchman, J. H., Zucker, K. J., Hood, J. E., daCosta, G. A., & Akman, D. (1992). A review of the short-term effects of child sexual abuse. *Child Abuse and Neglect, 15,* 537–556.

Browne, A., & Finkelhor, D. (1986). Impact of child sexual abuse: A review of research. *Psychological Bulletin, 99,* 66–77.

Burke, C. R. (1994). *Survivors journey.* Indianapolis, IN: Kidsright.

Cain, J. (2000). *The way I feel.* New York: Scholastic.

Center for the Future of Children. (1994). *The Future of Children: Sexual abuse of children, 4*(2). Los Altos, CA: David and Lucile Packard Foundation.

Chaiet, D., Russell, F., & Gee, L. (1998). *The safe zone: A kid's guide to personal safety.* New York: Harper Trophy

Chewning-Korpach, M. (1993). Sexual revictimization: A cautionary note. *Eating Disorders: The Journal of Treatment and Prevention, 1,* 287–297.

Cohen, J. A., Berliner, L., & Mannarino, A. (2003). Psychosocial and pharmacological interventions for child crime victims. *Journal of Traumatic Stress, 16,* 175–186.

Cohen, J. A., Deblinger, E., Mannarino, A. P., & Steer, R. (2004). A multi-site, randomized, controlled trial for children with sex abuse-related PTSD symptoms. *Journal of the American Academy of Child and Adolescent Psychiatry, 43,* 393–402.

Cohen, J. A., & Mannarino, A. P. (1996). A treatment outcome study for sexually abused preschool children: Initial findings. *Journal of the American Academy of Child and Adolescent Psychiatry, 35,* 42–50.

Cohen, J. A., & Mannarino, A. P. (1998). Interventions for sexually abused children: Initial treatment outcome findings. *Child Maltreatment, 3,* 17–26.

Cohen, J. A., & Mannarino, A. P. (2004). Treatment of childhood traumatic grief. *Journal of Clinical Child and Adolescent Psychology, 33,* 820–832.

Cohen, J. A., Mannarino, A. P., & Deblinger, E. (2001). *Child and parent trauma-focused cognitive behavioral therapy treatment manual.* Unpublished manuscript, MCP Hahnemann University, School of Medicine.

Cole, J (1988). *Asking about sex and growing up.* New York: Morrow.

Cunningham, J., Pearce, T., & Pearce, P. (1988). Childhood sexual abuse and medical complaints in adult women. *Journal of Interpersonal Violence, 3,* 131–144.

Curtis, J. L. (1998). *Today I feel silly.* New York: HarperCollins.

Deblinger, E., & Heflin, A. H. (1996). *Treating sexually abused children and their nonoffending parents: A cognitive behavioral approach.* Thousand Oaks, CA: Sage.

Deblinger, E., Lippmann, J., & Steer, R. (1996). Sexually abused children suffering posttraumatic stress symptoms: Initial treatment outcome findings. *Child Maltreatment, 1,* 310–321.

Deblinger, E., Mannarino, A., Cohen, J., & Steer, R. (2005). *A multisite, randomized, controlled trial for children with sexual abuse-related PTSD symptoms: A follow-up and examination of predictors of treatment response.* Manuscript submitted for publication.

Deblinger, E., McLeer, S. V., & Henry, D. E. (1990). Cognitive/behavioral treatment for sexually abused children suffering post-traumatic stress: Preliminary findings. *Journal of the American Academy of Child and Adolescent Psychiatry, 29,* 747–752.

Deblinger, E., Stauffer, L. B., & Steer, R. (2001). Comparative efficacies of supportive and cognitive-behavioral group therapies for young children who have been sexually abused and their non-offending mothers. *Child Maltreatment, 6,* 332–343.

Deblinger, E., Steer, B., & Lippmann, J. (1999). Maternal factors associated with sexually abused children's psychosocial adjustment. *Child Maltreatment, 4,* 13–20.

Dubowitz, H., & DePanfilis, D. (1999). *Handbook for Child Protection Practice*. Thousand Oaks, CA: Sage.

Faller, K. C. (1996). *Evaluating children suspected of having been sexually abused*. Thousand Oaks, CA: Sage.

Feiring, C., Taska, L., & Lewis, M. (2002). Adjustment following sexual abuse discovery: The role of shame and attributional style. *Developmental Psychology, 38*, 79–92.

Finkelhor, D. (1994). Current information on the scope and nature of child sexual abuse. *Future of Children, 4*, 31–53.

Finkelhor, D., Asdigian, N., & Dziuba-Leatherman, J. (1995). Victimization prevention programs for children: A follow-up. *American Journal of Public Health, 85*, 1684–1689.

Freeman, L. (1982). *It's my body*. Seattle, WA: Parenting Press.

Friedrich, W. N. (1994). Individual psychotherapy for child abuse victims. *Child and Adolescent Psychiatric Clinics of North America, 3*, 797–812.

Friedrich, W. N. (2002). An integrated model of psychotherapy for abused children. In J. E. B. Myers & L. Berliner, L. (Eds.), *The APSAC handbook on child maltreatment* (2nd ed., pp. 141–157). Thousand Oaks, CA: Sage.

Friedrich, W. N., Berliner, L., Urquiza, A. J., & Beilke, R. L. (1988). Brief diagnostic group treatment of sexually abused boys. *Journal of Interpersonal Violence, 3*, 331–343.

Friedrich, W. N., Grambsch, P., Damon, L., Hewitt, S. K., Koverola, C., Lang, R. A., et al. (1992). Child Sexual Behavior Inventory: Normative and clinical comparisons. *Psychological Assessment, 4*, 303–311.

Friedrich, W. N., & Luecke, W. J., Beilke, R. L., & Place, V. (1992). Psychotherapy outcome of sexually abused boys: An agency study. *Journal of Interpersonal Violence, 7*, 396–409.

Fry, R. (1993). Adult physical illness and childhood sexual abuse. *Journal of Psychosomatic Research, 37*, 89–103.

Gil, E. (1991). *The healing power of play: Working with abused children*. New York: Guilford Press.

Gil, E. (1996). *Systemic treatment of families who abuse*. San Francisco: Jossey-Bass.

Gladstone, G. L., Parker, G. B., Mitchell, P. B., Malhi, G. S., Wilhelm, K., & Austin, M. (2004). Implications of childhood trauma for depressed women: An analysis of pathways from childhood sexual abuse to deliberate self-harm and revictimization. *American Journal of Psychiatry, 161*, 1417–1425.

Hatcher, R. A., Wong, L., Wade, T. L., & Golden, S. D. (1993). *The Quest for Excellence*. Tiger, GA: Bridging the Gap Foundation.

James, B. (1989). *Treating traumatized children: New insights and creative interventions*. Lexington, MA: Lexington Books/Heath.

Jessie (1991). *Please tell! A child's story about sexual abuse*. Center City, MN: Hazelden.

Joseph, S. A., Williams, R., Yule, W., & Walker, A. (1992). Factor analysis of the Impact of Events Scale with survivors of two disasters at sea. *Personality and Individual Differences, 13*, 693–697.

Kaufman, J., Birmaher, B., & Brent D. (1997). Schedule for affective disorders and schizophrenia for school-age children—present and lifetime version (K-SADS-PL): Initial reliability and validity data. *Journal of the American Academy of Child and Adolescent Psychiatry, 36*, 980–988.

Kendall-Tackett, K. A., Williams, L. M., & Finkelhor, D. (1993). Impact of sexual abuse on children: A review and synthesis of recent empirical studies. *Psychological Bulletin, 113*, 164–180.

King, N., Tonge, B. J., Mullen, P., Myerson, N., Heyne, D., Rollings, S., et al. (2000). Treating sexually abused children with post-traumatic stress symptoms: A randomized clinical trial. *Journal of the American Academy of Child and Adolescent Psychiatry, 59*, 1347–1355.

Kovacs, M. (1985). The Children's Depression Inventory (CDI). *Psychopharmacology Bulletin, 113*, 164–180.

Lanktree, C. B., & Briere, J. (1995). Outcome of therapy for sexually abused children: A repeated measures study. *Child Abuse and Neglect, 19*, 1145–1155.

Laws, A. (1993). Does a history of sexual abuse in childhood play a role in women's medical problems? A review. *Journal of Women's Health, 2*, 165–172.

MacMillan, H. L., & Munn, C. (2001). The sequalae of child maltreatment. *Current Opinion in Psychiatry, 14*, 325–331.

Mannarino, A. P., & Cohen, J. A. (1996). A follow-up study of factors which mediate the development of psychological symptomatology in sexually abused girls. *Child Maltreatment, 1*, 246–260.

Mannarino, A., Cohen, J., & Berman, S. (1994). The Children's Attribution and Perceptions Scale: Methodological implications of a two-stage survey. *Child Abuse and Neglect, 16*, 399–407.

Marx, B. P., Calhoun, K. S., Wilson, A. E., & Meyerson, L. A. (2001). Sexual revictimization prevention: An outcome evaluation. *Journal of Consulting and Clinical Psychology, 69*, 25–32.

Mayle, P. (1995). *Where did I come from?* New York: Kensington.

McLeer, S., Deblinger, E., Henry, D., & Orvaschel, H. (1992). Sexually abused children at high risk for posttraumatic stress disorder. *Journal of the American Academy of Child and Adolescent Psychiatry, 31*, 875–879.

Myers, J. E. B., Berliner, L., Briere, J., Hendrix, C. T., Jenny, C., & Reid, T. A. (2002). *The APSAC handbook on child maltreatment* (2nd ed.). Thousand Oaks, CA: Sage.

National Center on Child Abuse and Neglect (NCCAN). (2002). *Child Maltreatment 2002.* Washington, DC: U.S. Department of Health and Human Services.

National Registry of Evidence-based Programs and Practices, Substance Abuse and Mental Health Services Administration. (2005). *Cognitive-behavioral therapy for child sexual abuse (CBT-CSA).* Washington, DC: Author. Available online at modelprograms. samhsa.gov/template_cf.cfm?page=model&pkProgramID=90

Planned Parenthood. (1986). *How to talk with your child about sexuality.* Available online at www.plannedparenthood.org/parents/howto_page1.html

Putnam, F. W. (2003). Ten-year research update review: Child sexual abuse. *Journal of the American Academy of Child and Adolescent Psychiatry, 42*, 269–278.

Rey, J. M., Schrader, E., & Morris-Yates, A. (1992). Parent–child agreement on children's behaviors reported by the Child Behavior Checklist (CBCL). *Journal of Adolescence, 15*, 219–230.

Reynolds, C. R., & Kamphaus, R.W. (1992). *Behavioral Assessment System for Children manual.* Circle Pines, MN: American Guidance Service.

Rodriguez, N., Steinberg, A. M., & Pynoos, R. S. (1999). *UCLA PTSD Index for DSM IV.* Unpublished measure, UCLA Trauma Psychiatry Service, Los Angeles.

Saunders, B. E., Berliner, L., & Hanson, R. F. (Eds.) (2003). *Child physical and sexual abuse: Guidelines for treatment* (Rev. report, April 26, 2004). Charleston, SC: National Crime Victims Research and Treatment Center. Available online at musc.edu/cvc/guide1.htm

Saywitz, K. J., Mannarino, A. P., Berliner, L., & Cohen, J. A. (2000). Treatment for sexually abused children and adolescents. *American Psychologist, 55*, 1040–1049.

Seligman, M. E. P. (1991). *Learned optimism.* New York: Knopf.

Spaccarelli, S. (1994). Stress, appraisal, and coping in child sexual abuse: A theoretical and empirical review. *Psychological Bulletin, 116*, 340–362.

Spielberger, C. D. (1973). *Preliminary manual for the State Trait Anxiety Inventory for Children.* Palo Alto, CA: Consulting Psychologists.

Stauffer, L. B., & Deblinger, E. (2003). *Let's talk about taking care of you: An educational book about body safety*. Hatfield, PA: Hope for Families, Inc.

Sternberg, K. J., Lamb, M. E., Hershkowitz, I., Yudilevitch, L., Orbach, Y., Esplin, P. W., & Hovav, M. (1997). Effects of introductory style on children's abilities to describe experiences of sexual abuse. *Child Abuse and Neglect, 21*, 1133–1146.

Sullivan, P. M., Scanlan, J. M., Brookhouser, P. E., Schulte, L. E., & Knutson, J. F. (1992). The effects of psychotherapy on behavior problems of sexually abused deaf children. *Child Abuse and Neglect, 16*, 297–307.

Thakkar, R. R., & McCanne, T. R. (2000). The effects of daily stressors on physical health in women with and without a childhood history of sexual abuse. *Child Abuse and Neglect, 24*, 209–221.

Wolfe, V. V., Gentile, C., & Wolfe, D. A. (1989). The impact of sexual abuse on children: A PTSD formulation. *Behavioral Therapy, 20*, 215–228.

Wyatt, G. E., Guthrie, D., & Notgrass, C. M. (1992). Differential effects of women's child sexual abuse and subsequent sexual revictimization. *Journal of Consulting and Clinical Psychology, 60*, 167–173.

SPECIAL TOPICS

CHAPTER 12

Cognitive-Behavioral Therapy with Adolescents

Guides from Developmental Psychology

GRAYSON N. HOLMBECK, KERRY O'MAHAR,
MONA ABAD, CRAIG COLDER, and ANNE UPDEGROVE

The literature on therapeutic interventions for adolescents has matured to the point where numerous volumes and special issues of journals have been devoted to the topic (e.g., Henggeler, Schoenwald, Borduin, Rowland, & Cunningham, 1998; Holmbeck & Kendall, 2002; Rose, 1998; Tolan & Cohler, 1993; Wolfe & Mash, 2006). Despite such attention, it is also noteworthy that there are roughly twice as many published treatment outcome studies on children versus adolescents, even though there are somewhat higher rates of psychopathology during adolescence (Weisz & Hawley, 2002). Moreover, most of the available interventions have focused on a relatively small number of psychopathologies (e.g., 60% of intervention studies focused on anxiety or conduct disorders in one review; Weisz & Hawley, 2002), with few interventions available for some of the psychopathologies that are relatively common during adolescence (e.g., eating disorders, substance use disorders, suicidality; Weisz & Hawley, 2002). Finally, of the many empirically supported treatments that have been applied to adolescents, most are either downward adaptations of interventions originally developed for adults or upward extensions of treatments originally developed for children. Indeed, at the time of Weisz and Hawley's (2002) review, only 1 of 14 empirically supported treatments for adolescents was designed specifically for adolescents (Henggeler et al., 1998). In short, there is a need for more empirically supported interventions that are designed specifically for use with adolescents.

As new interventions are developed, we argue that the quality of such treatments is likely to be enhanced if one develops such interventions by taking into account the important developmental milestones and changes of the adolescent stage of development (see also Holmbeck et al., 2000; Kendall, Lerner, & Craighead, 1984; Ollendick, Grills, & King, 2001; Shirk, 2001; Silverman & Ollendick, 1999; Weisz & Hawley, 2002). Unfortunately, however, a belief in the "developmental uniformity myth" (i.e., that children and adolescents are more alike than they are different; Kendall, 1984) is implicit in most interventions developed to date. But just as adolescents are more likely to prosper when there is a reasonable match between their developmental level and their social or school environment (e.g., Eccles et al., 1993), we expect that interventions that are matched to the developmental level of the treatment recipients are more likely to be effective (Kendall, 1993).

What do we mean by "developmental level"? An adolescent's developmental level can be conceptualized as a snapshot at one point in time of the accumulation of predictable age-related changes that occur in an individual's biological, cognitive, emotional, and social functioning (Feldman, 2001). Although developmental level comprises all of these domains of functioning, researchers in the area of adolescent treatment (and cognitive-behavioral therapy [CBT] in particular) have tended to focus on the cognitive domain, since many treatments designed for children and adolescents are predicated on the assumption that altering one's thinking is an important precursor to more adaptive functioning in the emotional, behavioral, or social domains (Shirk, 2001).

What makes a given treatment developmentally oriented? As we discuss in more detail, such a treatment takes into account the critical developmental tasks and milestones relevant to a particular adolescent's presenting problems (e.g., pubertal development, cognitive development, the development of behavioral autonomy and social perspective taking during adolescence). Such a treatment would also be flexible enough that therapists could choose which presenting symptoms to prioritize, depending on the degree to which each of the symptoms is developmentally atypical (Weisz & Hawley, 2002). For example, an adolescent might present with inappropriately low levels of behavioral self-control (e.g., poor anger management, high levels of risk taking) as well as moderate levels of parent–adolescent conflict. The therapist might determine that the former is more developmentally atypical and problematic than the latter, thus necessitating a focus on self-control difficulties in treatment.

A developmentally sensitive treatment would also be tailored to take into account the developmental level of the adolescent (Forehand & Wierson, 1993);

in fact, different versions of the same treatment may be needed for different groups of adolescents (see Kendall, Choudhury, Hudson, & Webb, 2002a, 2002b, for an example of this strategy). For example, it may be that a less complex version of a treatment would be provided for adolescents at lower cognitive developmental levels, with a more sophisticated version being provided for those at higher levels (Shirk, 2001). Indeed, many CBT treatments require that adolescents be able to evaluate and change their own thought processes as well as consider links between their own thinking and their subsequent emotional states—skills that require more advanced cognitive abilities (Shirk, 2001). Finally, a treatment that is developmentally oriented would take an adolescent's current social context into account (Forehand & Wierson, 1993). Thus, in early childhood, parents may be incorporated into the treatment, whereas during adolescence, relations with peers are more likely to be considered.

In this chapter, the focus is on the developmental changes and milestones of adolescence as they impact on the application of CBT. We begin by providing a rationale for why an exclusive focus on adolescents is justified. Next, we review findings of a literature search on CBT with adolescents, highlighting the general lack of attention paid to developmental factors in this literature. Third, we provide an overview of a developmental framework for understanding adolescent development and adjustment; in describing this framework, we also discuss intervention implications of each component of the model. Fourth, we discuss several developmental factors (e.g., normative development, developmental psychopathology) that clinicians will want to consider in their work with adolescent clients. Finally, we provide recommendations for therapists who seek to apply CBT strategies with adolescents.

WHY FOCUS ON ADOLESCENTS?

Adolescence is a transitional developmental period between childhood and adulthood that is characterized by more biological, psychological, and social role changes than any other stage of life except infancy (Feldman & Elliott, 1990; Holmbeck, 1994; Lerner, Villarruel, & Castellino, 1999; Steinberg, 2005). "Change" is the defining feature of the adolescent period, and there is considerable variability across individuals with respect to the onset, duration, and intensity of changes that adolescents experience. Moreover, there are two transition points during this single developmental period—the transition to early adolescence from childhood and the transition to adulthood from late adolescence (Steinberg, 2005).

Given the multitude of such changes, it is not surprising that there are also significant changes in the types and frequency of psychological disorders that are manifested during adolescence as compared to childhood (Cicchetti & Rogosch, 2002; Holmbeck, Friedman, Abad, & Jandasek, 2006). For some adolescents, it is a period of adaptation and improved mental health, but for others it is a period of maladaptation and increasing levels of psychopathology. In short, it is a critical period in a child's development when one's developmental trajectory can be dramatically altered in positive or negative directions.

In keeping with this developmental psychopathology perspective, many scholars have attempted to identify risk and protective processes that are predictive of such individual differences in developmental pathways (Cicchetti & Rogosch, 2002; Rolf, Masten, Cicchetti, Nuechterlein, & Weintraub, 1990). Protective and vulnerability processes may have their greatest impact during life transitions or periods of dramatic developmental change (Rutter, 1990). In fact, some have argued that "the transitional nature and disequilibrium of adolescence represents an opportune period for intervention, as times of developmental change may result in a greater receptivity to intervention" (Cicchetti & Toth, 1996, p. xiii). Furthermore, we would argue that such opportunities are likely to be missed if one does not take developmental issues into account. We believe that a focus on the adolescent period is a particularly effective way to demonstrate the importance and usefulness of a developmental perspective, given that *change* is the defining feature of adolescence and given the opportunities for having a positive impact on a system that is in a state of flux.

OVERVIEW OF RECENT RESEARCH ON CBT INTERVENTIONS WITH ADOLESCENTS

For a previous version of this chapter (Holmbeck et al., 2000), we examined the degree to which developmental factors had been considered in the design and evaluation of cognitive-behavioral interventions for adolescent clients. To do this, we conducted a computer search to identify relevant empirical journal articles, book chapters, and journal reviews or meta-analyses of the literature published between 1990 and 1998, inclusive. For this version of the chapter, we sought to update this literature review by conducting a similar search for the period from 1999 to 2004, inclusive. Criteria were consistent with the original search and involved the use of various combinations of the following keywords: "cognitive," "behavioral," "adolescent," "therapy," and "treatment." These searches yielded a total of 650 overlapping entries. From this larger list, we selected the following: (1) empirical treatment-outcome studies employing CBT with adolescents (*n* = 29; studies that focused on a mixed sample of children and adolescents and single cases were not included); (2) book chapters on CBT with adolescents (*n* = 9); and (3) journal reviews and meta-analyses of empirical outcome studies of CBT with adolescents (*n* = 20).

For the empirical journal articles, papers were coded for the following information (when relevant): (1) journal name, (2) title of publication, (3) authors, (4) year of publication, (5) age of participants (e.g., early, middle, late adolescence),

(6) type of disorder targeted, (7) type of study (e.g., treatment outcome), (8) nature of treatment (e.g., individual, group), (9) treatment specifics (e.g., whether a control group was employed, number of sessions, length of treatment), (10) whether the treatment was manualized, (11) treatment setting (e.g., university clinic, hospital), (12) statistical methods, and (13) whether (and what types of) developmental factors were discussed. Data from these questions are provided in Tables 12.1 and 12.2. Each document was reviewed to determine if developmental factors were taken into consideration.

The 29 empirical articles appeared in 12 different journals, with two or more papers coming from the following (number of papers in parentheses): (1) *Journal of the American Academy of Child and Adolescent Psychiatry* ($n = 10$) and (2) *Journal of Consulting and Clinical Psychology* ($n = 5$). As can be seen in Table 12.1, the most common targets of cognitive-behavioral interventions with adolescents were major depression ($n = 8$, or 28%), substance abuse ($n = 3$, or 10%), and school refusal ($n = 3$, or 10%). Interestingly, this result differs from that found by Weisz and Hawley (2002), where the most common targets of intervention for adolescents were anxiety disorders and conduct problems (although Weisz and Hawley reviewed studies published prior to 2000, and they did not restrict their review to studies of CBT). In fact, Weisz and Hawley (2002) recommended a more intense focus on depression and substance use; perhaps interventionists and investigators have begun to heed their call. The majority of studies in the current review focused on the early/middle adolescent period (83%), and the number of sessions was most often 11–15 (38%). A little more than a third used a control group (38%); roughly half employed group interventions (52%), and almost two-thirds employed manuals in their treatment (59%). The treatment setting was often not reported, but among those who did report this, secondary schools were the most common location (17%).

It was encouraging that approximately 70% of the empirical articles reviewed mentioned developmental issues when designing and evaluating the treatments. This percentage contrasts sharply with our earlier review of the literature from 1990 to 1998 (Holmbeck et al., 2000), where the percentage of empirical articles that focused on developmental issues was 26%. Does this mean that developmental issues are now being taken more seriously by interventionists who evaluate treatments for adolescents? We believe the answer to this question is both "yes" and "no."

With respect to the "yes" side of the answer, in our previous review (Holmbeck et al., 2000), 2 of 9 (22%) empirical articles "considered issues relevant to parent involvement." In the current review, 10 of 20 (50%) articles did so (see Table 12.2 for a listing of the developmental issues discussed). Although none of the studies in the previous review included treatments that focused on "the contexts in which adolescents interact" (i.e., family, peer, school, and other contexts; see a more complete description of "contexts" below), 3 of the 20 studies in this review did, in fact, focus on contexts. Thus, with respect to the

TABLE 12.1. Review of CBT Outcome Studies Conducted with Adolescents (1999–2004; N = 29 Empirical Journal Articles)

Dimensions and subcategories	No. of studies	% of total articles
Disorder targeted		
Major depression	8	28
Substance abuse	3	10
School refusal	3	10
Social phobia	2	7
Anxiety disorders	2	7
Incarcerated youth	2	7
Obsessive–compulsive disorder	2	7
Comorbid substance use and internalizing/externalizing disorder	2	7
Conduct disorder	1	3
Social skills deficits	1	3
Pregnant and parenting adolescents	1	3
Adolescents with impulse control deficits	1	3
Aggression in adolescents who were abused	1	3
Age of participants		
"Adolescents"	1	3
Early adolescence	0	0
Early/middle adolescence	24	83
Middle adolescence	1	3
Early/middle/late	3	10
Control group?		
Yes	11	38
No	18	62
Number of sessions		
1–5	0	0
6–10	7	24
11–15	11	38
16–20	6	21
Over 20	3	10
Not given	1	3
Varies	1	3
Length of treatment		
1–5 weeks	0	0
6–10 weeks	10	34
11–15 weeks	13	45
16–20 weeks	1	3
Over 20 weeks	3	10
Not given	1	3
Varies	1	3

(continued)

TABLE 12.1. *(continued)*

Dimensions and subcategories	No. of studies	% of total articles
Individual or group		
Individual	7	24
Group	15	52
Not Stated	7	24
Manualized treatment		
Yes	17	59
No	3	10
Not given	9	31
Treatment setting		
School	5	17
University clinic	2	7
Hospital	3	10
Correctional facility	2	7
Office-based	1	3
Not given	16	55
Developmental issues discussed?		
Yes	20	69
No	9	31

Note. Early, middle, and late adolescence were defined with respect to the following age ranges: 11–14, 15–18, and 19–21 years, respectively (Steinberg, 1996). Percentages may not add up to 100% due to rounding. For the 20 empirical journal articles where developmental issues were discussed, such issues are summarized in Table 12.2.

inclusion of contextual issues (and appropriate parental involvement, in particular), there has been an increase in attention to developmental issues since our earlier review.

On the other hand, and similar to the previous review, less than half of the studies that included a discussion of development "intepreted findings in relation to developmental issues" (33% in the previous review; 25% in the current review). Also, very few studies employed a developmental variable as a moderator of treatment effects (1 of 9 in the previous review; 2 of 9 in the current review). In the current review, "age" was the moderator in both instances (Kaminer, Burleson, & Goldberger, 2002; Rohde, Jorgensen, Seeley, & Mace, 2004). The failure to use developmental markers as moderators of treatment effectiveness was also noted in Weisz and Hawley's (2002) recent review of the larger literature on interventions with adolescents (i.e., only 6% of the studies they reviewed used age as a moderator even though *all* of the studies included information on the ages of the participants). There was also an apparent drop in

TABLE 12.2. Developmental Issues Discussed in Empirical Journal Articles (N = 20), Journal Reviews (N = 17), and Book Chapters (N = 8) on Cognitive-Behavioral Therapy with Adolescents (1999–2004)

Developmental issue	N
Empirical journal articles (N = 20)	
Considered issues relevant to parental involvement.	10
Treatments developed by considering developmental issues.	7
Interpreted findings in relation to developmental issues.	5
Treatments focused on contexts in which adolescents interact.	3
Employed a developmental variable as a moderator of treatment effects.	2
Discussed cognitive development or cognitive skills required for CBT.	1
Adapted manual for use with adolescents.	1
Journal reviews/book chapters (N = 25)	
Suggests that treatments focus on contexts in which adolescents interact.	11
Discusses issues relevant to parental involvement in treatment.	9
Discusses cognitive development or cognitive skills required for CBT.	9
Treatments developed by considering developmental issues.	7
Proposes treatment model that varies as a function of stages of development.	6
Differentiates between normative development and psychopathology.	5
Discusses adolescent developmental issues in relation to etiology.	4
Emphasizes developmental variability across adolescents.	4
Advocates adaptations of treatment manuals for use with adolescents.	5
Discusses developmentally based barriers to treatment of adolescents.	3
Development issues to consider in the selection and use of assessment strategies.	2
Section on "developmental issues" relevant to adolescents.	2
Emphasizes importance of maximizing match between developmental level and nature of CBT treatment.	2
Discusses importance of examining developmental status as a moderator of treatment effects.	2
Discusses adolescent developmental issues in relation to symptom presentation.	1
Acknowledges that CBT can foster development.	1

Note. This table summarizes data only for articles, reviews, and chapters that included some type of discussion of developmental issues (i.e., 20 of 29 empirical journal articles, 17 of 20 journal reviews, and 8 of 9 book chapters included such discussions).

the percentage of studies where the treatment was *developed* by considering developmental issues (56% in the previous review; 35% in the current review). Thus, when it comes to the application of developmental principles to the design of the intervention, the analysis of the data, and the interpretation of the findings, there has been no improvement over time within the literature on cognitive-behavior therapy with adolescents.

With respect to book chapters and journal reviews or meta-analyses, most authors took note of developmental issues when discussing the literature on CBT as applied to adolescents (86%, or 25 of 29). Again, this percentage is higher than in the earlier review (43%; Holmbeck et al., 2000). As was the case with the empirical articles, the increase appears to be at least partly attributable to the increase in the number of authors that consider contextual issues (in the current review, 44% of the papers considered contextual issues and 36% considered issues related to parental involvement, compared with 5% and 10%, respectively, in the earlier review).

As was true of the prior review, there were few concrete examples or methods for incorporating development concerns into treatment. In addition, specific tools for the assessment of development were generally not presented. Nevertheless, it does appear that authors are more often considering developmental factors when discussing interventions for adolescents, but these discussions are restricted to the consideration of contextual issues. Indeed, there have been few examples of treatments that were developed with developmental issues in mind and fewer still that have considered developmental variables as moderators of treatment outcomes. Moreover, developmental theory is rarely considered in the introductory or conclusion sections of empirical papers (Weisz & Hawley, 2002). Thus, the *integration* of the developmental psychology and treatment literatures remains a challenge.

A FRAMEWORK FOR UNDERSTANDING ADOLESCENT DEVELOPMENT AND ADJUSTMENT

Given the lack of attention paid to many of the important developmental issues in studies of CBT with adolescents, we provide an overview of a developmental framework for understanding adolescent adaptation and adjustment (see Figure 12.1). We believe that an appreciation for the rapid developmental changes of adolescence and the contexts of such development would aid the clinician and treatment outcome researcher.

This framework summarizes the major constructs that have been studied by researchers in this field and is based on earlier models presented by Hill (1980), Holmbeck (1996; Holmbeck et al., 2006; Holmbeck & Kendall, 1991; Holmbeck & Updegrove, 1995), Steinberg (2005), and Grotevant (1997). See these references for more complete descriptions of the constructs reviewed. An overview of each of the components of the model will be provided, and relevant clinical issues will be described. The model presented emphasizes the biological, psychological, and social changes of the adolescent developmental period (see Figure 12.1).

At the most general level, the framework presented in Figure 12.1 indicates that the primary developmental changes of adolescence have an impact on the developmental outcomes of adolescence *via* the interpersonal contexts in which adolescents develop. In other words, the developmental changes of adolescence

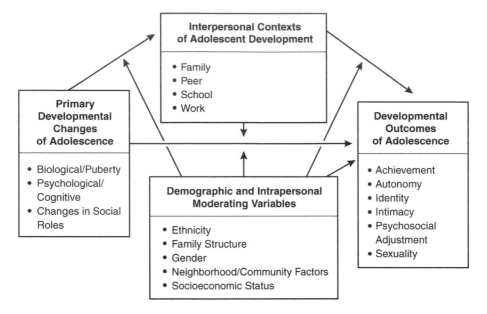

FIGURE 12.1. A framework for understanding adolescent development and adjustment. From Holmbeck and Shapera (1999). Copyright 1999 by John Wiley & Sons, Inc. Reprinted by permission.

have an impact on the behaviors of significant others, which, in turn, influence ways in which adolescents resolve the major issues of adolescence, namely, autonomy, sexuality, identity, and so on.

For example, suppose that a young preadolescent girl begins to physically mature much earlier than her age-mates. Such early maturity will likely affect her peer relationships, insofar as early maturing girls are more likely to date and initiate sexual behaviors at an earlier age than are girls who mature on time (American Psychological Association, 2002). Such dating and sexual experiences may influence her own self-perceptions in the areas of identity and sexuality. In this way, the behaviors of peers in response to the girl's early maturity could be said to *mediate* associations between pubertal change and sexual outcomes (and therefore account, at least in part, for these significant associations). We use the term mediation because of the proposed A→B→C relationship inherent in this example, whereby B is hypothesized to mediate associations between A and C (see Baron & Kenny, 1986, and Holmbeck, 1997, for a more thorough explanation of mediated effects).

Such causal and mediational influences may vary depending on the demographic and intrapersonal context in which they occur (see Figure 12.1, "Demographic and Intrapersonal Moderating Variables"). Specifically, associations between the primary developmental changes and the developmental outcomes may be *moderated* by demographic variables such as ethnicity, gender, socioeconomic status, and the like. We use the term "moderated" because it is expected that associations between the primary changes and developmental outcomes may *differ*, depending on the demographic status of the individual (see Baron & Kenny, 1986, and Holmbeck, 1997, for a more thorough explanation of moderated effects). For example, if associations between pubertal change and certain sexual outcomes *only* held for girls, we could infer that gender moderates such associations. In addition to serving a mediational role, as described above, the interpersonal contexts (i.e., family, peer, school, and work contexts) can also serve a moderational role in the association between the primary changes and the developmental outcomes. For example, early maturity may lead to poor adjustment outcomes *only* when families react to early pubertal development in certain ways (e.g., with increased restrictiveness and supervision); in this example, familial reactions to puberty moderate associations between pubertal development and adjustment.

Primary Developmental Changes of Adolescence

It can be seen in Figure 12.1 that there are three types of primary developmental changes that occur during adolescence: biological/puberty, psychological/cognitive, and social role redefinition. They are viewed as "primary" because (1) they are universal across culture, and (2) they occur temporally prior to the developmental outcomes of adolescence (i.e., changes in autonomy, identity, sexuality, etc.). Despite the universality and intensity of these changes, there has unfortunately been a decided lack of attention to these developmental issues in the adolescent clinical literature (Holmbeck, Greenley, & Franks, 2003; Holmbeck & Updegrove, 1995; Kazdin & Weisz, 1998; Kendall & Holmbeck, 1991; Kendall & Williams, 1986; Ollendick et al., 2001; Shirk, 1999; Weisz & Hawley, 2002; Weisz & Weersing, 1999).

Biological/Pubertal Changes

More than any other stage of life except the fetal/neonatal period, adolescence is a time of substantial physical growth and change (Brooks-Gunn & Reiter, 1990; Tanner, 1962). For boys, there are changes in body proportions, facial characteristics, voice, body hair, strength, and coordination. For girls, changes in body proportions, body hair, breast growth, and menarcheal status occur. Crucial to the understanding of this process is the knowledge that the peak of pubertal development occurs two years *earlier* in the modal female than in the modal male. *Intra*individual variation is also evident with respect to the onset of different pubertal changes (i.e., all pubertal events do not begin at the same time; for example, breast development typically occurs prior to menarche for girls). Moreover, there is substantial variation between individuals in the time of onset, duration, and termination of the pubertal cycle (Brooks-Gunn & Reiter, 1990). Thus, it is possible, for example, that two 14-year-old boys may be at very different stages of pubertal development, such that one boy has not yet begun pubertal changes and the other boy has experienced nearly all pubertal events.

Research also suggests that both *pubertal status* (an individual's placement in the sequence of predictable pubertal changes) and *pubertal timing* (timing of changes relative to one's age peers) have an impact on the quality of family relationships, an adolescent's mood and affective expression, and certain indicators of psychosocial adaptation (Buchanan, Eccles, & Becker, 1992; Holmbeck & Hill, 1991; Laursen, Coy, & Collins, 1998; Paikoff & Brooks-Gunn, 1991). With respect to pubertal timing, early maturing girls, for example, are at risk for a variety of adaptational difficulties, including depression, substance use, early sexual risk behaviors, eating problems and disorders, and family conflicts (American Psychological Association, 2002). Therapists working with such girls should be aware of their at-risk status. Early-developing boys, on the other hand, are favored over later-developing boys for involvement in athletic activities, dating, and social events (Richards, Abell, & Petersen, 1993). However, similar to girls, early-maturing boys may also be at-risk for deviant and risky activities and substance use (Steinberg, 2005). Late-maturing boys may be at-risk for depression and school problems (American Psychological Association, 2002).

Other links between physical development and psychopathology have been found in past research. For example, the rate of overweight and obese adolescents has increased dramatically since 1980 (American Psychological Association, 2002), with such rates being even higher in some ethnic groups (e.g., African American girls). Such overweight adolescents are at-risk for other health-related problems and social discrimination. Although concerns with physical appearance, such as weight dissatisfaction and body preoccupation, are normative during adolescence, some adolescents also develop eating disorders, with most cases being females (90%; American Psychological Association, 2002). Interestingly, the only studies of CBT with adolescents (or interventions of any kind) that have taken biological variables into account have been those that have focused on anorexia or obesity; none has focused on pubertal development (Weisz & Hawley, 2002).

Unlike the newborn, adolescents are aware of their physical changes, and this awareness can range from contentment to horror. Most of the psychological effects of pubertal changes are probably not direct but rather are moderated by responses of the individual or significant others to such changes (Holmbeck, 1996). For example, a lack of information about puberty/sexuality and a low frequency of parent–child discussions about puberty can contribute to emotional upset (e.g., Ruble & Brooks-Gunn, 1982).

Interestingly, there appear to be no links between physical development and cognitive development (e.g., an early-maturing boy who appears more mature than the majority of his peers is not necessarily able to think more abstractly or complexly than others his age). It is helpful for CBT therapists and others in the adolescent's life not to assume that physical changes are indicative of development in cognitive or psychological areas

Psychological/Cognitive Changes

Perhaps most relevant to the interface between developmental psychology and CBT is the potential moderating effect of the adolescent's psychological/cognitive changes on the efficacy of treatment interventions. Although some efforts have been made at taking cognitive development into account when designing treatments (e.g., Guerra, 1993; Kendall, 1984; Kendall, Lerner, & Craighead, 1984; Shirk, 1999; Temple, 1997), few investigators have attempted to examine whether available treatments are differentially effective, depending on adolescents' cognitive developmental level (Durlak, Fuhrman, & Lampman, 1991; Schleser, Cohen, Meyers, & Rodick, 1984). Thus, we have devoted extra space to this component of the model. (In this section, we focus only on cognitive development, to the exclusion of other forms of psychological development such as the development of emotional regulation abilities [Cole, Martin, & Dennis, 2004]. Because the latter have been virtually ignored by CBT therapists, it will be helpful if emotional development is integrated into future intervention protocols.)

A Historical Perspective: The Importance of "Cognition" in Theoretical Formulations. CBT developed in response to the apparent inadequacy of conditioning paradigms in explaining human behavior (Bandura, 1977; Rosenthal, 1982). For example, the success of classical conditioning appears to extend beyond behavioral factors to include personal, social, and cognitive variables. Moreover, in a therapy context, clients cannot be viewed as passive recipients of stimuli; instead, they actively interpret their environment (Ollendick et al., 2001).

All cognitive-behavioral approaches emphasize cognitive processes in the development, maintenance, and modification of behavior (Meichenbaum & Cameron, 1982). From a social learning perspective (e.g., Bandura, 1977), for example, behavior is the product of cognitive processes. These processes determine what we attend to, how events are perceived, whether events are remembered, one's degree of self-efficacy in performing a behavioral response, and the consequences we expect (Bandura, 1977). From this basic assumption several treatment goals follow, including (1) identification of the cognitive processes that underlie the problem behavior and (2) creation of learning experiences that will alter these processes, and in turn, behavioral patterns.

The Focus on "Cognition" in Treatment. CBT draws upon a number of techniques to change cognitive processes. Often a therapist will try to identify maladaptive thoughts or assumptions (e.g., attributions, outcome expectancies) through questioning, imagery, and role playing. New, more adaptive thoughts are encouraged and faulty assumptions are challenged. Another CBT technique is problem-solving training, which has been widely used to help adolescents develop adaptive responses during social conflicts. The training often includes skill development in self-monitoring, means–ends thinking, evaluation of probable consequences, selection of a solution, enactment, evaluation of the solution, and, if necessary, repeating the process to find an alternative solution (Temple, 1997).

In general, the techniques of CBT emphasize self-reflection (thinking about how one thinks), consequential thinking (reflecting on the impact of a particular pattern of thinking or behaving), and consideration of future possibilities (thinking about how a change in thinking or behaving might, in turn, impact on one's life in the future). Thus, the techniques of CBT rely on complex symbolic processes, which typically require a high level of cognitive development. As suggested by Harrington, Wood, and Verduyn (1998) in their discussion of CBT as applied to clinically depressed adolescents:

> For a patient to have cognitive therapy . . . it is necessary to have not only the ability to experience negative cognitions, but also the capabilities to reflect on these cognitions and to engage in complex reasoning in which hypotheses are evaluated and alternative solutions to problems are generated. . . . A key feature of many cognitive therapies . . . is the ability to reflect on one's psychological interior and to consider private attributes of the self such as thoughts and feelings. Some of these are real and concrete but others are hypothetical. (p. 163)

Of course, some clients may not be capable of advanced symbolic processing, particularly when the focus is on their specific areas of psychological difficulty. Although adolescence is often a time of dramatic cognitive development, there is also considerable interindividual variability in the degree to which such development has taken place. It follows, then, that an adolescent's level of cognitive development is likely to impinge on (or facilitate) the success of some CBT techniques (e.g., Bobbit & Keating, 1983; Kendall & Braswell, 1985; Schleser et al., 1984; Shirk, 1999). Indeed, a meta-analysis by Durlak and colleagues (1991) suggested that CBT is more likely to be effective with older (and, presumably, more cognitively mature) adolescents.

Cognitive Development During Adolescence. Specifically, what are the cognitive changes of adolescence? Piaget (1970) has provided a comprehensive stage theory of cognitive development, which has dominated this field of study. He identified adolescence as the period in which formal operational thinking emerges and when adult-level reasoning can take place. Adolescents who have achieved such thinking abilities are able to think more complexly, abstractly, and hypothetically. They are able to think in terms of possibilities, and many are able to think realistically about the future.

Although there is general agreement that a shift in thinking occurs during the transition from childhood to adolescence, critics of the Piagetian approach have suggested alternatives (Moshman, 1998). Proponents of the information processing perspective, for example, have attempted to identify specific changes in cognitive activity that may account for advances in thinking. They maintain that there are significant advances in the following areas during adolescence: (1) processing capacity or efficiency (e.g., working and long-term memory, processing speed); (2) organizational strategies (e.g., planfulness); (3) knowledge about their own thinking processes; and (4) cognitive self-regulation (e.g., selective attention, divided attention; Keating, 1990; Steinberg, 2005). It is important to note that the information processing and Piagetian perspectives are not necessarily mutually exclusive. Piaget's theory describes a qualitative shift in adolescent thinking that appears to begin around age 11 or 12, and the information processing perspective compliments this theory because it suggests possible cognitive features that underlie this shift.

In addition to the Piagetian and information processing perspectives, a third approach to understanding cognitive development during adolescence is the contextualist perspective. Vygotsky (1978) has suggested that psychological processes have a social basis. According to this approach, social interactions, particularly verbal communication, have an important influence on cognitive development. Of interest here are the child's socially relevant cognitions, such as one's understanding of significant others and their behaviors. Some of the social cognitive developmental tasks that may influence progress in therapy include the development of social perspective taking and empathy skills, the role of affect in understanding people, attributional processes in social situations, and prosocial behavior (Guerra, 1993; Nelson & Crick, 1999).

Overall, it appears that a fairly sophisticated way of thinking develops during adolescence, which is characterized by abstraction, consequential thinking, and hypothetical reasoning. Moreover, these cognitive processes are of central importance to many of the strategies used within CBT. That is, this approach to treatment emphasizes complex symbolic representation, which appears to become consolidated during adolescence. Although the processes that underlie the shift in adolescent thinking are not well understood, it appears that increases in efficiency, capacity, and attentional control are important factors. In addition, from a contextual point of view, environmental factors seem to be of importance.

Adolescents may benefit from treatment that initially focuses on changing or accelerating cognitive developmental processes (Shirk, 1999), which in turn may influence the effectiveness of treatment (e.g., Temple, 1997, discusses strategies for helping adolescents to develop means–ends thinking and perspective taking). That is, the therapist may find it necessary to promote the developmental changes that are necessary for the child to benefit from subsequent therapeutic interventions (provided, of course, that the child is developmentally ready to experience such changes and that there is adequate environmental support to maintain the changes). As with other forms of cognitive development, social cognitive development can also be fostered by the therapeutic intervention (as well as by the therapeutic relationship itself; Guerra, 1993). Interestingly, therapists may find that adolescents' maladaptive cognitive beliefs are not as well developed or consolidated as those of adults, thus making the former more amenable to treatment (Bowers, Evans, & Van Cleve, 1996).

In sum, basic knowledge of cognitive development and its application in therapy is likely to be very useful to CBT therapists. Weisz and Hawley (2002) have suggested that CBT therapists (and reseachers who study outcomes of CBT in this age group) can: (1) assess cognitive level prior to treatment, (2) include cognitively oriented approaches in work with adolescents, (3) examine whether outcome varies as a function of cognitive level, (4) examine whether one's young clients can grasp the cognitive concepts, and (5) determine whether advances in cognitive skills (e.g., problem-solving skills) are associated with positive changes in therapeutic outcome.

Have CBT therapists and researchers incorporated cognitive variables and outcomes into their work? Interestingly, Weisz and Hawley (2002) found that only 25% of the intervention studies they reviewed assessed any aspect of cognition, and even fewer (9%) tested any type of association between a cognitive variable and a therapy outcome. This lack of attention to cognitive variables in intervention studies with adolescents may be due, in part, to the lack of assessment measures available to measure cognitive processes (see discussion of such assessment techniques below).

Social Role Redefinition

A variety of changes in the social status of children occur during adolescence (Steinberg, 2005). Although such social redefinition is universal, the specific changes vary greatly across different cultures. In some nonindustrial societies, public rituals (i.e., rites of passage) take place soon after the onset of pubertal change. In Western industrialized societies, the transition is less clear, but analogous changes in social status do take place. Steinberg (2005) cites changes across four domains in Western cultures: *interpersonal* (e.g., changes in familial status), *political* (e.g., late adolescents are eligible to vote), *economic* (e.g., adolescents are allowed to work), and *legal* (e.g., late adolescents can sometimes be tried in adult court systems). In addition, adolescents are able to obtain a driver's permit and can get married. Leaving home in late adolescence (e.g., Moore, 1987) also serves to redefine one's social role. Finally, research suggests that stereotypical gender role expectations are intensified during the adolescent period (Galambos, Almeida, & Petersen, 1990; Gilligan, Lyons, & Hanmer, 1990).

Such changes in social role have clinical implications. Adolescents' abilities to adapt to changing societal expectations for acceptable behavior will vary.

Expected roles are less clear in this culture than is the case in less industrialized societies (Steinberg, 2005); there is little consensus about what constitutes "normal" behavior for adolescents in Western culture (e.g., conflicting messages concerning sexuality and substance abuse are frequently presented in the media). Indeed, psychopathology may be a frequent outcome of failure to sort through the conflicting role expectations.

Interpersonal Contexts of Adolescence

As indicated in Figure 12.1, there are four components included within the interpersonal context portion of the framework: (1) family, (2) peer, (3) school, and (4) work. As is clear from the work of Henggeler and colleagues (1998) on multisystemic treatment of antisocial behavior, the effectiveness of interventions can be enhanced by consideration of context. Adolescents are embedded within multiple systems to a greater degree than are children; clearly, these systems are appropriate targets for interventions and are likely to be amenable to change (Kazdin & Weisz, 1998; Shirk, 1999; Weisz & Weersing, 1999). As noted above, interventionists appear to be attending to "context" more extensively in recent years than previously.

Family Context

Adolescence is a time of transformation in family relationships (Collins, 1990; Holmbeck, 1996; Paikoff & Brooks-Gunn, 1991; Steinberg, 1990). Recent research involving large representative samples of adolescents (see Arnett, 1999) has *not* supported the extreme version of the early storm-and-stress perspective (Freud, 1958). Despite such disconfirming evidence, it appears that public policy and the public's beliefs are still in line with this out-of-date perspective (Buchanan et al., 1990; Holmbeck & Hill, 1988). For example, in a recent national survey of adults, 71% provided negative labels for the typical American teenager (e.g., "rude," "irresponsible"; Public Agenda, 1999).

Although serious parent–child relationship problems are not typical during early adolescence (Holmbeck, Paikoff, & Brooks-Gunn, 1995), a period of increased emotional distance in the parent–adolescent relationship appears at the peak of pubertal change (Holmbeck & Hill, 1991; Laursen, Coy, & Collins, 1998; Paikoff & Brooks-Gunn, 1991). For example, the amount of time spent with family members decreases from 35% to 14% from 5th grade to 12th grade; however, positive connections between adolescents and other family members continue to be present for the large majority of adolescents (Larson, Richards, Moneta, Holmbeck, & Duckett, 1996). Although there also may be an increase in conflict and negative affect, most adolescents negotiate this period *without* severing ties with parents or developing serious disorders (Collins & Laursen, 1992). Also, families with adolescents are more likely to experience conflict over mundane issues rather than basic values (Montemayor, 1983). Any discontinuities in the parent–child relationship during the transition to adolescence tend to occur against a backdrop of relational continuity (Holmbeck, 1996). Moreover, some have argued that the conflicts that arise during the transition to adolescence may serve an adaptive role; indeed, increases in conflicts may indicate that adjustments are needed in parenting and in the manner in which decisions are made and autonomy is granted in the family (Cooper, 1988; Holmbeck, 1996).

One of the major tasks for parents during this developmental period is to be responsive to adolescents' needs for increasing responsibility and decision-making power in the family while at the same time maintaining a high level of cohesiveness in the family environment, monitoring their offspring's behavior, and having clear developmentally appropriate expectations (American Psychological Association, 2002). Parents who lack flexibility and adaptability during this developmental period, particularly in areas of strictness and decision making, tend to have offspring with less adaptive outcomes (Fuligni & Eccles, 1993; Holmbeck et al., 1995). Treatments that include parents (or the family; Walsh & Scheinkman, 1993) can be used in combination with CBT to address this issue by facilitating such parental adaptability and developmental sensitivity.

It also appears that parent–adolescent relationships are altered by the cognitive changes discussed earlier. For example, adolescents are increasingly able and willing to discuss (and argue about) issues with their parents in more complex ways, to see the flaws in their parents' arguments and even to imagine what it would be like to have different parents (American Psychological Association, 2002). This type of advanced thinking is to be encouraged; yet, parents often feel threatened and challenged by this type of adolescent behavior. When faced with this situation, the CBT therapist may want to use "reframing" techniques by suggesting to parents that their adolescent offspring are actually "asking" their parents (in their own inimitable way, of course) to help them learn to think. Telling an adolescent to "just do it because I said so!" does not prepare the adolescent for the myriad choices and decisions they will face. However, a parent who is willing to engage in appropriate discussions with their adolescent concerning issues of rules, responsibilities, and decision making is communicating to the child that there are multiple ways to view the same issue. Cognitive development is likely to be facilitated by such discussions insofar as this type of communication promotes more complex thinking abilities. In short, the degree to which an adolescent has developed cognitively within the family context has clear implications for how a CBT intervention is implemented.

The CBT therapist will benefit from an awareness that transformations in attachments to parents are to be expected during adolescence and that some normative familial problems may arise because of difficulties in managing this transition. On the other hand, it is important for the therapist to evaluate whether or not an adolescent's adaptational difficulties are actually continuations of problems that began in early or middle childhood. Interestingly, of those families who have difficulties during the adolescent developmental period, roughly 80% of these families experienced difficulties during childhood as well (Steinberg, 2005). Although difficulties that develop in childhood as well as difficulties that develop anew in adolescence may be in need of therapeutic attention, the latter are more likely to represent difficulties in negotiating the transition to adolescence.

Peer Context

One of the most robust predictors of adult difficulties (e.g., dropping out of school, criminality) is poor peer relationships during childhood and adolescence (Parker & Asher, 1987). Most now agree that child–child relationships are necessities and not luxuries and that these relationships have positive effects on cognitive, social-cognitive, linguistic, sex role, and moral development (Berndt & Savin-Williams, 1993; Steinberg, 2005). Peers tend to select as friends individuals like themselves (selection effects), and they tend to subsequently influence one another over time (socialization effects; Dodge & Pettit, 2003).

Peer relationships during childhood and adolescence appear to evolve through a series of developmental stages (e.g., Brown, 1990; La Greca & Prinstein, 1999). Selman (1980, 1981), for example, presented a stage theory for the development of social perspective taking. Many adolescents are increasingly able to employ advanced levels of role-taking skills that serve to enhance the maturity of their relationships. Sullivan (1953) stressed differences between child–child and parent–child relationships and described his notion of "chumship"—a (typically) same-sex friendship that is viewed as a critical developmental accomplishment. It is with this relationship that the child presumably learns about intimacy, and this friendship serves as a basis for later close relationships. CBT therapists will want to facilitate the development of social skills and the development of such "chumship" relationships in young adolescents who have few friends either by increasing the adolescents' involvement in extracurricular activities or by including the adolescent in group therapy. Indeed, children need a new set of enhanced social skills as they move from childhood to adolescence and as the demands of social situations become more complex (Steinberg, 2005).

More generally, CBT therapists will benefit from an assessment of the status and quality of their clients' peer relationships (Kendall & MacDonald, 1993) as well as the manner in which the family and peer environments are intertwined. With respect to the latter, therapists may want to involve older siblings in treatment to provide opportunities for the adolescent to practice social skills that they will use in their interactions with peers (although the effectiveness of this strategy has not been tested). Moreover, parents should be encouraged to monitor their children's friendships (La Greca & Prinstein, 1999). Some have suggested that therapists should involve the adolescent's peers in the treatment (e.g., La Greca & Prinstein, 1999). Regardless of the specific strategy employed, friendship skills (e.g., conflict resolution) can be promoted via modeling and rehearsal (La Greca & Prinstein, 1999).

Cognitive-behavioral group therapy can often be a useful context when doing CBT with adolescents. As noted earlier, this is a commonly used intervention strategy with this age group, with roughly half of the studies we reviewed being of this type. Because peers play an important role in shaping adolescent psychosocial development, group therapy with adolescents can be an effective means of challenging maladaptive patterns of thinking and behaving as well as a powerful source of reinforcement for adaptive psychosocial skills. On the other hand, it is important to note that group-based interventions designed to decrease antisocial behaviors may actually have iatrogenic effects due to the "deviance training" that may take place when antisocial individuals have frequent contact with other antisocial peers (Dishion, McCord, & Poulin, 1999; Steinberg, 2005). Such iatrogenic effects may be attributable to a variety of factors (e.g., age of group members, severity of behavior problems, etc.); thus, group therapy for antisocial youth should be approached cautiously.

School Context

Another context of adolescent development is the school environment. Scholars have maintained that not only should we be interested in the school's impact on cognition and achievement but also that we should examine the role of the school environment in the development of an adolescent's personality, values, and social relationships (Entwisle, 1990), particularly given the number of hours children spend in this context.

With increasing age, children are exposed to more complex school environments (Steinberg, 2005; multiple teachers, increasing demands for autonomy, the need to switch classes more frequently). Movement between schools (such as between an elementary school and a junior high school) can be viewed as a stressor, with multiple school transitions producing more deleterious effects (Petersen & Hamburg, 1986; Simmons & Blyth, 1987). The physical setting, limitations in resources, philosophies of education, teacher expectations, curriculum characteristics, and interactions between teacher and student have been found to be related to a variety of child and adolescent outcomes (Minuchin & Shapiro, 1983). Also, the high rate of dropouts in some school districts may indicate that the school environment and the needs of the students have not been well matched (Eccles et al., 1993). More generally, recent research indicates that the best school environments have the following characteristics: an emphasis on intellectual activities, committed teachers who are granted autonomy from administrators, strategies in place to monitor the school's progress, a commitment to the surrounding community, and students who are active participants in their own education (Steinberg, 2005).

CBT therapists can benefit from assessing the nature and quality of their adolescent clients' school environments (Trickett & Schmid, 1993); practitioners can work to enhance or to minimize various aspects of the school environment, depending on their impact (e.g., CBT interventionists can provide referrals for special education classes when there is a poor fit between an adolescent's skills and the school's teaching methods). Interestingly, in Weisz and Hawley's (2002) review of interventions for adolescents, roughly 20% of all interventions involved the school context in some manner. But in no cases were associations between school factors and treatment outcome examined.

Work Context

The last context that we will consider is the work environment (Greenberger & Steinberg, 1986; Lewko, 1987). Although more than 80% of all high school students in this country work before they graduate (Steinberg, 2005) and many government agencies have recommended that adolescents work, little research has been done on the effects of such work on adolescent development and the adolescents' relationships with significant others.

Based on the research that has been done (e.g., Greenberger & Steinberg, 1986), however, it seems clear that the work environment has both positive *and* negative effects on adolescent development. Although adolescents who work tend to develop an increased sense of self-reliance, they also tend to (1) develop cynical attitudes about work, (2) spend less time with their families and peers, (3) be less involved in school, (4) be more likely to abuse drugs or commit delinquent acts, and (5) have less time for self-exploration and identity development. The primary problem seems to be the monotonous and stressful nature of many jobs performed by adolescents. CBT therapists will benefit from attending to the balance between work and other aspects of an adolescent's life, the quality and impact of the work environment itself, and the adolescent's attitudes and beliefs about work. In past work, some have used feedback from work settings to gauge adolescents' progress in treatment (Weisz & Hawley, 2002). Of course, it will be helpful if CBT therapists consider the necessity of the adolescents' work status for their family income level in making recommendations concerning adolescents' involvement with work.

Developmental Outcomes of Adolescence

As can be seen in Figure 12.1, the developmental changes of adolescence impact on the interpersonal contexts of adolescent development, which, in turn, impact on the developmental outcomes of adolescence. In this section, the primary developmental outcomes of adolescence will be discussed: achievement, autonomy, identity, intimacy, psychosocial adjustment, and sexuality (see Figure 12.1).

Achievement

Decisions made during adolescence can have serious consequences for future education, career, and choice of extracurricular activities (Henderson & Dweck, 1990). For those who remain in school, it is during high school that most adolescents are, for the first time, given the opportunity to make decisions about their education. Adolescence is also a time of preparation for adult work roles, a time when vocational training begins. Given the increase in choices, one might expect to see an increase in anxiety around "life decisions," particularly among those who are not cognitively ready to be able to manage such complex decision-making processes.

The CBT therapist can use a number of strategies to help adolescents manage these challenges. For example, a therapist can aid the parent in serving as a guide or a model for the adolescent around these issues. Given the complexity of achievement decisions, adolescents also may benefit from naturally evolving or intervention-induced advances in cognitive abilities (i.e., the ability to employ future-oriented thinking, abstract reasoning, and hypothetical thinking). Those who have developed these abilities are at an advantage when they begin to make education- and career-related decisions.

Autonomy

Autonomy is a multidimensional construct in the sense that there is more than one type of adolescent autonomy (Hill & Holmbeck, 1986; Steinberg, 1990). Emotional autonomy is the capacity to relinquish childlike dependencies on parents (Fuhrman & Holmbeck, 1995). Adolescents increasingly come to de-idealize their parents, see them as "people" rather than simply as parenting figures, and be less dependent on them for immediate emotional support. When adolescents are behaviorally autonomous, they have the capacity to make their own decisions and to be self-governing. Adolescents become increasingly able to recognize those situations where they have the ability to make their own decisions versus those situations where they will need to consult with a parent or peer for advice (Steinberg, 2005).

The CBT therapist will benefit from being attentive to the following autonomy-related issues as they arise during treatment: (1) the degree to which the adolescent is responsible in managing the level of autonomy he or she has been granted by parents, (2) whether the parent and the child have realistic expectations for the level of autonomy that should be granted in the future, (3) the degree to which there is a discrepancy between how much autonomy the parent is willing to grant and the amount of autonomy the adolescent is able to manage (Holmbeck & O'Donnell, 1991), (4) the parents' responses to their child's attempts to be autonomous, (5) the degree of flexibility demonstrated by parents in changing their parenting around autonomy issues (Holmbeck et al.,

1995), and (6) the degree to which the child is susceptible to peer pressure (Steinberg, 2005).

Autonomy development has implications for how parents and adolescents are involved in treatment (Forehand & Wierson, 1993; Shirk, 1999). For example, when conducting parent management training (PMT), such treatment "must be reconceptualized in terms of mutual rather than unilateral interventions" (Shirk, 1999, p. 64). Rather than parents being entirely in control of the intervention (as is the case with PMT as applied to *children*), parents *and* adolescents who are involved in PMT will learn negotiation skills, and adolescents will be instrumentally involved in the treatment (Shirk, 1999). Parents and therapists may want to utilize an approach where there is a balance between respecting and validating the input of the adolescent and maintaining some level of parental authority.

Identity

A major psychological task of adolescence is the development of an identity (Erikson, 1968; Harter, 1990). Adolescents develop an identity through role explorations and role commitments. One's identity is multidimensional and includes self-perceptions and commitments across a number of domains, including occupational, academic, religious, interpersonal, sexual, and political commitments. Although the notion that all adolescents experience identity crises appears to be a myth, identity development is recognized as an important adolescent issue (Harter, 1990).

Research in the area of identity development has isolated at least four identity statuses that are defined with respect to two dimensions: commitment and exploration (Steinberg, 2005). These identity statuses are as follows: identity moratorium (exploration with no commitment), identity foreclosure (commitment with no exploration), identity diffusion (no commitment and no systematic exploration), and identity achievement (commitment after extensive exploration). An adolescent's identity status can also vary depending on the domain under consideration (e.g., academic vs. interpersonal). It is helpful for the CBT therapist to recognize that the process of identity formation is different for males and females and that neither process is pathological. Identity development in males appears to involve struggles with autonomy and themes of separation, whereas identity development in females is more likely to be intertwined with the development and maintenance of intimate relationships (although both genders may experience either or both processes; Gilligan et al., 1990; Harter, 1990).

Intimacy

It is not until adolescence that one's friendships have the potential to become intimate (Savin-Williams & Berndt, 1990). An intimate relationship is characterized by trust, mutual self-disclosure, a sense of loyalty, and helpfulness. Intimate sharing with friends increases during adolescence, as does adolescents' intimate knowledge of their friends. All relationships become more emotionally charged during the adolescent period, and adolescents are more likely to engage in friendships with opposite-sex peers than are children. Girls' same-sex relationships are described as more intimate than are boys' same-sex relationships. Some scholars have proposed that friendships change during the adolescent period because of accompanying social cognitive changes. The capacity to exhibit empathy and adopt multiple perspectives in social encounters makes it more likely that friendships (and therapy relationships) will become similarly more mature, complex, and intimate.

Adolescents may benefit from a CBT intervention that focuses on the development of perspective-taking skills, given that such skills are precursors to the development of intimate relationships with others (Shirk, 1999). In the same way that there are changes in the nature of adolescent peer relationships, therapeutic relationships with adolescents are more likely to become intimate and emotionally charged than is the case with younger children. Issues of trust, loyalty, and self-disclosure (including a more intense focus on issues of confidentiality) also become salient therapeutic concerns during this developmental period.

Psychosocial Adjustment

A host of psychosocial adjustment outcomes have been of interest to researchers who study the adolescent period. Handbooks on the topic typically have chapters on a variety of diagnostic categories (e.g., Tolan & Cohler, 1993; Van Hasselt & Hersen, 1995; Weiner, 1992), namely, depression and anxiety disorders, suicidal behavior, conduct disorders and delinquency, substance use disorders, eating disorders (anorexia and bulimia), schizophrenia, and academic underachievement. Studies that examine potential predictors of adjustment typically focus on a single outcome (e.g., delinquency), given that predictors tend to vary across outcomes and because the outcomes themselves tend to be multidimensional (Loeber, Farrington, Stouthamer-Loeber, & Van Kammen, 1998; Tolan & Cohler, 1993). Psychopathology can be assessed with self-, parent-, and/or teacher-report on questionnaires or with adolescent-report in diagnostic clinical interviews (e.g., Diagnostic Interview for Children and Adolescents [DICA]; Reich, Shayka, & Taibleson, 1991).

As is true for all who work with adolescents, CBT therapists benefit from being aware that there are dramatic changes in the rates of disorders during the adolescent period (e.g., increases in rates of schizophrenia and alcohol/substance use, decreases in rates of enuresis), with some disorders becoming major psychiatric problems for the first time during this developmental period (Holmbeck et al., 2006). The features of certain childhood disorders change as the child moves into the adolescent years (e.g., attention-deficit/hyperactivity disorder [ADHD];

Barkley, 1997), and there are also dramatic gender differences for some disorders during adolescence (e.g., depression; Nolen-Hocksema, 1994). Many scholars have become interested in predictors of rates of change in disorders. For example, one might ask: Why do depression scores increase rapidly over time for some adolescents but not for others?

The various problem behaviors of adolescence tend to be intercorrelated, insofar as they tend to co-occur within the same individuals. One clustering scheme suggests that there are two broadband categories of psychopathology (Achenbach, 1982, 1985): *internalizing* problems (i.e., disorders that represent problems within the self, such as depression, anxiety, somatic complaints, and social withdrawal) and *externalizing* problems (i.e., disorders that represent conflicts with the external environment, such as delinquency, aggression, and other self-control difficulties). Alternatively, Jessor and colleagues (Jessor, Donovan, & Costa, 1991; Jessor & Jessor, 1977) have proposed that a "problem behavior syndrome" characterizes some adolescents, such that there tend to be high intercorrelations among several types of problem behavior (e.g., drug use, sexual intercourse, drinking, and aggression). According to problem behavior theory, such behaviors develop as a function of the same etiological factors and, therefore, tend to co-occur in the same individuals (findings that have been replicated in other laboratories; e.g., Farrell, Danish, & Howard, 1992; although see Loeber et al., 1998, for an alternative perspective). Finally, some adolescents have multiple disorders (i.e., comorbidity; Biederman, Newcorn, & Sprich, 1991; Loeber et al., 1998); treatment techniques often have to address multiple psychopathologies that may interact in various ways. For example, ADHD and conduct disorders (CD) often co-occur, and this combination of disorders is associated with more negative outcomes relative to either ADHD or CD alone (Lynam, 1996).

In sum, knowledge of the various psychopathologies of adolescence and how such pathologies change from childhood to adolescence can be helpful to the CBT therapist. Importantly, therapists benefit from knowledge about developmental variations in the onset and course of these different pathologies and the degree to which there is overlap or comorbidity among the various disorders.

Sexuality

Most children have mixed reactions to becoming a sexually mature adolescent. Parents also have conflicting reactions to such increasing maturity. Despite the high rates of sexual activity during adolescence (nearly 70% of adolescents have had sexual intercourse by age 18; Steinberg, 2005), we know very little about normal adolescent sexuality (whether heterosexual or homosexual), primarily due to the difficulty in conducting studies on this topic (Katchadourian, 1990). There are a host of factors that are associated with the onset and maintenance of sexual behaviors. Pubertal changes of adolescence have both direct (hormonal) and indirect (social stimulus) effects on sexual behaviors. Ethnic and religious differences in the onset of sexuality also exist. Finally, personality characteristics (e.g., the development of a sexual identity) and social factors (e.g., parent and peer influences) also serve as antecedents to the early onset of adolescent sexual behaviors. For example, McBride, Paikoff, and Holmbeck (2003) found that more advanced pubertal development, higher levels of family conflict, and lower levels of positive affect in observed family interactions were associated with earlier sexual debut in African American adolescents.

The increasing rates of sexually transmitted diseases among adolescents and the fact that many young adults with AIDS (acquired immune deficiency syndrome) probably became infected as adolescents would suggest that adolescent sexuality is deserving of considerable attention from researchers and mental health practitioners working with adolescents. Also, early onset of adolescent sexuality is often viewed as part of a more general adolescent problem behavior syndrome (Jessor & Jessor, 1977).

Given the often conflictive nature of adolescent, peer, and parental responses to sexuality, CBT therapists may be called upon to serve as educators about sexual matters (e.g., they may provide accurate information about transmission of HIV). Moreover, practitioners must be clear, direct, and thorough in their evaluation of adolescent sexual behaviors. Not surprisingly, this is best done when therapists are aware of any of their own conflicts or concerns around issues of sexuality.

Use of the Framework for Understanding Adolescent Development

Having reviewed the different components of the framework, we provide two brief examples of how this framework can be used to understand the behavior of individuals. Recall that the primary developmental changes of adolescence impact on the interpersonal contexts of adolescence, which, in turn, impact on the developmental outcomes of adolescence (see Figure 12.1).

Example 1

Suppose that a young adolescent boy is recently able to take multiple perspectives in social interactions, think hypothetically, and conceive of numerous possibilities for his own behaviors. Such newly developed cognitive skills will impact on his familial relationships insofar as he is now able to imagine how his relationships with his parents could be different. He begins to challenge the reasoning of his parents and requests more decision-making power in his family. These changes may either be welcomed by the family and serve to facilitate growth and change within the family system or may be received more negatively and result in conflict. The accompanying changes in his relationships with his parents will, in turn, impact his level of behavioral autonomy, the nature of his attachments to his parents, and his identity.

Example 2

A 16-year-old girl has just obtained a driver's license and has decided that she will look for her first job to earn some spending money. Because she is now 16 years old, she recently gained a number of privileges that she did not have before (i.e., her social role has been redefined). She takes a job in a fast-food restaurant several miles from home, and, because she now has a driver's license, she can get to work on her own. Her experiences at her job produce increases in feelings of autonomy and achievement as she begins to develop an occupational identity. Moreover, her peer group may become less school-based and more heterogeneous.

IMPLICATIONS OF DEVELOPMENTAL PSYCHOLOGY FOR THE USE OF CBT WITH ADOLESCENTS

As suggested by Shirk (1988), "The psychological treatment of children can be informed, and advanced, by the introduction of developmental principles into clinical concepts and techniques" (p. 14). This section will be divided into two subsections: (1) normative development and CBT with adolescents and (2) developmental psychopathology and CBT with adolescents.

Normative Development and CBT with Adolescents

Several issues related to the interface between the literatures on normative development during adolescence and the use of CBT with adolescent clients will be discussed. Specifically, we focus on (1) the developmental uniformity myth, (2) developmental norms, (3) developmental level as a moderator, (4) developmental level as a mediator, and (5) considering developmental level when selecting an intervention approach.

The Developmental Uniformity Myth

As mentioned earlier, it appears that therapists may inadvertently endorse the "developmental level uniformity myth" (Kendall, 1984; Kendall et al., 1984), which is the tendency of clinicians to view children and adolescents of different ages as more alike than different. The consequence of a belief in this myth is that treatments are more likely to be applied without consideration of the developmental level (i.e., the social, emotional, and/or cognitive developmental level) of the child or adolescent client.

Shirk (1999) has described a number of interrelated subtypes of the developmental level uniformity myth. First, there is the "developmental continuity myth." This myth involves the assumption that therapies that are applied to adults can be applied with little modification to children with similar presenting problems. A second myth ("the developmental invariance myth") involves the assumption that a given disorder has a single etiological pathway (Shirk, 1999; more will be said about etiological pathways later, in the section on developmental psychopathology). Third, the "developmental consistency myth" involves the assumption that the same developmental tasks are relevant across different ages. Contrary to this myth: (1) the clinical concerns that need to be addressed in treatment are likely to vary as a function of the developmental level of the child (e.g., the acquisition of certain conflict resolution skills may be more relevant at certain ages than at others); (2) the therapeutic interventions that will successfully redirect a child from a maladaptive trajectory to an adaptive trajectory are likely to vary developmentally (e.g., techniques to manage aggression in early childhood differ from those that are most useful in working with aggressive adolescents; Shirk, 1999); and (3) the presence of certain pathologies may make it more likely that a child will be off-time in the development of certain skills (e.g., an aggressive child with ADHD may not have developed appropriate social skills). An implication of the last issue is that the therapist may need to address not only the presenting symptoms (e.g., the ADHD and aggressiveness) but also the skills (e.g., social skills) that the child failed to develop as a consequence of having a severe behavior problem (Shirk, 1999).

Finally, "the myth of individual development" involves the assumption that treatment can proceed at the individual level without providing attention to contextual factors (Shirk, 1999). Contrary to this myth, Henggeler and colleagues (Henggeler et al., 1998) have documented the importance of attending to multiple systems (family, peer, school) in which the adolescent interacts. Similarly, if a family-oriented CBT approach is deemed optimal, the adjustment of the parents and the quality of parenting must be assessed prior to including the parents as part of the intervention (Kendall & MacDonald, 1993; Shirk, 1999).

Developmental Norms

The therapist who is knowledgeable about both normal and maladaptive adolescent development is likely at a great advantage when attempting to design a treatment, determine the conditions under which a treatment is efficacious, and/or apply a given treatment. Simply put, it is likely that the quality of adolescent treatment will "move up a notch or two" when the clinician is sensitive to adolescent developmental norms.

Knowledge of developmental norms serves as a basis for making sound diagnostic judgments, assessing the need for treatment, and selecting the appropriate treatment. In terms of diagnosis, both overdiagnosis and underdiagnosis can result from a lack of or erroneous knowledge of developmental norms. A CBT clinician who lacks the knowledge that a given behavior is typical of the adolescent age period (e.g., increases in adolescent questioning of parental authority due to advances in cognitive development, increases in time spent with peers at the expense of time with family) is much more prone to *overdiagnose* and to inappropriately refer such adolescents (and their families) for treatment.

With regard to *underdiagnosis*, it is a common belief that adolescents have extremely stormy and stressful relationships with their parents and that "detachment" from parents is the norm (Arnett, 1999; Holmbeck & Hill, 1988). On the other hand, research has not supported this notion—it appears that approximately 20% (rather than 100%) of adolescents have such detached relationships with their parents (Holmbeck & Hill, 1988). A problem results, then, when clinicians underdiagnose psychopathology during adolescence, owing to storm-and-stress beliefs. Underdiagnosis is also possible when the same diagnostic criteria are applied to children and adolescents. For example, March and Mulle (1998) suggested that children tend to exhibit developmentally appropriate levels of obsessive–compulsive symptoms (e.g., normal children often insist that certain activities follow rigid routines). Such obsessive compulsive behaviors are not typical of adolescents, however. Failure to recognize that such behaviors are developmentally inappropriate during the teenage years may lead to underdiagnosis.

Given the adolescent's normal developmental trend toward greater autonomous functioning (Steinberg & Silverberg, 1986), certain CBT treatments are more appropriate for this age group. Self-control strategies (e.g., Feindler & Ecton, 1986) are probably more useful with older adolescents than are behavioral programs where parents are employed as behavior change agents (Guerra, 1993; Kendall & Williams, 1986; Shirk, 1999). Even if a therapist's sense of what is normative is consistent with the research literature, a parent of an adolescent may need to be educated about typical adolescent behavior. Parents may use their own adolescence as "the norm," thus biasing their attributions about their child's behavior. Parents also have the additional task of integrating their own sense of what is normative with the norms and expectations of their child's peer group. Particularly for parents who are dealing with "adolescence" for the first time, the CBT therapist can help such parents bring their expectations in line with what is known about normative behavior during the adolescent period.

Developmental Level as a Moderator

The importance of cognitive developmental level as a moderator of treatment effectiveness has been stressed by many scholars in the field (e.g., Guerra, 1993; Holmbeck et al., 2003; Holmbeck & Updegrove, 1995; Kendall & Braswell, 1985; Shirk, 1999). By examining *moderators* of treatment effectiveness, we are interested in isolating conditions that determine when a treatment is particularly effective or ineffective (top of Figure 12.2). Given the list of cognitive changes presented earlier, it seems reasonable to propose that the degree to which a child has developed these skills will enhance or limit the potential effectiveness of a given psychotherapeutic intervention (Downey, 1995; Forehand & Wierson,

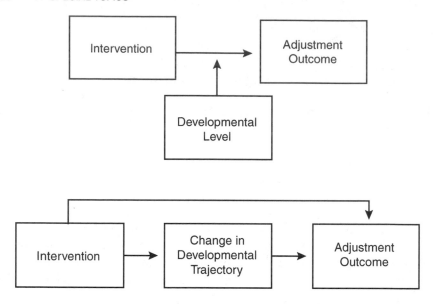

FIGURE 12.2. Moderational (top) and mediational (bottom) models of treatment outcome: The role of developmental level. From Holmbeck, Greenley, and Franks (2003). Copyright 2003 by The Guilford Press. Reprinted by permission.

1993; Wasserman, 1984; Weisz, Rudolph, Granger, & Sweeney, 1992). It is even possible that more advanced cognitive abilities may exacerbate some types of psychopathology (e.g., depressogenic cognitions; Eyberg, Schuhmann, & Rey, 1998). Research on cognitive-developmental moderator variables can be of use to those who develop new cognitively oriented treatments or to those who wish to develop alternative versions of treatments tailored to the needs of individuals at different developmental levels.

How might therapists assess the cognitive developmental level of their adolescent clients? Unfortunately, a straightforward user-friendly method of assessing level of cognitive development across different cognitive subdomains is not available. On the other hand, researchers in the area of cognitive development have been successful in developing several measures, some of which may be relevant within the therapeutic context. Some examples are as follows: (1) Fischhoff's measure of perceived consequences of risky behaviors (Beyth-Marom, Austin, Fischhoff, Palmgren, & Jacobs-Quadrel, 1993); (2) the Youth Decision-Making Questionnaire that assesses social decision making in various peer and parent approval conditions (Ford, Wentzel, Wood, Stevens, & Siesfeld, 1989); (3) the Selection Task (Chapell & Overton, 1998), which requires evaluation of 10 conditional "if . . . then" propositions that assess deductive reasoning abilities; (4) the Similarities subtest of the WISC-IV (Wechsler, 2003), which assesses abstract reasoning abilities; and (5) Dodge's measures of social information processing

(Dodge & Coie, 1987; see also Nelson & Crick, 1999, for other similar measures). Other more complex measures are also available but may be more useful to researchers than to clinicians (e.g., Flavell's and Selman's measures of role taking, perspective taking, and friendship development; Flavell, 1968; Selman, 1981).

More generally, it is recommended that clinicians informally assess the level of cognitive development in their adolescent clients. For example, clinicians could determine whether an adolescent is able to (1) consider future consequences, (2) generate alternative responses to complex social situations, (3) "think about his (or her) own thinking," (4) think in an organized and planful manner, or (5) consider the perspectives of others. Such an informal assessment will facilitate the matching of intervention to an adolescent's developmental level.

Of course, cognitive developmental variables are not the only developmentally oriented variables that can serve as moderators of treatment impact. Weisz and Hawley (2002; see also Shirk, 2001) highlight a different psychological moderator, namely, motivation. Here the focus is on the motivation to engage in treatment and the motivation for therapeutic change. This variable is "developmental" insofar as children of different ages may exhibit differing levels of motivation. As noted by Weisz and Hawley (2002), motivation may be lower in adolescence and particularly for those who are more peer-oriented (versus adult- or parent-oriented). On the other hand, therapists who work with adolescents may be more successful in using "future benefits" as a motivator than those who work with children (Piacentini & Bergman, 2001). Regarding biological development, interventions focusing on early sexual risk behaviors may prove to be more effective with adolescents who have begun to experience the changes of puberty because such interventions may be viewed as more salient by this subset of adolescents (although there are certain preventive benefits to providing such interventions in prepubertal children).

Developmental Level as a Mediator

Examining developmental level as a *mediator* addresses a different set of questions (bottom of Figure 12.2). If one has already established that a given treatment affects a given outcome, one is likely to pose questions regarding possible mechanisms by which the treatment affects the outcome of interest (Kazdin, 1997; Weersing & Weisz, 2002). From this perspective, a mediator is assumed to account for at least a portion of the treatment effect. Also, the mediator is viewed as causally antecedent to the outcome, such that change in the mediator is expected to be associated with subsequent changes in the outcome.

Interestingly, some may prefer to focus on the mediator (rather than the adjustment outcome) as the preferred target of treatment because of some known causal connection between the mediator and the outcome. First, we will provide an example involving a nondevelopmentally oriented mediator of treatment effectiveness. Treadwell and Kendall (1996) found that negative self-statements (or, more accurately, changes in self-statements) mediated the effect of treatment on anxiety severity. In this way, self-statements accounted for a portion of the treatment effect. Moreover, self-statements were not only a target of the treatment, but were also viewed as causally antecedent to anxiety severity. With respect to developmentally oriented mediators of treatment effects, Guerra and Slaby (1990) found that changes in problem-solving ability were associated with positive outcomes in delinquent behavior. Arbuthnot and Gordon (1986) have found similar results with moral reasoning as a mediator. Finally, changes in parenting skills (Forgatch & DeGarmo, 1999; Martinez & Forgatch, 2001), family relations (Eddy & Chamberlain, 2000; Huey, Henggeler, Brondino, & Pickrel, 2000), and deviant peer affiliation (Eddy & Chamberlain, 2000; Huey et al., 2000) have been examined as developmentally relevant mediators of treatment-adjustment effects.

Examining mediator models in the context of treatment outcome studies is a particularly useful research strategy because of the experimental (i.e., random assignment) aspects of the design. As noted by Collins, Maccoby, Steinberg, Hetherington, and Bornstein (2000), if the manipulated variable (i.e., treatment) is associated with changes in the mediator, which are, in turn, associated with changes in the outcome, there is significant support for the hypothesis that the mediator is a causal mechanism. To further support this hypothesis, it would be important to demonstrate (via the research design) that changes in the mediator *precede* changes in the treatment outcome (Kraemer, Stice, Kazdin, Offord, & Kupfer, 2001).

An important corollary of these findings and speculations is that developmental level can be the *focus* of treatment (Figure 12.2; Eyberg et al., 1998; Shirk, 1999). That is, if research suggests that children who have failed to master certain developmental tasks or successfully navigate certain developmental milestones are more likely to exhibit certain symptoms, the developmental level of the child could be the target of the intervention. To put it another way: One implication of this "developmental level as mediator" perspective is that therapists who work with adolescents may need to address not only a client's presenting symptoms (e.g., aggressiveness) but also the normative developmental skills (e.g., self-control, emotion regulation) that the child failed to develop as a consequence of having a severe behavior problem (Shirk, 1999).

As noted earlier, adolescents may benefit from treatment that initially focuses on changing or accelerating cognitive developmental processes (Shirk, 1999; Temple, 1997), particularly if lack of development in this domain has been linked with subsequent increases in symptoms. For example, treatment that affects children's perspective-taking abilities or their development of social-cognitive hostile attribution biases may ultimately produce a decrease in children's level of aggression, perhaps by facilitating their ability to regulate their emotions (Aber, Jones, Brown, Chaudry, & Samples, 1998). In this example, hostile attribution biases are mediators of the effects of the intervention on level of aggression. In the area of social anxiety, aiding adolescents in developing more intimate relationships with their same-age peers may affect socially anxious behavior. In the area of substance use, treatments that focus on an adolescent's level of decision-making autonomy or future-oriented thinking may facilitate their ability to make decisions that reduce health risks. For externalizing symptoms and ADHD, level of impulse control and self-regulation may be an appropriate mediator of treatment impact (Mezzacappa, Kindlon, & Earls, 1999). Finally, the stages of normative developmental change may guide the stages of treatment. When teaching a child increasingly complex levels of social interaction as part of social skills training, for example, the therapist can follow the developmental sequencing and stages of social play and social relationships (Selman, 1981) that may, in turn, impact on the adolescent's social skills.

Developmental Level: Selecting an Intervention Approach

Weisz and Weersing (1999) detailed ways in which the cognitive developmental level affects the process of therapy and the types of treatments that are selected. The degree to which a child is able to employ abstract reasoning or perspective-taking skills may determine, in part, whether certain cognitive or insight-oriented techniques as well as strategies that require hypothetical thinking (e.g., role-playing exercises) can be implemented (Weisz, 1997). If a child does not have such skills, other therapeutic techniques may be necessary (e.g., therapists may need to demonstrate how to identify maladaptive thoughts by talking aloud during role plays; Piacentini & Bergman, 2001).

As noted by Henggeler and Cohen (1984), when discussing different treatment options for children and adolescents who have experienced trauma (e.g., sexual abuse), consideration of the developmental stage is critical when selecting an appropriate treatment. For example, when working with an adolescent who has experienced a traumatic event, it is important that the therapist distinguish between recent traumatic events versus events that occurred during childhood that are now being revisited anew during adolescence. With a previously experienced event, an adolescent may view the event from a new perspective (e.g., he or she can comprehend the injustice of the events). Such a new perspective on an "old" event may necessitate additional therapeutic attention. Indeed, treatment for a given trauma (e.g., early child abuse, marital disruption) may need to be administered *intermittently* at different critical periods as the original trauma is "reexperienced" at new developmental stages. For example, if an adolescent was sexually abused as a child, new issues may arise for the adolescent as he or she develops physically and begins developing opposite-sex friendships.

Developmental Psychopathology and CBT with Adolescents

Developmental psychopathology is an extension of developmental psychology insofar as the former is concerned with variations in the course of normal development (Rutter & Garmezy, 1983). Research based on a developmental psychopathology perspective has informed us about the developmental precursors and future outcomes of adolescent psychopathology. Moreover, the field of developmental psychopathology has provided us with a vocabulary with which to explain phenomena that are relevant to therapists and that researchers seek to explain empirically (e.g., risk and protective processes, cumulative risk factors, equifinality, multifinality, heterotypic continuity, resilience, developmental trajectories, distinctions between factors that produce symptom onset versus those that serve to maintain or exacerbate existing symptoms; Cicchetti & Rogosch, 2002; Olin, 2001). Developmental psychopathologists have also informed us about boundaries between normal and abnormal and how such distinctions are often blurred at certain stages of development for certain symptoms (e.g., substance abuse versus normative experimentation with substances; Cicchetti & Rogosch, 2002). In fact, some symptoms may even be reflections of children's attempts to negotiate normative developmental tasks (Siegel & Scoville, 2000).

Research indicates that the frequency and nature of most disorders varies as a function of age. Regarding changes in frequencies, Loeber and colleagues (1998) have documented age shifts in the prevalence of certain disorders (e.g., delinquency, substance use, sexual behaviors, etc.). Loeber and his colleagues have also documented important differences between children and adolescents with early-onset problem behavior (i.e., life-course-persistent delinquency; Moffitt, 1993) versus those with later-onset problem behaviors (i.e., adolescent-limited delinquency). Rutter (1980) reviewed changes that occur in behavior disorders from childhood to adolescence and concluded that roughly half of all adolescent disorders are continuations of those seen in childhood. Those that emerge during adolescence (e.g., anorexia) tend to be quite different than those that began during childhood (e.g., ADHD), with the symptomatology of most child and adolescent disorders being manifestations of particular stages of development (e.g., for anorexia: pubertal and body image concerns during adolescence; for ADHD: self-regulation concerns during early childhood). The field of developmental psychopathology also addresses issues of continuity/discontinuity. Antisocial behavior tends toward continuity insofar as antisocial adults almost always have been antisocial children (Loeber et al., 1998), but many depressed adults tend not to have been depressed children. Similarly, schizophrenia is often not preceded by psychotic disorders during childhood and adolescence (Rutter, 1980).

A clinician's knowledge of developmental predictors has a number of implications for the treatment of adolescents, as illustrated by the following examples. First, if we know, based on longitudinal studies, that a specific set of behavioral deficits in early childhood (e.g., externalizing behavior symptoms, oppositional defiant disorder) is related to more serious pathology in adolescence (e.g., delinquency, conduct disorder), we can then treat the less severe antecedent disturbance before having to deal with the more serious subsequent disturbance. Early intervention is critical, since children with behavioral difficulties often "choose" environments that exacerbate psychopathology.

Second, some adolescents with certain developmental trajectories (e.g., girls who experience early pubertal development) may be at risk for subsequent behavioral symptoms (e.g., early sexual risk behaviors), and these individuals could be the targets of intervention. Third, the literature on peer relationships and later personal adjustment suggests that poor peer relationships early in childhood (e.g., peer rejection, aggressiveness, shyness, social withdrawal) place children at risk for developing adjustment difficulties in adolescence. Although individuals such as those just described are often the focus of both universal and targeted *group* prevention efforts, the "at-risk" status of a given individual is also relevant within the context of *individual* treatment. In addition to focusing on behaviors that are most likely to place the individual at risk for future psychopathology, therapists can also identify opportunities for "protection" in the adolescent's life (e.g., the availability of supportive nonparental adults) that can buffer the at-risk adolescent from developing later adaptational difficulties.

Equifinality, multifinality, and *heterotypic continuity* are also likely to be useful concepts for the clinician who works with adolescents. Interestingly, it appears that equifinality and multifinality are more the rule than the exception (Cicchetti & Rogosch, 2002). Specifically, equifinality is the process by which a single disorder is produced via different developmental pathways (adolescents "may share the same diagnosis but not the same pathogenic process," Shirk, 1999, p.65). For example, it is likely that two depressed adolescents will have very different etiological factors present in their backgrounds. Multifinality involves the notion that the same developmental events may lead to different adjustment outcomes (some adaptive, some maladaptive). For example, two young children who are sexually abused at the same level of severity may exhibit very different developmental trajectories during adolescence. Given past research support for the concepts of equifinality and multifinality (Cicchetti & Rogosch, 2002), it appears that therapists are best served by gathering as much developmental and historical information as possible about a given adolescent (in addition to what the therapist already knows about the etiology of the disorder in question). Put another way, if equifinality proves to be an adequate explanatory model for most adolescent psychopathologies, then treatments that are based on single causal/mediational models will likely not be effective for sizable proportions of affected adolescents (Cicchetti & Rogosch, 2002).

Finally, heterotypic continuity involves the notion that a given pathological process will be exhibited differently with continued development. For example, behavioral expression of an underlying conduct disorder may change over time even though the underlying disorder and meaning of the behaviors remain relatively unchanged (Cicchetti & Rogosch, 2002).

In sum, a therapist working with adolescents can use knowledge of developmental psychopathology to aid in generating hypotheses about the course of a given adolescent's disturbance. With such knowledge, one would be in a better position to answer such questions as: In the absence of treatment, is it likely that this adolescent's disturbance will increase, abate, or stay the same over time? Is the observed disturbance typical of the problems that are usually seen for an adolescent of this age? Without answers to these questions, the therapist may misdiagnose, be prone to apply inappropriate treatments, or be overly concerned about the presence of certain symptoms.

RECOMMENDATIONS FOR THERAPISTS

1. *Stay informed.* It is recommended that therapists subscribe to journals such as *Development and Psychopathology, Child Development, Developmental Psychology,* and the *Journal of Research on Adolescence* to stay up to date on research focusing on developmental issues during adolescence. Interestingly, all of these journals regularly publish papers that examine clinical issues within a developmental context. Similarly, outlets such as the *Journal of Consulting and Clinical Psychology* and the *Journal of the American Academy of Child and Adolescent Psychiatry* often publish papers that integrate developmental and clinical issues.

2. *Use developmentally sensitive techniques.* Make a developmentally oriented assessment a regular part of your initial evaluation of a child or adolescent. With respect to treatment, researchers who conduct interventions with young children (ages 4–8) often have success using techniques such as videotape modeling strategies or life-sized puppets rather than strict cognitive approaches (Eyberg et al., 1998). For example, most young children are unable to distinguish between different types of emotions; thus, drawings and pictures from media publications may be useful. The degree to which children are motivated by the possibility of acquiring future benefits of treatment also varies as a function of age and can be considered when addressing motivational issues (Piacentini & Bergman, 2001). Similarly, Kendall and colleagues (2002a, 2002b) have altered their CBT manuals for anxious adolescents by taking the developmental changes of adolescence into account.

3. *Focus on developmental tasks and milestones* that the adolescent is attempting to master (e.g., social skills; Forehand & Wierson, 1993; Weisz, 1997). Weisz and Hawley (2002) have argued that developmental research may not always be useful in guiding the treatment of a specific adolescent, since group trends that emerge in developmental research may not apply to a specific case. On the other hand, these authors also provide some useful suggestions for ways to incorporate knowledge of developmental tasks into one's clinical work with adolescents.

First, they suggest that knowledge of developmental findings can *alert* the therapist to specific domains of functioning that are likely salient at a given age. Second, findings from developmental research can aid therapists in *prioritizing* certain presenting complaints over others, depending on which are most developmentally atypical or pathological. Finally, developmental research data can help the therapist in *selecting* treatment strategies or modules that may be developmentally appropriate for a given individual. It is also recommended that CBT therapists begin to integrate developmental variables that have largely been ignored thus far within their intervention strategies (e.g., emotion regulation; see Stark et al., Chapter 5, this volume).

4. When working with older children and adolescents, *think multisystemically* and consider a child's context (Forehand & Wierson, 1993; Henggeler et al., 1998; Kazdin, 1997; Reid, 1993). As children mature during the adolescent stage of development, they are increasingly pulled into other contexts (e.g., peer, school, work). Such contexts can be taken into account when developing interventions for older adolescents.

5. *Help parents (and other relevant adults, such as teachers) to become developmentally sensitive* (Forehand & Wierson, 1993; Holmbeck & Updegrove, 1995). Adult reactions to the onset of adolescent developmental changes are critical to take into account; knowledge of such changes can increase the appropriateness of parent and teacher responses to developing adolescents.

6. To prevent exacerbation of symptomatology, *anticipate future developmental tasks and milestones* (Forehand & Wierson, 1993). For example, therapists can discuss the normative tasks of adolescence with a family seeking treatment for a preadolescent. Discussing how such future tasks may affect a particular child with certain vulnerabilities could be helpful. That is, it is helpful to educate parents about how events may be reexperienced at different ages (e.g., childhood sexual abuse).

7. *Consider the concept of equifinality* when conducting treatment (Cicchetti & Rogosch, 2002; Shirk, Talmi, & Olds, 2000). As noted earlier, different developmental pathways may lead to the same psychopathological outcome (i.e., equifinality). Thus, treatments may be unsuccessful for some children because the developmental precursors for their symptoms differ from the precursors of symptoms for children exhibiting successful treatment outcomes (Shirk et al., 2000).

8. *Consider alternative models of treatment delivery.* Kazdin (1997) has provided a useful discussion of how different types of psychopathology may require different types of treatment delivery. Some psychopathologies may require continued care, much like ongoing treatment for diabetes. Treatment is modified over time but is never discontinued. Other psychopathologies may be best treated with a "dental model." With this approach, treatment is discontinued, but the child is monitored at regular intervals (particularly during important developmental transition points).

9. *Begin to fill your therapeutic "toolbox"* with empirically supported treatment *"modules"* that can be used as needed (Shirk et al., 2000; Weisz & Hawley, 2002).

Rather than using a more rigidly defined set of therapeutic techniques, it may make more sense to have a set of empirically supported techniques ("tools") that can be used or not used, as indicated (see Weisz & Hawley, 2002, for an example involving youth depression).

SUMMARY AND CONCLUSIONS

Although it appears that many treatments for children and adolescents are not developmentally oriented (with most of them being downward or upward extensions of treatments for individuals of ages other than the target population), there is great potential for the integration of developmental research with clinical practice. In this chapter, we reviewed a framework for understanding adolescent development that illustrates the major developmental tasks of the adolescent period, and we discussed several developmental factors that are relevant to therapeutic interventions with adolescents. Knowledge of normative development and knowledge of psychological disorders can aid the therapist in formulating appropriate treatment goals, in providing a basis for designing alternative versions of the same treatment, and in guiding the stages of treatment. We have provided a number of recommendations for clinicians who wish to integrate developmental principles into their work. Although we argued that the quality of treatment is likely to be enhanced if therapists attend to developmental issues, this argument is mostly speculation as this point (Weisz, 1997). We hope that this chapter will serve as a "call" for more research on ways that "development" can influence treatment effectiveness.

ACKNOWLEDGMENTS

Completion of this chapter was supported in part by research grants from the March of Dimes Birth Defects Foundation (No. 12-FY01-98) and grants from the National Institutes of Health (Nos. R01-MH50423 and N01-HD-4-3363).

REFERENCES

Aber, J. L., Jones, S. M., Brown, J. L., Chaudry, N., & Samples, F. (1998). Resolving conflict creatively: Evaluating the developmental effects of a school-based violence prevention program in neighborhood and classroom context. *Development and Psychopathology, 10*, 187–213.

Achenbach, T. M. (1982). *Developmental psychopathology* (2nd ed.). New York: Wiley.

Achenbach, T. M. (1985). *Assessment and taxonomy of child and adolescent psychopathology: Vol. 3. Developmental clinical psychology and psychiatry*. Beverly Hills, CA: Sage.

American Psychological Association. (2002). *Developing adolescents: A reference for professionals*. Washington, DC: Author.

Arbuthnot, J., & Gordon, D. A. (1986). Behavioral and cognitive effects of a moral reasoning development intervention for high-risk behavior disordered adolescents. *Journal of Consulting and Clinical Psychology, 54*, 208–216.

Arnett, J. J. (1999). Adolescent storm and stress, reconsidered. *American Psychologist, 54*, 317–326.

Bandura, A. (1977). *Social learning theory*. Englewood Cliffs, NJ: Prentice Hall.

Barkley, R. A. (1997). *ADHD and the nature of self-control*. New York: Guilford Press.

Baron, R. M., & Kenny, D. A. (1986). The moderator–mediator variable distinction in social psychological research: Conceptual, strategic, and statistical considerations. *Journal of Personality and Social Psychology, 51*, 1173–1182.

Berndt, T. J., & Savin-Williams, R. C. (1993). Peer relations and friendships. In P. H. Tolan & B. J. Cohler (Eds.), *Handbook of clinical research and practice with adolescents* (pp. 203–220). New York: Wiley.

Beyth-Marom, R., Austin, L., Fischhoff, B., Palmgren, C., & Jacobs-Quadrel, M. (1993). Perceived consequences of risky behaviors: Adults and adolescents. *Developmental Psychology, 29*, 549–563.

Biederman, J., Newcorn, J., & Sprich, S. (1991). Comorbidity of attention-deficit hyperactivity disorder with conduct, depressive, anxiety, and other disorders. *American Journal of Psychiatry, 148*, 564–577.

Bobbitt, B. L., & Keating, D. P. A. (1983). A cognitive-developmental perspective for clinical research and practice. In P. C. Kendall (Ed.), *Advances in cognitive behavioral research and therapy* (Vol. 2, pp. 198–241). New York: Academic Press.

Bowers, W. A., Evans, K., & Van Cleve, L. (1996). Treatment of adolescent eating disorders. In M. A. Reinecke, F. M. Dattilio, & A. Freeman (Eds.), *Cognitive therapy with children and adolescents: A casebook for clinical practice*. New York: Guilford Press.

Brooks-Gunn, J., & Reiter, E. O. (1990). The role of pubertal processes. In S. S. Feldman & G. R. Elliott (Eds.), *At the threshold: The developing adolescent* (pp. 16–53). Cambridge, MA: Harvard University Press.

Brown, B. B. (1990). Peer groups and peer cultures. In S. S. Feldman & G. R. Elliott (Eds.), *At the threshold: The developing adolescent* (pp. 171–196). Cambridge, MA: Harvard University Press.

Buchanan, C. L., Eccles, J. E., Flanagan, C., Midgley, C., Feldlaufer, H., & Harold, R. (1990). Parents' and teachers' beliefs about adolescence: Effects of sex and experience. *Journal of Youth and Adolescence, 19*, 363–394.

Buchanan, C. M., Eccles, J. S., & Becker, J. B. (1992). Are adolescents the victims of raging hormones?: Evidence for activational effects of hormones on moods and behavior at adolescence. *Psychological Bulletin, 111*, 62–107.

Chapell, M. S., & Overton, W. F. (1998). Development of logical reasoning in the context of parental style and test anxiety. *Merrill-Palmer Quarterly, 44*, 141–156.

Cicchetti, D., & Rogosch, F. A. (2002). A developmental psychopathology perspective on adolescence. *Journal of Consulting and Clinical Psychology, 70*, 6–20.

Cicchetti, D., & Toth, S. L. (Eds.). (1996). *Adolescence: Opportunities and challenges*. Rochester, NY: University of Rochester Press.

Cole, P. M., Martin, S. E., & Dennis, T. A. (2004). Emotion regulation as a scientific construct: Methodological challenges and directions for child development research. *Child Development, 75*, 317–333.

Collins, W. A. (1990). Parent–child relationships in the transition to adolescence. Continuity and change in interaction, affect, and cognition. In R. Montemayor, G. Adams, & T. Gullotta (Eds.), *Advances in adolescent development: From childhood to adolescence: A transitional period?* (Vol. 2, pp. 85–106). Beverly Hills, CA: Sage.

Collins, W. A., & Laursen, B. (1992). Conflict and relationships during adolescence. In C. U.

Shantz & W. W. Hartup (Eds.), *Conflict in child and adolescent development* (pp. 216–241). New York: Cambridge University Press.

Collins, W. A., Maccoby, E. E., Steinberg, L., Hetherington, E. M., & Bornstein, M. H. (2000). Contemporary research on parenting: The case for nature and nurture. *American Psychologist, 55,* 218–232.

Cooper, C. R. (1988). Commentary: The role of conflict in adolescent–parent relationships. In M. R. Gunnar & W. A. Collins (Eds.), *21st Minnesota Symposium on Child Psychology* (pp. 181–187). Hillsdale, NJ: Erlbaum.

Dishion, T., McCord, J., & Poulin, F. (1999). When interventions harm: Peer groups and problem behavior. *American Psychologist, 54,* 755–764.

Dodge, K. A., & Coie, J. D. (1987). Social information-processing factors in reactive and proactive aggression in children's peer groups. *Journal of Personality and Social Psychology, 53,* 1146–1158.

Dodge, K. A., & Pettit, G. S. (2003). A biopsychosocial model of the development of chronic conduct problems in adolescence. *Developmental Psychology, 39,* 349–371.

Downey, J. (1995). Psychological counseling of children and young people. In R. Woolge & W. Dryden (Eds.), *The handbook of counseling psychology* (pp. 308–333). Thousand Oaks, CA: Sage.

Durlak, J. A., Fuhrman, T., & Lampman, C. (1991). Effectiveness of cognitive-behavior therapy for maladapting children: A meta-analysis. *Psychological Bulletin, 110,* 204–214.

Eccles, J. S., Midgley, C., Wigfield, A., Buchanan, C. M., Reuman, D., Flanagan, C., & MacIver, D. (1993). Development during adolescence: The impact of stage-environment fit in young adolescents' experiences in schools and in families. *American Psychologist, 48,* 90–101.

Eddy, J. M., & Chamberlain, P. (2000). Family management and deviant peer association as mediators of the impact of treatment condition on youth antisocial behavior. *Journal of Consulting and Clinical Psychology, 68,* 857–863.

Entwisle, D. R. (1990). Schools and the adolescent. In S. S. Feldman & G. R. Elliott (Eds.), *At the threshold: The developing adolescent* (pp. 197–224). Cambridge, MA: Harvard University Press.

Erikson, E. (1968). *Identity: Youth and crisis.* New York: Norton.

Eyberg, S., Schuhmann, E., & Rey, J. (1998). Psychosocial treatment research with children and adolescents: Developmental issues. *Journal of Abnormal Child Psychology, 26,* 71–81.

Farrell, A. D., Danish, S. J., & Howard, C. W. (1992). Relationship between drug use and other problem behaviors in urban adolescents. *Journal of Consulting and Clinical Psychology, 60,* 705–712.

Feindler, E. L., & Ecton, R. B. (1986). *Adolescent anger control: Cognitive-behavioral techniques.* New York: Pergamon.

Feldman, R. S. (2001). *Child development* (2nd ed.). Upper Saddle River, NJ: Prentice-Hall.

Feldman, S. S., & Elliott, G. R. (Eds.). (1990). *At the threshold: The developing adolescent.* Cambridge, MA: Harvard University Press.

Flavell, J. H. (1968). *The development of role-taking and communication skills in children.* New York: Wiley.

Ford, M. E., Wentzel, K. R., Wood, D., Stevens, E., & Siesfeld, G. A. (1989). Processes associated with integrative social competence: Emotional and contextual influences on adolescent social responsibility. *Journal of Adolescent Research, 4,* 405–425.

Forehand, R., & Wierson, M. (1993). The role of developmental factors in planning behavioral interventions for children: Disruptive behavior as an example. *Behavior Therapy, 24,* 117–141.

Forgatch, M. S., & DeGarmo, D. S. (1999). Parenting through change: An effective prevention program for single mothers. *Journal of Consulting and Clinical Psychology, 67,* 711–724.

Freud, A. (1958). Adolescence. *Psychoanalytic Study of the Child, 13,* 231–258.

Fuhrman, T., & Holmbeck, G. N. (1995). A contextual-moderator analysis of emotional autonomy and adjustment in adolescence. *Child Development, 66,* 793–811.

Fuligni, A. J., & Eccles, J. S. (1993). Perceived parent–child relationships and early adolescents' orientation toward peers. *Developmental Psychology, 29,* 622–632.

Galambos, N. L., Almeida, D. M., & Petersen, A. C. (1990). Masculinity, femininity, and sex role attitudes in early adolescence: Exploring gender intensification. *Child Development, 61,* 1905–1914.

Gilligan, C., Lyons, N. P., & Hanmer, T. J. (Eds.). (1990). *Making connections: The relational worlds of adolescent girls at Emma Willard School.* Cambridge, MA: Harvard University Press.

Greenberger, E., & Steinberg, L. (1986). *When teenagers work: The psychological and social costs of adolescent employment.* New York: Basic Books.

Grotevant, H. D. (1997). Adolescent development in family contexts. In W. Damon (Ed.), *Handbook of child psychology* (Vol. 3, pp. 1097–1149). New York: Wiley.

Guerra, N. G. (1993). Cognitive development. In P. H. Tolan & B. J. Cohler (Eds.), *Handbook of clinical research and practice with adolescents* (pp. 45–62). New York: Wiley.

Guerra, N. G., & Slaby, R. G. (1990). Cognitive mediators of aggression in adolescent offenders: II. Intervention. *Developmental Psychology, 26,* 269–277.

Harrington, R., Wood, A., & Verduyn, C. (1998). Clinically depressed adolescents. In P. Graham (Ed.), *Cognitive-behaviour therapy for children and families* (pp. 156–193). Cambridge, UK: Cambridge University Press.

Harter, S. (1990). Self and identity development. In S. S. Feldman & G. R. Elliott (Eds.), *At the threshold: The developing adolescent* (pp. 352–387). Cambridge, MA: Harvard University Press.

Henderson, V. L., & Dweck, C. S. (1990). Motivation and achievement. In S. S. Feldman & G. R. Elliott (Eds.), *At the threshold: The developing adolescent* (pp. 308–329). Cambridge, MA: Harvard University Press.

Henggeler, S. W., & Cohen, R. (1984). The role of cognitive development in the family–ecological systems approach to childhood psychopathology. In B. Gholson & T. L. Rosenthal (Eds.), *Applications of cognitive-developmental theory* (pp. 173–189). New York: Academic Press.

Henggeler, S. W., Schoenwald, S. K., Borduin, C. M., Rowland, M. D., & Cunningham, P. B. (1998). *Multisystemic treatment of antisocial behavior in children and adolescents.* New York: Guilford Press.

Hill, J. P. (1980). *Understanding early adolescence: A framework.* Carrboro, NC: Center for Early Adolescence.

Hill, J. P., & Holmbeck, G. N. (1986). Attachment and autonomy during adolescence. In G. J. Whitehurst (Ed.), *Annals of child development* (Vol. 3, pp. 145–189). Greenwich, CT: JAI Press.

Holmbeck, G. N. (1994). Adolescence. In V. S. Ramachandran (Ed.), *Encyclopedia of human behavior* (Vol.1, pp. 17–28). Orlando, FL: Academic Press.

Holmbeck, G. N. (1996). A model of family relational transformations during the transition to adolescence: Parent–adolescent conflict and adaptation. In J. A. Graber, J. Brooks-Gunn, & A. C. Petersen (Eds.), *Transitions through adolescence: Interpersonal domains and context* (pp. 167–199). Mahwah, NJ: Erlbaum.

Holmbeck, G. N. (1997). Toward terminological, conceptual, and statistical clarity in the study of mediators and moderators: Examples from the child-clinical and pediatric psychology literatures. *Journal of Consulting and Clinical Psychology, 65,* 599–610.

Holmbeck, G. N., Colder, C., Shapera, W., Westhoven, V., Kenealy, L., & Updegrove, A. (2000). Working with adolescents: Guides from developmental psychology. In P. C. Kendall (Ed.), *Child and adolescent therapy: Cognitive-behavioral procedures* (2nd ed., pp. 334–385). New York: Guilford Press.

Holmbeck, G. N., Friedman, D., Abad, M., & Jandasek, B. (2006). Development and psychopathology in adolescence. In D. A. Wolfe & E. J. Mash (Eds.), *Behavioral and emotional disorders in adolescents: Nature, assessment, and treatment* (pp. 21–55). New York: Guilford Press.

Holmbeck, G. N., Greenley, R. N., & Franks, E. A. (2003). Developmental issues and considerations in research and practice. In A. E. Kazdin & J. R. Weisz (Eds.), *Evidence-based psychotherapies for children and adolescents* (pp. 21–41). New York: Guilford Press.

Holmbeck, G. N., & Hill, J. P. (1988). Storm and stress beliefs about adolescence: Prevalence, self-reported antecedents, and effects of an undergraduate course. *Journal of Youth and Adolescence, 17*, 285–306.

Holmbeck, G. N., & Hill, J. P. (1991). Conflictive engagement, positive affect, and menarche in families with seventh-grade girls. *Child Development, 62*, 1030–1048.

Holmbeck, G. N., & Kendall, P. C. (1991). Clinical–childhood–developmental interface: Implications for treatment. In P. R. Martin (Ed.), *Handbook of behavior therapy and psychological science: An integrative approach* (pp. 73–99). New York: Pergamon.

Holmbeck, G. N., & Kendall, P. C. (2002). Introduction to the special section on clinical adolescent psychology: Developmental psychopathology and treatment. *Journal of Consulting and Clinical Psychology, 70*, 3–5.

Holmbeck, G. N., & O'Donnell, K. (1991). Discrepancies between perceptions of decision-making and behavioral autonomy. In R. L. Paikoff (Ed.), *Shared views in the family during adolescence: New directions for development* (No. 51, pp. 51–69). San Francisco: Jossey-Bass.

Holmbeck, G. N., Paikoff, R. L., & Brooks-Gunn, J. (1995). Parenting adolescents. In M. Bornstein (Ed.), *Handbook of parenting* (Vol. 1, pp. 91–118). Mahwah, NJ: Erlbaum.

Holmbeck, G. N., & Shapera, W. F. A. (1999). Research methods with adolescents. In P. C. Kendall, J. N. Butcher, & G. N. Holmbeck (Eds.), *Handbook of research methods in clinical psychology* (2nd ed., pp. 634–661). New York: Wiley.

Holmbeck, G. N., & Updegrove, A. L. (1995). Clinical-developmental interface: Implications of developmental research for adolescent psychotherapy. *Psychotherapy, 32*, 16–33.

Huey, S. J., Henggeler, S. W., Brondino, M. J., & Pickrel, S. G. (2000). Mechanisms of change in multisystemic therapy: Reducing delinquent behavior through therapist adherence and improved family and peer functioning. *Journal of Consulting and Clinical Psychology, 68*, 451–467.

Jessor, R., & Jessor, S. L. (1977). *Problem behavior and psychosocial development: A longitudinal study of youth.* New York: Academic Press.

Jessor, R., Donovan, J. E., & Costa, F. M. (1991). *Beyond adolescence: Problem behavior and young adult development.* New York: Cambridge University Press.

Kaminer, Y., Burleson, J. A., & Goldberger, R. (2002). Cognitive-behavioral coping skills and psychoeducation therapies for adolescent substance abuse. *Journal of Nervous and Mental Disease, 190*, 737–745.

Katchadourian, H. (1990). Sexuality. In S. S. Feldman & G. R. Elliott (Eds.), *At the threshold: The developing adolescent* (pp. 330–351). Cambridge, MA: Harvard University Press.

Kazdin, A. E. (1997). A model for developing effective treatments: Progression and interplay of theory, research, and practice. *Journal of Clinical Child Psychology, 26*, 114–129.

Kazdin, A. E., & Weisz, J. R. (1998). Identifying and developing empirically supported child and adolescent treatments. *Journal of Consulting and Clinical Psychology, 66*, 19–36.

Keating, D. P. (1990). Adolescent thinking. In S. S. Feldman & G. R. Elliott (Eds.), *At the threshold: The developing adolescent* (pp. 54–89). Cambridge, MA: Harvard University Press.

Kendall, P. C. (1984). Social cognition and problem solving: A developmental and child-clinical interface. In B. Gholson & T. L. Rosenthal (Eds.), *Applications of cognitive-developmental theory* (pp. 115–148). New York: Academic Press.

Kendall, P. C. (1993). Cognitive-behavioral therapies with youth: Guiding theory, current status, and emerging developments. *Journal of Consulting and Clinical Psychology, 61*, 235–247.

Kendall, P. C., & Braswell, L. (1985). *Cognitive-behavioral therapy for impulsive children.* New York: Guilford Press.

Kendall, P. C., Choudhury, M., Hudson, J., & Webb, A. (2002a). *The C.A.T. project therapist manual.* Ardmore, PA: Workbook Publishing.

Kendall, P. C., Choudhury, M., Hudson, J., & Webb, A. (2002b). *The C.A.T. project workbook for the cognitive-behavioral treatment of anxious adolescents.* Ardmore, PA: Workbook Publishing.

Kendall, P. C., & Holmbeck, G. N. (1991). Psychotherapeutic interventions for adolescents. In R. M. Lerner, A. C. Petersen, & J. Brooks-Gunn (Eds.), *Encyclopedia of adolescence* (pp. 866–874). New York: Pergamon.

Kendall, P. C., Lerner, R. M., & Craighead, W. E. (1984). Human development and intervention in childhood psychopathology. *Child Development, 55*, 71–82.

Kendall, P. C., & MacDonald, J. P. (1993). Cognition in the psychopathology of youth and implications for treatment. In K. S. Dobson & P. C. Kendall (Eds.), *Psychopathology and cognition.* San Diego, CA: Academic Press.

Kendall, P. C., & Williams, C. L. (1986). Therapy with adolescents: Treating the "Marginal Man." *Behavior Therapy, 17*, 522–537.

Kraemer, H. C., Stice, E., Kazdin, A., Offord, D., & Kupfer, D. (2001). How do risk factors work together? Mediators, moderators, and independent, overlapping, and proxy risk factors. *American Journal of Psychiatry, 158*, 848–856.

La Greca, A. M., & Prinstein, M. J. (1999). Peer group. In W. K. Silverman & T. H. Ollendick (Eds.), *Developmental issues in the clinical treatment of children* (pp. 171–198). Boston: Allyn & Bacon.

Larson, R. W., Richards, M. H., Moneta, G., Holmbeck, G., & Duckett, E. (1996). Changes in adolescents' daily interactions with their families from ages 10 to 18: Disengagement and transformation. *Developmental Psychology, 32*, 744–754.

Laursen, B., Coy, K. C., & Collins, W. A. (1998). Reconsidering changes in parent–child conflict across adolescence: A meta-analysis. *Child Development, 69*, 817–832.

Lerner, R. M., Villarruel, F. A., & Castellino, D. R. (1999). Adolescence. In W. K. Silverman & T. H. Ollendick (Eds.), *Developmental issues in the clinical treatment of children* (pp. 125–136). Boston: Allyn & Bacon.

Lewko, J. H. (Ed.). (1987). *How children and adolescents view the world of work* (New Directions for Child Development, No. 35). San Francisco: Jossey-Bass.

Loeber, R., Farrington, D. P., Stouthamer-Loeber, M., & Van Kammen, W. B. (1998). *Antisocial behavior and mental health problems: Explanatory factors in childhood and adolescence.* Mahwah, NJ: Erlbaum.

Lynam, D. R. (1996). Early identification of chronic offenders: Who is the fledgling psychopath? *Psychological Bulletin, 120*, 209–234.

March, J. S., & Mulle, K. (1998). *OCD in children and adolescents: A cognitive-behavioral treatment manual.* New York: Guilford Press.

Martinez, C. R., & Forgatch, M. S. (2001). Preventing problems with boys' noncompliance: Effects of a parent training intervention for divorcing mothers. *Journal of Consulting and Clinical Psychology, 69*, 416–428.

McBride, C. K., Paikoff, R. L., & Holmbeck, G. N. (2003). Individual and familial influences on the onset of sexual intercourse among urban African American adolescents. *Journal of Consulting and Clinical Psychology, 71*, 159–167.

Meichenbaum, D., & Cameron, R. (1982). Cognitive behavior modification: Current issues. In G. T. Wilson & C. M. Franks (Eds.), *Contemporary behavior therapy: Conceptual and empirical foundations* (pp. 310–338). New York: Guilford Press.

Mezzacappa, E., Kindlon, D., & Earls, F. (1999). Relations of age to cognitive and motivational elements of impulse control in boys with and without externalizing behavior problems. *Journal of Abnormal Child Psychology, 27*, 473–483.

Minuchin, P. P., & Shapiro, E. K. (1983). The school as a context for social development. In P. H. Mussen (Series Ed.) & E. M. Hetherington (Vol. Ed.), *Handbook of child psychology* (Vol. IV, pp. 197–274). New York: Wiley.

Moffitt, T. E. (1993). Adolescence-limited and life-course persistent anti-social behavior: A developmental taxonomy. *Psychological Review, 100*, 674–701.

Montemayor, R. (1983). Parents and adolescents in conflict: All families some of the time and some families most of the time. *Journal of Early Adolescence, 3*, 83–103.

Moshman, D. (1998). Cognitive development beyond childhood. In D. Kuhn & R. S. Siegler (Eds.), *Handbook of child psychology: Vol. 2. Cognition, perception, and language* (pp. 957–978). New York: Wiley.

Nelson, D. A., & Crick, N. R. (1999). Rose-colored glasses: Examining the social information-processing of prosocial young adolescents. *Journal of Early Adolescence, 19*, 17–38.

Nolen-Hoeksema, S. (1994). An interactive model for the emergence of gender differences in depression in adolescence. *Journal of Research on Adolescence, 4*, 519–534.

Olin, S. (2001). Blueprint for change: Research on child and adolescent mental health. *The Child, Youth, and Family Services Advocate, 24*, 1–5.

Ollendick, T. H., Grills, A. E., & King, N. J. (2001). Applying developmental theory to the assessment and treatment of childhood disorders: Does it make a difference? *Child Psychology and Psychotherapy, 8*, 304–314.

Paikoff, R. L., & Brooks-Gunn, J. (1991). Do parent–child relationships change during puberty? *Psychological Bulletin, 110*, 47–66.

Parker, J. G., & Asher, S. R. (1987). Peer relations and later personal adjustment: Are low-accepted children at risk? *Psychological Bulletin, 102*, 357–389.

Petersen, A. C., & Hamburg, B. A. (1986). Adolescence: A developmental approach to problems and psychopathology. *Behavior Therapy, 17*, 480–499.

Piacentini, J., & Bergman, R. L. (2001). Developmental issues in cognitive therapy for childhood anxiety disorders. *Journal of Cognitive Psychotherapy, 15*, 165–182.

Piaget, J. (1970). Piaget's theory. In P. H. Mussen (Ed.), *Manual of child psychology* (3rd ed., pp. 703–732). New York: Wiley.

Public Agenda. (1999). *Kids these days '99: What Americans really think about the next generation.* New York: Author.

Reich, W., Shayka, J. J., & Taibleson, C. (1991). *Diagnostic interview for children and adolescents (DICA-R-A; Adolescent version).* Unpublished interview, Washington University.

Reid, J. B. (1993). Prevention of conduct disorder before and after school entry: Relating interventions to developmental findings. *Development and Psychopathology, 5*, 243–262.

Richards, M., Abell, S. N., & Petersen, A. C. (1993). Biological development. In P. H. Tolan & B. J. Cohler (Eds.), *Handbook of clinical research and practice with adolescents* (pp. 21–44). New York: Wiley.

Richards, M., & Petersen, A. C. (1987). Biological theoretical models of adolescent development. In V. B. Van Hasselt & M. Hersen (Eds.), *Handbook of adolescent psychology* (pp. 34–52). New York: Pergamon.

Rohde, P., Jorgensen, J. S., Seeley, J. R., & Mace, D. E. (2004). Pilot evaluation of the coping course: A cognitive-behavioral intervention to enhance coping skills in incarcerated youth. *Journal of the American Academy of Child and Adolescent Psychiatry, 43*, 669–676.

Rolf, J., Masten, A. S., Cicchetti, D., Nuechterlein, K. H., & Weintraub, S. (1990). *Risk and protective factors in the development of psychopathology.* New York: Cambridge University Press.

Rose, S. D. (1998). *Group therapy with troubled youth: Cognitive behavioral interactive approach.* Thousand Oaks, CA: Sage.

Rosenthal, T. L. (1982). Social learning theory and behavior therapy. In G. T. Wilson & C. M. Franks (Eds.), *Contemporary behavior therapy: Conceptual and empirical foundations* (pp. 339–366). New York: Guilford Press.

Ruble, D. N., & Brooks-Gunn, J. (1982). The experience of menarche. *Child Development, 53*, 1557–1566.

Rutter, M. (1980). *Changing youth in a changing society: Patterns of adolescent development and disorder.* Cambridge, MA: Harvard University Press.

Rutter, M. (1990). Psychosocial resilience and protective mechanisms. In J. Rolf, A. S. Masten, D. Cicchetti, D., K. H. Nuechterlein, & S. Weintraub (Eds.), *Risk and protective factors in the development of psychopathology* (pp. 181–214). New York: Cambridge University Press.

Rutter, M., & Garmezy, N. (1983). Developmental psychopathology. In P. H. Mussen (Series Ed.) & E. M. Hetherington (Vol. Ed.), *Handbook of child psychology* (Vol. IV, pp. 775–912). New York: Wiley.

Savin-Williams, R. C., & Berndt, T. J. (1990). Friendship and peer relations. In S. S. Feldman & G. R. Elliott (Eds.), *At the threshold: The developing adolescent* (pp. 277–307). Cambridge, MA: Harvard University Press.

Schleser, R., Cohen, R., Meyers, A., & Rodick, J. D. (1984). The effects of cognitive level and training procedures on the generalization of self-instructions. *Cognitive Therapy and Research, 8*, 187–200.

Selman, R. L. (1980). *The growth of interpersonal understanding: Developmental and clinical analyses.* New York: Academic Press.

Selman, R. L. (1981). The child as a friendship philosopher. In S. R. Asher & J. M. Gottman (Eds.), *The development of children's friendships* (pp. 242–272). New York: Cambridge University Press.

Shirk, S. R. (Ed.). (1988). *Cognitive development and child psychotherapy.* New York: Plenum Press.

Shirk, S. R. (1999). Developmental therapy. In W. K. Silverman & T. H. Ollendick (Eds.), *Developmental issues in the clinical treatment of children* (pp. 60–73). Boston: Allyn & Bacon.

Shirk, S. R. (2001). Development and cognitive therapy. *Journal of Cognitive Psychotherapy, 15*, 155–163.

Shirk, S., Talmi, A., & Olds, D. (2000). A developmental psychopathology perspective on child and adolescent treatment policy. *Development and Psychopathology, 12*, 835–855.

Siegel, A. W., & Scoville, L. C. (2000). Problem behavior: The double symptom of adolescence. *Development and Psychopathology, 12*, 763–793.

Silverman, W. K., & Ollendick, T. H. (Eds.). (1999). *Developmental issues in the clinical treatment of children.* Boston: Allyn & Bacon.

Simmons, R. G., & Blyth, D. A. (1987). *Moving into adolescence: The impact of pubertal change and school context.* New York: Aldine de Gruyter.

Steinberg, L. (1990). Autonomy, conflict, and harmony in the family relationship. In S. S. Feldman & G. L. Elliott (Eds.), *At the threshold: The developing adolescent* (pp. 255–276). Cambridge, MA: Harvard University Press.

Steinberg, L. (2005). *Adolescence* (7th ed.). Boston: McGraw-Hill.

Steinberg, L., & Silverberg, S. (1986). The vicissitudes of autonomy in early adolescence. *Child Development, 57*, 841–851.

Sullivan, H. S. (1953). *The interpersonal theory of psychiatry.* New York: Norton.

Tanner, J. (1962). *Growth at adolescence* (2nd ed.). Springfield, IL: Thomas.

Temple, S. (1997). *Brief therapy for adolescent depression.* Sarasota, FL: Professional Resource Press.

Tolan, P. H., & Cohler, B. J. (1993). *Handbook of clinical research and practice with adolescents.* New York: Wiley.

Treadwell, K. R. H., & Kendall, P. C. (1996). Self-talk in youth with anxiety disorders: States of mind, content specificity, and treatment outcome. *Journal of Consulting and Clinical Psychology, 64*, 941–950.

Trickett, E. J., & Schmid, J. D. (1993). The school as a social context. In P. H. Tolan & B. J. Cohler (Eds.), *Handbook of clinical research and practice with adolescents* (pp. 173–202). New York: Wiley.

Van Hasselt, V. B., & Hersen, M. (Eds.). (1995). *Handbook of adolescent psychopathology.* New York: Lexington Books.

Vygotsky, L. (1978). *Mind in society: The development of higher psychological processes.* Cambridge, MA: Harvard University Press.

Walsh, F., & Scheinkman, M. (1993). The family context of adolescence. In P. H. Tolan & B. J. Cohler (Eds), *Handbook of clinical research and practice with adolescents* (pp. 149–172). New York: Wiley.

Wasserman, T. H. (1984). The effects of cognitive development on the use of cognitive behavioral techniques with children. *Child and Family Behavior Therapy, 5*, 37–50.

Wechsler, D. (2003). *Wechsler Intelligence Scale for Children: Fourth Edition.* San Antonio, TX: Psychological Corporation.

Weersing, V. R., & Weisz, J. R. (2002). Mechanisms of action in youth psychotherapy. *Journal of Child Psychology and Psychiatry, 43*, 3–29.

Weiner, I. B. (1992). *Psychological disturbance in adolescence.* New York: Wiley.

Weisz, J. R. (1997). Effects of interventions for child and adolescent psychological dysfunction: Relevance of context, developmental factors, and individual differences. In S. S. Luthar, J. A. Burack, D. Cicchetti, & J. R. Weisz (Eds.), *Developmental psychopathology: Perspectives on adjustment, risk, and disorder.* (pp. 3–22). Cambridge, UK: Cambridge University Press.

Weisz, J. R., & Hawley, K. M. (2002). Developmental factors in the treatment of adolescents. *Journal of Consulting and Clinical Psychology, 70*, 21–43.

Weisz, J. R., Rudolph, K. D., Granger, D. A., & Sweeney, L. (1992). Cognition, competence, and coping in child and adolescent depression: Research findings, developmental concerns, therapeutic implications. *Development and Psychopathology, 4*, 627–653.

Weisz, J. R., & Weersing, V. R. (1999). Developmental outcome research. In W. K. Silverman & T. H. Ollendick (Eds.), *Developmental issues in the clinical treatment of children* (pp. 457–469). Boston: Allyn & Bacon.

Wolfe, D. A., & Mash, E. J. (Eds.). (2006). *Behavioral and emotional disorders in adolescents: Nature, assessment, and treatment.* New York: Guilford Press.

CHAPTER 13

Process Issues in Cognitive-Behavioral Therapy for Youth

STEPHEN SHIRK and MARC KARVER

Some years ago, the therapy process was described as "everything that can be observed to occur between and within the patient and therapist during their work together" (Orlinsky & Howard, 1986, pp. 311–312). This broad domain of inquiry has received substantial attention in the adult psychotherapy literature, but as Kazdin (1995) has noted, process research is "perhaps the area of work that is most discrepant between child and adult therapy" (p. 268). Recent reviews have revealed little change (Kazdin & Nock, 2003; Weersing & Weisz, 2002). Not only is process research sparse in the child literature, but also much of the published research fails to link treatment *processes* with treatment *outcomes*— or, when such linkages are made, they frequently are within treatments of no known efficacy (Shirk & Russell, 1998). If the central goal of process research is to clarify *how* a therapy works, then it is critical to know, first, *if* the therapy works. This perspective is consistent with the view that process research *follows* outcome research, and that the aim of process research is to understand why and how efficacious treatments work (Kazdin & Kendall, 1998; Kendall & Choudhury, 2003). Process research, then, should be in the service of improving treatment outcomes.

In process research, the core question shifts from "Which treatment works for what disorder?" to "How do treatment processes change pathogenic mechanisms that result in improved outcomes?" (Shirk & Russell, 1996). Implicit in this view are two interrelated sets of processes; the first involves specific treatment processes or procedures, and the second involves specific treatment targets, namely, the postulated pathogenic mechanisms that account for the development, maintenance, or desistance of the disorder. Growing interest in *mediators* of outcome in youth treatment (e.g., Weersing & Weisz, 2002) has focused on the latter set of processes, that is, on the pathogenic mechanisms contributing to the disorder. Insofar as child treatments, including cognitive-behavioral therapy (CBT), do not solely target manifest symptoms of a disorder, but rather address mechanisms assumed to contribute to symptoms, the association between treatment and outcome is presumably mediated by changes in pathogenic processes. For example, in the treatment of depression, CBT typically addresses information-processing biases and cognitive distortions, as well as skills deficits, in emotion regulation and interpersonal relations. Changes in these treatment targets are hypothesized to result in corresponding changes in symptoms of the disorder, such as sad mood and low self-esteem, as depicted in Figure 13.1.

Certainly, identifying and measuring change in pathogenic processes is a critical component of understanding how treatments work, but it is only half of the equation. Missing from the figure are the corresponding therapeutic processes that account for change in the pathogenic mechanisms. Virtually all "stand-alone" treatments are composed of multiple therapeutic procedures (Shirk, 1999). Consequently, from a process perspective it is not sufficient to relate whole treatments to outcomes through pathogenic mechanisms. Instead, analyses are based on increased specificity of both therapeutic processes and pathogenic mechanisms. The unit of analysis shifts from "brand-name" therapies, or treatment packages, to specific treatment procedures, and from diagnostic entities to pathogenic mechanisms (Shirk & Russell, 1996). Understanding *how* therapy works ultimately involves establishing linkages between the delivery of specific treatment procedures such as relaxation training and changes in mechanisms such

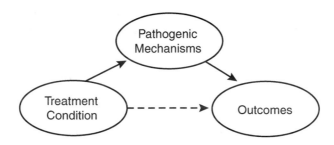

FIGURE 13.1. Mediation of treatment outcomes.

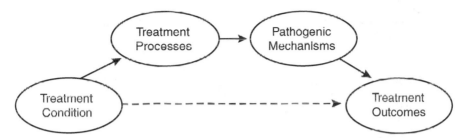

FIGURE 13.2. Treatment process mediation model.

as physiological reactivity (though pathogenic processes do not have to be defined biologically). Further, this set of associations should be embedded in the mediation model linking treatment status to outcomes, as depicted in Figure 13.2.

Although it is recognized that both sets of mediators are critical for understanding how therapy works, and that the two processes are closely linked, because of their relative neglect this chapter will focus on postulated change processes, that is, the therapeutic procedures that contribute to outcomes in CBT. The aim is to move the field toward the identification of active ingredients in CBT for different youth disorders. As Kazdin and Nock (2003) observed, the study of change mechanisms is "probably the best short-term and long-term investment for improving clinical practice and patient care" (p. 1117). Identification of mechanisms of therapeutic action will allow us to distill and refine our treatments, to increase the emphasis on active ingredients, and to pare unnecessary procedures from our protocols. Thus, process research could enhance efficacy and facilitate the transport of treatments to real-world settings.

RESEARCH ON CHANGE PROCESSES IN YOUTH CBT

Despite a substantial and growing body of evidence for the efficacy of CBT for many youth disorders, remarkably little research has addressed the mechanisms of therapeutic action. In their review of mediators of outcome in empirically supported treatments for youth, Weersing and Weisz (2002) found that over half of the studies, roughly 67, included potential mediators, but that only a half-dozen actually attempted formal mediation tests. Further, most of the studies that conducted mediation analyses measured the mediator and outcome at the same time point, thus making interpretation of direction of effect ambiguous (Kazdin & Nock, 2003). Of equal importance, none of the candidate mediators involved specific treatment processes or procedures. Instead, it appears that what little research is available has focused solely on pathogenic mechanisms, and in many cases has not done it very well. How, then, are we to understand the lack of evidence on treatment processes?

Multicomponent Treatments

As the chapters in this volume illustrate, virtually all CBT treatments for youth involve multiple components and procedures. For example, Kendall, Kane, Howard, and Sequeline's (1990) CBT intervention for childhood anxiety disorders, Coping Cat, involves a core set of components including emotion identification and self-monitoring, relaxation training, cognitive restructuring, coping skills training, and exposure. Although it is evident that this package yields significant treatment effects (Kendall, 1994; Kendall et al., 1997), it is not clear if all components contribute to outcome, or if some components primarily serve the function of preparing the child for participation in other active components of treatment. As this example implies, a treatment component may be active, inert, or an indirect contributor to outcome. In the case of Coping Cat, active participation in demanding exposure activities may depend on acquisition of basic cognitive and relaxation skills, as well as the development of a strong alliance with the therapist. If this is the case, then initial cognitive interventions may indirectly affect outcome by facilitating involvement in exposure. Alternatively, both components might independently contribute to outcome such that behavioral components reduce arousal while cognitive components modify maladaptive schema, and both may have an incremental effect on symptom change. For the most part, these types of issues have yet to be addressed in CBT treatments for virtually all child and adolescent disorders.

Even for the same disorder, treatments grouped under the umbrella of CBT typically involve a package of treatment techniques offered in alternative sequences and permutations (Durlak, Fuhrman, & Lampman, 1991). For example, in their review treatments for adolescent depression, Lewinsohn and Clarke (1999) showed that CBT treatment packages exhibit a strong *family resemblance*, but that no two treatment packages are identical twins. For example, most packages include cognitive restructuring and social problem-solving training, but vary in terms of emphasis, sequence, and therapeutic approach, e.g., how the treatment component is actually presented to adolescents. Conversely, not all CBT treatment packages for depression include relaxation training despite sharing most other treatment components. In essence, what gets dubbed the "same" treatment may differ along many important dimensions. The fact that CBT treatment packages with somewhat different components produce beneficial effects raises the important question of which components are essential and which are not. Furthermore, given variation across treatment manuals in how specific treatment components are presented (e.g., there can be substantial variation in how problem-solving training is presented in various CBT packages for depression), it is unclear whether these variations are equally effective or whether some are more engaging than others. To complicate matters further, it is possible that some variations will work better for some therapists or for some patients. The current literature recognizes the need for greater specificity but in some instances provides clinicians with few guidelines on such matters.

Design Issues

A second, but equally important, factor contributing to the dearth of evidence on how treatments work is the prevailing research design for outcome studies. The randomized controlled trial with pre- and postassessments has been the primary method for establishing a causal relation between treatment and change in outcomes. From the perspective of understanding treatment process, this design is not optimal, principally because assessments conducted prior to and following treatment provide limited access to processes presumed to occur during the course of treatment. In fairness, the first wave of child intervention research was directed toward a different question, and the randomized controlled trial with pre- and postassessment is well suited for identifying overall treatment effects. But an understanding of process necessitates assessment over the course of treatment and moving beyond the evaluation of whole therapies. To be sure, the randomized controlled trial is compatible with process research and provides the best framework for ensuring that associations between specific treatment procedures and changes in outcomes are truly a function of treatment. But for a trial to shed light on how treatment produces change, components of treatment must be isolated and compared across conditions, or the degree to which specific therapy procedures are utilized must be assessed over the course of therapy. Furthermore, such assessments of treatment procedures and their use need to precede assessments of change in pathogenic mechanism (mediator) and treatment outcomes. Two approaches to evaluating treatment processes, components analysis and process-outcome designs, provide a window on how treatments work.

Component Analysis Studies

Component analysis designs are experimental designs that isolate some of the specific ingredients in a therapeutic approach and provide information on which of these ingredients/components contributes to therapeutic outcomes. Two alternative designs have been used in component analysis studies, with each design providing a window on how treatments work (Ahn & Wampold, 2001). The first is the additive design, in which a treatment component is added onto an existing treatment approach. This type is the most common. The second design that has been used much less frequently but tells us more about existing treatments is the dismantling design, in which treatment components of an existing treatment are isolated or removed and systematically varied across conditions. The component analysis approaches allow the investigator to differentiate active from inert components, stronger from weaker components, and the relative effect of components on varied outcomes (assuming more than one type of outcome is assessed).

Ahn and Wampold (2001) conducted a meta-analysis of component analysis studies, but, as often happens in the mental health literature, child treatment studies were neglected (only two studies were undertaken). In fact, Chronis, Chacko, Fabiano, Wymbs, and Pelham (2004) identified 16 enhancement studies just with behavioral parent training for ADHD. Our own review of the literature identified over 30 component analysis studies of behavioral approaches for parents and/or their children, and this does not even include studies looking at combined treatments with medication or school intervention.

The CBT literature for youth is not as well advanced as the behavioral literature, despite initial component analysis studies dating back to the early 1980s. However, an increasing number of component analysis studies have appeared in recent years (see Table 13.1). We were able to identify 21 additive studies involving cognitive-behavioral therapy as a primary treatment approach but only 2 dismantling studies. The additive studies tend to have a broad unit of analysis such that the components being studied really represent "stand-alone" treatments being added to one another. Across the additive studies that involve treatments to a wide range of different children (anxious, ADHD, conduct-disordered, oppositional, sexually abused, etc.), there is no clear pattern of what components should or should not be added. In eight studies, cognitive-behavioral treatment was found sufficient to deliver effective treatment to youth. There was no gain found by adding a parent component. On the other hand, there were seven studies in which the combined effects of a youth cognitive-behavioral approach and a parent-focused intervention were additive relative to either component in isolation.

A study by Kazdin, Siegel, and Bass (1992) provides a good example of this. These investigators compared the separate and combined effects of parent management training (PMT) and problem-solving skills training (PSST) for youth ages 7–13 with clinically elevated antisocial behavior. Youngsters and their parents were randomly assigned to receive PMT, PSST, or PSST and PMT. Duration of treatment was comparable across conditions. Briefly, results indicated that both PSST and PMT alone produced significant improvements in overall child dysfunction, prosocial competence, and aggressive antisocial behavior. The combined treatment yielded greater effects on child aggression, antisocial behavior, and delinquency than either PMT or PSST alone. These results indicate that both PMT and PSST actively contribute to outcomes, and that their combination provides an additive effect. In terms of relative efficacy, there was a slight advantage for PSST in improving social competence at school and self-reported aggression and delinquency compared to PMT alone, hardly a basis for prescribing one component over another. With regard to differential impact on sets of outcomes, it was somewhat surprising that PMT alone, a parent-focused inter-

TABLE 13.1. Studies in the Youth CBT Component Analysis Review

Study	Type of treatment	Mean age (yr)	n	Results
Azrin et al. (2001)	Cognitive-behavioral therapy (CBT) Contingency management (CMT)	12–17	56	CBT = CBT + CMT
Baum et al. (1986)	Systematic training for effective parenting (STEP) Child self-control (CSC) Parent discussion and child attention control (PDCA)	6–10	34	STEP + CSC > STEP > PDCA
Barrett et al. (1996, 2001)	CBT Family management (FAM) Waiting-list control (WLC)	8.2–10.1	79	CBT + FAM > CBT > WLC Follow up: CBT + FAM = CBT > WLC
Cobham et al. (1998)	CBT Parent anxiety management (PAM)	9.6	67	CBT + PAM > CBT
Deblinger et al. (1996, 1999)	CBT—child (CBT-C) CBT—parent (CBT-P) Community comparison (treatments as ususal [TAU])	9.9	100	CBT C + CBT-P > CBT-P > CBT-C > TAU
Dishion & Andrews (1995)	Parent family management (PFM) CBT—teen focus Self-directed parent and teen change (SDC) Control (CON)	12.4	158	PFM > CBT = PFM + CBT = SDC = CON
Heyne et al. (2002)	CBT Parent/teacher training (PTT)	11.5	61	CBT = PTT = CBT + PTT
Horn et al. (1987)	Behavioral parent training (BPT) Self-control training (SCT)	9 years, 7 months	24	SCT = BPT = SCT + BPT
Horn et al. (1990)	BPT SCT	8.45–9.18	42	SCT = BPT = SCT + BPT
Jaycox et al. (1994)	Cognitive therapy (CT) Social problem solving (SPS) CON	5th and 6th grades	143	CT + SPS = CT = SPS > CON
Kazdin et al. (1989)	Problem-solving skills training (PSST) In vivo practice (PRA) Client-centered relationship therapy (CCR)	11	112	PRA + PSST = PSST > CCR

(continued)

TABLE 13.1. *(continued)*

Study	Type of treatment	Mean age (yr)	n	Results
Kazdin et al. (1992)	PSST Parent management training (PMT)	10.3	97	PSST + PMT > PSST > PMT
Kendall & Braswell (1982)	CBT Behavioral therapy (BEH) Attention (ATT)	8–12	27	CBT + BEH + ATT > BEH + ATT > ATT
King et al. (2000)	CBT Family CBT (FCBT) WLC	11.4	36	CBT = FCBT > WLC
Lewinsohn et al. (1990)	Coping with Depression Course to adolescents (CWD-A) CWD to parents (CWD-P) WLC	16.15–16.28	69	CWD-A + CWD-P = CWD-A > WLC
Lochman & Curry (1986)	Anger coping program (ACP) Self-instructional training (SIT)	9–11	20	ACP = ACP + SIT
Lochman & Wells (2004)	ACP Parent coping/management program (PCP) TAU in the school	5th or 6th grade	183	ACP + PCP > ACP > TAU
Mendlowitz et al. (1999)	Coping Bear (CBT) Parenting your anxious child (PAC)	9.8	68	CBT + PAC > CBT = PAC
Nauta et al. (2001)	CBT-C CBT-P	10.2	18	CBT-C = CBT-C + CBT-P
Nauta et al. (2003)	CBT-C CBT-P WLC	7–18	79	CBT-C = CBT-C + CBT-P > WLC
Spence et al. (2000)	CBT Parent involvement (PI) WLC	9.9–11	50	CBT + PI = CBT > WLC
Stolberg & Garrison (1985)	CBT Parent skill building (PSB) No-treatment CON	10.7	82	CBT > PSB = CBT + PSB = CON
Stolberg & Mahler (1994)	Child support group (SUP) Skills training (CBT) Transfer procedures with parents (TRA) No-treatment CON	9.8	103	CBT + SUP = CBT + SUP + TRA > SUP = CON

vention, did not produce greater improvements in parenting stress and parental psychopathology than PSST alone, a child-focused intervention. Interestingly, the combined treatment resulted in greater improvements on parental variables than each of the component treatments. Thus, focus of intervention (who was seen) appeared to be less important than magnitude of change in child antisocial behavior for improving parental functioning.

A second study by Kazdin and colleagues (Kazdin, Bass, Siegel, & Thomas, 1989) provides one of the few examples of an additive study in which a treatment component as opposed to a "stand-alone" treatment is added in a component analysis study. These investigators compared the combined effects of PSST and *in vivo* practice (PRA) versus PSST for youth ages 7–13 with clinically elevated antisocial behavior. Youth were randomly assigned to receive PSST and PRA, PSST, or client-centered relationship therapy (CCR) to control for treatment gains due to therapeutic contact. Duration of treatment was comparable across conditions (25 sessions), as the treatment addition was incorporated into the PSST treatment. The results indicated that PSST and PSST plus PRA produced significantly greater improvements in overall behavioral problems, prosocial behavior, and antisocial behavior as compared to CCR. The addition of PRA contributed to greater improvements in school functioning as compared to PSST alone. These results suggest that adding the practice component to PSST enhanced the generalizability of the treatment, and thus it is a useful added component. On the other hand, the authors were disappointed that more children were not removed from the clinical range of scores due to the treatment. This suggested that some additional treatment component that was not provided might be necessary. This likely formed the basis for the aforementioned Kazdin and colleagues (1992) additive study.

As opposed to additive studies that attempt to add small or larger components to an existing treatment, dismantling studies attempt to find out which parts of an existing treatment are necessary and which can be removed to make the treatment more efficient. These studies are considered the "gold standard" of component analysis studies. We were able to identify two youth CBT dismantling studies. Each of these studies helps to demonstrate the value of this type of design. In one study, each of the components of CBT was found to be equivalent, with no gain in having more than one component. Jaycox, Reivich, Gillham, and Seligman (1994) tested the Penn Prevention Program, which was developed to intervene with middle-school-age children (10–13 years) at risk due to elevated depressive symptoms or family conflict. This depression prevention program utilized a cognitive component (CT) that was focused on teaching children how to interpret problem situations in more adaptive ways by identifying negative beliefs, evaluating the evidence for beliefs, and generating alternatives. The second component of the program, a social problem-solving and coping component (SPS), focused on the children's actions for solving their problems by teaching social problem solving and adaptive coping. The authors simultaneously evaluated the overall prevention intervention and the specific components of the intervention. Control group youths were in one school; and intervention youths in other schools were paired with control youths based on risk scores. The intervention youths were randomly assigned to CT, SPS, or the complete treatment (CT + SPS). Results of the study failed to identify the active component of treatment, as each of the three intervention groups were equally superior to the control group relative to depressive symptoms and classroom behavior. Despite not finding evidence for the superiority of a specific component, and not finding evidence that more than one component in the intervention was necessary, the investigators combined the three intervention groups into one in comparing results with the control group and concluded that the prevention effort was successful. Follow-up studies of this sample continued to combine the three groups and to treat them as one intervention (Gillham & Reivich, 1999; Gillham, Reivich, Jaycox, & Seligman, 1995). Even more problematic, relative to the purpose of component analysis studies, is that other researchers (e.g. Roberts, Kane, Thomson, Bishop, & Hart, 2003) have implemented the Penn Prevention Program by continuing to use all of the components in the treatment despite the evidence that all of the components are not necessary.

In the other dismantling study, each of the CBT components was found to make an important contribution to treatment outcomes for youth 8–12 years old. Kendall and Braswell (1982) dismantled the cognitive-behavioral package that had been found efficacious in treating non-self-controlled children (Kendall & Wilcox, 1980; Kendall & Zupan, 1981). This CBT treatment utilized a cognitive component (CT) focused on self-instructional training and cognitive modeling of problem resolution. The second component of the program, a behavioral component (BEH), focused on the use of behavioral contingencies and therapist modeling of appropriate behavior. The authors attempted to discover the contribution of the various components of the CBT treatment by simultaneously evaluating the overall CBT intervention against the intervention with specific components removed. Youth were randomly assigned to CBT (CT + BEH +ATT); to BT, which was CBT with the cognitive component removed (BEH + ATT); or to ATT, which was CBT with the cognitive and behavioral components removed but use of the same therapy materials, comparable duration treatment, use of a credible rationale, and rewards yoked to treatment children. The results indicated that CT + BEH + ATT and BEH + ATT produced significantly greater improvements in teacher ratings of child hyperactivity and child academic achievement and decreases in off-task behavior as compared to ATT. The addition of CT contributed to greater improvements in teacher ratings of child self-control and child reports of their self-concept as compared to BEH + ATT alone. These results suggest that each component of the CBT treatment enhances the impact of the intervention. On the other hand, the authors were disappointed that improvement was not seen on parent-report measures, and improvements were not maintained at 1-year follow-up. This suggested that some additional treatment component that was not provided might be necessary. Perhaps this was the reason for conducting additive studies specifically involving parental components of treatment. Ideally, future youth CBT dismantling studies will be completed (there is a dearth of these studies) in which it is discovered that some but not all components of a treatment are necessary for successful treatment outcomes, as this will lead to more efficient delivery of treatments.

Process-Outcome Studies

Although additive and dismantling studies allow us to isolate the relative contribution of different treatment components, the unit of analysis is typically a treatment "module." At the level of specific techniques, procedures, and transactions that occur within sessions, the process-outcome design represents the most widely used approach for examining treatment processes. Essentially, the process-outcome design utilizes longitudinal analyses in the context of a randomized controlled trial. Although some investigators have evaluated process-outcome associations in open trials, one weakness of this design is that additional variance might be attributed to therapeutic processes that are, in fact, due to non-therapeutic factors such as maturation or the passage of time. In process-outcome studies, facets of therapy process are measured during the course of therapy (or coded afterward) and used as predictors of variation in treatment response. Strong associations between process variables and outcomes measured prospectively can provide important leads concerning change mechanisms, though causal status depends on subsequent control and manipulation of candidate variables. Longitudinal data provide evidence for direction of effect, but can be misleading. For example, there is growing evidence for rapid symptom reduction in CBT for adult and adolescent depression (Gaynor et al., 2003; Tang & DeRubeis, 1999). Process variables that appear to be collected early in treatment might actually *follow* rapid symptom reduction. Consequently, it is critical to account for changes in outcomes that potentially precede the measurement of process variables.

Within the youth CBT literature, studies of process-outcome relations are just beginning to emerge, and most tend to focus on more molar constructs than those found in the adult literature. For example, Huey, Henggeler, and Brondine (2000) examined the association between one dimension of process, therapist adherence to treatment principles, and changes in hypothesized pathogenic mechanisms—in this case, parental monitoring and delinquent peer affiliation—among youth treated with multisystemic therapy (MST). To be sure, MST is not equivalent to CBT, but the study is highlighted because MST includes some CBT procedures, and the study is unique in its linking of, first, treatment processes to pathogenic mechanisms, and then mechanisms to treatment outcomes. In brief, therapist adherence to the MST protocol, measured from multiple participant perspectives, was predictive of changes in family functioning (family cohesion, parent monitoring) at the end of treatment. In turn, changes in family functioning were both directly and indirectly related to changes in delinquent behavior. Although therapist adherence had both a direct and indirect association with outcome, adherence principally operated on delinquency through the more proximal mechanism of improved family functioning.

The study does have a number of limitations. First, the process variable was assessed during the fourth and sixth week of treatment; consequently, an early change in treatment, or initial family characteristics, could be driving therapist adherence. Second, measures of change in pathogenic mechanisms did not precede measures of change in outcomes, thereby making it difficult to disentangle the direction of effect. Nevertheless, the study is unique in the child literature in that it actually demonstrated an association between therapist adherence and treatment outcomes. Again, there are some limitations regarding the measurement of adherence in this study; for example, actual observations were not used, and mean level of adherence was derived from multiple sessions. Research on the relation between adherence and outcome would benefit from a sharper focus on adherence to specific treatment tasks. In fact, establishing a gradient between adherence to specific therapy tasks (how completely were they delivered?) and treatment outcomes represents a type of dose–response relation. Dose–response relations represent one piece of evidence for making the case that a specific task or treatment procedure is an active mechanism of change (Kazdin & Nock, 2003).

Surprisingly few studies of youth CBT report associations between treatment adherence and treatment outcome. Although one might expect some restriction in range in randomized clinical trials (RCTs) in which therapists are closely supervised, it is likely that therapists vary to some degree in the delivery of manual-guided treatments. For example, in our own study of CBT for adolescent depression, we coded adherence across all sessions for all therapists. Although overall adherence was quite high and 89% of the specific components of treatment were delivered, adherence ranged from 72 to 97% across cases; moreover, some sessions were carried out more faithfully than others. Despite a well- developed manual, protocol-trained, doctoral level clinicians, session recordings with adherence checks, and weekly supervision, there still was variation in adherence. From a process perspective, this is actually fortunate insofar as variations in adherence provide a window on process–outcome relations. First, if one finds overall adherence to be related to outcome, it provides some evidence for the therapeutic action of the specified components as a whole. If not, one must certainly consider other processes not defined by the adherence checklist, or check for problems with restricted range. Again, if adherence represents the degree to which a treatment component is delivered, then one should expect dose–response relations similar to those found by Huey and colleagues (2000). Strong associations between adherence to a specific component and variations in outcome would suggest that the component is critical for change.

Although therapist adherence is critical for ensuring delivery of a protocol, CBT requires more from a therapist than reading skill! Certainly critics of manualized treatments have expressed concern that manuals rigidify the process of therapy (Strupp & Anderson, 1997) and potentially dilute the truly essential ingredient of therapy, the therapeutic relationship. In our meta-analysis of relationship predictors of outcomes in child and adolescent therapy, we found that relationship variables were equally related to outcomes in manualized and nonmanualized treatments (Shirk & Karver, 2003). Furthermore, recent studies of manual-guided CBT for youth anxiety do not support these concerns. In their 3-year follow-up of anxious youth treated with manual-guided CBT, Kendall and Southam-Gerow (1996) found a majority of youth mentioned the therapeutic relationship as the "most important" part of therapy, with a substantial number of youth indicating that the relationship was what they liked best about therapy. In fact, child reports of the therapeutic relationship in Kendall and colleagues' (1997) second CBT trial for anxious youth showed rather low variability in relationship scores; most were highly positive! Taken together, these findings suggest that manuals and relationships may be compatible, after all. Of course, manuals can be administered in a rigid, inflexible manner, and it would not be surprising if such an approach undermined the therapeutic relationship. Our own research on therapist engagement behaviors and the development of a working alliance in CBT showed that therapists who followed the manual without acknowledging adolescents' emotional expressions tended to have poorer alliances (Shirk & Karver, 2003). But advocates of manual-guided therapy *do not* promote rigid adherence to the text. As Kendall, Chu, Gifford, Hayes, and Nauta (1998) warn, overly close adherence to the manual risks turning the therapist into a teacher. Instead, therapists must flexibly apply the manual's concepts and procedures to fit the individual child or, as the authors suggest, "breathe life" into the manual (Kendall et al., 1998). Research on therapist flexibility in CBT for anxious youth found that therapists rated themselves as using a full range of flexibility, and used supervision to adapt modules to specific cases (Kendall & Chu, 2000). Although most youth in this trial had favorable outcomes, therapist self-rated flexibility was not associated with change in symptoms. It is possible that therapist flexibility has a more proximal effect on the therapy relationship or youth involvement in the tasks of therapy.

Youth CBT is not a passive, receptive experience. Although therapists come to sessions with an agenda and a plan for presenting concepts and activities, youth CBT resembles "coaching" far more than teaching (see Kendall, Chapter 1, this volume). Few coaches have won many games by simply telling their players what to do. Instead, they model behaviors, drill execution, combine simple behaviors into complex plays, coordinate them with the demands of situations, and practice them, usually in live scrimmages, before taking the court or field. And, as many coaches will tell you, the outcome of contests seems to hinge on the players' level of involvement during practice. With its skills building and active problem-solving focus, youth CBT hinges on client involvement as well. Emerging process–outcome research (see Braswell, Kendall, Braith, Carey, & Vye, 1985; Chu & Kendall, 2004), reviewed in the last section of this chapter, indicates that youth involvement in CBT is pivotal for treatment outcomes.

Summary of Emerging Youth CBT Process Research

Our harvest of youth CBT process studies is rather meager—not because youth CBT is infertile ground, but because our energy has been directed toward other tasks. As mentioned at the start of this chapter, process research serves outcome research through identifying mechanisms of action. The limited number of dismantling and process-outcome studies of youth CBT represents a step, albeit a first step, in this effort. We have yet to identify the essential active ingredients of most of our multicomponent treatments. Early results suggest that therapist adherence is important for outcomes, though few studies have evaluated this association. Recent evidence also suggests that child involvement in the tasks of CBT is pivotal for outcome. But, again, evidence is just beginning to emerge. And finally, there is some evidence indicating that manual-guided therapy for youth does not undermine the therapeutic relationship. In fact, most children, at least children with anxiety, appear to form a positive, and memorable, relationship with their CBT therapist.

　　If the first wave of child treatment research was to demonstrate the efficacy of specific cognitive-behavioral therapies for specific disorders, the second wave of research should involve an analysis of the processes that contributed to beneficial effects. Although it is possible that different processes will account for change in effectiveness trials in real-world settings (Weisz, 2000), identification of active therapeutic processes will enable us to refine and distill our treatments so that they may be efficiently delivered in real-world contexts. This means that investigators are faced with the challenge of looking inside the therapy sessions of their original randomized controlled trials. Though the task of coding sessions is labor-intensive, it could yield a bountiful harvest of leads for the next generation of outcome studies.

ENGAGEMENT, ALLIANCE, AND INVOLVEMENT IN YOUTH CBT

As the chapters in this volume show, mounting evidence supports the efficacy of CBT procedures for a range of child and adolescent disorders. Although we have yet to isolate the active ingredients of our treatment packages, it is evident that exposure to CBT protocols beats the passage of time and, in many cases, the provision of therapeutic support (Brent et al., 1997; Kazdin et al., 1992). But as any practitioner will tell you, treatment is not merely exposure to a protocol. Instead, at the heart of effective treatment is engagement and involvement of the child, adolescent, or parent in the therapeutic tasks defined by the protocol. We propose that this process variously labeled "engagement," "alliance," "involvement," "collaboration," "adherence," and "compliance" is the most fundamental process issue for youth CBT. First, it is one of the most prominent questions raised by practitioners, usually presented as a variation of "Yes, but how do I get my clients to *do* these procedures?" Second, early attrition, sporadic attendance, and marginal participation are likely to undermine treatment efficacy by diluting treatment dose, and diminished effects from intent-to-treat analyses underscore the importance of treatment completion. Third, one major obstacle to the successful transportation of efficacious cognitive-behavioral treatments to service clinics involves the widely reported pattern of early attrition and inconsistent appointment keeping in such clinics. Together, these concerns suggest that youth CBT is likely to be enhanced by a greater understanding of the processes of engagement, alliance, and involvement.

Issues pertaining to engagement, alliance, and involvement have often been discussed under the rubric of therapeutic relationship processes. Although the importance of forming a good working relationship has been acknowledged by CBT developers for some time (e.g., Kendall, 1991), relationship processes have been viewed as nonspecific factors that all youth receive in treatment. Thus, in order to isolate the impact of specific cognitive-behavioral processes, relationship processes have been the target of control conditions, and largely isolated from other technical interventions in our models. The lack of clear definitions and measurable indicators of core constructs has undoubtedly impeded progress in integrating relationship processes into a cognitive-behavioral model of change. Therefore, we offer the following distinctions as a starting point for framing process issues in this area.

We distinguish three core constructs—engagement, alliance, and involvement. *Engagement* refers to actions, strategies, and behaviors to promote treatment alliance, involvement, and completion. Conceptualized in this manner, engagement processes refer to interventions delivered to promote treatment involvement and completion and, indirectly through involvement and completion, a reduction in psychopathology or an improvement in functioning. *Treatment involvement* refers to the client's active participation in the tasks of therapy. Involvement goes well beyond mere treatment attendance and includes participation in therapeutic "work." A child who attends a session and only participates in peripheral activities such as board games would be viewed as low on treatment involvement (though such activities might promote subsequent involvement in treatment tasks). As this example implies, the concept of treatment involvement is contingent on the specification of therapeutic tasks, that is, the activities that are viewed as essential for change. In the context of manualized treatments, tasks are readily identified as the activities such as generating alternative solutions to social problems, deep-breathing exercises, or cognitive restructuring that constitute our treatments.

Finally, *alliance* may be the most difficult to define, in part because it has been imbued with different meanings in the adult psychotherapy literature (see Martin, Graske, & Davis, 2000). Bordin's (1976) pantheoretical model of the alliance has informed much of this work and posits the alliance to be a multidimensional construct involving bond, tasks, and goals. To distinguish the alliance from involvement in treatment tasks and the process of agreeing on treatment goals (a potentially critical part of engagement), we highlight the bond component of the alliance. Specifically, we propose that alliance refers to *the client's experience of the therapist as someone that can be counted on for help in overcoming problems or distress.* In this respect, the alliance involves the experience of the therapist as being on "your side" and allied against the problems that require treatment. In essence, therapist and client are part of the "same team," and the opponent is the problems that distress or impair the client. This definition of alliance goes beyond mere liking of the therapist and is consistent with Luborsky's (1975) view of the alliance as involving the experience of the therapist as supportive and helpful, and allied in a joint effort against problems. It also distinguishes the alliance from other relationship constructs such as therapist warmth, genuineness, or structuring. These constructs are viewed as potential predictors of the alliance and may be critical for engagement processes.

Two dimensions of experience are implicit in our definition of alliance. The first involves the perception of the therapist as reliable, as someone you can count on. This dimension is consistent with views of the alliance as involving a relationship of trust and respect. It is possible that this aspect of the alliance emerges from interactions that demonstrate consistency, responsiveness, support, and understanding. The second dimension involves the experience of the therapist as a helper. This dimension of the alliance has deep roots in the child therapy literature (A. Freud, 1947) and distinguishes the alliance from other close relationships that involve different aims. Therapy involves collaborating on specific tasks to attain specific goals in the context of a helping relationship. If the therapist is not viewed as a guide, coach, or general helper in the therapy endeavor, a positive relationship may exist, but not a therapeutic alliance.

There are developmental implications for this view of alliance. It is unclear whether young children, in particular, understand the relationship between treatment goals, therapy activities, and the role of the therapist. In some of our early work (Shirk & Saiz, 1992), we proposed that children might differ developmentally in terms of the degree to which they recognize and acknowledge problems, understand the causes of their problems, and view the therapist as a potential source of relief from problems. The perception of the therapist as a credible and potentially effective helper might both contribute to and follow from involvement and outcome. If so, alliance formation might be facilitated by achieving small but salient goals early in treatment. However, at this point, it is not known if a positive therapy *relationship*, defined largely in terms of bond, or a therapeutic *alliance*, involving both the experience of therapist as reliable and a helper, is a better predictor of involvement in therapy and, ultimately, treatment outcome.

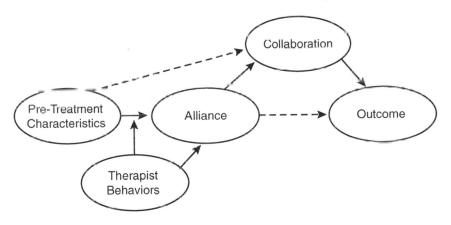

FIGURE 13.3. Relationship processes in youth CBT

Hypothesized relations among the core constructs in our model are presented in Figure 13.3. Both child pretreatment characteristics and therapist engagement strategies are hypothesized to contribute to the development of the alliance. In turn, treatment involvement is predicted from the alliance, and potentially from therapist engagement strategies. As the model suggests, the alliance is viewed as a catalyst for treatment involvement, that is, collaboration with treatment tasks. Although there may be a direct relationship between alliance and outcome, we propose that most of this association will be mediated by treatment involvement in CBT. Other possible relations may exist among constructs; for example, youth pretreatment characteristics may influence therapist engagement strategies, and treatment involvement may feed back on the alliance at later sessions. However, as a starting point, we offer this linear model as a heuristic.

Emerging Evidence on Relational Processes in CBT

What evidence is available to support the proposed associations in this model? Our recent meta-analysis of therapy relationship–outcome associations revealed an overall pattern of association between relationship variables and outcomes that is consistent with findings from the adult literature (Shirk & Karver, 2003). That is, across age of youth, relationship variables were consistent but modest predictors of outcomes (mean $r = .24$). One of the major drawbacks of the existing literature is that the therapy relationship has been conceptualized and measured in diverse ways. In fact, only one study in this sample would have met the criteria for inclusion in the adult reviews (individual therapy, alliance as the construct, and prospective relations with outcomes). Recently, however, two papers have appeared that explicitly assess the alliance in child treatment, and both indicate that the child–therapist alliance, measured either by self-report (Hawley & Weisz, 2005), or by observation (McCleod & Weisz, 2005) predict outcomes in youth treatment as usual (TAU). In both studies the alliance was conceptualized as both bond and task collaboration, and this variable, measured early in treatment, predicted changes in internalizing symptoms. A unique feature of both studies was the inclusion of a measure of parent alliance with the therapist, an important addition given the role of parents in managing child treatment initiation and continuation. In both studies, parent alliance predicted changes in symptoms and was a better predictor of cancellations, no shows, and treatment persistence than child–therapist alliance (Hawley & Weisz, 2005). This finding suggests that alliance formation with parents may be especially important for treatment continuation. This result is consistent with the findings of Garcia and Weisz (2002), who found that the number-one reason for ending treatment involved relationship problems between parents and therapists.

But what is the association between relationship variables and outcomes in cognitive-behavioral therapy for youth? In the meta-analytic sample, strength of association for behavioral and nonbehavioral treatments did not differ. Of the six behavioral studies that included a measure of relationship, three were explicitly cognitive-behavioral, child-focused therapy (Braswell et al., 1985; Kendall, 1994; Kendall et al., 1997). The average correlation across these studies was .18, slightly lower than the estimate for the full sample. However, there was significant variability in results across studies, ranging from .00 to .41. Interestingly, the latter result came from a study in which relationship process was conceptualized as treatment involvement (Braswell et al., 1985). Thus, at present, there is little evidence for a direct link between alliance and outcome in youth CBT. However, the proposed model hypothesizes that treatment involvement is a more proximal predictor of outcomes in CBT than therapy alliance.

A small but growing set of studies indicates that treatment involvement is predictive of change in youth CBT. In an early study, Braswell and colleagues (1985) coded child verbal behavior (e.g., self-disclosure, off-task comments) during cognitive-behavioral therapy sessions for children with disruptive classroom behavior. A measure of positive involvement was derived from process codes. In brief, verbal indicators of active, positive involvement with therapy tasks were associated with improvements in classroom behavior as rated by teachers. This finding reminds us that it is not our protocol that produces change, but the child's *involvement* with our protocol that is critical.

More recently, Chu and Kendall (2004) evaluated the association between child involvement and treatment outcome in CBT for anxious children. Level of child involvement in therapy was based on ratings of two 10-minute segments of therapy sessions. Raters coded child "enthusiasm for the task," "self-disclosure," "verbal initiation," and "verbal elaboration" as indicators of positive involvement. Negative involvement codes included "child withdrawal or passivity" and "child inhibition or avoidance." Good-to-excellent reliability was demonstrated for the *Child Involvement Rating Scale*. Level of child involvement measured at midtreatment was predictive of positive treatment outcomes as indexed by the absence of an anxiety disorder diagnosis and reduction in impairment. Early involvement in therapy tasks during sessions 2 5 may signal to the therapist that strategies to reengage the child may be required (p. 827). Early involvement did not predict outcomes, but significant shifts in involvement by midtreatment were highly predictive of diagnostic improvement. Interestingly, most youth showed a negative shift in involvement over the course of therapy. Those who showed a large negative shift were far more likely to retain their anxiety diagnosis. It is possible that the early tasks of therapy are less demanding and treatment involvement less challenging than later sessions, when resistance may emerge. These results suggest that *maintenance* of a working relationship that includes the child's active involvement may be as critical, or more so, than the initial building of the relationship. As Chu and Kendall (2004) observe, "Growing signs of withdrawal, avoidance, and diminished participation may signal to the therapist that strategies to re-engage the child may be required." Chu and Kendall are quick to point out that their correlational design does not permit causal inferences about involvement despite evidence for prospective associations. Although the case is strengthened by the absence of associations between pretreatment child characteristics and involvement, early symptom change might have preceded variation in involvement, and/or involvement could be correlated with causal processes not isolated by the study.

Consistent with the foregoing results, Shirk, Karver, and Spirito (2003) reported associations between youth involvement, measured as collaboration with problem-solving training, and change in depressive symptoms in a small controlled trial with suicidal adolescents. A unique feature of this study involved the measurement of involvement in terms of adolescents' responses to a specific therapy task, namely, generating alternative solutions for social problems. This approach to assessing involvement has the advantage of gauging participation across different components of therapy, a strategy that could aid in the identification of active ingredients of treatment. Taken together, the results of these initial studies are consistent across three types of problems, and are congruent with the theory guiding CBT for youth; emotional and behavioral change is based on the acquisition or reactivation of cognitive and behavioral skills through active involvement in therapy.

Is there evidence for the therapy bond to function as a catalyst for treatment involvement? Results suggest that the two constructs are closely related. In an early study, Shirk and Saiz (1992) found bond and collaboration, their measure of involvement, to be moderately related within both child and therapist reports. More recently, McLeod and Weisz (2005) found substantial overlap between observational ratings of bond and collaboration for both child and parent relationships with the therapist. Together these studies could indicate that bond and collaboration or involvement are not distinct constructs, a finding that has some parallels in the adult literature (Horvath, 1994). However, it should be noted that both studies involved treatment as usual, and both measured bond and collaboration at the same time. In order to address the hypothesis that the therapy bond functions as a catalyst for involvement, minimally prospective relations need to be assessed. In the only study thus far, Shirk and colleagues (2003) reported moderate relations between the alliance (bond) measured both by adolescent report and by observational rating in session 3 and treatment collaboration measured in session 4. Although this finding is consistent with the hypothesis that alliance (bond) promotes treatment involvement, involvement was not measured prior to alliance, and early outcomes were not assessed. Consequently, it is possible that involvement in tasks influences therapy bond and/or that early changes in symptoms drive both processes. In addition, the small sample size in the study by Shirk and colleagues did not allow for a test of the hypothesis that involvement mediates the association between alliance and outcome. Further research is needed to evaluate the contribution of these relational processes to treatment progress and outcome in CBT for youth.

Relatively little attention has been directed to therapist behaviors or actions that facilitate or impede therapy alliance and involvement. Although many treatment manuals acknowledge the importance of establishing rapport and a good working relationship with the child and parent, few empirically based guidelines have been established for these processes. A new line of research is emerging that focuses on therapist behaviors or strategies for alliance building. Creed and Kendall (2005) examined a set of therapist behaviors hypothesized to promote or interfere with alliance formation during the first three sessions of CBT for anxious children. Child and therapist reports were used to assess the alliance at Sessions 3 and 7. Child-reported alliance at session 3 was positively associated with therapist collaboration strategies, including presenting therapy as a team effort, building a sense of togetherness by using words like "we," "us," and "let's," and by helping the child set goals for treatment. "Pushing the child to talk" about anxiety and "emphasizing common ground"—that is, where the therapist makes comments like "me, too!"—predicted weaker child-reported alliance. At Session 7, "pushing the child to talk" about anxiety continued to predict a poorer alliance. For therapist–reported alliance, none of the therapist behaviors predicted alliance scores at session 3, but collaborative strategies predicted better alliances at session 7, and being "overly formal"—that is, talking to the child in a way that is overly didactic, stuffy, or patronizing—predicted a weaker alliance. Other therapist behaviors were not predictive of child or therapist reports of alliance, including being playful, providing hope and encouragement, and general conversations.

The results from this study point to a connection between early therapist behavior and subsequent levels of therapy alliance. Two findings seem especially important. Therapist collaborative behavior, including the establishment of treatment goals with the child, may be critical for alliance formation with children. Although most CBT manuals include some discussion of treatment goals, it may be particularly important to elicit the child's perspective on goals and to include the child's goals in the overall treatment plan. This finding is consistent with results suggesting that self-generated statements about participation and motivation are predictive of better adherence (Nock & Kazdin, 2003). This issue takes on added significance when considered in the context of treatment as usual, where there is often little agreement about treatment goals (Hawley & Weisz, 2003) and outcomes are far from optimal (Weisz, Huey, & Weersing, 1998). Of course, given the correlational nature of the evidence, it is possible that children who are easily allied elicit collaborative behaviors from their therapists. Interestingly, pretreatment characteristics did not predict alliance ratings in this sample.

Pushing the child to talk about anxiety who was not ready was a significant negative predictor of alliance and merits further consideration. Unlike play therapy, CBT is an active, problem-focused treatment and as such revolves around addressing specific problems such as anxiety or depression. Certainly the finding of a negative relationship between "pushing" and alliance should not be used as a justification for problem avoidance in CBT. It should be noted that "pushing" refers to the therapist continuing to ask about anxiety beyond the point where the child seems interested or comfortable (Creed & Kendall, 2005). This suggests that therapists must be mindful of the child's level of tolerance and must work to gradually shape the child's ability to talk about anxiety through verbal reinforcement. The finding also suggests that therapists may need to be flexible in the *pace* of CBT for anxiety, and not be overly rigid about the prescribed schedule of activities.

A second study has been reported on therapist alliance-building strategies in CBT, but with a different age group and target problem. Shirk and colleagues (2003) presented initial results linking therapist behaviors and early alliance in CBT for depressed adolescents who made a suicide attempt. To evaluate the therapist contribution to alliance formation, Shirk and colleagues proposed a heuristic model that organized therapist behaviors into four broad clusters: experience focused, motivation-focused, negotiation-focused, and efficacy-focused interventions. Experience-focused interventions emphasize the provision of empathy, validation, and support, and tend to focus on eliciting event descriptions and internal state responses. Motivation-focused interventions involve strategies for mobilizing the adolescent's intent to change, and tend to involve eliciting self-motivating statements. Negotiation-focused interventions revolve around the establishment of treatment goals and linking these goals to treatment participation. Finally, efficacy-focused interventions involve establishing positive expectations for change, including the provision of a recovery model and statements about the utility of the treatment for adolescents.

Initial results based on coding the first two sessions of therapy for 22 depressed adolescents showed that the specific behavioral codes could be reliably rated, but that some behaviors were quite rare, e.g., eliciting self-motivating statements. Of equal importance, close analysis of the tapes revealed a set of *therapist lapses* that occurred despite careful training of these doctoral-level therapists

Three lapses were identified: therapist criticizes, therapist fails to understand, and therapist fails to respond to expressed emotion. Although criticism was quite rare, the other two lapses were the best predictors of adolescent alliance at session 3. In brief, none of the positive alliance-building behaviors reliably predicted strength of alliance, but both therapists' misunderstanding of adolescents' comments and therapists' failure to respond when teens expressed emotion were associated with poorer alliances. Interestingly, therapists' failure to respond to expressed emotion was predicted by the adolescent's level of pretreatment hostility, thus suggesting that therapists may have the most difficulty responding to anger. These results suggest that core interviewing skills involving active listening and accurate acknowledgment of expressed emotion cannot be overlooked in the engagement process, at least with depressed adolescents.

Results from a study of therapist verbal behavior in the early phase of parent–child interaction therapy also indicate that basic interviewing skills are critical for engagement. Harwood and Eyberg (2004) found that therapist-expressed support—but not facilitating behaviors (one-word utterances like "uh-huh" and "right")—predicted treatment completion. In fact, higher rates of facilitating behaviors were predictive of premature termination. Furthermore, higher use of closed-ended questions (e.g., "When did the problem start?") was associated with early termination. Although such basic interviewing skills are rarely addressed in treatment manuals, given emerging evidence for their connection with alliance and continuation, these fundamentals cannot be overlooked in clinical training.

CONCLUSION

There has been substantial progress in the first wave of treatment research on CBT for childhood disorders. A growing number of treatment packages has been identified as promising or efficacious treatments. A new wave of research is just beginning to emerge that examines links between treatment processes and outcomes in CBT. This research is guided by the question "How do treatment processes alter pathogenic mechanisms that result in improved outcomes?" (Shirk & Russell, 1996). This wave of research will require the identification and potentially the manipulation of specific treatment components or procedures within CBT treatment packages. Further, these treatment processes will need to be examined in a model that connects process with outcome through pathogenic mechanisms. As our review has shown, this wave of research is currently a ripple rather than a swell.

One area of process research that is beginning to attract attention is research on treatment engagement, alliance, and involvement. To the degree that CBT requires the active involvement of children, adolescents, and parents, this line of research may provide us with important insights about the processes that enhance or impede outcomes. Empirically supported treatments should be complemented with empirically supported strategies for engagement and alliance formation. Such research appears to be especially critical for the transportation of CBT to community settings where early attrition, sporadic attendance, and marginal involvement may be endemic to clinical practice. It is likely that treatment involvement and participation define the boundaries of treatment effectiveness. The degree to which we are able to engage children and their parents in therapies of known efficacy will strongly influence the generalizability of efficacious treatments.

Although initial process research is beginning to identify therapist behaviors that predict alliance formation, this line of work would benefit from an analysis of therapist–client transactions. There is some suggestion that therapist behaviors are partially shaped by clients' pretreatment characteristics, and that therapists' responses, in turn, may affect the client's experience of alliance. Thus, the unit of analysis may need to be expanded to patterns of interactions rather than frequencies of therapist behaviors in isolation. There is precedence for this type of research in the child treatment literature. Patterson and Forgatch (1985) evaluated the conditional probabilities of client resistance and therapist behaviors in the context of parent management training, and Stoolmiller, Duncan, Bank, and Patterson (1993) showed that patterns of resistance over the course of treatment were better predictors of outcome than a static measure of early resistance. This type of approach to therapy process holds significant promise for identifying interactions that contribute to treatment completion, involvement, and outcome.

In conclusion, the tide of process research on youth CBT appears to be coming in. We invite CBT investigators to ride this new wave of treatment research and to reexamine variations in treatment processes in relation to treatment outcomes in the first wave of randomized trials. A focus on specific therapy processes, their variation in treatment, and their relation to outcomes will help us refine and strengthen our cognitive-behavioral interventions for youth.

REFERENCES

Ahn, H., & Wampold, B. E. (2001). Where oh where are the specific ingredients?: A meta-analysis of component studies in counseling and psychotherapy. *Journal of Counseling Psychology, 48,* 251–257.

Azrin, N. H., Donohue, B., Teichner, G. A., Crum, T., Howell, J., & DeCato, L. H. (2001). A controlled evaluation and description of individual-cognitive problem solving and family-behavior therapies in dually diagnosed conduct-disordered and substance-dependent youth. *Journal of Child and Adolescent Substance Abuse, 11,* 1–43.

Baum, C. G., Reyna-McGlone, C. L., & Ollendick, T. H. (1986, November). *The efficacy of behavioral parent training, behavioral parent training plus clinical self-control training, and a modified STEP program with children referred for noncompliance.* Paper presented at the annual meeting of the Association for the Advancement of Behavior Therapy, Chicago.

Barrett, P. M., Dadds, M. R., & Rapee, R. M. (1996). Family treatment of childhood anxiety: A controlled trial. *Journal of Consulting and Clinical Psychology, 64,* 333–342.

Barrett, P. M., Duffy, A. L., Dadds, M. R., & Rapee, R. M. (2001). Cognitive-behavioral treatment of anxiety disorders in children: Long-term (6-year) follow up. *Journal of Consulting and Clinical Psychology, 69,* 135–141.

Bordin, E. (1976). The generalizability of the psychoanalytic concept of the working alliance. *Psychotherapy, Theory, Research, and Practice, 16,* 252–260.

Braswell, L., Kendall, P., Braith, J., Carey, M., & Vye, C. (1985). "Involvement" in cognitive-behavioral therapy with children: Process and its relationship with outcome. *Cognitive therapy and research, 9,* 611–630.

Brent, D., Holder, D., Kolko, D., Birmaher, B., Baugher, M., Roth, C., et al. (1997). A clinical psychotherapy trial for adolescent depression comparing cognitive, family, and supportive therapy. *Archives of General Psychiatry, 54,* 877–885.

Chronis, A. M., Chacko, A., Fabiano, G. A., Wymbs, B. T., & Pelham, W. E. (2004). Enhancements to the Behavioral Parent Training Paradigm for Families of Children with ADHD: Review and future directions. *Clinical Child and Family Psychology Review, 7*(1), 1–27.

Chu, B., & Kendall, P. (2004). Positive association of child involvement and treatment Outcome within a manual-based cognitive-behavioral treatment for children with anxiety. *Journal of Consulting and Clinical Psychology, 72,* 821–829.

Cobham, V. E., Dadds, M. R., & Spence, S. H. (1998). The role of parental anxiety in the treatment of childhood anxiety. *Journal of Consulting and Clinical Psychology, 66,* 893–905.

Creed, T., & Kendall, P. (2005). Therapist alliance building behavior within a cognitive Behavioral treatment for anxiety in youth. *Journal of Consulting and Clinical Psychology, 73,* 498–505.

Deblinger, E., Lippman, J., & Steer, R. (1996). Sexually abused children suffering posttraumatic stress symptoms: Initial treatment outcome findings. *Child Maltreatment: Journal of the American Professional Society on the Abuse of Children, 1,* 310–321.

Deblinger, E., Steer, R. A., & Lippmann, J. (1999). Two-year follow-up study of cognitive behavioral therapy for sexually abused children suffering post-traumatic stress symptoms. *Child Abuse and Neglect, 23,* 1371–1378.

Dishion, T. J., & Andrews, D. W. (1995). Preventing escalation in problem behaviors with high-risk young adolescents: Immediate and 1-year outcomes. *Journal of Consulting and Clinical Psychology, 63,* 538–548.

Durlak, J., Fuhrman, T., & Lampman, C. (1991). Effectiveness of cognitive-behavioral therapy for maladapting children: A meta-analysis. *Psychological Bulletin, 110,* 204–214.

Freud, A. (1947). *The psychoanalytic treatment of children.* New York: International Universities Press.

Garcia, J., & Weisz, J. (2002). When youth mental health care stops: Therapeutic relationship problems and other reasons for ending youth outpatient treatment. *Journal of Consulting and Clinical Psychology, 70,* 439–443.

Gaynor, S., Weersing, R., Kolko, D., Birmaher, B., Heo, J., & Brent, D. (2003). The prevalence and impact of sudden large improvements during adolescent therapy for depression: A comparison across cognitive-behavioral, family, and supportive therapy. *Journal of Consulting and Clinical Psychology, 71,* 386–393.

Gillham, J. E., & Reivich, K. J. (1999). Prevention of depressive symptoms in school children: A research update. *Psychological Science, 10,* 461–462.

Gillham, J. E., Reivich, K. J., Jaycox, I. H., & Seligman, M. E. P. (1995). Prevention of depressive symptoms in schoolchildren: Two-year follow-up. *Psychological Science, 6,* 343–351.

Harwood, M., & Eyberg, S. (2004). Therapist verbal behavior early in treatment: Relation to successful completion of Parent-Child Interaction Therapy. *Journal of Clinical Child and Adolescent Psychology, 33*, 601–612.

Hawley, K., & Weisz, J. (2003). Child, parent, and therapist (dis)agreement on target problems in outpatient therapy: The therapist dilemma and its implications. *Journal of Consulting and Clinical Psychology, 71*, 62–70.

Hawley, K, & Weisz, J. (2005). Youth versus parent working alliance in usual clinical care: Distinctive associations with retention, satisfaction, and treatment outcome. *Journal of Clinical Child and Adolescent Psychology, 34*, 117–128.

Heyne, D., King, N. J., Tonge, B. J., Rollings, S., Young, D., Pritchard, M., & Ollendick, T. H. (2002). Evaluation of child therapy and caregiver training in the treatment of school refusal. *Journal of the American Academy of Child and Adolescent Psychiatry, 41*(6), 687–695.

Horn, W. F., Ialongo, N. S., Greenberg, G., Packard, T., & Smith-Winberry, C. (1990). Additive effects of behavioral parent training and self-control therapy with ADHD children. *Journal of Clinical Child Psychology, 19*, 98–110.

Horn, W. F., Ialongo, N., Popovich, S., & Peradotto, D. (1987). Behavioral parent training and cognitive-behavioral self-control therapy with ADD-H children: comparative and combined effects. *Journal of Clinical Child Psychology, 16*(1), 57–68.

Horvath, A. (1994). Empirical validation of Bordin's pantheoretical model of the alliance: The working alliance inventory perspective. In A. Horvath & L. Greenberg (Eds.), *Working alliance: Theory, research, and practice* (pp. 109–128). Oxford, UK. Wiley.

Huey, S., Henggeler, S., & Brondino, M. (2000). Mechanisms of change in multisystemic therapy: Reducing delinquent behavior through therapist adherence and improved family and peer functioning. *Journal of Consulting and Clinical Psychology, 68*, 451–467.

Horvath, A. (1994). Empirical validation of Bordin's pantheoretical model of the alliance: The Working Alliance Inventory perspective. In A. O. Horvath & L. S. Greenberg (Eds.), *Working alliance: Theory, research, and practice* (pp. 109–128). New York: Wiley.

Jaycox, L. H., Reivich, K. J., Gillham, J. E., & Seligman, M. E. (1994). Prevention of depressive symptoms in school children. *Behaviour Research Therapy, 32*(8), 801–816.

Kazdin, A. (1995). Bridging child, adolescent, and adult psychotherapy: Directions for research. *Psychotherapy Research, 5*, 258–277.

Kazdin, A. E., Bass, D., Siegel, T., & Thomas, C. (1989). Cognitive-behavioral therapy and relationship therapy in the treatment of children referred for antisocial behavior. *Journal of Consulting and Clinical Psychology, 57*, 522–535.

Kazdin, A., Esveldt-Dawson, K., & French, N. (1987). Problem-solving skills training and relationship therapy in the treatment of anti-social child behavior. *Journal of Consulting and Clinical Psychology, 55*, 76–85.

Kazdin, A., & Kendall, P. (1998). Current progress and future plans for developing effective treatments: Comments and perspectives. *Journal of Clinical Child Psychology, 27*, 217–226.

Kazdin, A., & Nock, M. (2003). Delineating mechanisms of change in child and adolescent therapy: Methodological issues and research recommendations. *Journal of Child Psychology and Psychiatry, 44*, 1116–1129.

Kazdin, A., Siegel, T., & Bass, D. (1992). Cognitive problem-solving skills training and parent managent training in the treatment of antisocial behavior in children. *Journal of Consulting and Clinical Psychology, 60*, 733–747.

Kendall, P. C. (1991). *Child and adolescent therapy: Cognitive-behavioral procedures.* New York: Guilford Press.

Kendall, P. C. (1994). Treating anxiety disorders in youth: Results of a randomized clinical trial. *Journal of Consulting and Clinical Psychology, 61*, 235–247.

Kendall, P. C., & Braswell, L. (1982). Cognitive-behavioral self-control therapy for children: A components analysis. *Journal of Consulting and Clinical Psychology, 50*, 672–689.

Kendall, P, & Choudbury, M. (2003). Children and adolescents in cognitive-behavioral therapy: Some past efforts and current advances, and the challenges of the future. *Cognitive Therapy and Research, 27,* 89–104.

Kendall, P. C., & Chu, B. (2000). Retrospective reports of therapist flexibility in manual-based treatment for youths with anxiety disorders. *Journal of Clinical Child Psychology, 29,* 209–220.

Kendall, P. C., Chu, B., Gifford, A., Hayes, C., & Nauta, M. (1998). Breathing life into a manual: Flexibility and creativity with manual-based treatments. *Cognitive and Behavioral Practice, 5,* 177–198.

Kendall, P. C., Flannery-Schroeder, E., Panichelli-Mindel, S., Southam-Gerow, M., Henin, A., & Warman, M. (1997). Therapy for youths with anxiety disorders: A second randomized trial. *Journal of Consulting and Clinical Psychology, 64,* 724–730.

Kendall, P. C., Kane, M., Howard, B., & Sequeline, L. (1990). *Cognitive-behavioral therapy for anxious children: Treatment manual.* Ardmore, PA: Workbook Publishing.

Kendall, P. C., & Southam-Gerow, M. (1996). Long-term follow up of a cognitive-behavioral therapy for anxiety disordered youth. *Journal of Consulting and Clinical Psychology, 64,* 724–730.

Kendall, P. C., & Wilcox, L. E. (1980). A cognitive-behavioral treatment for impulsivity: Concrete versus conceptual training with non-self-controlled problem children. *Journal of Consulting and Clinical Psychology, 48,* 80–91.

Kendall, P. C., & Zupan, B. A. (1981). Individual versus group application of cognitive-behavioral self-control procedures with children. *Behavior Therapy, 12,* 344–359.

King, N. J., Tonge, B. J., Mullen, P., Myerson, N., Heyne, D., Rollings, S., et al. (2000). Treating sexually abused children with posttraumatic stress symptoms: A randomized clinical trial. *Journal of the American Academy of Child and Adolescent Psychiatry, 39*(11), 1347–1355.

Lewinsohn, P., & Clarke, G. (1999). Psychosocial treatments for adolescent depression. *Clinical Psychology Review, 19,* 329–342.

Lewinsohn, P. M., Clarke, G. N., Hops, H., & Andrews, J. A. (1990). Cognitive-behavioral treatment for depressed adolescents. *Behavior Therapy, 21,* 385–401.

Lochman, J. E., & Wells, K. C. (2004). The Coping Power program for preadolescent aggressive boys and their parents: Outcome effects at the one-year follow-up. *Journal of Consulting and Clinical Psychology, 72,* 571–578.

Luborsky, L. (1995). Helping alliances in psychotherapy. In J. Creighorn (Ed.), *Successful psycyhotherapy* (pp. 92–116). New York: Brunner/Mazel.

Martin, D. J., Graske, J. P., & Davis, M. K. (2002). Relation of the therapeutic alliance with outcome and other variables: A meta-analytic review. *Journal of Consulting and Clinical Psychology, 68,* 438–450.

McLeod, B., & Weisz, J. (2005). The Therapy Process Observational Coding Scale: Measure characteristics and prediction of outcome in usual clinical practice. *Journal of Consulting and Clinical Psychology, 73,* 323–333.

Mendlowitz, S. L., Manassis, K., Bradley, S., Scapillato, D., Miezitis, S., & Shaw, B. F. (1999). Cognitive-behavioral group treatments in childhood anxiety disorders: The role of parental involvement. *Journal of the American Academy of Child and Adolescent Psychiatry, 38,* 1223–1229.

Nauta, M. H., Scholing, A., Emmelkamp, P. M. G., & Minderaa, R. B. (2001), Cognitive-behavioural therapy for anxiety disordered children in a clinical setting: Does additional cognitive parent training enhance treatment effectiveness? *Clinical Psychology and Psychotherapy, 8,* 330–340.

Nauta, M. H., Scholing, A., Emmelkamp, P. M., & Minderaa, R. B. (2003), Cognitive-behavioral therapy for children with anxiety disorders in a clinical setting: No additional effect of a cognitive parent training. *Journal of the American Academy of Child and Adolescent Psychiatry, 42*, 1270–1278.

Nock, M., & Kazdin, A. (2001). Parent expectations for child therapy: Assessment and relation to participation in treatment. *Journal of Child and Family Studies, 10*, 155–180.

Orlinski, D., & Howard, K. (1986). Process and outcome in psychotherapy. In S. L. Garfield & A. E. Bergin (Eds.), *Handbook of psychotherapy and behavior change* (3rd ed., pp. 477–502). New York: Wiley.

Patterson, G., & Forgatch, M. (1985). Therapist behavior as a determinant of client noncompliance: A paradox for the behavior modifier. *Journal of Consulting and Clinical Psychology, 53*, 846–851.

Roberts, C., Kane, R., Thomson, H., Bishop, B., & Hart, B. (2003). The prevention of depressive symptoms in rural school children: A randomized controlled trial. *Journal of Consulting and Clinical Psychology, 71*, 622–628.

Shirk, S., & Karver, M. (2003). Prediction of treatment outcome from relationship variables in child and adolescent therapy. *Journal of Consulting and Clinical Psychology, 71*, 462–471.

Shirk, S., Karver, M., & Spirito, A. (2003, November). *Relationship processes in youth CBT: Measuring alliance and collaboration.* Paper presented at the annual meeting of the Association for the Advancement of Behavior Therapy, Boston.

Shirk, S. R., & Russell, R. L. (1996). *Change processes in child psychotherapy: Revitalizing treatment and research.* New York: Guilford Press.

Shirk, S., & Russell, R. (1998). Process issues in child psychotherapy. In A. Bellack & M. Hersen (Eds.), *Comprehensive clinical psychology* (Vol. 5, pp. 57–82). Oxford, UK: Pergamon Press.

Shirk, S., & Saiz, C. (1992). The therapeutic alliance in child therapy: Clinical, empirical and developmental perspectives. *Development and Psychopathology, 31*, 713–728.

Spence, S. H., Donovan, C., & Brechman-Toussaint, M. (2000). The treatment of childhood social phobia: The effectiveness of a social skills training-based, cognitive-behavioral intervention, with and without parental involvement. *Journal of Child Psychology and Psychiatry, 41*(6), 713–726.

Stolberg, A. L., & Garrison, K. M. (1985). Evaluating a primary prevention program for children of divorce: The Divorce Adjustment project. *American Journal of Community Psychology, 13*, 111–124.

Stolberg, A. L., & Mahler, J. L. (1994). Enhancing treatment gains in a school-based intervention for children of divorce through skill training, parental involvement, and transfer procedures. *Journal of Consulting and Clinical Psychology, 62*, 147–156.

Stoolmiller, M, Duncan, T., Bank, L., & Patterson, G. (1993). Some problems and solutions to the study of change: Significant patterns of client resistance. *Journal of Consulting and Clinical Psychology, 61*, 920–928.

Strupp, H., & Anderson, T. (1997). On the limitations of therapy manuals. *Clinical Psychology: Science and Practice, 4*, 76–82.

Tang, T., & DeRubeis, R. (1999). Sudden gains and critical sessions in cognitive-behavioral therapy for depression. *Journal of Consulting and Clinical Psychology, 67*, 894–904.

Weersing, V. R., & Weisz, J. (2002). Mechanisms of action in youth psychotherapy. *Journal of Child Psychology and Psychiatry, 43*, 3–29.

Weisz, J. (2000, Spring). Lab-clinic differences and what we can do about them: The clinic-based treatment development model. *Clinical Child Psychology Newsletter, 15*, 1–3.

Weisz, J., Huey, S., & Weersing, R. (1998). Psychotherapy outcome research with children and adolescents: The state of the art. *Advances in Clinical Child Psychology, 20*, 49–91.

CHAPTER 14

Empirically Supported Treatments for Children and Adolescents

THOMAS H. OLLENDICK, NEVILLE J. KING, and BRUCE F. CHORPITA

A little over 50 years ago, Eysenck (1952) published his now (in)famous review of the effects of adult psychotherapy. Boldly, he asserted that psychotherapy practices in vogue at that time were no more effective than the simple passage of time (i.e., spontaneous remission). Subsequently, Levitt (1957, 1963) reviewed the child psychotherapy literature and offered a similar conclusion. These reviews were unsettling inasmuch as they led many clinicians and researchers to question the continued viability of the psychotherapy enterprise for both adults and children.[1]

Fortunately, as noted by Kazdin (2000), these reviews also served as a wake-up call to the professions of child psychiatry and clinical child psychology. Advances in the study of developmental psychopathology, psychiatric diagnostic nomenclature, assessment and treatment practices, and experimental designs for the evaluation of treatment process and outcome all have occurred subsequent to those reviews. These developments, in turn, resulted in well over 1,500 studies (Durlak, Wells, Cotton, & Johnson, 1995, Kazdin, 2000) and four major meta-analyses examining the effects of child therapy (Casey & Berman, 1985; Kazdin, Bass, Ayers, & Rodgers, 1990; Weisz, Weiss, Alicke, & Klotz, 1987; Weisz, Weiss, Han, Granger, & Morton, 1995). As noted by Weersing and Weisz (2002), there is little doubt these days that child psychotherapy results in beneficial impacts on the lives of children and their families. Consistently, reviews of the literature now show that therapy for children outperforms waiting-list and attention–placebo conditions; moreover, in several studies, it is becoming clear that some forms of therapy work better than other forms. As a result, much progress has been made, and we can conclude that the fields of clinical child psychology and child psychiatry have moved beyond the question "Does psychotherapy work for children?" to identify the efficacy of *specific* treatments for children who present with *specific* behavioral, emotional, and social problems. The field has moved from the generic question of whether psychotherapy "works" at all for children to a more specific one that seeks to determine the evidence base for various treatments and the conditions under which they are effective. These times are exciting for the field of child therapy research, and the various chapters in this volume attest to what we know and what we need yet to learn in treating various problems and disorders of youth.

This chapter reviews some of the early work undertaken to identify empirically supported psychosocial treatments for children and raises a series of critical issues attendant to this movement. First, it is acknowledged that this movement is part of the larger zeitgeist referred to as "evidence-based medicine" (Sackett, Richardson, Rosenberg, & Haynes, 1997, 2000), which we refer to here as "evidence-based practice." Evidence-based practice is at its core an approach to knowledge and a strategy for improving performance outcomes (Ollendick & King, 2004). It is not wedded to any one theoretical position or orientation. Rather, it holds that treatments, of whatever theoretical orientation, need to be based on objective and scientifically credible evidence—evidence that is obtained largely from randomized clinical trials (RCTs). In an RCT, children with a specific presenting problem are randomly assigned to one treatment or another or to a control condition, such as a waiting list or attention–placebo condition, and the effects of these conditions are compared. Although such a design is not fail-safe, it appears to be the best strategy for ruling out biases and expectations (on the part of the child, the child's parents, and the therapist) that can result in misleading findings. By its nature, evidence-based practice also values, albeit less highly, information or opinions obtained from observational studies, logical intuition, personal experiences, and the testimony of experts. Such evidence is not necessarily "wrong" or "undesired," but it is less credible and acceptable from a scientific, evidentiary-based standpoint (i.e., it occupies a lower rung on the ladder of evidentiary support).

The movement to develop, identify, disseminate, and use empirically supported psychosocial treatments (initially referred to as empirically "validated" treatments; see Chambless, 1996; Chambless & Hollon, 1998) has been a controversial one. On the surface, it hardly seemed possible that anyone could or would object to the initial report developed by the Society of Clinical Psychology (Division 12) of the American Psychological Association in 1995 or that the movement associated with it would be contested. Surely, identifying, developing, and disseminating treatments that "work" and possess empirical support should be encouraged, not discouraged, especially by a profession that is committed to the welfare of those whom it serves.

Sensible as this may seem, the task force report not only was controversial, but also, unfortunately, served to foster a divide within the profession of clinical psychology and allied mental health disciplines (Ollendick & King, 2000, 2004). In this chapter, we first define empirically supported treatments and then briefly examine the current status of such treatments. In doing so, we hope to illustrate the potential value of these treatments. Other chapters in this volume provide in-depth detail on the efficacy of these treatments for specific problems and disorders. We also illustrate and discuss some of the lingering and contentious issues associated with empirically supported treatments and their development and promulgation. Finally, we conclude our discourse by offering recommendations for future research and practice.

ON THE NATURE OF EMPIRICALLY SUPPORTED TREATMENTS

In 1995, the Society of Clinical Psychology Task Force on Promotion and Dissemination of Psychological Procedures published its report on empirically validated psychological treatments. The task force comprised members who represented a number of theoretical orientations, including psychodynamic, interpersonal, cognitive-behavioral, and systemic points of view. This diversity in membership was an intentional step taken by the committee to emphasize a commitment to identifying and promulgating *all* psychotherapies of proven worth, not just those emanating from one particular school of thought. Defining empirically validated treatments proved to be a difficult task, however. Of course, from a scientific standpoint no treatment is ever fully validated, and, as noted in the task force report, there are always more questions to ask about any treatment, including questions about the essential components of treatments, client characteristics that predict treatment outcome, and the mechanisms or processes that account for behavior change. In recognition of this state of affairs, the term "empirically supported" was adopted subsequently to describe treatments of scientific value—a term that many agreed was more felicitous than "empirically validated."

Three categories of treatment efficacy were proposed in the 1995 report: (1) *well-established treatments*, (2) *probably efficacious treatments*, and (3) *experimental treatments* (see Table 14.1). The primary distinction between *well-established* and *probably efficacious* treatments was that a well-established treatment should have been shown to be superior to a psychological placebo, pill, or another treatment, whereas a probably efficacious treatment should be shown to be superior only to a waiting-list or no-treatment control condition. In addition, effects supporting a well-established treatment should be demonstrated by at least two different

TABLE 14.1. Criteria for Empirically Validated Treatments

I. Well-established treatments
   A. At least two good between-group design experiments demonstrating efficacy in one or more of the following ways:
      1. Superior to pill or psychological placebo or to another treatment.
      2. Equivalent to an already established treatment in experiments with adequate statistical power (about 30 per group).

   or

   B. A large series of single-case design experiments ($n > 9$) demonstrating efficacy. These experiments must have:
      1. Used good experimental designs.
      2. Compared the intervention to another treatment in A.1.

Further criteria for both A and B:
   C. Experiments must be conducted with treatment manuals.
   D. Characteristics of the client samples must be clearly specified.
   E. Effects must have been demonstrated by at least two different investigators or investigatory teams.

II. Probably efficacious treatments
   A. Two experiments showing the treatment is more effective than a waiting-list control group

   or

   B. One or more experiments meeting the well-established treatment criteria A, C, D, but not E

   or

   C. A small series of single-case design experiments ($n > 3$) otherwise meeting well-established treatment criteria B, C, and D.

---

investigatory teams, whereas the effects of a probably efficacious treatment need not be (the effects might be demonstrated in two studies from the same investigator, for example). For both types of empirically supported treatments, characteristics of the clients should be well specified (e.g., age, sex, ethnicity, diagnosis), and the clinical trials should be conducted with treatment manuals. Furthermore, it was required that the outcomes of treatment should be demonstrated in "good" group design studies or a series of controlled single-case design studies. "Good" designs were those in which it was reasonable to conclude that the benefits observed were due to the effects of treatment and not due to chance or confounding factors such as the passage of time, the effects of psychological assessment, or the presence of different types of clients in the various treatment conditions (Chambless & Hollon, 1998; see also Kazdin, 1998, and Kendall, Flannery-Schroeder, & Ford, 1999, for a fuller discussion of research design issues). Ideally, and as noted earlier, treatment efficacy should be demonstrated in RCTs—designs in which patients are assigned randomly to treatment or comparison conditions—or carefully controlled single-case experiments and their group analogues. Finally, *experimental* treatments were those treatments not yet shown to be at least probably efficacious. This category was intended to capture treatments frequently used in clinical practice but that had not yet been fully evaluated or newly developed ones not yet put to the test of scientific scrutiny. The development of new treatments was strongly encouraged. It was also noted that treatments could "move" from one category to another dependent on the empirical support available for that treatment *over time*. For example, an experimental procedure might move into probably efficacious or well-established status as new findings became available. The categorical system was intended to be a dynamic one, not a static or fixed one.

EMPIRICALLY SUPPORTED PSYCHOSOCIAL TREATMENTS FOR CHILD BEHAVIOR PROBLEMS AND DISORDERS

The 1995 Task Force Report identified 18 well-established treatments and 7 probably efficacious treatments, using the criteria described earlier and presented in Table 14.1. Of these 25 efficacious treatments, only *three* well-established treatments for children (behavior modification for developmentally disabled individuals, behavior modification for enuresis and encopresis, and parent training programs for children with oppositional behavior) and *one* probably efficacious treatment for children (habit reversal and control techniques for children with tics and related disorders) were identified. As noted in that report, the list of empirically supported treatments was intended to be representative of efficacious treatments, not exhaustive. In recognition of the need to identify additional psychosocial treatments that were effective with children, concurrent task forces were set up by the Society of Clinical Psychology and its offspring, the Society of Clinical Child and Adolescent Psychology (Division 53 of the American Psychological Association). The two independent task forces joined efforts and in 1998 published their collective reviews in the *Journal of Clinical Child Psychology*. Reviews of empirically supported treatments for children with autism, anxiety disorders, attention-deficit/hyperactivity disorder (ADHD), depression, and oppositional and conduct problem disorders were included in the special issue. As noted by Lonigan, Elbert, and Johnson (1998), the goal was not to generate an exhaustive list of treatments that met criteria for empirically supported treatments; rather, the goal was to focus on a number of high-frequency problems encountered in clinical and other settings serving children with mental health problems. As such, a number of problem areas were not reviewed (e.g., bipolar disorder, childhood schizophrenia), and the identification of empirically supported treatments for these problem areas remains to be accomplished, even to this day. Overall, the goal was to identify effective psychosocial treatments for a limited number of frequently occurring disorders in childhood.

In a recent review of empirically supported psychological interventions for adults *and* children published in the *Annual Review of Psychology*, Chambless and Ollendick (2001) noted that other work groups have also been instrumental in identifying empirically supported treatments for children and adults. Roth and Fonagy (1996) and Nathan and Gorman (1998) have identified other treatments and evaluated many of the same ones identified by the Society of Clinical Psychology and the Society of Clinical Child and Adolescent Psychology. In general, the criteria used by the various groups have been similar to those used by Division 12, although some relatively minor differences are evident (see Chambless & Ollendick, 2001, for details). In Table 14.2, we present a summary of interventions for children with various problems and disorders found to be empirically supported by at least one of these four review groups. In many if not most instances, the same treatments were identified as effective by two or more of these groups.

As shown in Table 14.2, many well-established and probably efficacious treatments have been identified. Yet, we must be somewhat modest inasmuch as, according to these guidelines, no well-established treatments have been identified for the treatment of such common problems as autism, childhood depression, or childhood anxiety. Although a host of interventions appear highly promising and can be described as probably efficacious, it is evident that support for them is relatively modest at this time. Rarely did any one treatment have more than the two requisite studies to support its well-established or probably efficacious status (with the exception of parenting programs for oppositional and conduct problem children and for children with ADHD). It should also be evident that nearly all of these probably efficacious and well-established treatments are based on behavioral and cognitive-behavioral principles (with the notable exception of interpersonal psychotherapy for the treatment of depression). As a result, using these criteria, we do not really know whether frequently practiced treatments from other orientations work or do not work (e.g., play therapy, psychodynamic psychotherapy, family therapy); in many instances, they simply have not been evaluated sufficiently. Still, the value of identifying and promulgating treatments that do have support for their use is apparent. Demonstration of the efficacy of treatments in well-controlled randomized trials may point the way to determining the effectiveness of the treatments in real-life clinical settings (see Chorpita et al., 2002).

ON EMPIRICALLY SUPPORTED TREATMENTS: ISSUES OF CONCERN

As noted by Ollendick (1999), three major concerns about the movement to identify, develop, disseminate, and use empirically supported psychosocial treatments have been raised:

TABLE 14.2. Well-Established and Probably Efficacious Psychosocial Treatments for Children

Problem/ disorder	Psychosocial treatments	
	Well established	Probably efficacious
ADHD	Behavioral parent training Behavior modification in classroom	Cognitive-behavioral therapy
Anxiety	None	Cognitive-behavioral therapy Cognitive-behavioral therapy plus family anxiety management
Autism	None	Contingency management
Depression	None	Behavioral self-control therapy Cognitive-behavioral coping skills
Enuresis	Behavior modification	
Encopresis	Behavior modification	
OCD	None	Exposure/response prevention
ODD/CD	Behavioral parent training Functional family therapy Multisystemic therapy Videotape modeling	Anger control training with stress inoculation Anger coping therapy Assertiveness training Cognitive-behavioral therapy Delinquency prevention program Parent–child interaction therapy Problem-solving skills training Rational-emotive therapy Time out plus signal seat treatment
Phobias	Graduated exposure Participant modeling Reinforced practice	Imaginal desensitization *In vivo* desensitization Live modeling Filmed modeling Cognitive-behavioral therapy

Note. "Anxiety" includes generalized anxiety disorder, separation anxiety disorder, and social phobia; OCD, obsessive–compulsive disorder; ODD, oppositional defiant disorder; CD, conduct disorder. Data from Chambless and Ollendick (2001) and Ollendick and King (2000).

1. Some treatments have been shown to be more effective than others and, as a result, the "Dodo Bird" effect (i.e., no treatment is superior to another) that has long been used to characterize the state of psychosocial treatment interventions can no longer be asserted.
2. Use of treatment manuals might lead to mechanical, inflexible interventions, and "manually driven" treatments might stifle creativity and innovation in the therapy process.
3. Treatments shown to be effective in randomized clinical trials and based

largely in university-based research settings might not generalize or transport to "real-life" clinical practice settings.

What is the status of these concerns for empirically supported treatments for children, and how might they be addressed? In the sections that follow, we address these issues in some detail.

Differential Effectiveness of Psychosocial Treatments

Regarding the first issue, our previous reviews of the literature (Ollendick & King, 1998, 2000) as well as the present one reveals a rather alarming set of findings. It is obvious that interventions other than behavioral or cognitive-behavioral ones have not been examined adequately in the controlled treatment outcome literature and therefore cannot be said to be well-established or probably efficacious. For example, across such frequently occurring problem areas as depression, phobias, anxiety, ADHD, oppositional behaviors, and conduct problems, *no* randomized controlled trials using "good" experimental designs have been identified for psychodynamic psychotherapies or family systems therapies (with the exception of research in the area of oppositional behavior, in which psychodynamic and family systems interventions have been shown to be *less* efficacious than behavioral parenting programs; see Brestan & Eyberg, 1998). In addition, the efficacy of interpersonal psychotherapy (Mufson et al., 1994; Mufson, Weissman, Moreau, & Garfinkel, 1999; Rosello & Bernal, 1999) has only been established in the treatment of depression in adolescents. Inasmuch as these and many other treatments have not been evaluated systematically, we simply do not know whether or not they are effective.

Although behavioral and cognitive-behavioral treatment (CBT) procedures have been shown to be effective and to fare better than other interventions (a conclusion identical to that arrived at in meta-analytic studies of treatment outcomes with children; see Weisz et al., 1987, 1995, for reviews indicating the superiority of behavioral over "nonbehavioral" treatments), a word of caution needs to be inserted, because the evidence base for these conclusions is limited and not as strong as we would like. For example, we were able to identify only two well-established psychosocial treatments for specific phobias in children (participant modeling, reinforced practice), two well-established psychosocial treatments for ADHD (behavioral parent training, operant classroom management), and two well-established psychosocial treatments for oppositional and conduct problems (Webster-Stratton's videotape modeling parent training, Patterson's social learning parent training program). Granted, and as summarized in Table 14.2, additional support for the treatment of these and other disorders is available from treatments designated as "probably efficacious," including CBT for the anxiety disorders and interpersonal psychotherapy and CBT for the mood disorders. Still, the corpus of research is not strong at this time.

Given the somewhat limited state of evidence for empirically supported psychosocial treatments, we pose the obvious question for continued use of frequently practiced treatments in clinical settings: "What is the current status of 'treatment as usual' in clinical practice settings, and should such treatments continue to be used until more empirical support is available? How effective is treatment as usual? Weisz, Huey, and Weersing (1998) examined this question in a reanalysis of their 1995 meta-analytic study. They searched for studies that involved treatment of clinic-referred children who were treated in service-oriented clinics or clinical agencies and who were treated by practicing clinicians. Nine candidate studies, spanning a period of 50 years, were identified that compared treatment as usual to a control condition in a clinical setting. Effect sizes associated with these nine studies were computed. They ranged from -.40 to +.29, with a mean effect size of .01, falling well below the average effect size (+.70) obtained in their overall meta-analyses of research- and clinic-based treatments. The effect size of .01 indicates that the treated children were no better off than the untreated children following treatment. Clearly, based on these analyses, outcomes associated with treatment as usual are disquieting, if not alarming.

Bickman and his colleagues reported similar outcomes in their examination of a comprehensive mental health services program for children (Bickman, 1996; Bickman et al., 1995). Popularly known as the Fort Bragg Project, the U.S. Army spent over $80 million to provide an organized continuum of mental health care (organized and coordinated by a case manager) to children and their families and to test its cost–effectiveness relative to a more conventional and less comprehensive intervention (treatment as usual) in a matched comparison site. Although there was good evidence that the program produced better access to treatment and higher levels of client satisfaction, the program was significantly more costly, and it failed to demonstrate clinical and functional outcomes superior to those in the comparison site. In brief, the Fort Bragg children and their families received more interventions at a higher cost, but their outcomes were not improved by the increased intensity of treatment and cost. Moreover, neither treatment produced gains that approached those found in clinical trials reported by Weisz and colleagues (1995) in their meta-analytic review.

Finally, in a study conducted by Weiss, Catron, Harris, and Phung (1999), an RCT was used to ascertain the effectiveness of child psychotherapy as typically delivered ("treatment as usual") in a school setting. A total of 160 children who presented with problems of anxiety, depression, aggression, and attention were randomly assigned to treatment and control conditions. Children were enrolled in normal elementary and middle schools, and their mean age was 10.3 years. Treatment was provided by mental health professionals hired through regular clinic practices (six were master's-level clinicians and one was a doctoral-level clinical psychologist); therapists reported favoring psychodynamic–humanistic approaches over cognitive and behavioral ones. Treatment itself was open-ended (i.e., not guided by manuals) and delivered over an extended 2-year period on an "as-needed" and individualized basis. Overall, results of the trial provided little support for the effectiveness of "treatment as usual" in this setting. In fact, treatment produced an overall effect size of -0.08, indicating that the treatment was no better than the control condition in which children simply received academic tutoring. Even so, parents of children who received treatment reported higher levels of satisfaction with the services than parents of children in the academic tutoring condition.

These results along with those of Bickman and colleagues, in addition to those summarized by Weisz and colleagues (1998) in their meta-anlaytic review, argue for the importance of developing, validating, and transporting effective treatments to clinical settings. Apparently, "treatment as usual" is not very effective treatment when it is compared to nontherapy alternatives (e.g., tutoring) or no treatment—such "treatments" have little support for their ongoing use and remind us of the conclusions derived by Levitt (1957, 1963)—namely, "treatment as usual" may be no more effective than the mere passage of time. In fact, these findings suggest that, for some children, treatment may be detrimental to their ongoing functioning.

One final comment should be offered about the ethics of continuing to provide treatments that have not been shown to be helpful to children and their families and, in fact, in some instances have been shown to be harmful (recall that the effect sizes for the nine clinic-based studies reviewed by Weisz and colleagues (1998) ranged from -.40 to +.29 and that the effect size reported was -.08). As psychologists, the identification, promulgation, and use of empirically supported treatments is certainly in accord with ethical standards asserting that psychologists "should rely on scientifically and professional derived knowledge when making scientific or professional judgments" (Canter, Bennett, Jones, & Nagy, 1994, p. 36). Yet, as noted in a lively debate on this issue (Eifert, Schulte, Zvolensky, Lejuez, & Lau, 1998; Persons, 1998; Zvolensky & Eifert, 1998, 1999), the identification and use of empirically supported treatments represent a two-edged sword. On the one hand, it might seem unethical to use a treatment that has not been empirically supported; on the other hand, inasmuch as few empirically supported treatments have been developed, it might be unethical to delimit or restrict practice to those problem areas and disorders for which treatment efficacy has been established (Ollendick & Davis, 2004). What, after all, should we do in instances in which children and their families present with problems for which empirically supported treatments have not yet been developed? Quite obviously, there are no easy answers here. In the final analysis, though, we are supportive of the conclusions reached by Kinscherff (1999):

> Generally, clinicians should develop a formulation of the case and select the best approaches for helping a client from among the procedures in which the clinician is competent. Clinicians should remain informed about advances in treatment, including empirically-supported treatments, and maintain their own clinical skills by learn-

ing new procedures and strengthening their skills in areas in which they are already accomplished. Because there are limitations to how many treatments any one clinician can master, a key professional competence is knowing when to refer for a treatment approach that may be more effective for the client. This, in turn, requires at least a basic ongoing familiarity with the evolution of psychotherapeutic treatments and the scientific basis for them in clinical populations. (p. 4)

We concur.

Until such evidence becomes available, Chorpita and his colleagues have proposed an alternative model to consider regarding how to proceed with selection and evaluation of interventions in the face of insufficient evidentiary support. They suggest an "evidence-based decision-making" model, a model recently implemented in the Hawaii Child and Adolescent Mental Health Division (Chorpita & Donkervoet, 2005; Daleiden & Chorpita, 2005). In the instance in which little or no evidence for a particular treatment is available to the clinician, the therapist is encouraged to use case-specific evidence to guide and test clinical choices. Regular measurement of clinical progress has the potential to provide support for the clinical choices made when evidence from RCTs is not available to us (e.g., Ollendick & Hersen, 1984). This model allows for services to continue in the face of minimal supportive evidence, insofar as clinical and functional improvements are evident *in that individual case*. More generally, this model might also prevent disrupting a "non evidence-based" service plan that might be working, only to bring the service plan more in line with the treatment literature. Given that "usual" care is poorly understood at this time, there is certainly the possibility that a reasonable minority of youths would improve with some of these interventions, and, moreover, they might be adversely affected if switched to a different treatment—even an empirically-supported one without proper clinical justification. Only preliminary evaluation of this alternative model is available at this time (Daleiden, 2004), but it appears to offer promise and accountability.

Manualization of Psychosocial Treatments

The recommendation that well-established and probably efficacious treatments require a treatment manual was the second major source of controversy identified by Ollendick (1999). As noted by Chambless (1996), there were two reasons for this requirement. First, inclusion of a treatment manual leads to the standardization of treatment. In experimental design terms, the manual provides an operational definition of the treatment. That is, a treatment manual provides a description of the treatment that makes it possible to determine whether the treatment, as intended, was actually delivered (i.e., the treatment possesses "integrity"). Second, use of a manual allows other mental health professionals and researchers to know what the treatment actually consisted of and therefore what procedures were supported in the efficacy trial. Manualization (as it has come to be called) is especially important to clarify the many types or variants of therapy. For example, there are many types of cognitive-behavioral therapy or psychodynamic therapy. To say that cognitive-behavioral therapy or psychodynamic therapy is efficacious is largely meaningless. What type of psychodynamic therapy was used in this study? What form of cognitive-behavior therapy was used in that study? There are many interventions and there are many variations of those interventions that fall under any one type of psychotherapy. As Chambless (1996, p. 6) noted, "Brand names are not the critical identifiers. The manuals are."

In response to this controversy about the use of manuals, Chorpita, Daleiden, and Weisz (in press) proposed an alternative model to understanding how to define a treatment protocol. These authors reviewed a set of issues related to the manualization requirement, including the following three primary concerns. First, the requirement that a treatment is defined by its manual implies that revisions to a manual require empirical justification to begin afresh every time a manual is changed or altered in some way. For example, although the Coping Cat (Kendall, Kane, Howard, & Siqueland, 1990) enjoys at least two good randomized clinical trials for the treatment of childhood anxiety disorders (Kendall, 1994; Kendall et al., 1997), the currently available Coping Cat manual (Kendall, 2002) is an updated version of the original. Strict adherence to the manualization principle would indicate that the latter manual is not empirically supported in its present form, a conclusion which seems inappropriate and counterintuitive to good clinical practice (i.e., manuals change based on feedback obtained in using them). Relaxing the manualization standard might allow for small revisions to continue resting on prior empirical support, but then the issue becomes one of defining a boundary. How much change is too much?

The second concern raised by Chorpita and colleagues (in press) is one facing most practice systems and involves the unavailability of manuals for particular problems. For example, there are currently no empirically supported treatment manuals for childhood panic disorder (although a treatment approach based on the work with adults with panic disorder has been proposed and evaluated by Ollendick, 1995b, and Mattis & Ollendick, 2002, with single-case but not RCT support). Under strict interpretation of the Division 12 guidelines, this would imply that any treatment for childhood panic is as good as any other (i.e., none has strong empirical support). Again, this is a conclusion that could be potentially misleading, especially given the strong support for cognitive-behavioral interventions with adults with panic disorder (see Barlow, Gorman, Shear, & Woods, 2000).

Third, Chorpita and colleagues (in press) raised the opposite issue of what to do when more than one manual exists for a given disorder and how clinicians might go about selecting one of them for use. For example, for childhood depression, there are several probably efficacious treatment manuals (Brent,

Kolko, Birmaher, Baugher, & Bridge, 1999; Kaslow & Thompson, 1998), although most are variations of cognitive behavioral approaches. How does a therapist determine which one or ones to use? There are few extant guidelines for how one selects one of the many available treatments, which can inhibit successful adoption of the approaches.

The model proposed to address these concerns involves a new methodology for the identification and selection of "common elements" of evidence-based protocols. Chorpita and colleagues (in press) demonstrated that "practice elements" (e.g., "time out," "exposure") could be reliably coded and then empirically "factored" into groupings representing particular approaches. Each factor yields a practice element profile, which denotes the relative frequency of the occurrence of different practice elements for a particular problem. For example, the practice element profile for childhood anxiety showed that exposure was universally present in the evidence-based protocols coded, and other practice elements such as psychoeducation, relaxation, and self-monitoring were highly common. Such a "common elements" approach represents an alternative to the strict definition of manuals at the level of individual manuals, allowing the grouping of manuals empirically determined to be similar in content. In that manner, the model addresses the three concerns reviewed above, in that the similarity of revised manuals can be empirically defined (e.g., the revised Coping Cat would share the support of the original), unavailability of manuals can be addressed through the construction of a profile averaging across similar problem areas (e.g., a cognitive-behavioral protocol for childhood anxiety would be recommended for panic disorder), and overavailability of manuals can be addressed by creating a master profile that represents the aggregate frequency of approaches (e.g., a clinician could select the manual that is most similar to the depression profile, or could develop a new approach including the elements outlined in the profile). Although this model offers some promising alternatives, its use as an intervention selection or development algorithm awaits additional empirical investigation.

Not surprisingly, the developing model proposed by Chorpita and colleagues (in press) arose in the context of considerable controversy regarding the use of manuals. In recent years, a flood of commentaries—some commendatory, others derogatory—have filled the pages of several major journals, including the *American Psychologist, Australian Psychologist, Journal of Clinical Psychology, Journal of Consulting and Clinical Psychology, Clinical Psychology: Science and Practice, Clinical Psychology Review,* and *Psychotherapy.* Some authors have viewed manuals as "promoting a cookbook mentality" (Smith, 1995), "paint by numbers" (Silverman, 1996), "more of a straightjacket than a set of guidelines" (Goldfried & Wolfe, 1996), "somewhat analogous to cookie cutters" (Strupp & Anderson, 1997), and a "hangman of life" (Lambert, 1998). Others have viewed them in more positive terms (e.g., Chambless & Hollon, 1998; Craighead & Craighead, 1998; Heimberg, 1998; Kendall, 1998; King & Ollendick, 1998; Ollendick, 1995b,

1999; Strosahl, 1998; Wilson, 1996a, 1996b, 1998). Wilson (1998, p. 363), for example, suggested that "the use of standardized, manual-based treatments in clinical practice represents a new and evolving development with far-reaching implications for the field of psychotherapy."

In its simplest form, a treatment manual can be defined as a set of guidelines that instruct or inform the user as to "how to do" a certain treatment (Ollendick, 1999). They specify and, at the same time, standardize treatment. Although many opponents of manual-based treatment support efforts for greater accountability with respect to the effects of psychotherapy, they are concerned that treatments evaluated in research settings will not generalize to "real-life" clinical settings and that manual-based treatments will need to be implemented in a lockstep fashion with little opportunity for flexibility or clinical judgement in implementation of the procedures. Seligman (1995, p. 967), for example, indicated that, unlike the manual-based treatment of controlled laboratory research—in which "a small number of techniques, all within one modality" are delivered in fixed order for a fixed duration—clinical practice is, by necessity, "self-correcting. If one technique is not working, another technique—or even modality—is usually tried." As noted by Wilson (1998), this characterization or depiction of manual-based treatment is simply wrong. A variety of treatments have been "manualized," including those embedded in psychodynamic (e.g., Strupp & Binder, 1984), interpersonal (e.g., Klerman, Weissman, Rounsaville, & Chevron, 1984), and behavioral (Patterson & Gullion, 1968) and cognitive-behavioral theory (e.g., Beck, Rush, Shaw, & Emery, 1979); moreover, these manuals allow for flexible use and, for the most part, are responsive to progress or regress in treatment.

It should be recalled that the movement to manualization of treatment practices existed long before the Task Force issued its report in 1995. Almost 30 years earlier, Patterson and Gullion (1968) published their now-classic book *Living with Children: New Methods for Parents and Teachers*, a "how to" parent and teacher manual that has served as the foundation for many behavioral treatments of oppositional, defiant, and conduct problem children. Not surprisingly, treatment based on this "manual" was one of the first treatments designated as "evidence based." Over a decade prior to the issue of the Task Force Report, Luborsky and DuRubeis (1984) commented upon the potential use of treatment manuals in a paper titled "The Use of Psychotherapy Treatment Manuals: A Small Revolution in Psychotherapy Research Style." Similarly, Lambert and Ogles (1988) indicated that manuals were not new; rather, they noted, manuals have been used to train therapists and define treatments since the 1960s. It seems to us that the 1995 Task Force Report simply reaffirmed a movement that had been present for some years and that had become the unofficial, if not official, policy of the National Institute of Mental Health for funding studies designed to explore the efficacy of various psychotherapies. On the other hand—and this is where its actions became contentious—the Task Force Report asserted that psychotherapies described and operationalized by manuals should not only be identified but also be disseminated to clinical training programs, practicing mental health professionals, the public, and to third-party payors (i.e., insurance companies, health maintenance organizations). Many authors were concerned that such actions were premature and that they would prohibit or, in the least, constrain the practice of those psychotherapies that had not yet been manualized or not yet shown to be efficacious. They also were concerned that the development of new psychotherapies would be curtailed, if not stifled totally. Although these are possible outcomes of the movement to manualize and evaluate psychotherapies, they need not be the inevitable or only outcome. In fact, some have argued that these developments can serve to stimulate additional treatments by systematically examining the parameters of effective treatments as well as the therapeutic mechanisms of change (see Kendall, 1998, and Wilson, 1998, for examples), a position in which we are in full accord.

What is the current status of this movement toward manualization in the treatment of children? First, it should be clear that the studies summarized in our recent reviews of empirically supported treatments for children either used manuals, or the procedures were described in sufficient detail as to not require manuals (as originally suggested by the Task Force Report on Promotion and Dissemination, 1995, and by Chambless et al., 1996). As we noted earlier, manuals are simply guidelines that describe treatment procedures and therapeutic strategies, and in some instances provide an underlying theory of change on which the procedures or techniques are based. Kendall and his colleagues (Kendall, 1998; Kendall & Chu, 2000; Kendall, Chu, Gifford, Hayes, & Nauta, 1998) have addressed some of the issues surrounding use of treatment manuals and have recommended that we undertake systematic research of the issues identified. They identified six (mis)perceptions that plague manual-based treatments: How flexible are they? Do they replace clinical judgment? Do manuals detract from the creative process of therapy? Does a treatment manual reify therapy in a fixed and stagnant fashion, and thereby stifle improvement and change? Are manual-based treatments effective with patients who present with multiple diagnoses or clinical problems? And, are manuals primarily designed for use in research programs, with little or no use or application in service-providing clinics? Although answers to each of these penetrating questions are not yet available, Kendall and his colleagues submit that careful research is needed to explore each of these perceptions. In addition, they provide evidence from their own work with children who have anxiety disorders that at least some of these issues or questions may be pseudo ones. For example, flexibility of treatment implementation is an issue that many critics have raised; accordingly, it should be investigated empirically to determine whether the degree to which a manual is implemented flexibly affects treatment outcome. Does it really make a difference? A recent study by Kendall and Chu (2000) undertook to answer that question.

Flexibility can be defined in a variety of ways; in their research, it was defined as a construct that measures the therapist's adaptive stance to the *specific* situation at hand while adhering *generally* to the instructions and suggestions in the manual. Ratings on the degree to which the manual was implemented in a flexible manner were obtained from 18 different therapists who had implemented their cognitive-behavioral, manual-based treatment for anxious children (Kendall et al., 1992). Flexibility ratings were obtained retrospectively on a 13-item questionnaire, with each item rated on a 1- to 7-point scale as to the extent of flexibility used in implementing treatment (e.g., "The manual suggests that clinicians spend 40–45 minutes of the session teaching the outlined skills to the child and 10–15 minutes of the session playing games. How flexible with this were you?" And, "During therapy sessions, how flexible were you in discussing issues not related to anxiety or directly related to the child's primary diagnoses?"). First of all, results revealed that therapists reported being flexible in their implementation of the treatment plan (both in general and with specific strategies). Second, and perhaps unexpectedly, the indices of flexibility were *not* related to whether the children were comorbid with other disorders *or* to the treatment outcome. The important point here is that flexibility, however defined, is amenable to careful and systematic inquiry. Kendall (1998) asserts that other issues raised by the manualization of treatment are also amenable to empirical investigation, and they need not remain in the area of "heated" speculation.

One additional example may help to illustrate how issues such as flexibility might be addressed empirically. In these studies, primarily conducted with adults, manual-based treatments have been "individualized" in a flexible manner by matching certain characteristics or profiles of the individuals being treated to specific elements or components of previously established effective treatments. These efforts have been labeled "prescriptive matching" by Acierno, Hersen, Van Hasselt, and Ammerman (1994). At the core of this approach is the assumption that an idiographic approach to treatment is more effective in producing positive treatment outcomes than a nomothetic approach (e.g., not all patients who receive the same diagnosis or who present with similar behavior problems are *really* the same—the homogeneity myth put forth some years ago by Kiesler, 1966). For example, in one of these studies, Jacobson and colleagues (1989) designed individually tailored marital therapy treatment plans where the number of sessions and the specific modules selected in each case were determined by the couple's specific needs and presenting problems. Individualized treatments were compared to a standard CBT program. Each was manualized. Although couples treated with individually tailored protocols could not be distinguished from those receiving standardized protocols at posttreatment, a greater proportion of couples receiving standardized treatment showed decrements in marital satisfaction at 6-month follow-up, whereas a majority of those in the individually tailored program maintained their treatment gains. These findings suggest individually tailored programs may help to reduce treatment relapse.

Similar beneficial findings have been obtained in the treatment of adults with depression (Nelson-Gray, Herbert, Herbert, Sigmon, & Brannon, 1990).

In this study, Nelson-Gray et al. assigned adult depressed patients to treatment protocols (e.g., cognitive treatment, social skills treatment) that were either matched or mismatched to presenting problems (e.g., irrational cognitions, social skills problems). Those in the matched conditions fared better than those in the mismatched conditions upon completion of treatment. Similarly, Ost, Jerremalm, and Johansson (1981) examined the efficacy of social skills training and applied relaxation in the treatment of adults with social phobia who were categorized as either "behavioral" or "physiological" responders. Physiological responders benefited most clearly from the applied relaxation training, whereas behavioral responders showed the most benefit from the social skills program. Not all studies with individualized treatments have produced such positive results, however. For example, Schulte, Kunzel, Pepping, and Schulte-Bahrenberg (1992) found that standardized treatment, contrary to expectations, proved more successful than either matched or mismatched treatments in an investigation of adults with agoraphobia or specific phobias. Mersch, Emmelkamp, Bogels and van der Sleen (1989) also failed to demonstrate the value of categorizing adults with social phobia into those with primarily cognitive or behavioral deficiencies and assigning them to matched or mismatched treatments. Matched treatments were not found to be superior to mismatched ones.

In the child arena, Eisen and Silverman (1993, 1998) provided preliminary support for the value of prescriptive matching in the treatment of fearful and anxious children. In the first study, the efficacy of cognitive therapy, relaxation training, and their combination was examined with four overanxious children, 6–15 years of age, using a multiple baseline design across subjects. The children received both relaxation training and cognitive therapy (counterbalanced), followed by a combined treatment that incorporated elements of both treatments. Results suggested that interventions were most effective when they matched the specific problems of the children. That is, children with primary symptoms of worry responded more favorably to cognitive therapy, whereas children with primary symptoms of somatic complaints responded best to relaxation treatment. Similar findings were obtained in the second study (Eisen & Silverman, 1998) with four children between 8 and 12 years of age who were diagnosed with overanxious disorder. The interventions that were prescribed on the basis of a match between the treatment and the response class (cognitive therapy for cognitive symptoms, relaxation therapy for somatic symptoms) produced the greatest changes and resulted in enhanced treatment effectiveness. These findings must be considered preliminary because of limitations associated with the single-case designs used to evaluate their efficacy; to our knowledge, no controlled group design studies have been conducted examining these issues. Nonetheless, these studies and those conducted with adults show yet another possible way of individualizing treatment and exploring flexibility in the use of empirically supported treatment manuals.

In a related vein, Chorpita, Taylor, Francis, Moffitt, and Austin (2004) recently demonstrated the successful application of a "modular" intervention for childhood anxiety that allowed for systematic adaptation of the protocol to client characteristics. The modular approach involved defining each practice technique as an independent module integrated with all others through a coordinating flowchart that served to guide module selection. In that investigation, seven youth with anxiety disorders were successfully treated using a multiple-baseline design. Data on patterns of use suggested that the protocol administration was highly individualized. For example, although all children participated in psychoeducation, exposure, and maintenance exercises, only 29% participated in differential reinforcement strategies, 29% were administered rewards, and 43% participated in formal cognitive exercises. Twenty-nine percent received only the four core components of the manual (self-monitoring, psychoeducation, exposure, and maintenance). The sessions delivered ranged from 5 to 17, and occurred in durations ranging from 7 to 30 weeks (Chorpita, Taylor, et al., 2004).

Although modularity is in some senses compatible with the notion of flexibility, the two properties should not be conflated. For example, Chorpita, Daleiden, and Weisz (2004) outlined a definition of modularity as it applies to intervention design. The authors argued that, although modularity provided a framework for flexibility, a modular protocol could just as easily be static in its delivery, were the data to support such an approach to implementation. The issues are beyond the scope of the present chapter, but it appears that modularity in design has the potential to offer multiple benefits to the intervention development paradigm, including possible improvements to clinical utility and design efficiency.

One final comment on manualization seems important. Recently, some have reminded us that manuals are only a small part of defining the proper treatment operations. For example, Henggeler and Schoenwald (2002) argued that practitioner behavior needs to be examined within a social ecological framework: "Practitioners are embedded in quality assurance systems (e.g., manuals, supervision), which are embedded within organizations, which are embedded within community contexts" (p. 419). These authors demonstrate that the successful implementation of an intervention requires all of these dimensions to work in concert. Thus, although a manual can arguably define the specific treatment operations, the proper implementation of these operations is not guaranteed simply because a manual is present.

If the spirit of the manual requirement is held as true (i.e., it is important to assure proper implementation), then perhaps the specification of these other dimensions bears additional consideration. For example, one should perhaps outline the supervision protocol used for many of the current evidence-based treatments, as each manual was surely tested within a richly supported supervision model relative to community-based usual care. The requirement that the manual only details the clinical operations and not the supervision or quality-assurance operations might falsely imply the primacy of the treatment over its delivery context. We know of no research demonstrating that treatment alone (or supervision alone) universally accounts for successful clinical outcomes.

Along these lines, some have argued that detailed specification of a quality-improvement infrastructure represents similar and perhaps complementary advantages to the use of manuals. Indeed, many of these models support the use of immediate, client-specific evidence in guiding intervention, and consider this "evidence base" as important as the treatment literature evidence base, at least in some contexts (Bickman & Noser, 1999; Daleiden & Chorpita, 2005). Whether future considerations of evidence-based treatments will consider these additional dimensions related to implementation, feasibility, and quality remains to be seen. Ultimately the real answers to these issues await research that examines the use of manualized treatments under different levels of supervision, or conversely examines an "evidence-based" supervision structure with and without the accompanying treatment manual. Only then will the relative importance, necessity, and sufficiency of codified treatment operations become better understood.

Issues with Efficacy and Effectiveness: The Transportability of Treatments

A third concern about the empirically supported or evidence-based treatment movement is evident in differences between what have come to be called *efficacy* studies and *effectiveness* studies (Hibbs, 1998; Hoagwood, Hibbs, Brent, & Jensen, 1995; Ollendick, 1999). Basically, efficacy studies demonstrate that the benefits obtained from a given treatment administered in a fairly standard way (with a treatment manual) are due to the treatment and not due to chance factors or to a variety of other factors that threaten the internal validity of the demonstration of efficacy. These studies are conducted under tightly controlled conditions, typically in laboratory or university settings. Most consist of RCTs and provide clear specification of sample characteristics, features reflective of "good" experimental designs. Appropriate concern has been raised about the exportability of these "laboratory-based" treatments to the real world—the world of clinical practice. Arguments have been mustered that the "subjects" in randomized clinical trials do not represent real-life "clients" or that the "experimenters" in these trials do not represent "clinical therapists" in applied practice settings. Moreover, or so it is argued, the settings themselves are significantly different—ranging from tightly controlled laboratory conditions to ill-defined and highly variable conditions in practice settings. Weisz and colleagues (1995) have referred to practice settings as the "real test," or the "proving ground," of interventions. To many of us, this distinction raises the ever-present concern about the need to build a strong bridge between science and practice, a bridge recommended over 50 years ago and embodied in the Boulder model of clinical training. Building this bridge is admittedly not easy, and a gap between efficacy and effectiveness studies remains.[2]

Nonetheless, it is evident that effectiveness studies that demonstrate the external validity of psychotherapies are very important; moreover, they need to be conducted in a way that will allow us to conclude that the treatments are responsible for the changes observed in our clients, not chance or other extraneous factors. Demonstration of both internal and external validity is important. One should not be viewed as more important than the other (Ollendick & King, 2000). Of course, not all treatments shown to be efficacious in clinical trials research will necessarily be shown to be effective in clinical settings. Such failures may be associated with a host of difficulties, including problems in implementing the treatment procedures in less-controlled clinical settings and the "acceptability" of the efficacious treatments to clients and therapists alike. In the final analysis, whether the effects found in RCTs and conducted in research-based settings generalize to "real-world" clinical settings is an empirical question that awaits additional research (see Kendall & Southam-Gerow, 1995, and Persons & Silberschatz, 1998, for further discussion of these issues).

The issues surrounding transportability and efficacy versus effectiveness studies are numerous (e.g., training of therapists, supervision of therapists, homogeneous/heterogeneous samples, development of manuals, adherence to manuals, competence in executing manual-based treatment, and the acceptability of manual-based treatments to clinicians and clients, among others). Weisz and colleagues (1998) examined these issues in some detail and have identified a set of characteristics frequently associated with child psychotherapy outcome research that distinguishes efficacy from effectiveness research. They are reproduced in Table 14.3 under the headings of "research therapy" and "clinic therapy." As evident in Table 14.3, Weisz and colleagues characterize "research" therapy as serving a relatively homogeneous group of children who exhibit less severe forms of child psychopathology and who present with single-focus problems. More-

TABLE 14.3. Some Characteristics Frequently Associated with Child Psychotherapy in Outcome Research (Research Therapy) and in Clinics (Clinic Therapy)

Research therapy	Clinic therapy
• Recruited cases (less severe, study volunteers)	• Clinic-referred cases (more severe, some coerced into treatment)
• Homogeneous groups	• Heterogeneous groups
• Narrow or single-problem focus	• Broad, multiproblem focus
• Treatment in lab, school settings	• Treatment in clinic, hospital settings
• Researcher as therapist	• Professional career therapists
• Very small caseloads	• Very large caseloads
• Heavy pretherapy preparation	• Little/light pretherapy preparation
• Preplanned, highly structured treatment (manualized)	• Flexible, adjustable treatment (no treatment manual)
• Monitoring of therapist behavior	• Little monitoring of therapist behavior
• Behavioral methods	• Nonbehavioral methods

over, they suggest that such studies are conducted in research laboratories or school settings with clinicians who are "really" researchers, who are carefully trained and supervised, and who have "light" client loads. Finally, such studies typically use manualized treatments of a behavioral or cognitive-behavioral nature. In contrast, "clinic" therapy is characterized by heterogeneous groups of children who are frequently referred for treatment and who have a large and diverse range of clinical problems. Treatment in such settings is of course delivered in a clinic, school, or hospital setting by "real" therapists who have "heavy" caseloads, little pretherapy training, and who are not carefully supervised or monitored. Finally, treatment manuals are rarely used, and the primary form of treatment is nonbehavioral.

Clearly, a number of differences are evident. Although such distinctions are important to make, in our opinion they tend to be broad generalizations that may or may not be true for various studies conducted in laboratory *or* clinical settings. Moreover, they may serve to accentuate differences in types of studies rather than to define areas of rapprochement and, inadvertently, create a chasm, rather than a bridge, between laboratory and clinic research. We shall illustrate how these distinctions become blurred by describing three studies: (1) a "research" therapy studied conducted by Kendall and colleagues (1997), (2) a "clinic" therapy study conducted by Weiss and colleagues (1999), and (3) a study examining the transportability of effective treatment into a practice setting (Tynan, Schuman, & Lampert, 1999).

In the Kendall and colleagues (1997) study, the efficacy of CBT for anxious children was compared to a wait-list condition. Efficacy of treatment was determined at posttreatment and at 1-year follow-up. An RCT was undertaken, detailed but flexible manuals were used, and the therapists were well trained and supervised graduate clinicians who carried "light" clinical loads. Treatment was conducted in a university-based clinic. Ninety-four children (ages 9–13 years) and their parents, referred from multiple community sources (not volunteers or normal children in school settings), participated. All received primary anxiety disorder diagnoses (attesting to the relative severity of their problems), and the majority were comorbid with other disorders (affirming multiple problems in these children, including other anxiety disorders, affective disorders, and disruptive behavior disorders). In short, a relatively heterogeneous sample of children with an anxiety disorder was treated. Treatment was found to be highly effective both at posttreatment and 1-year follow-up. In reference to Table 14.3, it is evident that some of the characteristics associated with "research" therapy obtained and that in at least some respects "clinic" therapy was enacted.

In the Weiss and colleagues (1999) study previously described, treatment as routinely practiced in an outpatient setting (a school setting) was evaluated by comparing it to an attention control placebo (academic tutoring). The seven therapists were hired through standard clinic practices (six were master's-level clinicians and one was a doctoral-level clinical psychologist) and were allowed to select and use whatever interventions they believed were necessary (most selected and used psychodynamic–humanistic or cognitive strategies). No manuals were used. They received no additional clinical training as part of the clinical trial and were provided with a minimal amount of supervision. One hundred and sixty children participated and were randomly assigned to one of the two "experimental" conditions. Children were identified in the school setting and presented with problems of anxiety, depression, aggression, and inattention. Diagnostic data were not obtained; however, the identified children were thought to represent a heterogeneous sample of children with multiple and serious problems. As noted earlier, traditional therapy, as implemented in this study, was determined to be largely ineffective. In reference to Table 14.3, it is evident that only some of the characteristics of "clinic" therapy obtained and that at least in some respects "research" therapy was examined.

Finally, in the study undertaken by Tynan and colleagues (1999), the transportability of a well-established treatment for oppositional defiant disorder and ADHD in children between 5 and 11 years of age (behavioral parent management training and child social skills training) was examined in a "real-life" clinical setting (a child psychiatry outpatient clinic). Therapy was conducted in a group format. All children who were referred for ADHD or oppositional defiant disorder were assigned to the groups as the first line of treatment. Parents and children were treated in separate groups. Diagnostic interviews were conducted, and the children met diagnostic criteria for disruptive behavior disorders; a majority were comorbid with other disorders. Problems were judged by the clinicians to be serious. Treatment was manualized and therapists in this clinical setting were carefully trained and supervised by the primary author. No control condition was used and no follow-up data were reported. Nonetheless, the treatment was reported to be highly efficacious at posttreatment (effect size of .89 from pretreatment to posttreatment). Although several methodological problems exist with this "uncontrolled" clinical trial, it nicely illustrates the potential to extend findings from laboratory settings to clinical settings. This study also illustrates characteristics of "research" therapy and "clinic" therapy. To which is it more similar? These three studies illustrate that demarcations between efficacy and effectiveness studies are not always easy or true to form. Perhaps more importantly, they illustrate the types of studies that need to be conducted that will bridge the gap between research and clinic settings.

Chorpita (2003) has argued that the efficacy–effectiveness distinction involves at least four different levels of consideration. With true efficacy research, the point is to determine the relation between therapeutic practices or strategies and outcomes (e.g., Chambless & Hollon, 1998; Chambless & Ollendick, 2001). With such research, "upstream" elements are typically controlled (i.e., children and families are carefully screened and selected, therapists are highly trained and have explicit allegiance to the investigator, and supervision is intensive and often provided by a national expert). Under conditions that maximize these upstream elements, we have some confidence that fidelity to a particular protocol matched to a certain problem is related to positive results.

The second type of research, which would be considered effectiveness research by many and has been termed "transportability research" by Schoenwald and Hoagwood (2001), speaks to whether a particular intervention might be promising for delivery in a true practice setting. Essentially, transportability research allows for inferences about the performance of a protocol under a wider range of client conditions that closely approximate or are equivalent to client conditions in true practice settings, but at the same time still maximizing therapist and supervisor performance in a contrived laboratory setting. This approach would allow us to say, for example, that "parent training is a promising approach for real-world cases of oppositional youth."

A third type of approach to be considered involves the use of system employees (e.g., school counselors, private practitioners) as therapists (Chorpita, 2003). Schoenwald and Hoagwood (2001) termed this approach "dissemination" research, in that it relates to the performance of a protocol once deployed into a system. This research is likely what is most commonly implied when one encounters the term "effectiveness," and it allows for inferences about the performance of the intervention under highly naturalistic conditions (e.g., Henggeler, Schoenwald, Borduin, Rowland, & Cunningham, 1998). Nevertheless, in such research the supervision is still provided by the investigator team, and thus questions remain about whether the same practice standards would be maintained after the investigator team withdrew from the system.

The final question regarding system independence can only be addressed directly by "system evaluation" research, in which the system to be evaluated and the investigative team are fully independent. This strategy would allow the final inference to be made: whether treatment operations can lead to positive outcomes when a system stands entirely on its own. Although studies of entire systems do exist (Bickman, 1996; Bickman, Lambert, Andrade, & Penaloza, 2000; Burns, Farmer, Angold, Costello, & Behar, 1996), these do not truly represent evidence-based system evaluation research (Chorpita, 2003), because they have not specified evidence-based interventions in one of the experimental conditions but rather have traditionally compared different arrangements of "usual care." Consequently, the outcomes of these studies primarily show differences in practice patterns (e.g., access to system, dropout rates) but are unsupportive with respect to differential outcomes at the level of the child (Bickman, 1999).

This absence of favorable child outcomes noted earlier in TAU practices such as the Fort Bragg Demonstration and other similar investigations is perhaps due to the fact that such "systems" studies have not controlled and specified the "downstream" elements involving specific therapeutic practices. Thus, there is no guarantee that strategies at the higher level (e.g., care coordination, quality assurance) will not be neutralized or compromised by poor strategies at the lower level (see Weisz, Han, & Valeri, 1997). Ultimately, the understanding of what works in system contexts awaits not only new research but also new paradigms of research, in which treatments and systems are simultaneously manipulated.

CONCLUSIONS

We have discussed salient issues associated with empirically supported treatments and determined their significance for psychosocial treatments with children and adolescents. We concluded that some treatments are more effective than others, that manualization need not be a stumbling block to providing effective therapy in both research and clinic settings, and that the transportability of treatments from the laboratory setting to the practice setting is feasible (although still being tested). We have also noted that tensions remain about each of these issues, and we have illustrated various avenues that might lead to a possible rapprochement.

Somewhat unexpectedly, however, our present review of empirically supported psychosocial treatments for children reveals that our armamentarium is relatively "light" and that much more work remains to be done. We really do not have very many psychosocial treatments that possess well-established status in *research* settings, let alone clinical settings. This is an exciting time, however, and we have the tools in our armamentarium to close the often lamented gap between laboratory and clinic studies and to arrive at a rapprochement between clinical research and clinical practice. Children and their families presenting at our clinics deserve our concerted attention to further the true synthesis of these approaches and to transform our laboratory findings into rich and clinically sensitive practices.

NOTES

1. The term "children" is used throughout to refer to both children and adolescents, unless otherwise specified.
2. Although the gap is being closed, as has been illustrated in this chapter.

REFERENCES

Acierno, R., Hersen, M., Van Hasselt, V. B., & Ammerman, R. T. (1994). Remedying the Achilles heel of behavior research and therapy: Prescriptive matching of intervention and psychopathology. *Journal of Behavior Therapy and Experimental Psychiatry, 25*, 179–188.

Barlow, D. H., Gorman, J. M., Shear, M. K., & Woods, S. W. (2000). Cognitive-behavioral therapy, imipramine, or their combination for panic disorder: A randomized controlled trial. *Journal of the American Medical Association, 283*, 2529–2536.

Beck, A. T., Rush, A. J., Shaw, B. F., & Emery, G. (1979). *Cognitive therapy of depression*. New York: Guilford Press.

Bickman, L. (1996). A continuum of care: More is not always better. *American Psychologist, 51*, 689–701.

Bickman, L. (1999). Practice makes perfect and other myths about mental health services. *American Psychologist, 54,* 965–977.

Bickman, L., Guthrie, P. R., Foster, E. M., Lambert, E. W., Summerfelt, W. T., Breda, C. S., & Heflinger, C. A. (1995). *Evaluating managed mental health services: The Fort Bragg experiment.* New York: Plenum Press.

Bickman, L., Lambert, E. W., Andrade, A. R., & Penaloza, R. V. (2000). The Fort Bragg continuum of care for children and adolescents: Mental health outcomes over 5 years. *Journal of Consulting and Clinical Psychology, 68,* 710–716.

Bickman, L., & Noser, K. (1999). Meeting the challenges in the delivery of child and adolescent mental health services in the next millennium: The continuous quality improvement approach. *Applied and Preventive Psychology, 8,* 247–255.

Burns, B. J., Farmer, E. M. Z., Angold, A., Costello, E. J., & Behar, L. (1996). A randomized trial of case management for youths with serious emotional disturbance. *Journal of Clinical Child Psychology, 25,* 476–486.

Brent, D. A., Kolko, D. J., Birmaher, B., Baugher, M., & Bridge, J. (1999). A clinical trial for adolescent depression: Predictors of additional treatment in the acute and follow-up phases of the trial. *Journal of the American Academy of Child and Adolescent Psychiatry, 38,* 263–270.

Brestan, E. V., & Eyberg, S. M. (1998). Effective psychosocial treatments of conduct-disordered children and adolescents: 29 years, 82 studies, and 5,272 kids. *Journal of Clinical Child Psychology, 27,* 179–188.

Canter, M. B., Bennett, B. E., Jones, S. E., & Nagy, T. F. (1994). *Ethics for psychologists: A commentary on the APA ethics code.* Washington, DC: American Psychological Association.

Casey, R. J., & Berman, J. S. (1985). The outcome of psychotherapy with children. *Psychological Bulletin, 98,* 388–400.

Chambless, D. L. (1996). In defense of dissemination of empirically supported psychological interventions. *Clinical Psychology: Science and Practice, 3,* 230–235.

Chambless, D. L., & Hollon, S. D. (1998). Defining empirically supported therapies. *Journal of Consulting and Clinical Psychology, 66,* 7–18.

Chambless, D. L., & Ollendick, T. H. (2001). Empirically supported psychological interventions: Controversies and evidence. *Annual Review of Psychology, 52,* 685–716.

Chorpita, B. F. (2003). The frontier of evidence-based practice. In A. E. Kazdin & J. R. Weisz (Eds.), *Evidence-based psychotherapies for children and adolescents* (pp. 42–59). New York: Guilford Press.

Chorpita, B. F., Daleiden, E., & Weisz, J. R. (2005). Identifying and selecting the common elements of evidence based interventions: A distillation and matching model. *Mental Health Services Research, 7,* 5–20.

Chorpita, B. C., Daleiden, E., & Weisz, J. R. (in press). Modularity in the design and application of therapeutic interventions. *Applied and Preventive Psychology.*

Chorpita, B. F., & Donkervoet, C. M. (2005). Implementation of the Felix Consent Decree in Hawaii: The impact of policy and practice development efforts on service delivery. In R. G. Steele & M. C. Roberts (Eds.), *Handbook of mental health services for children, adolescents, and families* (pp. 317–332). New York: Kluwer.

Chorpita, B. F., Taylor, A. A., Francis, S. E., Moffitt, C. E., & Austin, A. A. (2004). Efficacy of modular cognitive behavior therapy for childhood anxiety disorders. *Behavior Therapy, 35,* 263–287.

Chorpita, B. F., Yim, L. M., Donkervoet, J. C., Arensdorf, A., Amundsen, M. J., McGee, C., et al. (2002). Toward large-scale implementation of empirically supported treatments for children: A review and observations by the Hawaii Empirical Basis to Services Task Force. *Clinical Psychology: Science and Practice, 9,* 165–190.

Craighead, W. E., & Craighead, L. W. (1998). Manual-based treatments: Suggestions for improving their clinical utility and acceptability. *Clinical Psychology: Science and Practice, 5,* 403–407.

Daleiden E. (2004). *Child status measurement: System performance improvements during Fiscal Years 2002–2004.* Honolulu: Hawaii Department of Health Child and Adolescent Mental Health Division. Available online at www.hawaii.gov/health/mental-health/camhd/resources/rpteval/ge/library/pdf/er-ge/ge010.pdf

Daleiden, E., & Chorpita, B. F. (2005). From data to wisdom: Quality improvement strategies supporting large-scale implementation of evidence based services. In B. J. Burns & K. E. Hoagwood (Eds.), *Child and adolescent psychiatric clinics of North America* (pp. 329–349). Philadelphia: W. B. Saunders.

Durlak, J. A., Wells, A. M., Cotton, J. K., & Johnson, S. (1995). Analysis of selected methodological issues in child psychotherapy research. *Journal of Clinical Child Psychology, 24,* 141–148.

Eiffert, G. H., Schulte, D., Zvolensky, M. J., Lejuez, C. W., & Lau, A. W. (1998). Manualized behavior therapy: Merits and challenges. *Behavior Therapy, 28,* 499–509.

Eisen, A. R., & Silverman, W. K. (1993). Should I relax or change my thoughts? A preliminary examination of cognitive therapy, relaxation training, and their combination with overanxious children. *Journal of Cognitive Psychotherapy, 7,* 265–279.

Eisen, A. R., & Silverman, W. K. (1998). Prescriptive treatment for generalized anxiety disorder in children. *Behavior Therapy, 29,* 105–121.

Eysenck, H. J. (1952). The effects of psychotherapy: An evaluation. *Journal of Consulting Psychology, 16,* 319–324.

Goldfried, M. R., & Wolfe, B. E. (1996). Psychotherapy practice and research: Repairing a strained alliance. *American Psychologist, 51,* 1007–1016.

Heimberg, R. G. (1998). Manual-based treatment: An essential ingredient of clinical practice in the 21st century. *Clinical Psychology: Science and Practice, 5,* 387–390.

Henggeler, S. W., & Schoenwald, S. K. (2002). Treatment manuals: Necessary, but far from sufficient. *Clinical Psychology: Science and Pratcice, 9,* 419–420.

Henggeler, S. W., Schoenwald, S. K., Borduin, C. M., Rowland, M. D., & Cunningham, P. B. (1998). *Multisystemic treatment of antisocial behavior in children and adolescents.* New York: Guilford Press.

Hibbs, E. D. (1998). Improving methodologies for the treatment of child and adolescent disorders: Introduction. *Journal of Abnormal Child Psychology, 26,* 1–6.

Hoagwood, K., Hibbs, E., Brent, D., & Jensen, P. (1995). Introduction to the special section: Efficacy and effectiveness in studies of child and adolescent psychotherapy. *Journal of Consulting and Clinical Psychology, 63,* 683–687.

Jacobson, N. S., Schmaling, K. B., Holtzworth-Munroe, A., Katt, J. L., Wood, L. F., & Follette, V. M. (1989). Research-structured vs clinically flexible versions of social learning-based marital therapy. *Behaviour Research and Therapy, 27,* 173–180.

Kaslow, N. J., & Thompson, M. P. (1998). Applying the criteria for empirically supported treatments to studies of psychosocial interventions for child and adolescent depression. *Journal of Clinical Child Psychology, 27,* 146–155.

Kazdin, A. E. (1998). *Research design in clinical psychology* (3rd ed.). Boston: Allyn & Bacon.

Kazdin, A. E. (2000). Developing a research agenda for child and adolescent psychotherapy. *Archives of General Psychiatry, 57,* 829–836.

Kazdin, A. E., Bass, D., Ayers, W. A., & Rodgers, A. (1990). Empirical and clinical focus of child and adolescent psychotherapy research. *Journal of Consulting and Clinical Psychology, 58,* 729–740.

Kendall, P. C. (1994). Treating anxiety disorders in children: Results of a randomized clinical trial. *Journal of Consulting and Clinical Psychology, 62,* 100–110.

Kendall, P. C. (1998). Directing misperceptions: Researching the issues facing manual-based treatments. *Clinical Psychology: Science and Practice, 5,* 396–399.

Kendall, P. C. (2002). *Coping Cat therapist manual.* Ardmore, PA: Workbook Publishing.

Kendall, P. C., Chansky, T. E., Kane, M. T., Kim, R. S., Kortlander, E., Ronan, K. R., et al. (1992). *Anxiety disorders in youth: Cognitive-behavioral interventions.* Needham Heights, MA: Allyn & Bacon.

Kendall, P. C., & Chu, B. C. (2000). Retrospective self-reports of therapist flexibility in a manual-based treatment for youths with anxiety disorders. *Journal of Clinical Child Psychology, 29,* 209–220.

Kendall, P. C., Chu, B., Gifford, A., Hayes, C., & Nauta, M. (1998). Breathing life into a manual: Flexibility and creativity with manual-based treatments. *Cognitive and Behavioral Practice, 5,* 177–198.

Kendall, P. C., Flannery-Schroeder, E., & Ford, J. D. (1999). Therapy outcome research methods. In P. C. Kendall, J. N. Butcher, & G. N. Holmbeck (Eds.), *Handbook of research methods in clinical psychology* (2nd ed., pp. 330–363). New York: Wiley.

Kendall, P. C., Flannery-Schroeder, E., Panichelli-Mindel, S. M., Southam-Gerow, M., Henin, A., & Warman, M. (1997). Therapy for youths with anxiety disorders: A second randomized clinical trial. *Journal of Consulting and Clinical Psychology, 65,* 366–380.

Kendall, P. C., Kane, M., Howard, B., & Siqueland, L. (1990). *Cognitive-behavioral treatment of anxious children: Treatment manual.* Ardmore, PA: Workbook Publishing.

Kendall, P. C., & Southam-Gerow, M. A. (1995). Issues in the transportability of treatment: The case of anxiety disorders in youth. *Journal of Consulting and Clinical Psychology, 63,* 702–708.

Kiesler, D. J. (1966). Some myths of psychotherapy research and the search for a paradigm. *Psychological Bulletin, 65,* 110–136.

King, N. J., & Ollendick, T. H. (1998). Empirically validated treatments in clinical psychology. *Australian Psychologist, 33,* 89–95.

Kinscherff, R. (1999). Empirically supported treatments: What to do until the data arrive (or now that they have)? *Clinical Child Psychology Newsletter, 14,* 4–6.

Klerman, G. L., Weissman, M. M., Rounsaville, B. J., & Chevron, E. S. (1984). *Interpersonal psychotherapy for depression.* New York: Basic Books.

Lambert, M. J. (1998). Manual-based treatment and clinical practice: Hangman of life or promising development? *Clinical Psychology: Science and Practice, 5,* 391–395.

Lambert, M. J., & Ogles, B. M. (1988). Treatment manuals: Problems and promise. *Journal of Integrative and Eclectic Psychotherapy, 7,* 187–204.

Levitt, E. E. (1957). The results of psychotherapy with children: An evaluation. *Journal of Consulting and Clinical Psychology, 21,* 189–196.

Levitt, E. E. (1963). Psychotherapy with children: A further evaluation. *Behaviour Research and Therapy, 60,* 326–329.

Lonigan, C. J., Elbert, J. C., & Johnson, S. B. (1998). Empirically supported psychosocial interventions for children: An overview. *Journal of Clinical Child Psychology, 27,* 138–145.

Luborsky, L., & DuRubeis, R. (1984). The use of psychotherapy treatment manuals: A small revolution in psychotherapy research style. *Clinical Psychology Review, 4,* 5–14.

Mattis, S. G., & Ollendick, T. H. (2002). *Panic disorder and anxiety in adolescence.* Oxford, UK: Blackwell.

Mersch, P. P. A., Emmelkamp, P. M. G., Bogels, S. M., & van der Sleen, J. (1989). Social phobia: Individual response patterns and the effects of behavioral and cognitive interventions. *Behaviour Research and Therapy, 27,* 421–434.

Mufson, L., Moreau, D., Weissman, M. M., Wickramaratne, P., Martin, J., & Samoilov, A. (1994). Modification of interpersonal psychotherapy with depressed adolescents (IPT-A):

Phase I and II studies. *Journal of the American Academy of Child and Adolescent Psychiatry, 33*, 695–705.

Mufson, L., Weissman, M. M., Moreau, D., & Garfinkel, R. (1999). Efficacy of interpersonal psychotherapy for depressed adolescents. *Archives of General Psychiatry, 56*, 573–579.

Nathan, P. E., & Gorman, J. M. (1998). *A guide to treatments that work.* New York: Oxford University Press.

Nelson-Gray, R. O., Herbert, J. D., Herbert, D. L., Sigmon, S. T., & Brannon, S. E. (1990). Effectiveness of matched, mismatched, and package treatments of depression. *Journal of Behavior Therapy and Experimental Psychiatry, 20*, 281–294.

Ollendick, T. H. (1995a). AABT and empirically validated treatments. *The Behavior Therapist, 18*, 81–82.

Ollendick, T. H. (1995b). Cognitive-behavior treatment of panic disorder with agoraphobia in adolescents: A multiple baseline analysis. *Behavior Therapy, 26*, 517–531.

Ollendick, T. H. (1999). Empirically supported treatments: Promises and pitfalls. *The Clinical Psychologist, 52*, 1–3.

Ollendick, T. H., & Davis, T. E., III. (2004). Empirically supported treatments for children and adolescents: Where to from here? *Clinical Psychology: Science and Practice, 11*, 289–294.

Ollendick, T. H., & Hersen, M. (1984). *Child behavioral assessment: Principles and procedures.* New York: Pergamon Press.

Ollendick, T. H., & King, N. J. (1998). Empirically supported treatments for children with phobic and anxiety disorders: Current status. *Journal of Clinical Child Psychology, 27*, 156–167.

Ollendick, T. H., & King, N. J. (2000). Empirically supported treatments for children and adolescents. In P. C. Kendall (Ed.), *Child and adolescent therapy: Cognitive behavioral procedures* (2nd ed., pp. 386–425). New York: Guilford Press.

Ollendick, T. H., & King, N. J. (2004). Empirically supported treatments for children and adolescents: Advances toward evidence-based practice. In P. M. Barrett & T. H. Ollendick (Eds.), *Handbook of interventions that work with children and adolescents: Prevention and treatment* (pp. 1–26). Chichester, UK: Wiley.

Ost, L. G., Jerremalm, A., & Johansson, J. (1981). Individual response patterns and the effects of different behavioral methods in the treatment of claustrophobia. *Behaviour Research and Therapy, 20*, 445–560.

Patterson, G. R., & Gullion, M. E. (1968). *Living with children: New methods for parents and teachers.* Champaign, IL: Research Press.

Persons, J. B. (1998). Paean to data. *The Behavior Therapist, 21*, 123.

Persons, J. B., & Silberschatz, G. (1998). Are results of randomized controlled trials useful to psychotherapists? *Journal of Consulting and Clinical Psychology, 66*, 126–135.

Rossello, J., & Bernal, G. (1999). The efficacy of cognitive-behavioral and interpersonal treatments for depression in Puerto Rican adolescents. *Journal of Consulting and Clinical Psychology, 67*, 734–745.

Roth, A., & Fonagy, P. (1996). *What works for whom?: A critical review of psychotherapy research.* New York: Guilford Press.

Sackett, D., Richardson, W., Rosenberg, W., & Haynes, B. (1997). *Evidence-based medicine.* London: Churchill Livingstone.

Sackett, D., Richardson, W., Rosenberg, W., & Haynes, B. (2000). *Evidence-based medicine* (2nd ed.). London: Churchill Livingstone.

Schoenwald, S. K., & Hoagwood, K. (2001). Effectiveness, transportability, and dissemination of interventions: What matters when? *Psychiatric Services, 52*, 1190–1197.

Schulte, D., Kunzel, R., Pepping, G., & Schulte-Bahrenberg, T. (1992). Tailor-made versus standardized therapy of phobic patients. *Advances in Behaviour Research and Therapy, 14,* 67–92.

Seligman, M. E. P. (1995). The effectiveness of psychotherapy. *American Psychologist, 50,* 965–974.

Silverman, W. H. (1996). Cookbooks, manuals, and paint-by-numbers: Psychotherapy in the 90's. *Psychotherapy, 33,* 207–215.

Smith, E. W. L. (1995). A passionate, rational response to the "manualization" of psychotherapy. *Psychotherapy Bulletin, 33*(2), 36–40.

Strosahl, K. (1998). The dissemination of manual-based psychotherapies in managed care: Promises, problems, and prospects. *Clinical Psychology: Science and Practice, 5,* 382–386.

Strupp, H. H., & Binder, J. L. (1984). *Psychotherapy in a new key: A guide to time-limited dynamic psychotherapy.* New York: Basic Books.

Strupp, H. H., & Anderson, T. (1997). On the limitations of therapy manuals. *Clinical Psychology: Science and Practice, 4,* 76–82.

Task Force on Promotion and Dissemination. (1995). Training in and dissemination of empirically validated treatments: Report and recommendations. *The Clinical Psychologist, 48,* 3–23.

Tynan, W. D., Schuman, W., & Lampert, N. (1999). Concurrent parent and child therapy groups for externalizing disorders: From the laboratory to the world of managed care. *Cognitive and Behavioral Practice, 6,* 3–9.

Weiss, B., Catron, T., Harris, V., & Phung, T. M. (1999). The effectiveness of traditional child psychotherapy. *Journal of Consulting and Clinical Psychology, 67,* 82–94.

Weisz, J. R., Donenberg, G. R., Han, S. S., & Weiss, B. (1995). Bridging the gap between laboratory and clinic in child and adolescent psychotherapy. *Journal of Consulting and Clinical Psychology, 63,* 688–701.

Weisz, J. R., Han, S. S., & Valeri, S. M. (1997). More of what? Issues raised by the Fort Bragg Study. *American Psychologist, 52,* 541–545.

Weisz, J. R., Huey, S. J., & Weersing, V. R. (1998). Psychotherapy outcome research with children and adolescents: The state of the art. In T. H. Ollendick & R. J. Prinz (Eds.), *Advances in clinical child psychology* (Vol. 20, pp. 49–91). New York: Plenum Press.

Weisz, J. R., Weiss, B., Alicke, M. D., & Klotz, M. L. (1987). Effectiveness of psychotherapy with children and adolescents: A meta-analysis for clinicians. *Journal of Consulting and Clinical Psychology, 55,* 542–549.

Weisz, J. R., Weiss, B., Han, S. S., Granger, D. G., & Morton, T. (1995). Effects of psychotherapy with children and adolescents revisited: A meta-analysis of treatment outcome studies. *Psychological Bulletin, 117,* 450–468.

Wilson, G. T. (1996a). Empirically validated treatments: Reality and resistance. *Clinical Psychology: Science and Practice, 3,* 241–244.

Wilson, G. T. (1996b). Manual-based treatments: The clinical application of research findings. *Behaviour Research and Therapy, 34,* 295–314.

Wilson, G. T. (1998). Empirically validated treatments: Reality and resistance. *Clinical Psychology: Science and Practice, 3,* 241–244.

Zvolensky, M. J., & Eiffert, G. H. (1998). Standardized treatments: Potential ethical issues for behavior therapists? *The Behavior Therapist, 21,* 1–3.

Zvolensky, M. J., & Eiffert, G. H. (1999). Potential ethical issues revisited: A reply to Persons. *The Behavior Therapist, 22,* 40.

Index